Atlas of Human Anatomy

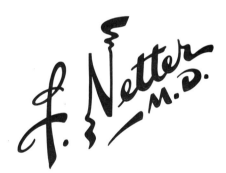

Atlas

Human

of Anatomy

Third Edition

by Frank H. Netter, M.D.

John T. Hansen, Ph.D., *Consulting Editor*
University of Rochester School of Medicine and Dentistry
Rochester, New York

Icon Learning Systems · Teterboro, New Jersey

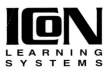

Fourth printing, 2004

NOTICE

Executive Editor: Paul Kelly
Editorial Director: Greg Otis
Managing Editor: Jennifer Surich
Director of Manufacturing: Mary Ellen Curry
Manager, Production Editing: Stephanie Klein
Graphic Artist: Colleen Quinn

ISBN 1-929007-11-6 (paperback)
ISBN 1-929007-12-4 (case bound)
ISBN 1-929007-15-9 (paperback/CD combo)
ISBN 1-929007-21-3 (case bound/CD combo)
ISBN 1-929007-17-5 (International Student Edition)
Library of Congress Control No: 2002110663

Printed and bound in USA by Quebecor World, Kingsport

To my dear wife, Vera

PREFACE TO THE FIRST EDITION

I have often said that my career as a medical artist for almost 50 years has been a sort of "command performance" in the sense that it has grown in response to the desires and requests of the medical profession. Over these many years, I have produced almost 4,000 illustrations, mostly for *The CIBA (now Netter) Collection of Medical Illustrations* but also for *Clinical Symposia*. These pictures have been concerned with the varied subdivisions of medical knowledge such as gross anatomy, histology, embryology, physiology, pathology, diagnostic modalities, surgical and therapeutic techniques and clinical manifestations of a multitude of diseases. As the years went by, however, there were more and more requests from physicians and students for me to produce an atlas purely of gross anatomy. Thus, this atlas has come about, not through any inspiration on my part but rather, like most of my previous works, as a fulfillment of the desires of the medical profession.

It involved going back over all the illustrations I had made over so many years, selecting those pertinent to gross anatomy, classifying them and organizing them by system and region, adapting them to page size and space and arranging them in logical sequence. Anatomy of course does not change, but our understanding of anatomy and its clinical significance does change, as do anatomical terminology and nomenclature. This therefore required much updating of many of the older pictures and even revision of a number of them in order to make them more pertinent to today's ever-expanding scope of medical and surgical practice. In addition, I found that there were gaps in the portrayal of medical knowledge as pictorialized in the illustrations I had previously done, and this necessitated my making a number of new pictures that are included in this volume.

In creating an atlas such as this, it is important to achieve a happy medium between complexity and simplification. If the pictures are too complex, they may be difficult and confusing to read; if oversimplified, they may not be adequately definitive or may even be misleading. I have therefore striven for a middle course of realism without the clutter of confusing minutiae. I hope that the students and members of the medical and allied professions will find the illustrations readily understandable, yet instructive and useful.

At one point, the publisher and I thought it might be nice to include a foreword by a truly outstanding and renowned anatomist, but there are so many in that category that we could not make a choice. We did think of men like Vesalius, Leonardo da Vinci, William Hunter and Henry Gray, who of course are unfortunately unavailable, but I do wonder what their comments might have been about this atlas.

Frank H. Netter, M.D.
(1906–1991)

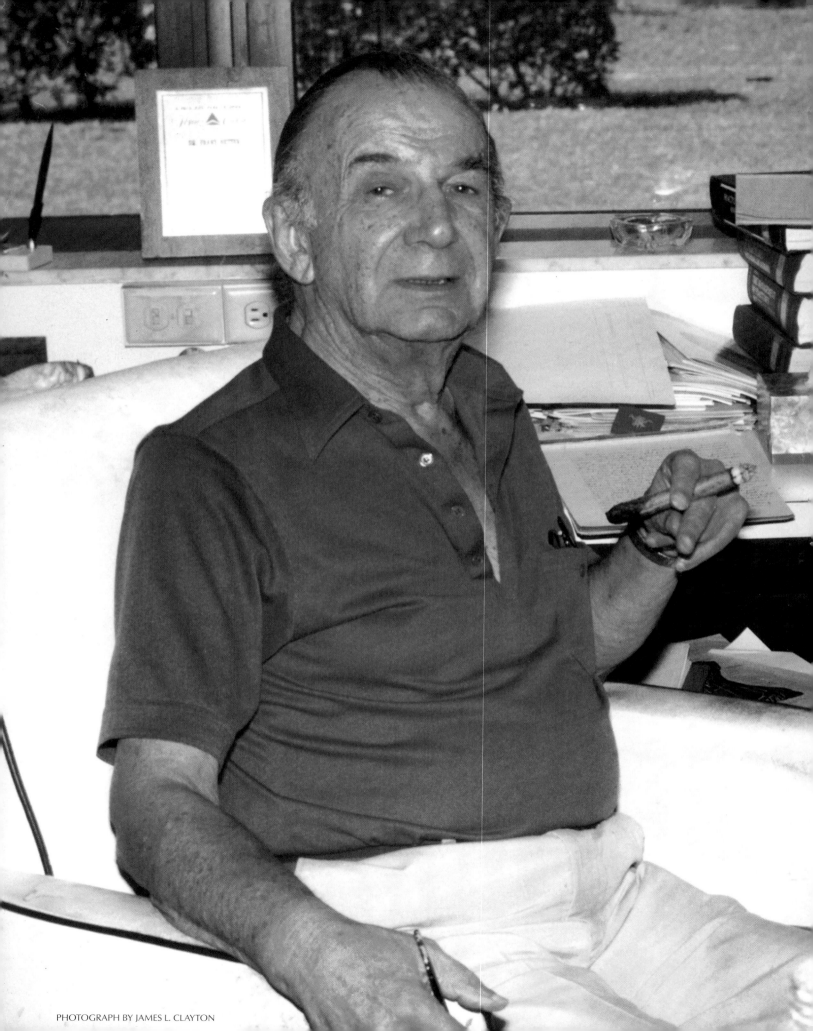

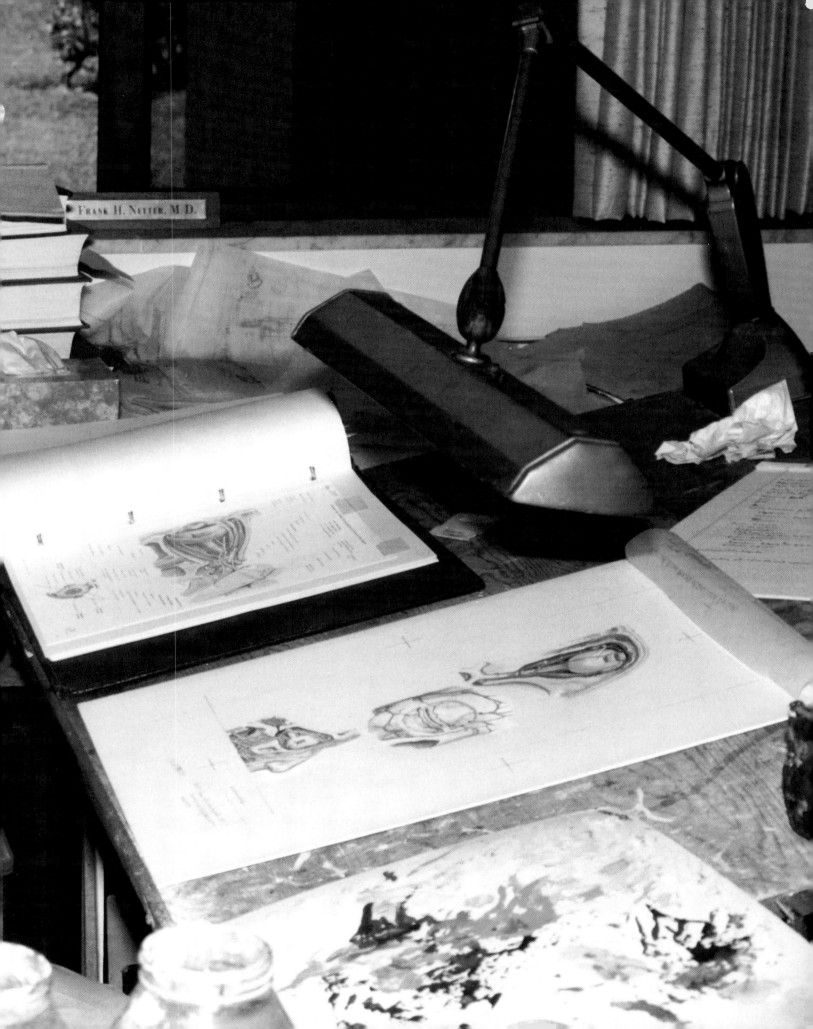

FOREWORD

"The release in 1989 of the first edition of Dr. Frank Netter's 'personal Sistine Chapel'—the Atlas of Human Anatomy—was a major event in the history of the teaching and learning of anatomy. Almost instantly, the Atlas of Human Anatomy became the top-selling anatomical atlas in the world and clearly became the students' choice universally." This quotation from the second edition of the *Atlas of Human Anatomy* still resonates today as the beautifully conceived and rendered artwork of Dr. Netter continues to capture the admiration of students and healthcare professionals.

The skillful editing and publishing teamwork of Novartis Medical Education, in consultation with many of the 20th century's outstanding anatomists and physicians, have made the first and second editions of the *Atlas* the standard against which all other atlases are compared. This third edition owes much to the Consulting Editors of the earlier editions, Drs. Sharon Colacino (Oberg) (first edition) and Arthur F. Dalley II (second edition), who shepherded their editions with great skill and uncompromising professionalism and thus made my task significantly easier. I am honored to serve as the Consulting Editor of the third edition and to continue the Netter tradition in partnership with Icon Learning Systems as the *Atlas of Human Anatomy* enters the new century.

Perceptive student and faculty response to the earlier editions prompted greater attention to several concepts that are critical to the anatomical basis of clinical practice. Notably, each regional section now begins with a surface anatomy plate, skillfully drawn by Carlos A.G. Machado, M.D. These surface anatomy plates remind us of the value of careful observation in clinical medicine and draw attention to surface features that portend the underlying anatomy.

We also have included a significant number of normal radiographic images in this edition, reflecting the importance of diagnostic imaging in clinical anatomy and medicine. These new images are not meant to be comprehensive of the radiographic knowledge available to today's clinicians, but rather are starting points for further exploration into the richness of anatomical detail that imaging can provide. I am grateful to Matthew Cham, M.D., and John Wandtke, M.D., of our Department of Radiology for selecting these images and permitting us to use them in this edition.

We balanced the addition of new surface and radiographic anatomy plates largely by eliminating several plates that contributed little to the quality of the *Atlas*. Several plates from *The Netter* (formerly *CIBA*) *Collection of Medical Illustrations* were added and several plates were altered slightly to correct anatomical errors consistent with our current knowledge. In sum, the third edition has grown by 30 images. Finally, the References and the Index have been updated.

The anatomical terminology is consistent throughout the *Atlas* and conforms to the International Anatomical Terminology (*Terminologia Anatomica*) approved in 1998 by the International Federation of Associations of Anatomists. Common eponyms are retained parenthetically, and the leader lines and labels have been checked and, where necessary, corrected to ensure their accuracy. For reviewing this material I thank Wojciech Pawlina, M.D., Leonard J. Cleary, Ph.D., Daniel O. Graney, Ph.D., and Brian R. MacPherson, Ph.D. Their meticulous examination of each plate has greatly enhanced the accuracy of this atlas.

For the proofreading, editing and designing, I am indebted to Jennifer Surich, Erika Gehringer and Greg Otis at Icon Learning Systems; their keen eyesight, dedication and professionalism buoyed me when I began to drift. A special thank you is reserved for Paul Kelly, Executive Editor, who continues to listen patiently and is a true believer in the power of the visual image to teach.

To all students, past, present and future, the legacy of Dr. Netter's artwork lives in you; his unique ability to "clarify rather than intimidate" is his gift to you. I am both privileged and humbled to have the opportunity to carry forward this tradition of excellence and to contribute to your understanding of human anatomy.

Finally, to my wife, Paula, thank you for giving me the freedom to write and the support to sustain me—in those respects, this book was co-edited.

John T. Hansen, Ph.D.
Professor of Neurobiology and Anatomy
University of Rochester School of Medicine and Dentistry
Rochester, New York

CONTENTS

Section I
HEAD AND NECK

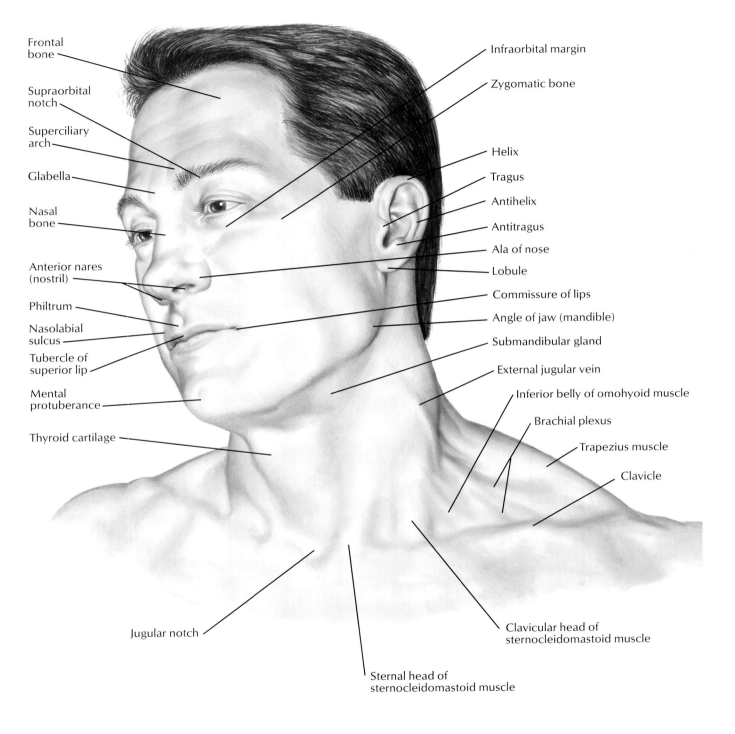

Frontal bone

Supraorbital notch

Superciliary arch

Glabella

Nasal bone

Anterior nares (nostril)

Philtrum

Nasolabial sulcus

Tubercle of superior lip

Mental protuberance

Thyroid cartilage

Jugular notch

Sternal head of sternocleidomastoid muscle

Infraorbital margin

Zygomatic bone

Helix

Tragus

Antihelix

Antitragus

Ala of nose

Lobule

Commissure of lips

Angle of jaw (mandible)

Submandibular gland

External jugular vein

Inferior belly of omohyoid muscle

Brachial plexus

Trapezius muscle

Clavicle

Clavicular head of sternocleidomastoid muscle

SURFACE ANATOMY

PLATE 1

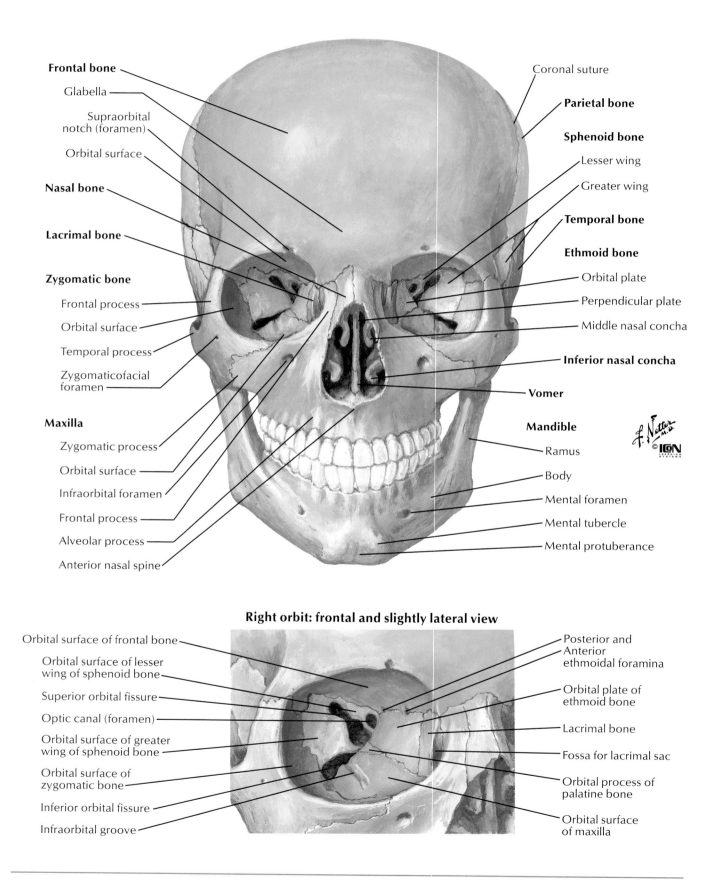

Frontal bone

Glabella

Supraorbital
notch (foramen)

Orbital surface

Nasal bone

Lacrimal bone

Zygomatic bone

Frontal process

Orbital surface

Temporal process

Zygomaticofacial
foramen

Maxilla

Zygomatic process

Orbital surface

Infraorbital foramen

Frontal process

Alveolar process

Anterior nasal spine

Coronal suture

Parietal bone

Sphenoid bone

Lesser wing

Greater wing

Temporal bone

Ethmoid bone

Orbital plate

Perpendicular plate

Middle nasal concha

Inferior nasal concha

Vomer

Mandible

Ramus

Body

Mental foramen

Mental tubercle

Mental protuberance

Right orbit: frontal and slightly lateral view

Orbital surface of frontal bone

Orbital surface of lesser
wing of sphenoid bone

Superior orbital fissure

Optic canal (foramen)

Orbital surface of greater
wing of sphenoid bone

Orbital surface of
zygomatic bone

Inferior orbital fissure

Infraorbital groove

Posterior and
Anterior
ethmoidal foramina

Orbital plate of
ethmoid bone

Lacrimal bone

Fossa for lacrimal sac

Orbital process of
palatine bone

Orbital surface
of maxilla

PLATE 2

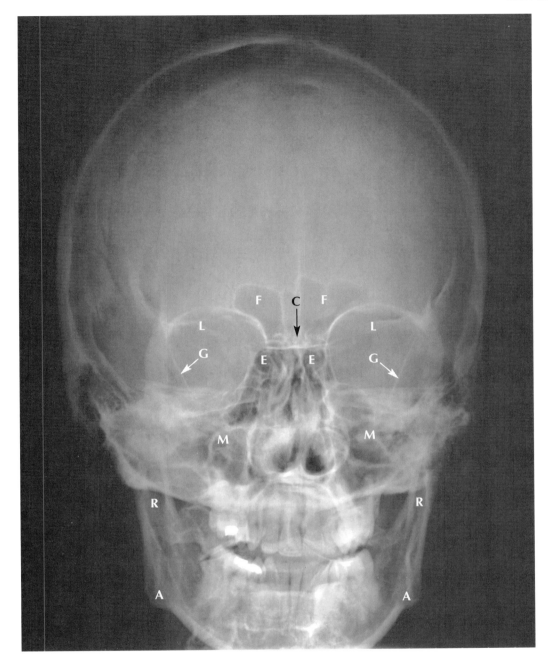

A Angle of mandible
C Crista galli
E Ethmoid sinus
F Frontal sinus
G Greater wing of sphenoid
L Lesser wing of sphenoid
M Maxillary sinus
R Ramus of mandible

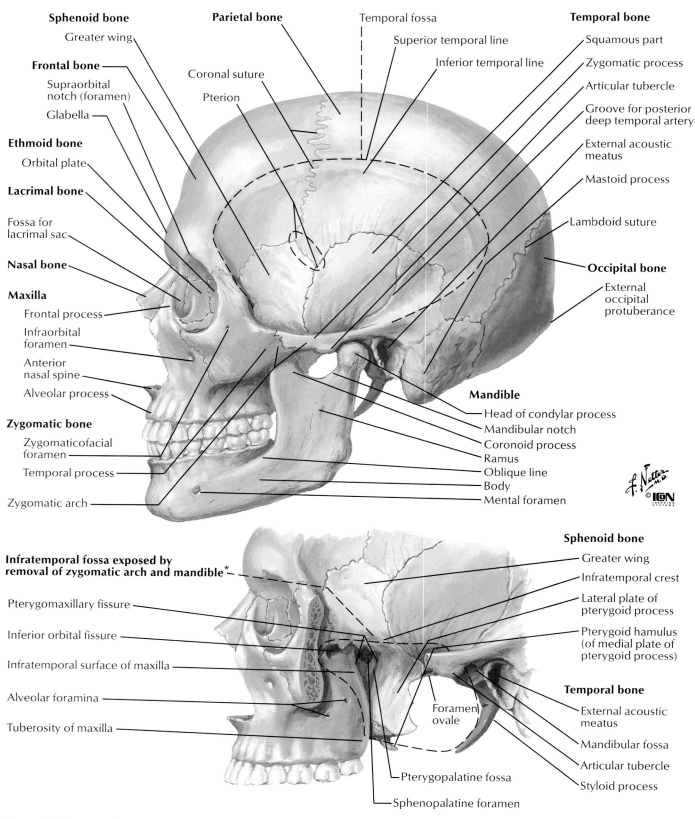

Sphenoid bone
Greater wing

Parietal bone
Temporal fossa

Temporal bone
Squamous part

Coronal suture

Superior temporal line
Inferior temporal line

Zygomatic process

Frontal bone
Supraorbital notch (foramen)
Glabella

Pterion

Articular tubercle

Groove for posterior deep temporal artery

External acoustic meatus

Ethmoid bone
Orbital plate

Mastoid process

Lacrimal bone
Fossa for lacrimal sac

Lambdoid suture

Nasal bone

Occipital bone
External occipital protuberance

Maxilla
Frontal process
Infraorbital foramen
Anterior nasal spine
Alveolar process

Mandible
Head of condylar process
Mandibular notch
Coronoid process
Ramus
Oblique line
Body
Mental foramen

Zygomatic bone
Zygomaticofacial foramen
Temporal process
Zygomatic arch

Sphenoid bone
Greater wing
Infratemporal crest
Lateral plate of pterygoid process
Pterygoid hamulus (of medial plate of pterygoid process)

Infratemporal fossa exposed by removal of zygomatic arch and mandible *

Pterygomaxillary fissure
Inferior orbital fissure
Infratemporal surface of maxilla
Alveolar foramina
Tuberosity of maxilla

Foramen ovale

Temporal bone
External acoustic meatus
Mandibular fossa
Articular tubercle
Styloid process

Pterygopalatine fossa
Sphenopalatine foramen

*Superficially, mastoid process forms posterior boundary

PLATE 4

HEAD AND NECK

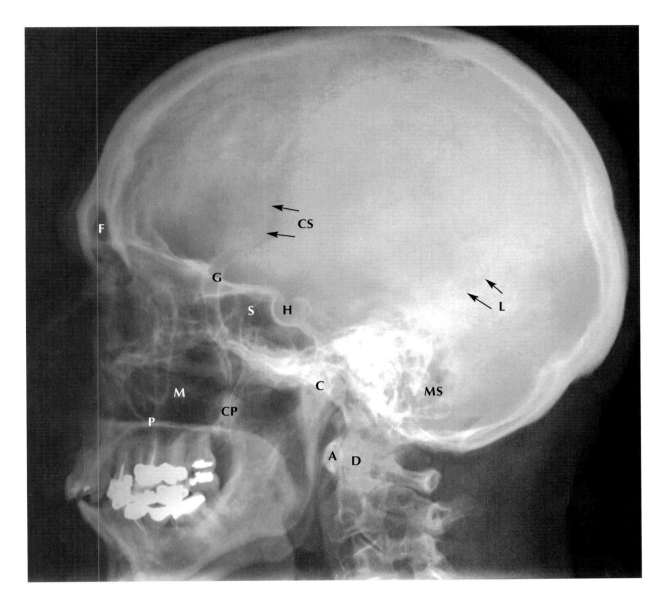

A	Anterior arch of atlas (CI vertebra)	**G**	Greater wing of sphenoid
C	Condyle of mandible	**H**	Hypophyseal fossa
CP	Coronoid process of mandible	**L**	Lambdoid suture
		M	Maxillary sinus
CS	Coronal suture	**MS**	Mastoid air cells
D	Dens of axis (C2 vertebra)	**P**	Palatine process of maxilla
F	Frontal sinus	**S**	Sphenoid sinus

Skull: Midsagittal Section

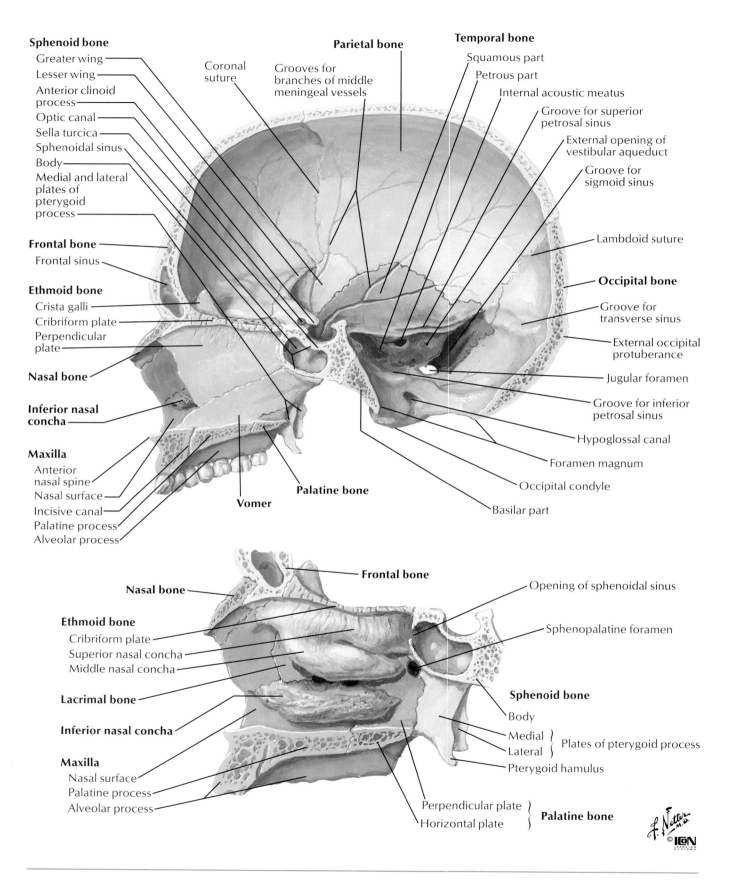

Sphenoid bone
Greater wing
Lesser wing
Anterior clinoid process
Optic canal
Sella turcica
Sphenoidal sinus
Body
Medial and lateral plates of pterygoid process

Frontal bone
Frontal sinus

Ethmoid bone
Crista galli
Cribriform plate
Perpendicular plate

Nasal bone

Inferior nasal concha

Maxilla
Anterior nasal spine
Nasal surface
Incisive canal
Palatine process
Alveolar process

Coronal suture

Parietal bone
Grooves for branches of middle meningeal vessels

Temporal bone
Squamous part
Petrous part
Internal acoustic meatus
Groove for superior petrosal sinus
External opening of vestibular aqueduct
Groove for sigmoid sinus

Lambdoid suture

Occipital bone
Groove for transverse sinus
External occipital protuberance
Jugular foramen
Groove for inferior petrosal sinus
Hypoglossal canal
Foramen magnum
Occipital condyle
Basilar part

Palatine bone

Vomer

Nasal bone

Ethmoid bone
Cribriform plate
Superior nasal concha
Middle nasal concha

Lacrimal bone

Inferior nasal concha

Maxilla
Nasal surface
Palatine process
Alveolar process

Frontal bone
Opening of sphenoidal sinus

Sphenopalatine foramen

Sphenoid bone
Body
Medial ⎫
Lateral ⎬ Plates of pterygoid process
Pterygoid hamulus

Perpendicular plate ⎫
Horizontal plate ⎬ **Palatine bone**

PLATE 6

HEAD AND NECK

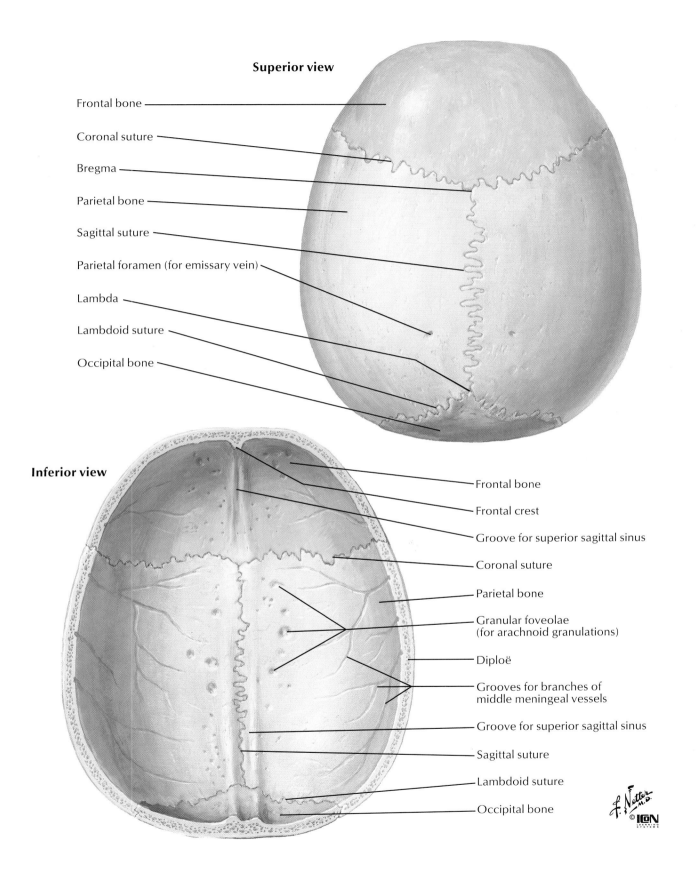

Superior view

Frontal bone

Coronal suture

Bregma

Parietal bone

Sagittal suture

Parietal foramen (for emissary vein)

Lambda

Lambdoid suture

Occipital bone

Inferior view

Frontal bone

Frontal crest

Groove for superior sagittal sinus

Coronal suture

Parietal bone

Granular foveolae
(for arachnoid granulations)

Diploë

Grooves for branches of
middle meningeal vessels

Groove for superior sagittal sinus

Sagittal suture

Lambdoid suture

Occipital bone

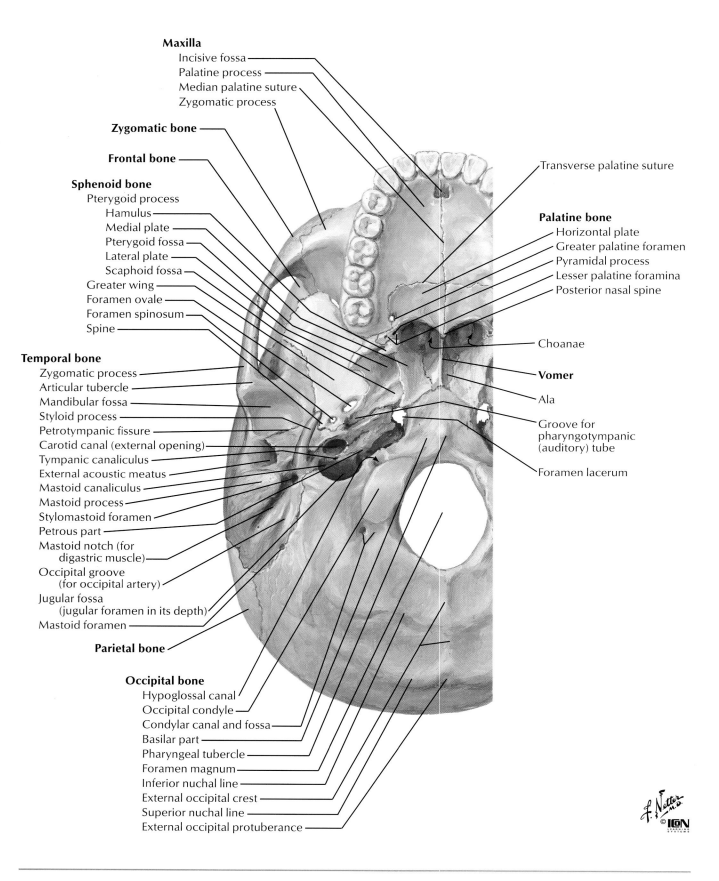

Maxilla
Incisive fossa
Palatine process
Median palatine suture
Zygomatic process

Zygomatic bone

Frontal bone

Sphenoid bone
Pterygoid process
Hamulus
Medial plate
Pterygoid fossa
Lateral plate
Scaphoid fossa
Greater wing
Foramen ovale
Foramen spinosum
Spine

Temporal bone
Zygomatic process
Articular tubercle
Mandibular fossa
Styloid process
Petrotympanic fissure
Carotid canal (external opening)
Tympanic canaliculus
External acoustic meatus
Mastoid canaliculus
Mastoid process
Stylomastoid foramen
Petrous part
Mastoid notch (for
    digastric muscle)
Occipital groove
    (for occipital artery)
Jugular fossa
    (jugular foramen in its depth)
Mastoid foramen

Parietal bone

Occipital bone
Hypoglossal canal
Occipital condyle
Condylar canal and fossa
Basilar part
Pharyngeal tubercle
Foramen magnum
Inferior nuchal line
External occipital crest
Superior nuchal line
External occipital protuberance

Transverse palatine suture

Palatine bone
Horizontal plate
Greater palatine foramen
Pyramidal process
Lesser palatine foramina
Posterior nasal spine

Choanae

Vomer

Ala

Groove for
pharyngotympanic
(auditory) tube

Foramen lacerum

PLATE 8

HEAD AND NECK

Frontal bone
    Groove for superior sagittal sinus
    Frontal crest
    Groove for anterior meningeal vessels
    Foramen cecum
    Superior surface of orbital part

Ethmoid bone
    Crista galli
    Cribriform plate

Sphenoid bone
    Lesser wing
        Anterior clinoid process
    Greater wing
        Groove for middle meningeal
        vessels (frontal branches)
    Body
        Jugum
        Prechiasmatic groove
    Sella   { Tuberculum sellae
    turcica   { Hypophyseal fossa
              { Dorsum sellae
              { Posterior clinoid process
    Carotid groove (for int. carotid a.)
    Clivus

Temporal bone
    Squamous part
    Petrous part
        Groove for lesser petrosal nerve
        Groove for greater petrosal nerve
        Arcuate eminence
        Trigeminal impression
        Groove for superior petrosal sinus
        Groove for sigmoid sinus

Parietal bone
    Groove for middle meningeal
    vessels (parietal branches)
    Mastoid angle

Occipital bone
    Clivus
    Groove for inferior petrosal sinus
    Basilar part
    Groove for posterior meningeal vessels
    Condyle
    Groove for transverse sinus
    Groove for occipital sinus
    Internal occipital crest
    Internal occipital protuberance
    Groove for superior sagittal sinus

**Anterior
cranial
fossa**

**Middle
cranial
fossa**

**Posterior
cranial
fossa**

f. Netter
©ICN
LEARNING SYSTEMS

Foramina of Cranial Base: Superior View

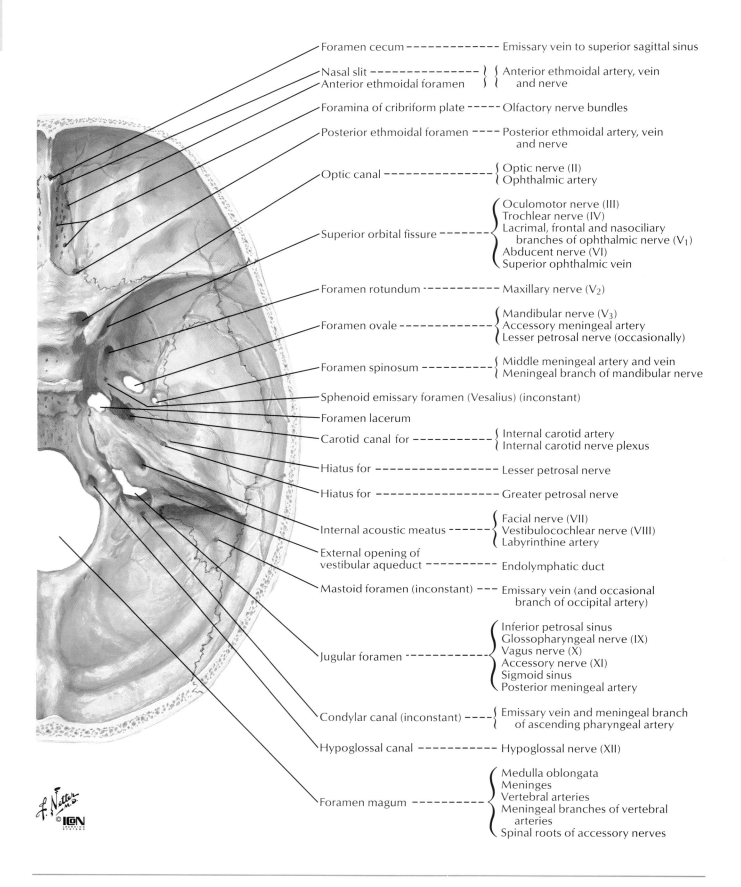

Foramen cecum ------------ Emissary vein to superior sagittal sinus

Nasal slit --------------- } { Anterior ethmoidal artery, vein
Anterior ethmoidal foramen } {   and nerve

Foramina of cribriform plate ----- Olfactory nerve bundles

Posterior ethmoidal foramen ---- Posterior ethmoidal artery, vein
                                   and nerve

Optic canal --------------- { Optic nerve (II)
                            { Ophthalmic artery

Superior orbital fissure ------- { Oculomotor nerve (III)
                                 { Trochlear nerve (IV)
                                 { Lacrimal, frontal and nasociliary
                                 {   branches of ophthalmic nerve (V₁)
                                 { Abducent nerve (VI)
                                 { Superior ophthalmic vein

Foramen rotundum --------- Maxillary nerve (V₂)

Foramen ovale ------------ { Mandibular nerve (V₃)
                           { Accessory meningeal artery
                           { Lesser petrosal nerve (occasionally)

Foramen spinosum --------- { Middle meningeal artery and vein
                           { Meningeal branch of mandibular nerve

Sphenoid emissary foramen (Vesalius) (inconstant)

Foramen lacerum

Carotid canal for ---------- { Internal carotid artery
                             { Internal carotid nerve plexus

Hiatus for --------------- Lesser petrosal nerve

Hiatus for --------------- Greater petrosal nerve

Internal acoustic meatus ------ { Facial nerve (VII)
                                { Vestibulocochlear nerve (VIII)
                                { Labyrinthine artery

External opening of
vestibular aqueduct --------- Endolymphatic duct

Mastoid foramen (inconstant) --- Emissary vein (and occasional
                                   branch of occipital artery)

Jugular foramen ----------- { Inferior petrosal sinus
                            { Glossopharyngeal nerve (IX)
                            { Vagus nerve (X)
                            { Accessory nerve (XI)
                            { Sigmoid sinus
                            { Posterior meningeal artery

Condylar canal (inconstant) ---- { Emissary vein and meningeal branch
                                 {   of ascending pharyngeal artery

Hypoglossal canal ---------- Hypoglossal nerve (XII)

Foramen magum ---------- { Medulla oblongata
                         { Meninges
                         { Vertebral arteries
                         { Meningeal branches of vertebral
                         {   arteries
                         { Spinal roots of accessory nerves

PLATE 10   HEAD AND NECK

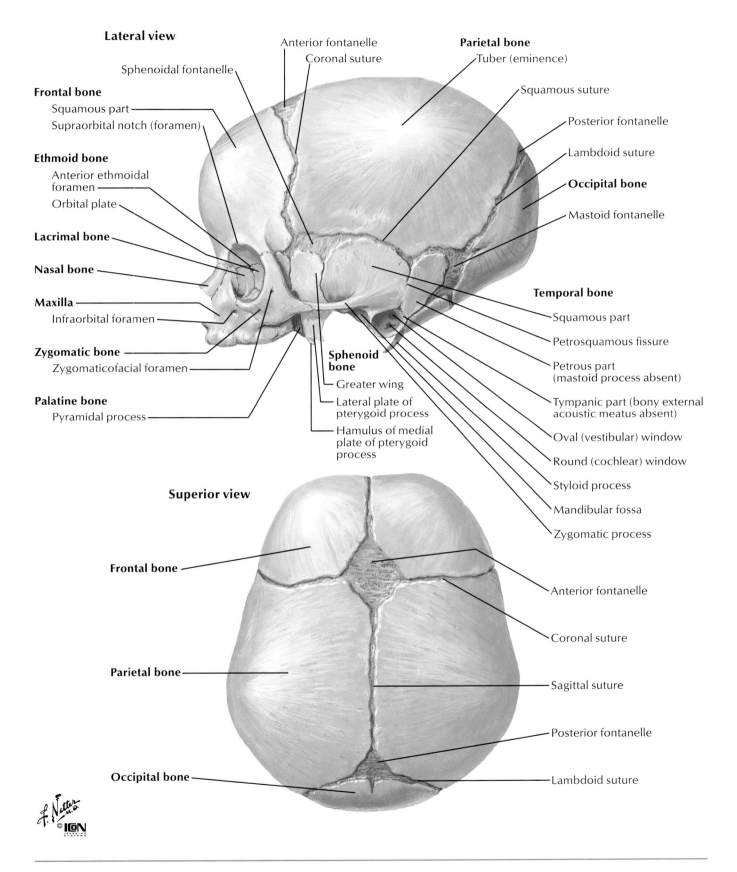

Lateral view

Anterior fontanelle
Coronal suture

Sphenoidal fontanelle

Parietal bone
Tuber (eminence)

Frontal bone
Squamous part
Supraorbital notch (foramen)

Squamous suture

Posterior fontanelle

Lambdoid suture

Ethmoid bone
Anterior ethmoidal foramen
Orbital plate

Occipital bone

Mastoid fontanelle

Lacrimal bone

Nasal bone

Temporal bone

Maxilla
Infraorbital foramen

Squamous part

Petrosquamous fissure

Zygomatic bone
Zygomaticofacial foramen

Sphenoid bone
Greater wing
Lateral plate of pterygoid process
Hamulus of medial plate of pterygoid process

Petrous part (mastoid process absent)

Tympanic part (bony external acoustic meatus absent)

Oval (vestibular) window

Round (cochlear) window

Styloid process

Mandibular fossa

Zygomatic process

Palatine bone
Pyramidal process

Superior view

Frontal bone

Anterior fontanelle

Coronal suture

Parietal bone

Sagittal suture

Posterior fontanelle

Occipital bone

Lambdoid suture

Bony Framework of Head and Neck

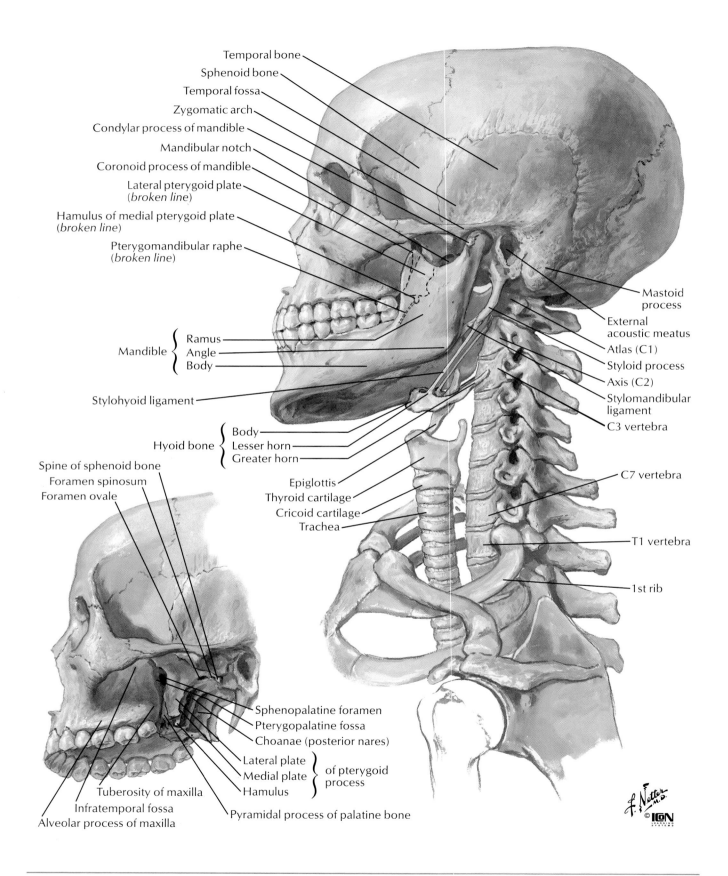

Temporal bone

Sphenoid bone

Temporal fossa

Zygomatic arch

Condylar process of mandible

Mandibular notch

Coronoid process of mandible

Lateral pterygoid plate
(*broken line*)

Hamulus of medial pterygoid plate
(*broken line*)

Pterygomandibular raphe
(*broken line*)

Mastoid process

External acoustic meatus

Atlas (C1)

Styloid process

Axis (C2)

Stylomandibular ligament

C3 vertebra

Mandible { Ramus
Angle
Body

Stylohyoid ligament

Hyoid bone { Body
Lesser horn
Greater horn

Epiglottis

Thyroid cartilage

Cricoid cartilage

Trachea

C7 vertebra

T1 vertebra

1st rib

Spine of sphenoid bone

Foramen spinosum

Foramen ovale

Sphenopalatine foramen

Pterygopalatine fossa

Choanae (posterior nares)

Lateral plate } of pterygoid
Medial plate   process
Hamulus

Tuberosity of maxilla

Infratemporal fossa

Alveolar process of maxilla

Pyramidal process of palatine bone

PLATE 12

HEAD AND NECK

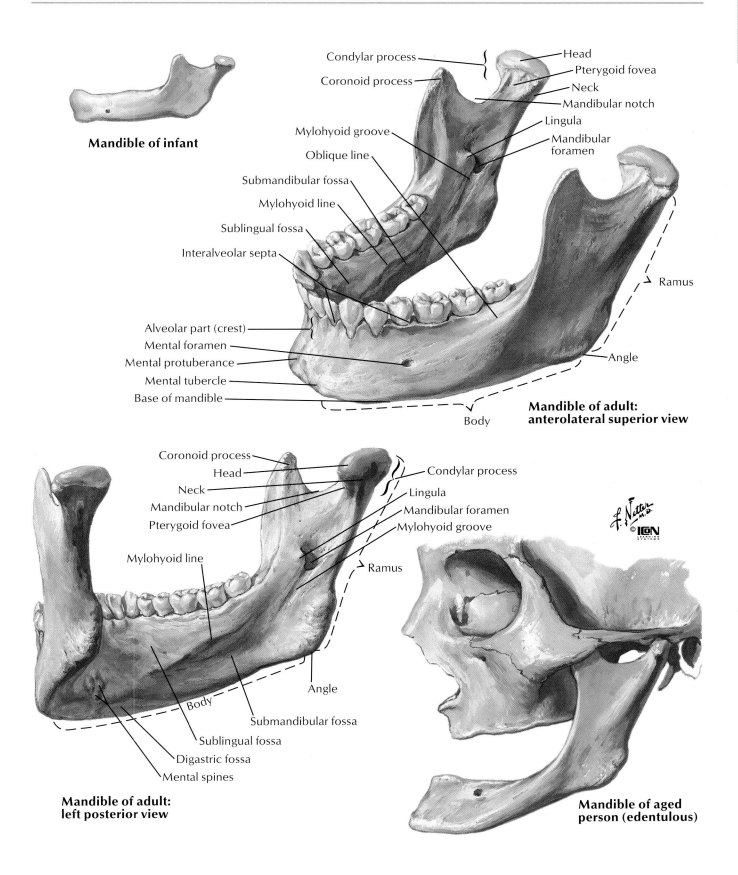

Mandible of infant

Condylar process — Head

Coronoid process — Pterygoid fovea

— Neck

— Mandibular notch

Mylohyoid groove — Lingula

Oblique line — Mandibular foramen

Submandibular fossa

Mylohyoid line

Sublingual fossa

Interalveolar septa

Alveolar part (crest)

Mental foramen — Ramus

Mental protuberance

Mental tubercle — Angle

Base of mandible

Body

**Mandible of adult:
anterolateral superior view**

Coronoid process

Head — Condylar process

Neck — Lingula

Mandibular notch — Mandibular foramen

Pterygoid fovea — Mylohyoid groove

Mylohyoid line — Ramus

Angle

Body

Submandibular fossa

Sublingual fossa

Digastric fossa

Mental spines

**Mandible of adult:
left posterior view**

**Mandible of aged
person (edentulous)**

Temporomandibular Joint

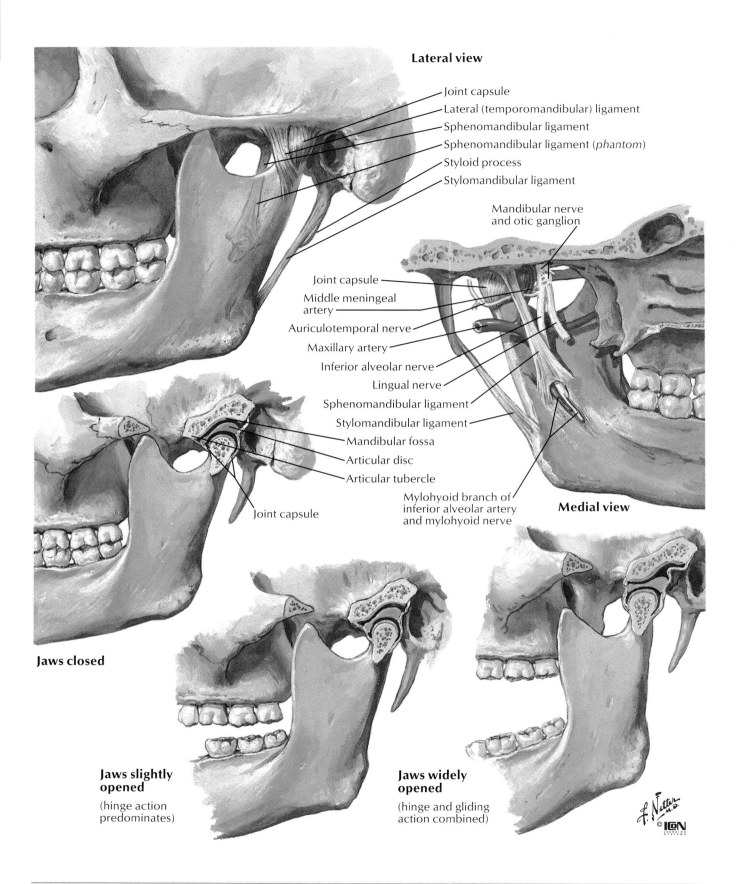

Lateral view

Joint capsule
Lateral (temporomandibular) ligament
Sphenomandibular ligament
Sphenomandibular ligament (*phantom*)
Styloid process
Stylomandibular ligament

Mandibular nerve and otic ganglion

Joint capsule
Middle meningeal artery
Auriculotemporal nerve
Maxillary artery
Inferior alveolar nerve
Lingual nerve
Sphenomandibular ligament
Stylomandibular ligament
Mandibular fossa
Articular disc
Articular tubercle

Joint capsule

Mylohyoid branch of inferior alveolar artery and mylohyoid nerve

Medial view

Jaws closed

Jaws slightly opened

(hinge action predominates)

Jaws widely opened

(hinge and gliding action combined)

PLATE 14

HEAD AND NECK

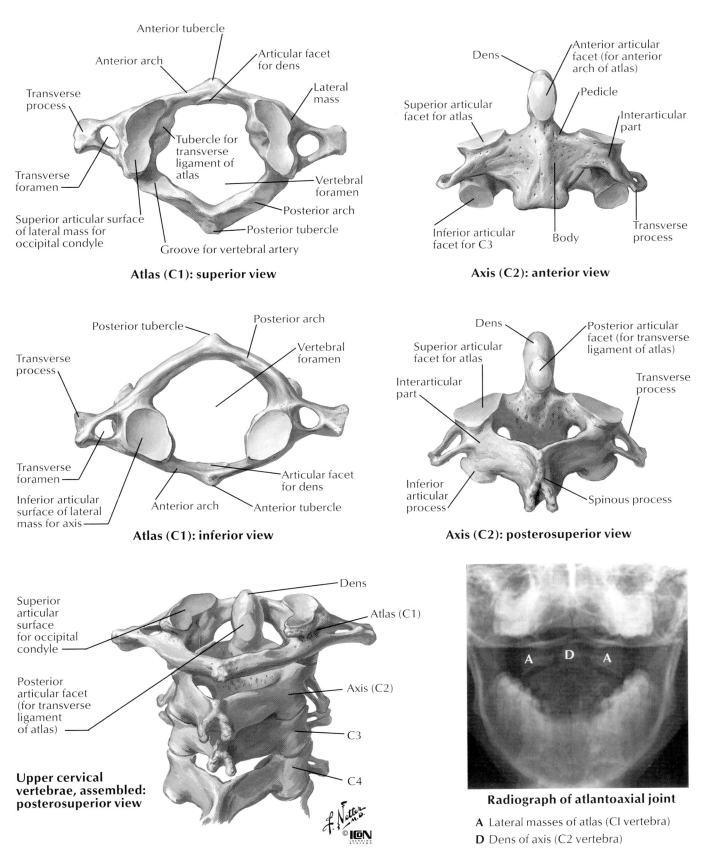

Atlas (C1): superior view

Anterior tubercle
Anterior arch
Articular facet for dens
Lateral mass
Transverse process
Tubercle for transverse ligament of atlas
Transverse foramen
Vertebral foramen
Superior articular surface of lateral mass for occipital condyle
Posterior arch
Posterior tubercle
Groove for vertebral artery

Axis (C2): anterior view

Dens
Anterior articular facet (for anterior arch of atlas)
Superior articular facet for atlas
Pedicle
Interarticular part
Inferior articular facet for C3
Body
Transverse process

Atlas (C1): inferior view

Posterior tubercle
Posterior arch
Vertebral foramen
Transverse process
Transverse foramen
Inferior articular surface of lateral mass for axis
Anterior arch
Articular facet for dens
Anterior tubercle

Axis (C2): posterosuperior view

Dens
Posterior articular facet (for transverse ligament of atlas)
Superior articular facet for atlas
Interarticular part
Transverse process
Inferior articular process
Spinous process

Upper cervical vertebrae, assembled: posterosuperior view

Superior articular surface for occipital condyle
Posterior articular facet (for transverse ligament of atlas)
Dens
Atlas (C1)
Axis (C2)
C3
C4

Radiograph of atlantoaxial joint

A Lateral masses of atlas (CI vertebra)
D Dens of axis (C2 vertebra)

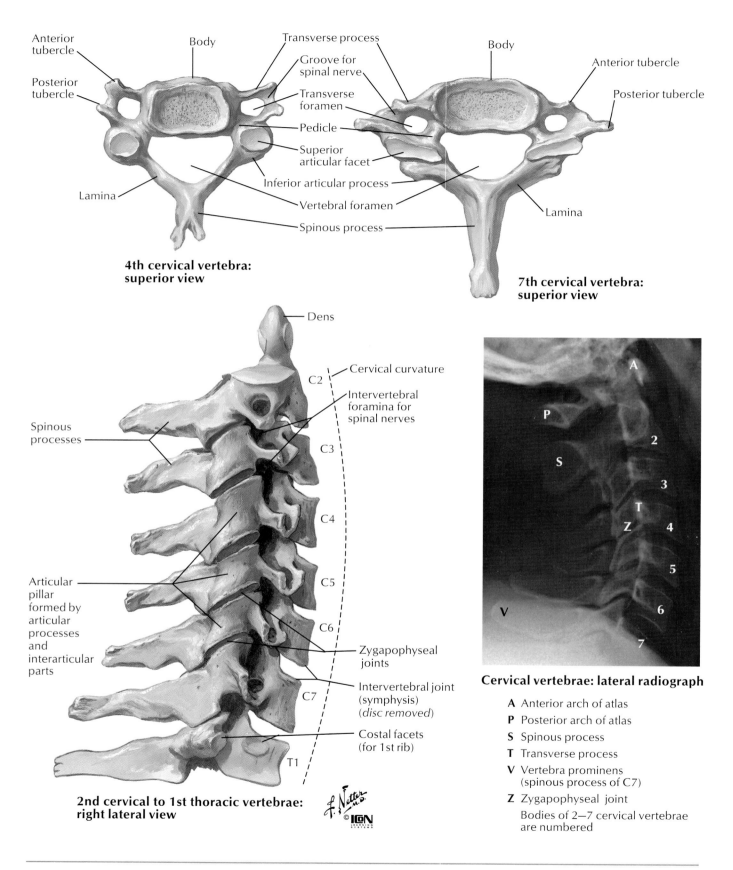

4th cervical vertebra: superior view

Anterior tubercle — Body — Transverse process — Groove for spinal nerve — Transverse foramen — Pedicle — Superior articular facet — Inferior articular process — Vertebral foramen — Spinous process — Posterior tubercle — Lamina

7th cervical vertebra: superior view

Body — Anterior tubercle — Posterior tubercle — Lamina

2nd cervical to 1st thoracic vertebrae: right lateral view

Dens — Cervical curvature — C2 — Intervertebral foramina for spinal nerves — C3 — Spinous processes — C4 — C5 — Articular pillar formed by articular processes and interarticular parts — C6 — Zygapophyseal joints — Intervertebral joint (symphysis) (disc removed) — C7 — Costal facets (for 1st rib) — T1

Cervical vertebrae: lateral radiograph

A Anterior arch of atlas
P Posterior arch of atlas
S Spinous process
T Transverse process
V Vertebra prominens (spinous process of C7)
Z Zygapophyseal joint
Bodies of 2—7 cervical vertebrae are numbered

PLATE 16

HEAD AND NECK

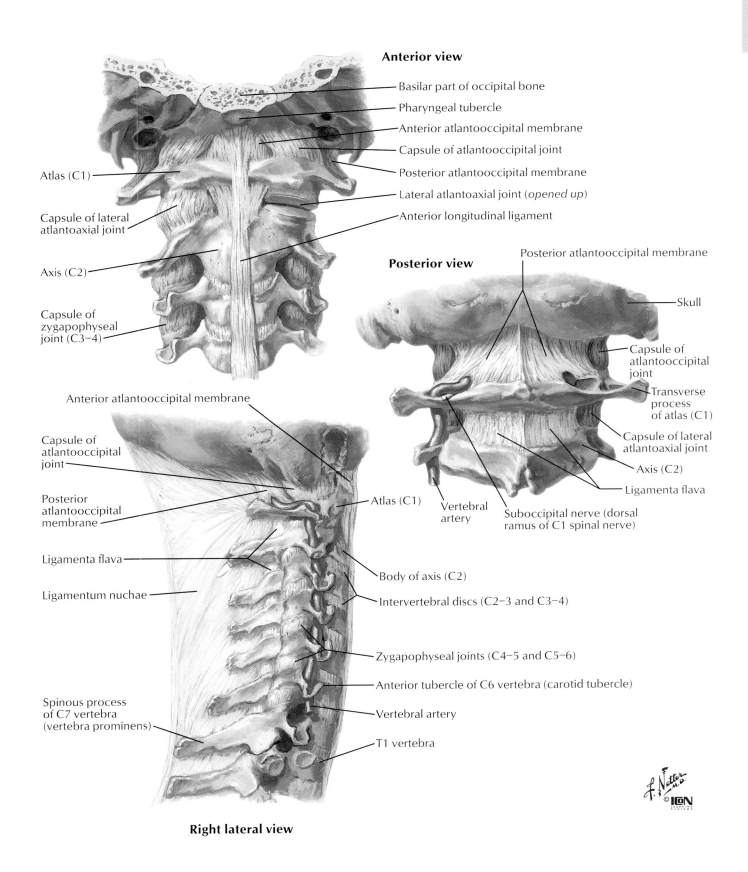

Anterior view

Basilar part of occipital bone

Pharyngeal tubercle

Anterior atlantooccipital membrane

Capsule of atlantooccipital joint

Posterior atlantooccipital membrane

Lateral atlantoaxial joint (*opened up*)

Anterior longitudinal ligament

Atlas (C1)

Capsule of lateral atlantoaxial joint

Axis (C2)

Capsule of zygapophyseal joint (C3–4)

Posterior view

Posterior atlantooccipital membrane

Skull

Capsule of atlantooccipital joint

Transverse process of atlas (C1)

Capsule of lateral atlantoaxial joint

Axis (C2)

Ligamenta flava

Vertebral artery

Suboccipital nerve (dorsal ramus of C1 spinal nerve)

Anterior atlantooccipital membrane

Capsule of atlantooccipital joint

Posterior atlantooccipital membrane

Ligamenta flava

Ligamentum nuchae

Spinous process of C7 vertebra (vertebra prominens)

Atlas (C1)

Body of axis (C2)

Intervertebral discs (C2–3 and C3–4)

Zygapophyseal joints (C4–5 and C5–6)

Anterior tubercle of C6 vertebra (carotid tubercle)

Vertebral artery

T1 vertebra

Right lateral view

Internal Craniocervical Ligaments

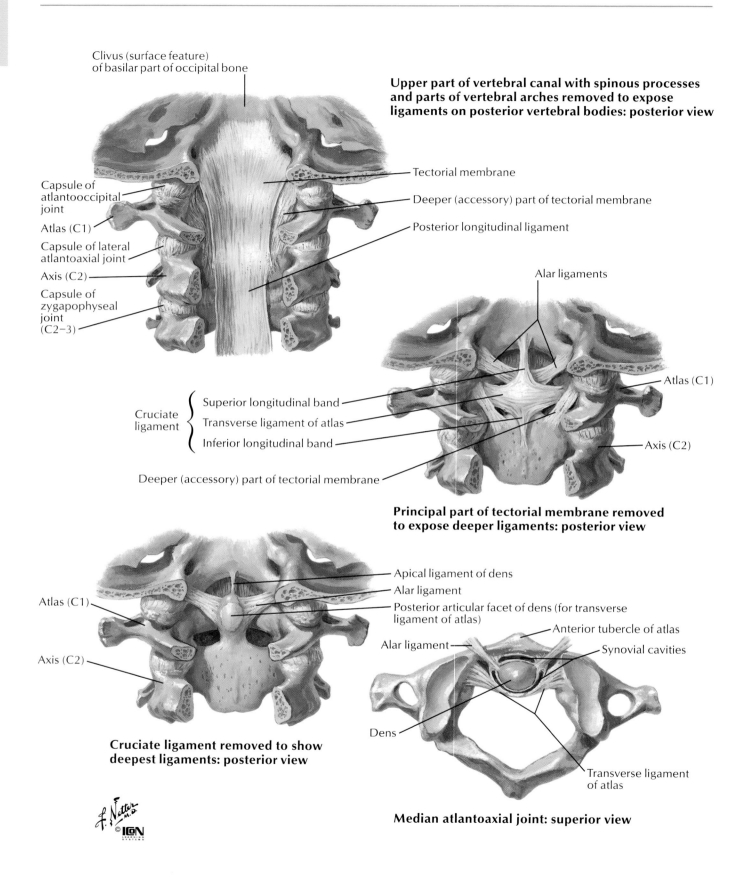

Clivus (surface feature) of basilar part of occipital bone

Upper part of vertebral canal with spinous processes and parts of vertebral arches removed to expose ligaments on posterior vertebral bodies: posterior view

Capsule of atlantooccipital joint

Atlas (C1)

Capsule of lateral atlantoaxial joint

Axis (C2)

Capsule of zygapophyseal joint (C2–3)

Tectorial membrane

Deeper (accessory) part of tectorial membrane

Posterior longitudinal ligament

Alar ligaments

Atlas (C1)

Axis (C2)

Cruciate ligament

Superior longitudinal band

Transverse ligament of atlas

Inferior longitudinal band

Deeper (accessory) part of tectorial membrane

Principal part of tectorial membrane removed to expose deeper ligaments: posterior view

Atlas (C1)

Axis (C2)

Apical ligament of dens

Alar ligament

Posterior articular facet of dens (for transverse ligament of atlas)

Anterior tubercle of atlas

Synovial cavities

Alar ligament

Dens

Transverse ligament of atlas

Cruciate ligament removed to show deepest ligaments: posterior view

Median atlantoaxial joint: superior view

PLATE 18

HEAD AND NECK

SEE ALSO PLATES 30, 36, 65, 66, 81, 98

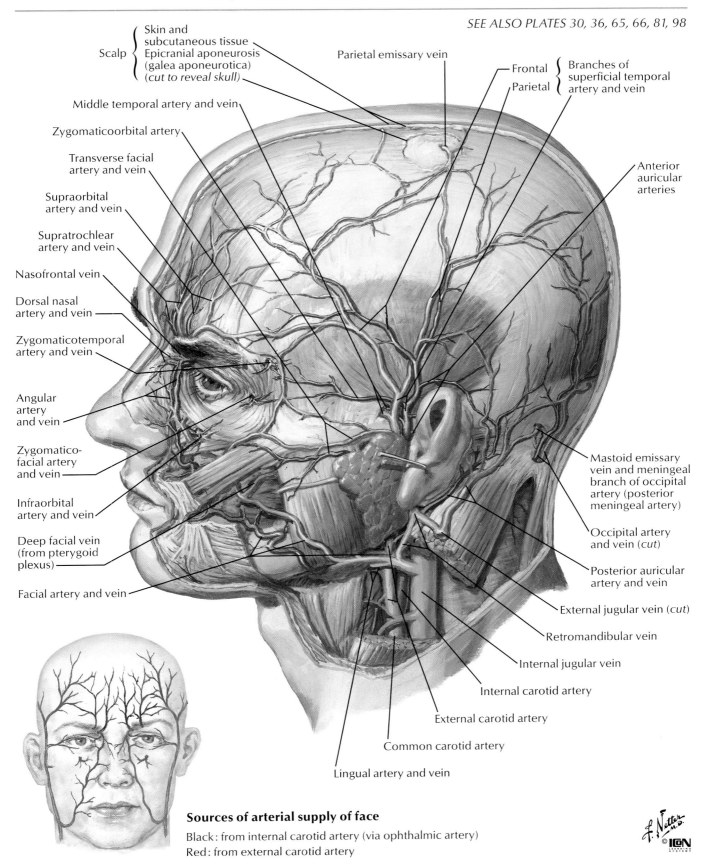

Scalp {
Skin and subcutaneous tissue
Epicranial aponeurosis (galea aponeurotica) (*cut to reveal skull*)

Parietal emissary vein

Frontal
Parietal } Branches of superficial temporal artery and vein

Middle temporal artery and vein

Zygomaticoorbital artery

Anterior auricular arteries

Transverse facial artery and vein

Supraorbital artery and vein

Supratrochlear artery and vein

Nasofrontal vein

Dorsal nasal artery and vein

Zygomaticotemporal artery and vein

Angular artery and vein

Zygomatico-facial artery and vein

Infraorbital artery and vein

Deep facial vein (from pterygoid plexus)

Facial artery and vein

Mastoid emissary vein and meningeal branch of occipital artery (posterior meningeal artery)

Occipital artery and vein (*cut*)

Posterior auricular artery and vein

External jugular vein (*cut*)

Retromandibular vein

Internal jugular vein

Internal carotid artery

External carotid artery

Common carotid artery

Lingual artery and vein

Sources of arterial supply of face

Black: from internal carotid artery (via ophthalmic artery)
Red: from external carotid artery

Cutaneous Nerves of Head and Neck

SEE ALSO PLATES 28, 32, 41, 42, 116

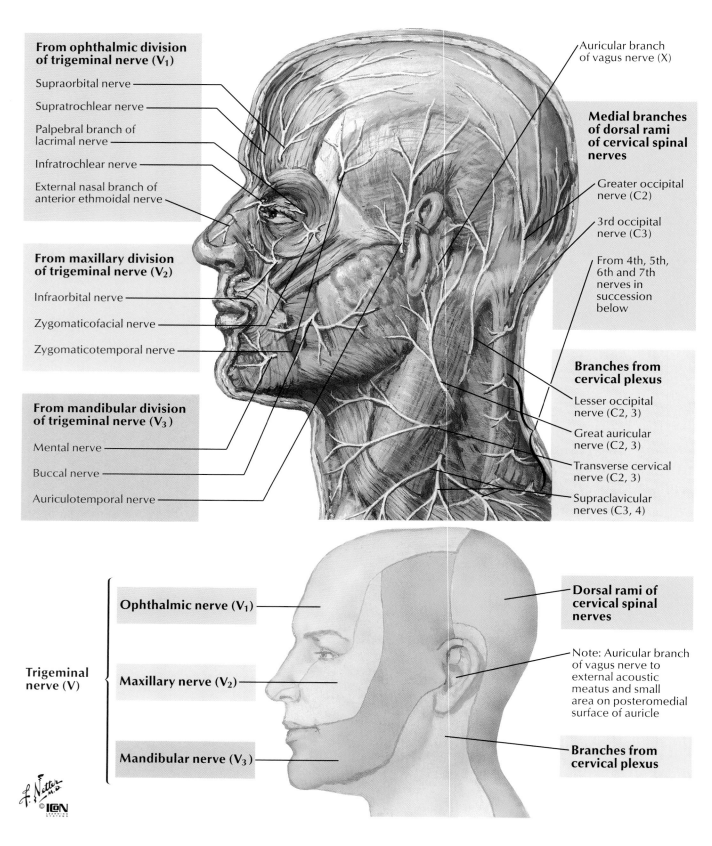

From ophthalmic division of trigeminal nerve (V₁)

Supraorbital nerve

Supratrochlear nerve

Palpebral branch of lacrimal nerve

Infratrochlear nerve

External nasal branch of anterior ethmoidal nerve

From maxillary division of trigeminal nerve (V₂)

Infraorbital nerve

Zygomaticofacial nerve

Zygomaticotemporal nerve

From mandibular division of trigeminal nerve (V₃)

Mental nerve

Buccal nerve

Auriculotemporal nerve

Auricular branch of vagus nerve (X)

Medial branches of dorsal rami of cervical spinal nerves

Greater occipital nerve (C2)

3rd occipital nerve (C3)

From 4th, 5th, 6th and 7th nerves in succession below

Branches from cervical plexus

Lesser occipital nerve (C2, 3)

Great auricular nerve (C2, 3)

Transverse cervical nerve (C2, 3)

Supraclavicular nerves (C3, 4)

Ophthalmic nerve (V₁)

Trigeminal nerve (V)

Maxillary nerve (V₂)

Mandibular nerve (V₃)

Dorsal rami of cervical spinal nerves

Note: Auricular branch of vagus nerve to external acoustic meatus and small area on posteromedial surface of auricle

Branches from cervical plexus

PLATE 20

HEAD AND NECK

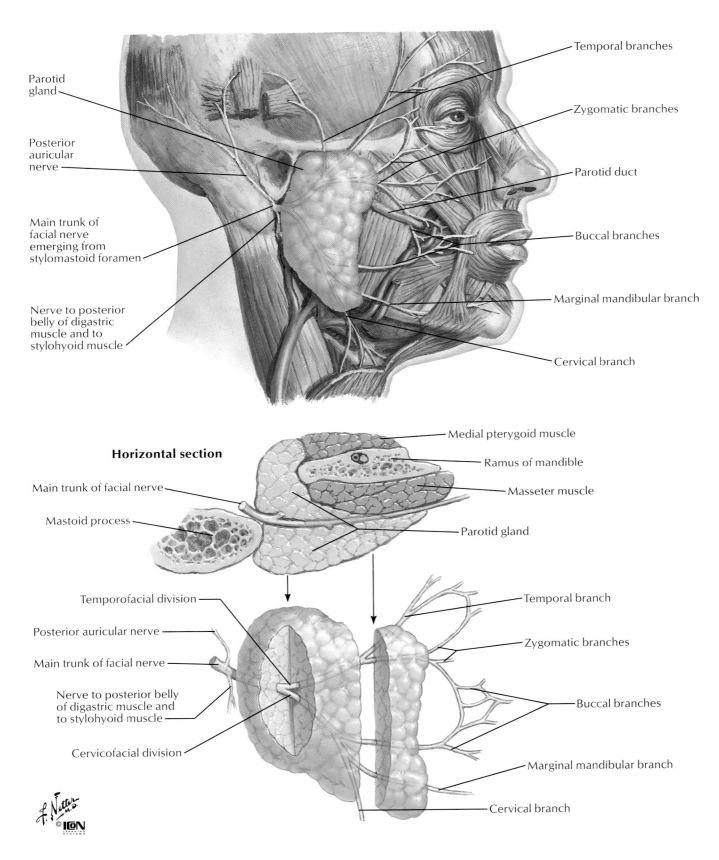

Parotid gland

Posterior auricular nerve

Main trunk of facial nerve emerging from stylomastoid foramen

Nerve to posterior belly of digastric muscle and to stylohyoid muscle

Temporal branches

Zygomatic branches

Parotid duct

Buccal branches

Marginal mandibular branch

Cervical branch

Horizontal section

Main trunk of facial nerve

Mastoid process

Medial pterygoid muscle

Ramus of mandible

Masseter muscle

Parotid gland

Temporofacial division

Posterior auricular nerve

Main trunk of facial nerve

Nerve to posterior belly of digastric muscle and to stylohyoid muscle

Cervicofacial division

Temporal branch

Zygomatic branches

Buccal branches

Marginal mandibular branch

Cervical branch

Muscles of Facial Expression: Lateral View

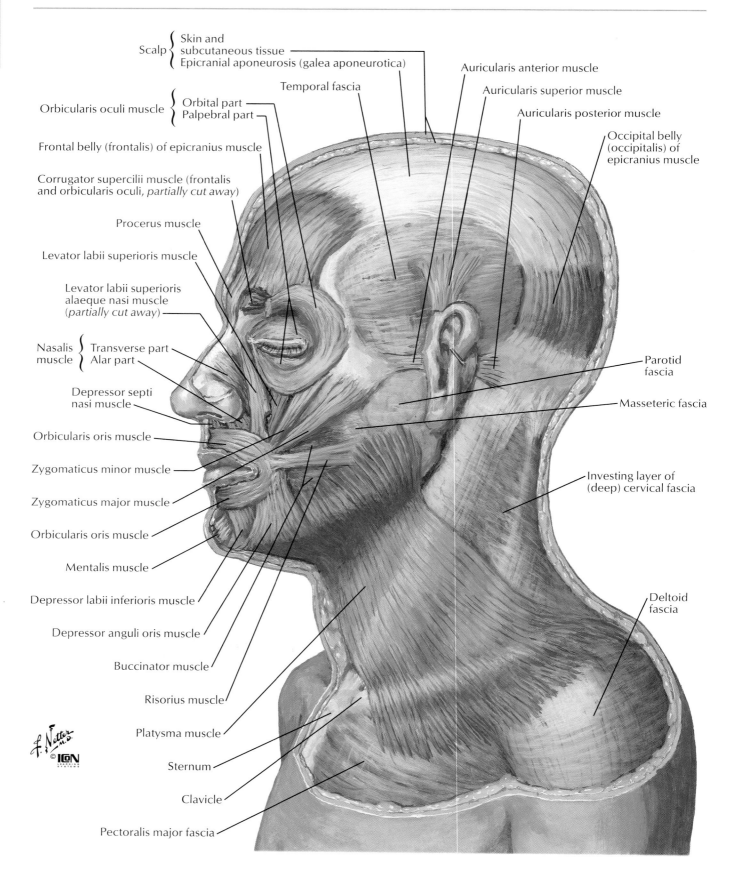

Scalp { Skin and subcutaneous tissue
Epicranial aponeurosis (galea aponeurotica)

Temporal fascia

Auricularis anterior muscle

Auricularis superior muscle

Auricularis posterior muscle

Occipital belly (occipitalis) of epicranius muscle

Orbicularis oculi muscle { Orbital part
Palpebral part

Frontal belly (frontalis) of epicranius muscle

Corrugator supercilii muscle (frontalis and orbicularis oculi, *partially cut away*)

Procerus muscle

Levator labii superioris muscle

Levator labii superioris alaeque nasi muscle (*partially cut away*)

Nasalis muscle { Transverse part
Alar part

Depressor septi nasi muscle

Orbicularis oris muscle

Zygomaticus minor muscle

Zygomaticus major muscle

Orbicularis oris muscle

Mentalis muscle

Depressor labii inferioris muscle

Depressor anguli oris muscle

Buccinator muscle

Risorius muscle

Platysma muscle

Sternum

Clavicle

Pectoralis major fascia

Parotid fascia

Masseteric fascia

Investing layer of (deep) cervical fascia

Deltoid fascia

PLATE 22

HEAD AND NECK

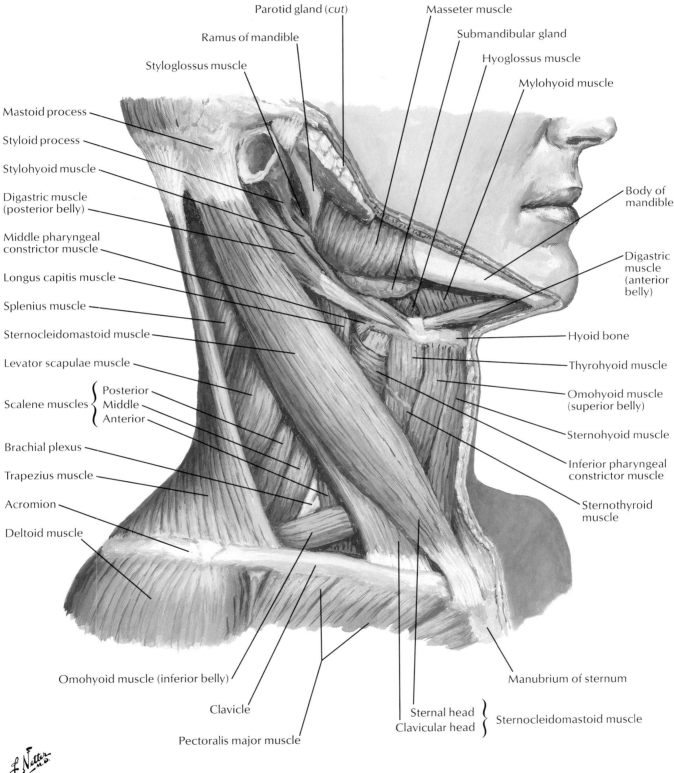

Parotid gland (*cut*)

Ramus of mandible

Styloglossus muscle

Masseter muscle

Submandibular gland

Hyoglossus muscle

Mylohyoid muscle

Mastoid process

Styloid process

Stylohyoid muscle

Digastric muscle (posterior belly)

Middle pharyngeal constrictor muscle

Longus capitis muscle

Splenius muscle

Sternocleidomastoid muscle

Levator scapulae muscle

Scalene muscles { Posterior / Middle / Anterior

Brachial plexus

Trapezius muscle

Acromion

Deltoid muscle

Body of mandible

Digastric muscle (anterior belly)

Hyoid bone

Thyrohyoid muscle

Omohyoid muscle (superior belly)

Sternohyoid muscle

Inferior pharyngeal constrictor muscle

Sternothyroid muscle

Omohyoid muscle (inferior belly)

Clavicle

Pectoralis major muscle

Sternal head } Sternocleidomastoid muscle
Clavicular head

Manubrium of sternum

Muscles of Neck: Anterior View

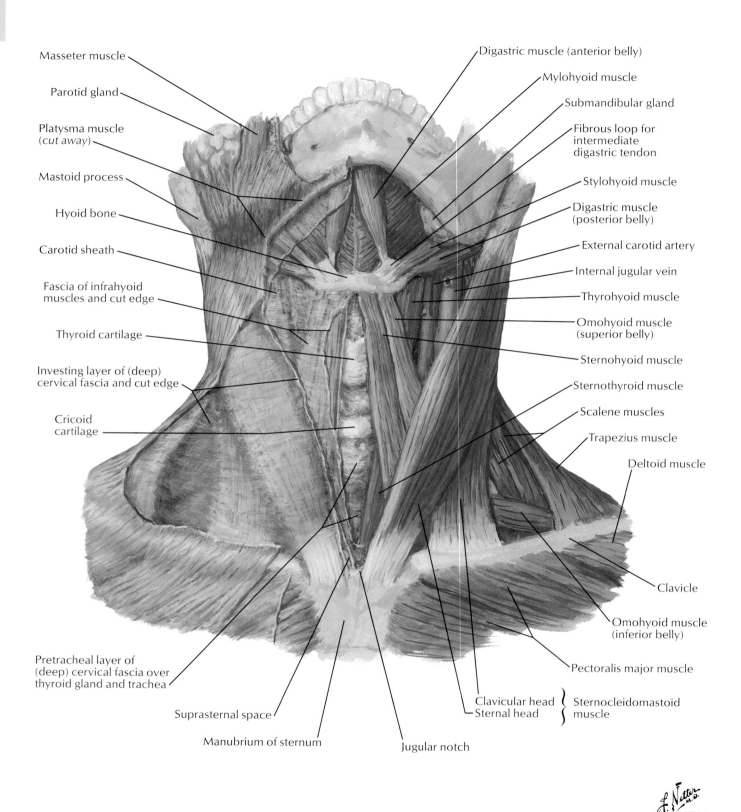

Masseter muscle

Parotid gland

Platysma muscle (*cut away*)

Mastoid process

Hyoid bone

Carotid sheath

Fascia of infrahyoid muscles and cut edge

Thyroid cartilage

Investing layer of (deep) cervical fascia and cut edge

Cricoid cartilage

Pretracheal layer of (deep) cervical fascia over thyroid gland and trachea

Suprasternal space

Manubrium of sternum

Jugular notch

Digastric muscle (anterior belly)

Mylohyoid muscle

Submandibular gland

Fibrous loop for intermediate digastric tendon

Stylohyoid muscle

Digastric muscle (posterior belly)

External carotid artery

Internal jugular vein

Thyrohyoid muscle

Omohyoid muscle (superior belly)

Sternohyoid muscle

Sternothyroid muscle

Scalene muscles

Trapezius muscle

Deltoid muscle

Clavicle

Omohyoid muscle (inferior belly)

Pectoralis major muscle

Clavicular head
Sternal head } Sternocleidomastoid muscle

PLATE 24

HEAD AND NECK

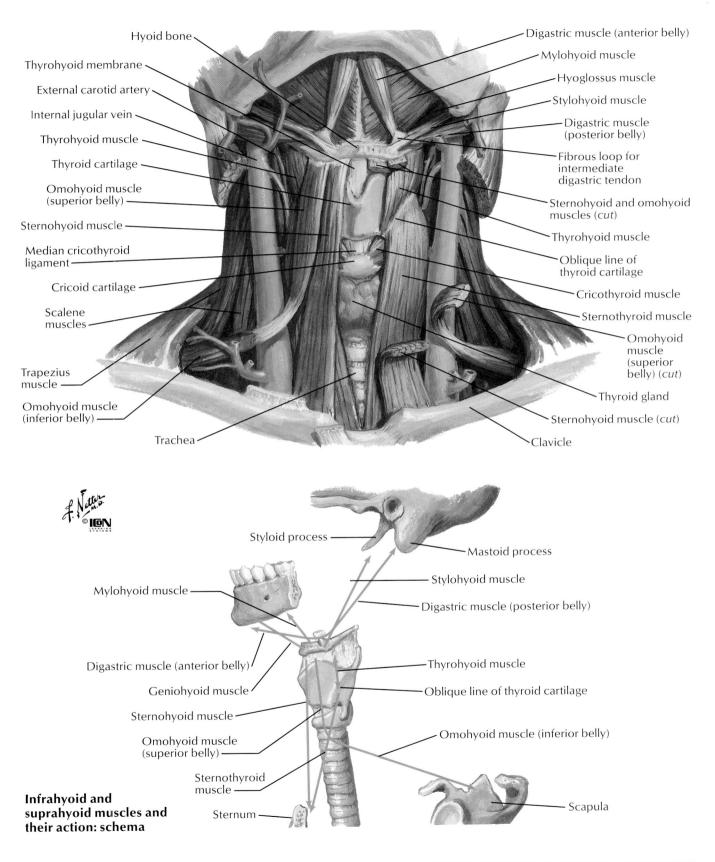

Hyoid bone

Thyrohyoid membrane

External carotid artery

Internal jugular vein

Thyrohyoid muscle

Thyroid cartilage

Omohyoid muscle (superior belly)

Sternohyoid muscle

Median cricothyroid ligament

Cricoid cartilage

Scalene muscles

Trapezius muscle

Omohyoid muscle (inferior belly)

Trachea

Digastric muscle (anterior belly)

Mylohyoid muscle

Hyoglossus muscle

Stylohyoid muscle

Digastric muscle (posterior belly)

Fibrous loop for intermediate digastric tendon

Sternohyoid and omohyoid muscles (*cut*)

Thyrohyoid muscle

Oblique line of thyroid cartilage

Cricothyroid muscle

Sternothyroid muscle

Omohyoid muscle (superior belly) (*cut*)

Thyroid gland

Sternohyoid muscle (*cut*)

Clavicle

Styloid process

Mastoid process

Stylohyoid muscle

Digastric muscle (posterior belly)

Mylohyoid muscle

Digastric muscle (anterior belly)

Geniohyoid muscle

Sternohyoid muscle

Omohyoid muscle (superior belly)

Thyrohyoid muscle

Oblique line of thyroid cartilage

Omohyoid muscle (inferior belly)

Sternothyroid muscle

Sternum

Scapula

Infrahyoid and suprahyoid muscles and their action: schema

Scalene and Prevertebral Muscles

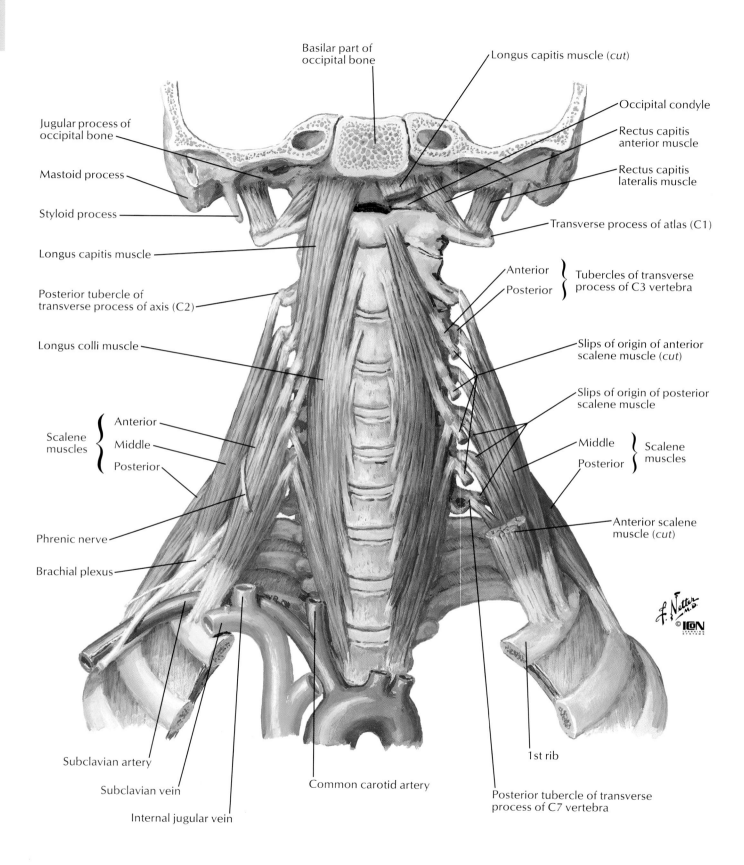

Basilar part of occipital bone

Longus capitis muscle (*cut*)

Occipital condyle

Rectus capitis anterior muscle

Rectus capitis lateralis muscle

Transverse process of atlas (C1)

Jugular process of occipital bone

Mastoid process

Styloid process

Longus capitis muscle

Posterior tubercle of transverse process of axis (C2)

Longus colli muscle

Anterior

Posterior

} Tubercles of transverse process of C3 vertebra

Slips of origin of anterior scalene muscle (*cut*)

Slips of origin of posterior scalene muscle

Scalene muscles { Anterior
Middle
Posterior

Middle

Posterior

} Scalene muscles

Anterior scalene muscle (*cut*)

Phrenic nerve

Brachial plexus

1st rib

Subclavian artery

Subclavian vein

Internal jugular vein

Common carotid artery

Posterior tubercle of transverse process of C7 vertebra

PLATE 26

HEAD AND NECK

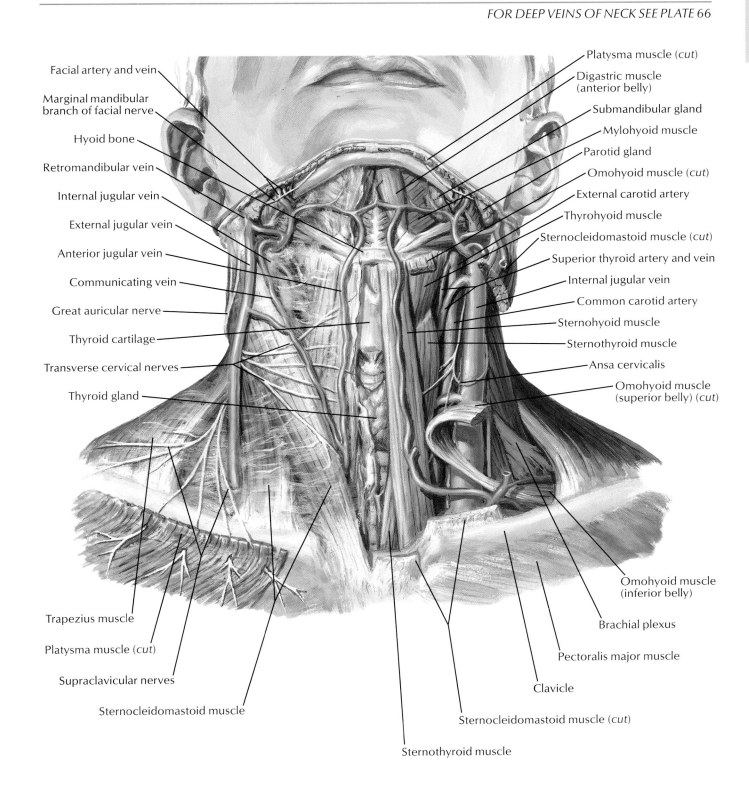

Facial artery and vein

Marginal mandibular branch of facial nerve

Hyoid bone

Retromandibular vein

Internal jugular vein

External jugular vein

Anterior jugular vein

Communicating vein

Great auricular nerve

Thyroid cartilage

Transverse cervical nerves

Thyroid gland

Trapezius muscle

Platysma muscle (*cut*)

Supraclavicular nerves

Sternocleidomastoid muscle

Platysma muscle (*cut*)

Digastric muscle (anterior belly)

Submandibular gland

Mylohyoid muscle

Parotid gland

Omohyoid muscle (*cut*)

External carotid artery

Thyrohyoid muscle

Sternocleidomastoid muscle (*cut*)

Superior thyroid artery and vein

Internal jugular vein

Common carotid artery

Sternohyoid muscle

Sternothyroid muscle

Ansa cervicalis

Omohyoid muscle (superior belly) (*cut*)

Omohyoid muscle (inferior belly)

Brachial plexus

Pectoralis major muscle

Clavicle

Sternocleidomastoid muscle (*cut*)

Sternothyroid muscle

SEE ALSO PLATES 121–123, 190

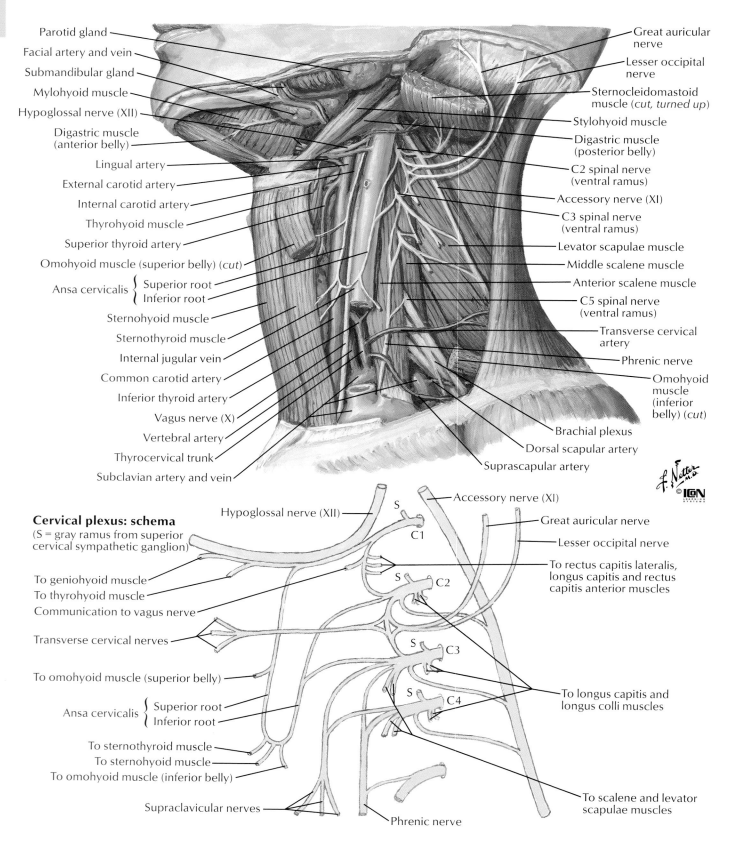

Parotid gland
Facial artery and vein
Submandibular gland
Mylohyoid muscle
Hypoglossal nerve (XII)
Digastric muscle (anterior belly)
Lingual artery
External carotid artery
Internal carotid artery
Thyrohyoid muscle
Superior thyroid artery
Omohyoid muscle (superior belly) (cut)
Ansa cervicalis { Superior root / Inferior root
Sternohyoid muscle
Sternothyroid muscle
Internal jugular vein
Common carotid artery
Inferior thyroid artery
Vagus nerve (X)
Vertebral artery
Thyrocervical trunk
Subclavian artery and vein

Great auricular nerve
Lesser occipital nerve
Sternocleidomastoid muscle (cut, turned up)
Stylohyoid muscle
Digastric muscle (posterior belly)
C2 spinal nerve (ventral ramus)
Accessory nerve (XI)
C3 spinal nerve (ventral ramus)
Levator scapulae muscle
Middle scalene muscle
Anterior scalene muscle
C5 spinal nerve (ventral ramus)
Transverse cervical artery
Phrenic nerve
Omohyoid muscle (inferior belly) (cut)
Brachial plexus
Dorsal scapular artery
Suprascapular artery

Cervical plexus: schema
(S = gray ramus from superior cervical sympathetic ganglion)

Hypoglossal nerve (XII)
To geniohyoid muscle
To thyrohyoid muscle
Communication to vagus nerve
Transverse cervical nerves
To omohyoid muscle (superior belly)
Ansa cervicalis { Superior root / Inferior root
To sternothyroid muscle
To sternohyoid muscle
To omohyoid muscle (inferior belly)
Supraclavicular nerves

Accessory nerve (XI)
Great auricular nerve
Lesser occipital nerve
To rectus capitis lateralis, longus capitis and rectus capitis anterior muscles
To longus capitis and longus colli muscles
To scalene and levator scapulae muscles
Phrenic nerve

S
C1
S C2
S C3
S C4

PLATE 28   **HEAD AND NECK**

Right anterior dissection

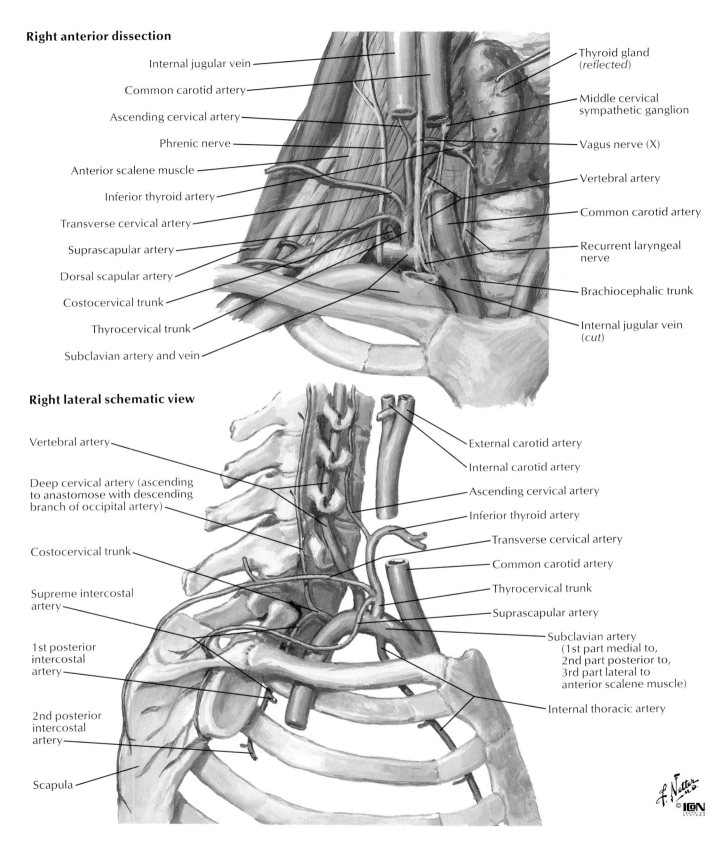

Internal jugular vein

Common carotid artery

Ascending cervical artery

Phrenic nerve

Anterior scalene muscle

Inferior thyroid artery

Transverse cervical artery

Suprascapular artery

Dorsal scapular artery

Costocervical trunk

Thyrocervical trunk

Subclavian artery and vein

Thyroid gland (*reflected*)

Middle cervical sympathetic ganglion

Vagus nerve (X)

Vertebral artery

Common carotid artery

Recurrent laryngeal nerve

Brachiocephalic trunk

Internal jugular vein (*cut*)

Right lateral schematic view

Vertebral artery

Deep cervical artery (ascending to anastomose with descending branch of occipital artery)

Costocervical trunk

Supreme intercostal artery

1st posterior intercostal artery

2nd posterior intercostal artery

Scapula

External carotid artery

Internal carotid artery

Ascending cervical artery

Inferior thyroid artery

Transverse cervical artery

Common carotid artery

Thyrocervical trunk

Suprascapular artery

Subclavian artery (1st part medial to, 2nd part posterior to, 3rd part lateral to anterior scalene muscle)

Internal thoracic artery

Carotid Arteries

SEE ALSO PLATES 130, 131

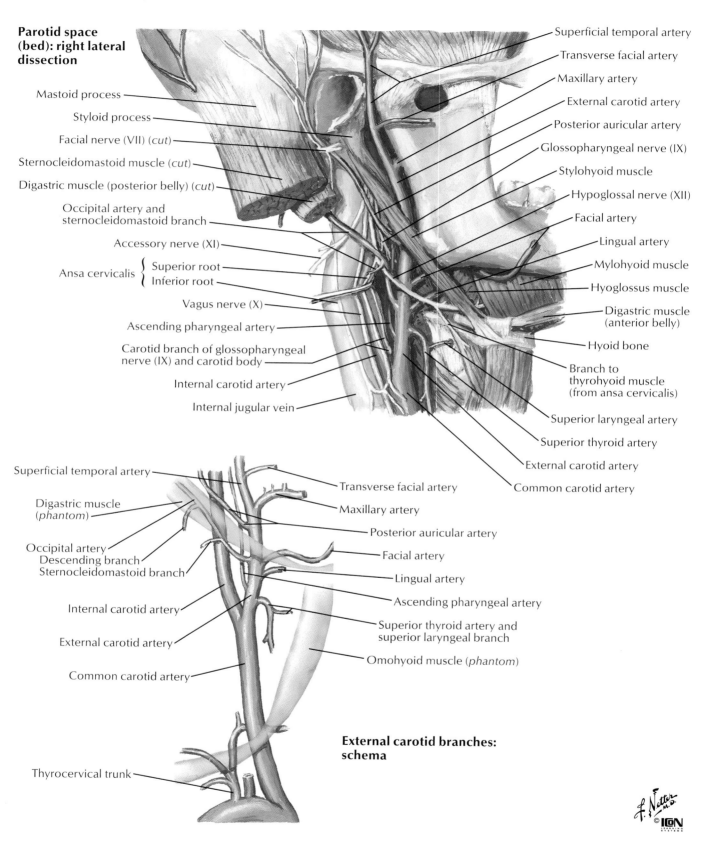

Parotid space (bed): right lateral dissection

Mastoid process

Styloid process

Facial nerve (VII) (*cut*)

Sternocleidomastoid muscle (*cut*)

Digastric muscle (posterior belly) (*cut*)

Occipital artery and sternocleidomastoid branch

Accessory nerve (XI)

Ansa cervicalis { Superior root / Inferior root

Vagus nerve (X)

Ascending pharyngeal artery

Carotid branch of glossopharyngeal nerve (IX) and carotid body

Internal carotid artery

Internal jugular vein

Superficial temporal artery

Transverse facial artery

Maxillary artery

External carotid artery

Posterior auricular artery

Glossopharyngeal nerve (IX)

Stylohyoid muscle

Hypoglossal nerve (XII)

Facial artery

Lingual artery

Mylohyoid muscle

Hyoglossus muscle

Digastric muscle (anterior belly)

Hyoid bone

Branch to thyrohyoid muscle (from ansa cervicalis)

Superior laryngeal artery

Superior thyroid artery

External carotid artery

Common carotid artery

Superficial temporal artery

Digastric muscle (*phantom*)

Occipital artery

Descending branch

Sternocleidomastoid branch

Internal carotid artery

External carotid artery

Common carotid artery

Thyrocervical trunk

Transverse facial artery

Maxillary artery

Posterior auricular artery

Facial artery

Lingual artery

Ascending pharyngeal artery

Superior thyroid artery and superior laryngeal branch

Omohyoid muscle (*phantom*)

External carotid branches: schema

PLATE 30

HEAD AND NECK

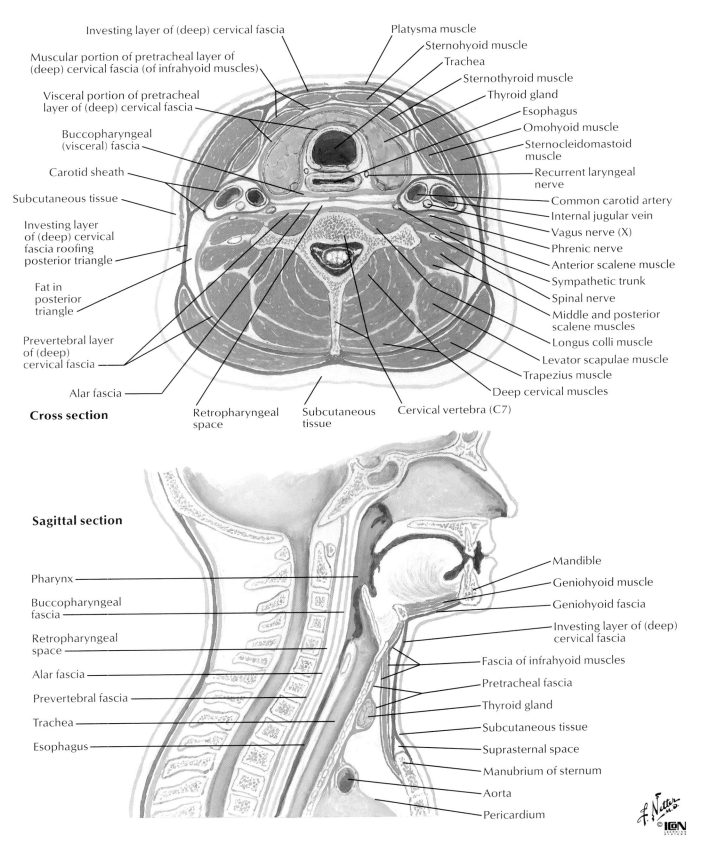

Investing layer of (deep) cervical fascia

Muscular portion of pretracheal layer of (deep) cervical fascia (of infrahyoid muscles)

Visceral portion of pretracheal layer of (deep) cervical fascia

Buccopharyngeal (visceral) fascia

Carotid sheath

Subcutaneous tissue

Investing layer of (deep) cervical fascia roofing posterior triangle

Fat in posterior triangle

Prevertebral layer of (deep) cervical fascia

Alar fascia

Cross section

Platysma muscle

Sternohyoid muscle

Trachea

Sternothyroid muscle

Thyroid gland

Esophagus

Omohyoid muscle

Sternocleidomastoid muscle

Recurrent laryngeal nerve

Common carotid artery

Internal jugular vein

Vagus nerve (X)

Phrenic nerve

Anterior scalene muscle

Sympathetic trunk

Spinal nerve

Middle and posterior scalene muscles

Longus colli muscle

Levator scapulae muscle

Trapezius muscle

Deep cervical muscles

Retropharyngeal space

Subcutaneous tissue

Cervical vertebra (C7)

Sagittal section

Pharynx

Buccopharyngeal fascia

Retropharyngeal space

Alar fascia

Prevertebral fascia

Trachea

Esophagus

Mandible

Geniohyoid muscle

Geniohyoid fascia

Investing layer of (deep) cervical fascia

Fascia of infrahyoid muscles

Pretracheal fascia

Thyroid gland

Subcutaneous tissue

Suprasternal space

Manubrium of sternum

Aorta

Pericardium

Nose

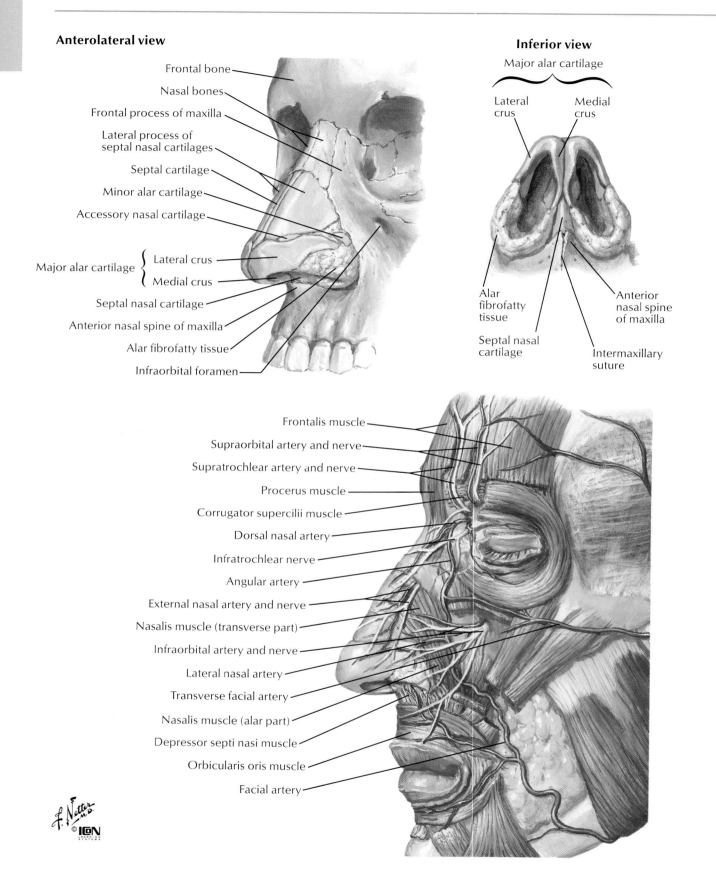

Anterolateral view

Frontal bone

Nasal bones

Frontal process of maxilla

Lateral process of septal nasal cartilages

Septal cartilage

Minor alar cartilage

Accessory nasal cartilage

Major alar cartilage { Lateral crus

Medial crus

Septal nasal cartilage

Anterior nasal spine of maxilla

Alar fibrofatty tissue

Infraorbital foramen

Inferior view

Major alar cartilage

Lateral crus

Medial crus

Alar fibrofatty tissue

Septal nasal cartilage

Anterior nasal spine of maxilla

Intermaxillary suture

Frontalis muscle

Supraorbital artery and nerve

Supratrochlear artery and nerve

Procerus muscle

Corrugator supercilii muscle

Dorsal nasal artery

Infratrochlear nerve

Angular artery

External nasal artery and nerve

Nasalis muscle (transverse part)

Infraorbital artery and nerve

Lateral nasal artery

Transverse facial artery

Nasalis muscle (alar part)

Depressor septi nasi muscle

Orbicularis oris muscle

Facial artery

PLATE 32

HEAD AND NECK

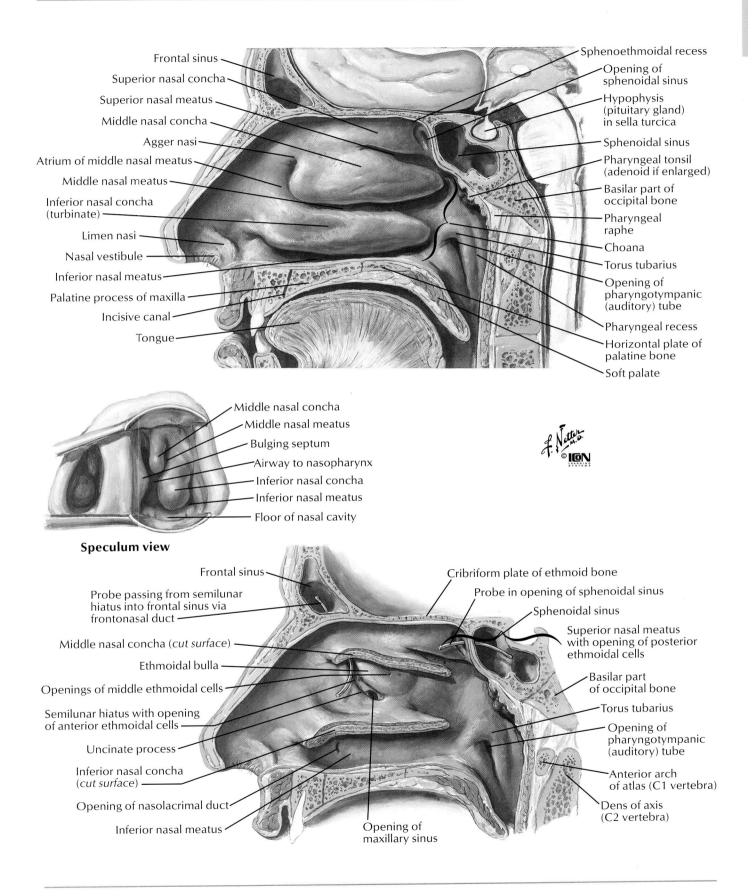

Frontal sinus

Superior nasal concha

Superior nasal meatus

Middle nasal concha

Agger nasi

Atrium of middle nasal meatus

Middle nasal meatus

Inferior nasal concha (turbinate)

Limen nasi

Nasal vestibule

Inferior nasal meatus

Palatine process of maxilla

Incisive canal

Tongue

Sphenoethmoidal recess

Opening of sphenoidal sinus

Hypophysis (pituitary gland) in sella turcica

Sphenoidal sinus

Pharyngeal tonsil (adenoid if enlarged)

Basilar part of occipital bone

Pharyngeal raphe

Choana

Torus tubarius

Opening of pharyngotympanic (auditory) tube

Pharyngeal recess

Horizontal plate of palatine bone

Soft palate

Middle nasal concha

Middle nasal meatus

Bulging septum

Airway to nasopharynx

Inferior nasal concha

Inferior nasal meatus

Floor of nasal cavity

Speculum view

Frontal sinus

Probe passing from semilunar hiatus into frontal sinus via frontonasal duct

Middle nasal concha (*cut surface*)

Ethmoidal bulla

Openings of middle ethmoidal cells

Semilunar hiatus with opening of anterior ethmoidal cells

Uncinate process

Inferior nasal concha (*cut surface*)

Opening of nasolacrimal duct

Inferior nasal meatus

Cribriform plate of ethmoid bone

Probe in opening of sphenoidal sinus

Sphenoidal sinus

Superior nasal meatus with opening of posterior ethmoidal cells

Basilar part of occipital bone

Torus tubarius

Opening of pharyngotympanic (auditory) tube

Anterior arch of atlas (C1 vertebra)

Dens of axis (C2 vertebra)

Opening of maxillary sinus

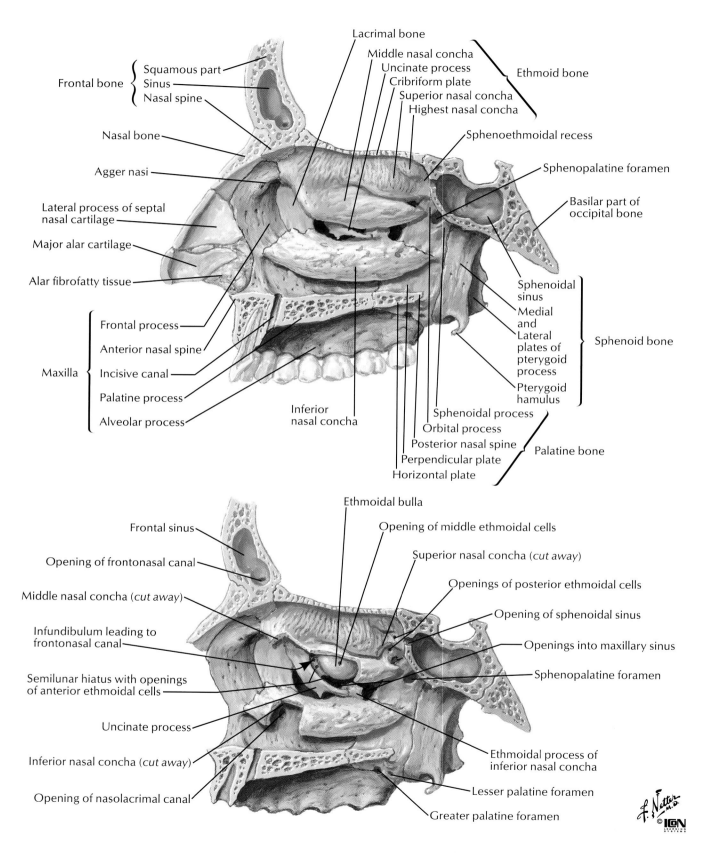

Lacrimal bone
Middle nasal concha
Uncinate process
Cribriform plate
Superior nasal concha
Highest nasal concha
Ethmoid bone

Frontal bone
Squamous part
Sinus
Nasal spine

Nasal bone

Agger nasi

Lateral process of septal nasal cartilage

Major alar cartilage

Alar fibrofatty tissue

Maxilla
Frontal process
Anterior nasal spine
Incisive canal
Palatine process
Alveolar process

Sphenoethmoidal recess

Sphenopalatine foramen

Basilar part of occipital bone

Sphenoidal sinus
Medial and Lateral plates of pterygoid process
Pterygoid hamulus
Sphenoid bone

Inferior nasal concha

Sphenoidal process
Orbital process
Posterior nasal spine
Perpendicular plate
Horizontal plate
Palatine bone

Ethmoidal bulla

Frontal sinus

Opening of frontonasal canal

Middle nasal concha (*cut away*)

Infundibulum leading to frontonasal canal

Semilunar hiatus with openings of anterior ethmoidal cells

Uncinate process

Inferior nasal concha (*cut away*)

Opening of nasolacrimal canal

Opening of middle ethmoidal cells

Superior nasal concha (*cut away*)

Openings of posterior ethmoidal cells

Opening of sphenoidal sinus

Openings into maxillary sinus

Sphenopalatine foramen

Ethmoidal process of inferior nasal concha

Lesser palatine foramen

Greater palatine foramen

PLATE 34

HEAD AND NECK

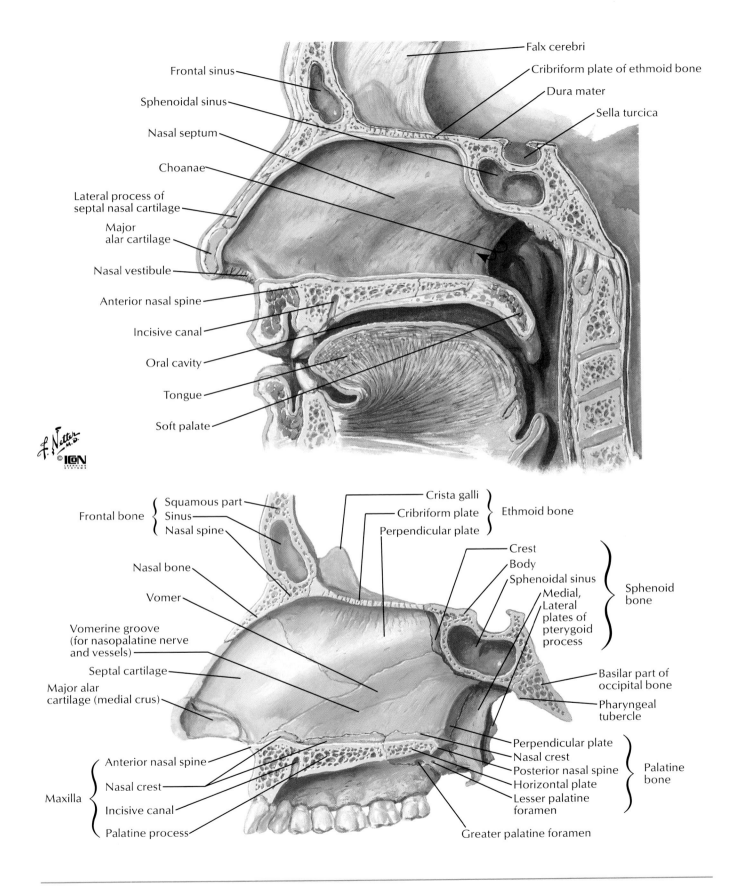

Falx cerebri

Frontal sinus

Cribriform plate of ethmoid bone

Spheroidal sinus

Dura mater

Nasal septum

Sella turcica

Choanae

Lateral process of
septal nasal cartilage

Major
alar cartilage

Nasal vestibule

Anterior nasal spine

Incisive canal

Oral cavity

Tongue

Soft palate

Crista galli

Frontal bone
{
Squamous part
Sinus
Nasal spine
}

Cribriform plate

Ethmoid bone

Perpendicular plate

Crest

Body

Nasal bone

Sphenoidal sinus

Vomer

Medial,
Lateral
plates of
pterygoid
process

Sphenoid
bone

Vomerine groove
(for nasopalatine nerve
and vessels)

Septal cartilage

Basilar part of
occipital bone

Major alar
cartilage (medial crus)

Pharyngeal
tubercle

Anterior nasal spine

Perpendicular plate
Nasal crest
Posterior nasal spine
Horizontal plate
Lesser palatine
foramen

Palatine
bone

Nasal crest

Maxilla
{

Incisive canal

Palatine process

Greater palatine foramen

Maxillary Artery

SEE ALSO PLATE 30

Lateral pterygoid artery and muscle
Supraorbital artery
Supratrochlear artery
Ophthalmic artery
Dorsal nasal artery
Angular artery
Infraorbital artery
Superior alveolar arteries { Posterior / Middle / Anterior
Buccal artery and nerve
Medial pterygoid artery and muscle
Pterygomandibular raphe
Lingual nerve
Facial artery
Mental branch of inferior alveolar artery
Submental artery

Anterior / Posterior } Deep temporal arteries and nerves
Masseteric artery and nerve
Lateral ligament of temporomandibular joint
Middle meningeal artery
Auriculotemporal nerve
Maxillary artery
Superficial temporal artery
Posterior auricular artery
Facial nerve
Inferior alveolar artery and nerve
Sphenomandibular ligament
Mylohyoid nerve and branch of inferior alveolar artery
Digastric muscle (posterior belly)
Stylohyoid muscle
External carotid artery
Facial artery
Lingual artery

Sphenopalatine artery
Posterior lateral nasal branch
Infraorbital artery
Posterior superior alveolar artery
Sphenopalatine artery
Posterior septal branches
Descending palatine artery in pterygo-palatine fossa
Buccal artery
Anastomosis in incisive canal
Left and right greater palatine arteries
Left and right lesser palatine arteries

Artery of pterygoid canal
Pharyngeal artery
Sphenopalatine foramen

Anterior / Posterior } Deep temporal arteries and nerves
Accessory meningeal artery
Middle meningeal artery
Anterior tympanic artery
Deep auricular artery
Auriculo-temporal nerve
Superficial temporal artery
Ascending pharyngeal artery
Ascending palatine artery
Tonsillar branches
Tonsillar artery
External carotid artery
Facial artery

Pterygoid arteries
Masseteric artery
Inferior alveolar artery
Superior pharyngeal constrictor muscle
Styloglossus muscle

f. Netter M.D.
© ICON

PLATE 36   **HEAD AND NECK**

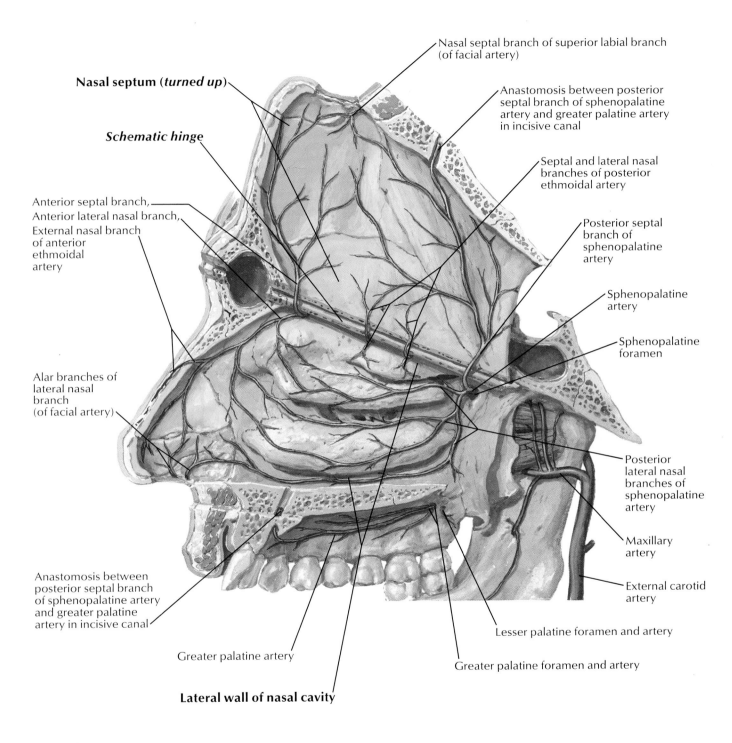

Nasal septal branch of superior labial branch (of facial artery)

Nasal septum (*turned up*)

Anastomosis between posterior septal branch of sphenopalatine artery and greater palatine artery in incisive canal

Schematic hinge

Septal and lateral nasal branches of posterior ethmoidal artery

Anterior septal branch,
Anterior lateral nasal branch,
External nasal branch of anterior ethmoidal artery

Posterior septal branch of sphenopalatine artery

Sphenopalatine artery

Sphenopalatine foramen

Alar branches of lateral nasal branch (of facial artery)

Posterior lateral nasal branches of sphenopalatine artery

Maxillary artery

Anastomosis between posterior septal branch of sphenopalatine artery and greater palatine artery in incisive canal

External carotid artery

Greater palatine artery

Lesser palatine foramen and artery

Greater palatine foramen and artery

Lateral wall of nasal cavity

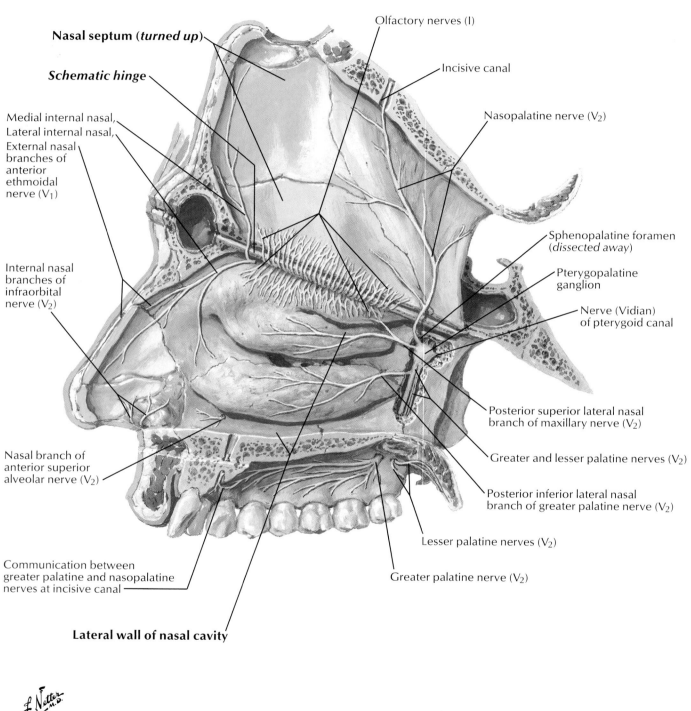

Nasal septum (*turned up*)

Schematic hinge

Medial internal nasal,
Lateral internal nasal,
External nasal
branches of
anterior
ethmoidal
nerve (V₁)

Internal nasal
branches of
infraorbital
nerve (V₂)

Nasal branch of
anterior superior
alveolar nerve (V₂)

Communication between
greater palatine and nasopalatine
nerves at incisive canal

Lateral wall of nasal cavity

Olfactory nerves (I)

Incisive canal

Nasopalatine nerve (V₂)

Sphenopalatine foramen
(*dissected away*)

Pterygopalatine
ganglion

Nerve (Vidian)
of pterygoid canal

Posterior superior lateral nasal
branch of maxillary nerve (V₂)

Greater and lesser palatine nerves (V₂)

Posterior inferior lateral nasal
branch of greater palatine nerve (V₂)

Lesser palatine nerves (V₂)

Greater palatine nerve (V₂)

PLATE 38

HEAD AND NECK

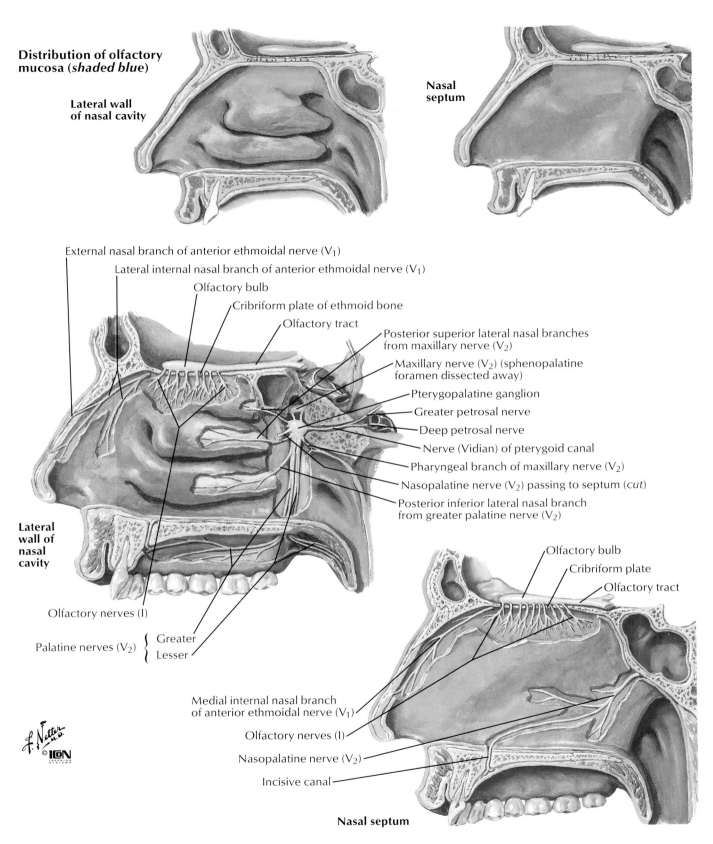

Distribution of olfactory mucosa (*shaded blue*)

Lateral wall of nasal cavity

Nasal septum

External nasal branch of anterior ethmoidal nerve (V_1)

Lateral internal nasal branch of anterior ethmoidal nerve (V_1)

Olfactory bulb

Cribriform plate of ethmoid bone

Olfactory tract

Posterior superior lateral nasal branches from maxillary nerve (V_2)

Maxillary nerve (V_2) (sphenopalatine foramen dissected away)

Pterygopalatine ganglion

Greater petrosal nerve

Deep petrosal nerve

Nerve (Vidian) of pterygoid canal

Pharyngeal branch of maxillary nerve (V_2)

Nasopalatine nerve (V_2) passing to septum (*cut*)

Posterior inferior lateral nasal branch from greater palatine nerve (V_2)

Lateral wall of nasal cavity

Olfactory nerves (I)

Palatine nerves (V_2) { Greater / Lesser }

Olfactory bulb

Cribriform plate

Olfactory tract

Medial internal nasal branch of anterior ethmoidal nerve (V_1)

Olfactory nerves (I)

Nasopalatine nerve (V_2)

Incisive canal

Nasal septum

SEE ALSO PLATES 116, 125, 127

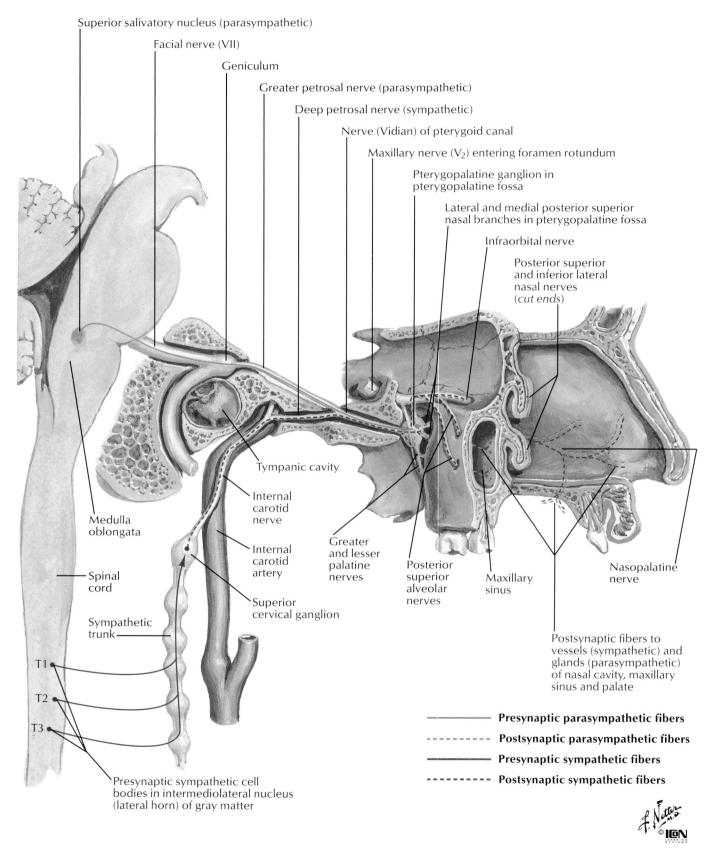

Superior salivatory nucleus (parasympathetic)

Facial nerve (VII)

Geniculum

Greater petrosal nerve (parasympathetic)

Deep petrosal nerve (sympathetic)

Nerve (Vidian) of pterygoid canal

Maxillary nerve (V$_2$) entering foramen rotundum

Pterygopalatine ganglion in pterygopalatine fossa

Lateral and medial posterior superior nasal branches in pterygopalatine fossa

Infraorbital nerve

Posterior superior and inferior lateral nasal nerves (*cut ends*)

Medulla oblongata

Spinal cord

Sympathetic trunk

T1

T2

T3

Presynaptic sympathetic cell bodies in intermediolateral nucleus (lateral horn) of gray matter

Tympanic cavity

Internal carotid nerve

Internal carotid artery

Superior cervical ganglion

Greater and lesser palatine nerves

Posterior superior alveolar nerves

Maxillary sinus

Nasopalatine nerve

Postsynaptic fibers to vessels (sympathetic) and glands (parasympathetic) of nasal cavity, maxillary sinus and palate

———————— **Presynaptic parasympathetic fibers**

- - - - - - - - **Postsynaptic parasympathetic fibers**

———————— **Presynaptic sympathetic fibers**

- - - - - - - - **Postsynaptic sympathetic fibers**

PLATE 40

HEAD AND NECK

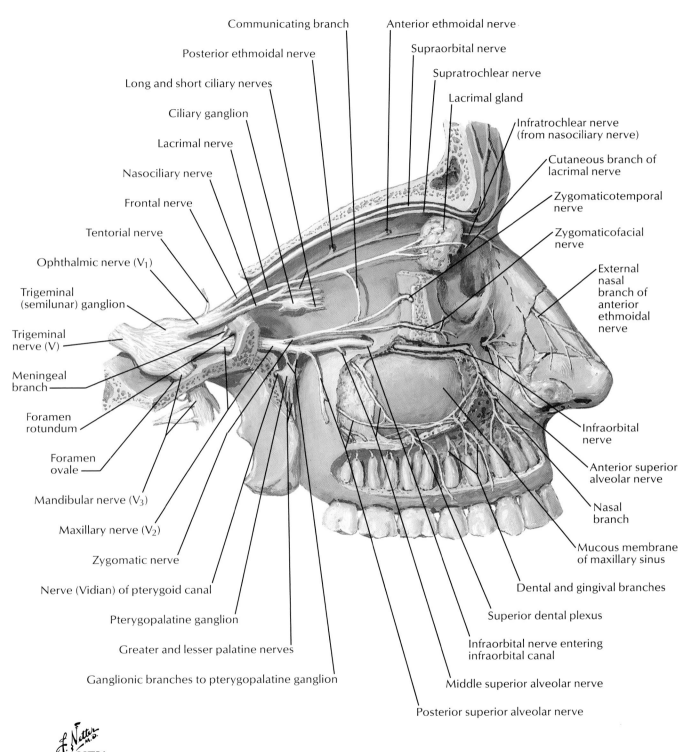

Communicating branch

Posterior ethmoidal nerve

Long and short ciliary nerves

Ciliary ganglion

Lacrimal nerve

Nasociliary nerve

Frontal nerve

Tentorial nerve

Ophthalmic nerve (V₁)

Trigeminal (semilunar) ganglion

Trigeminal nerve (V)

Meningeal branch

Foramen rotundum

Foramen ovale

Mandibular nerve (V₃)

Maxillary nerve (V₂)

Zygomatic nerve

Nerve (Vidian) of pterygoid canal

Pterygopalatine ganglion

Greater and lesser palatine nerves

Ganglionic branches to pterygopalatine ganglion

Anterior ethmoidal nerve

Supraorbital nerve

Supratrochlear nerve

Lacrimal gland

Infratrochlear nerve (from nasociliary nerve)

Cutaneous branch of lacrimal nerve

Zygomaticotemporal nerve

Zygomaticofacial nerve

External nasal branch of anterior ethmoidal nerve

Infraorbital nerve

Anterior superior alveolar nerve

Nasal branch

Mucous membrane of maxillary sinus

Dental and gingival branches

Superior dental plexus

Infraorbital nerve entering infraorbital canal

Middle superior alveolar nerve

Posterior superior alveolar nerve

Mandibular Nerve (V₃)

SEE ALSO PLATES 67, 116

Lateral view

Anterior division

Posterior division

Foramen ovale

Meningeal branch

Foramen spinosum

Middle meningeal artery

Auriculotemporal nerve

Posterior auricular nerve

Facial nerve (VII)

Chorda tympani nerve

Lingual nerve

Inferior alveolar nerve (cut)

Nerve to mylohyoid

Medial pterygoid muscle (cut)

Digastric muscle (posterior belly)

Stylohyoid muscle

Hypoglossal nerve

Submandibular gland

Sublingual nerve

Temporal fascia and temporalis muscle

Posterior / Anterior } Deep temporal nerves

Masseteric nerve

Lateral pterygoid nerve and muscle

Buccal nerve and buccinator muscle (cut)

Submandibular ganglion

Sublingual gland

Mylohyoid muscle (cut)

Mental nerve

Inferior alveolar nerve (cut)

Digastric muscle (anterior belly)

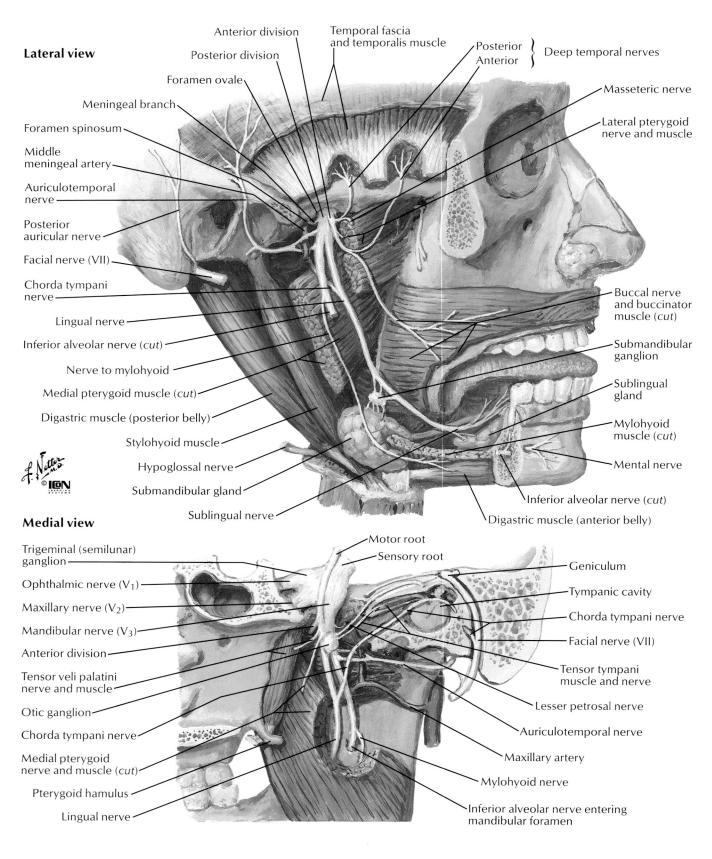

Medial view

Trigeminal (semilunar) ganglion

Ophthalmic nerve (V₁)

Maxillary nerve (V₂)

Mandibular nerve (V₃)

Anterior division

Tensor veli palatini nerve and muscle

Otic ganglion

Chorda tympani nerve

Medial pterygoid nerve and muscle (cut)

Pterygoid hamulus

Lingual nerve

Motor root

Sensory root

Geniculum

Tympanic cavity

Chorda tympani nerve

Facial nerve (VII)

Tensor tympani muscle and nerve

Lesser petrosal nerve

Auriculotemporal nerve

Maxillary artery

Mylohyoid nerve

Inferior alveolar nerve entering mandibular foramen

F. Netter MD. ©ICON

PLATE 42

HEAD AND NECK

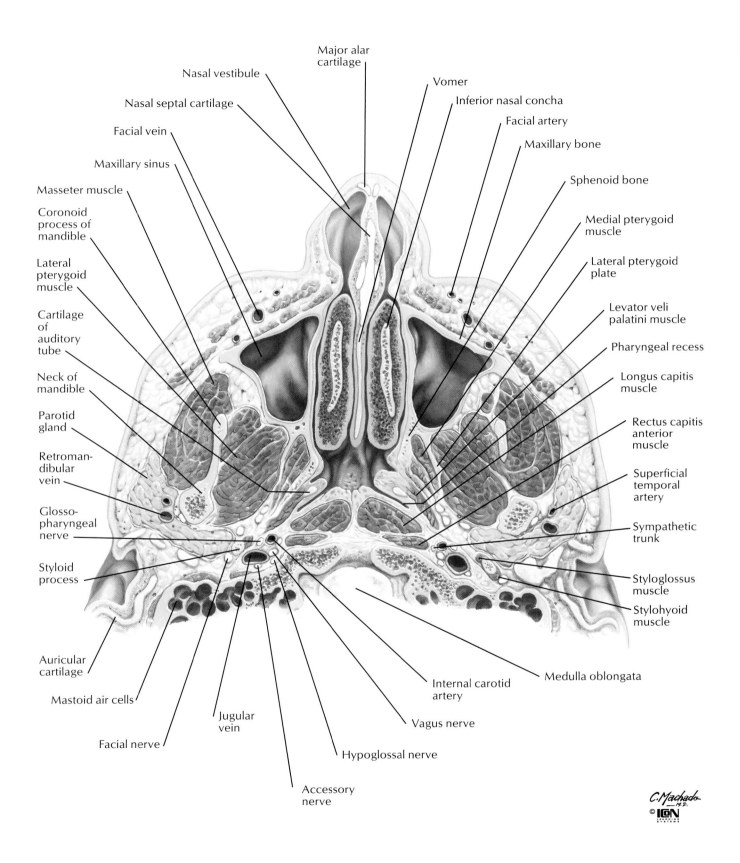

Major alar cartilage

Nasal vestibule

Nasal septal cartilage

Facial vein

Maxillary sinus

Masseter muscle

Coronoid process of mandible

Lateral pterygoid muscle

Cartilage of auditory tube

Neck of mandible

Parotid gland

Retromandibular vein

Glosso-pharyngeal nerve

Styloid process

Auricular cartilage

Mastoid air cells

Facial nerve

Jugular vein

Accessory nerve

Hypoglossal nerve

Vagus nerve

Internal carotid artery

Medulla oblongata

Vomer

Inferior nasal concha

Facial artery

Maxillary bone

Sphenoid bone

Medial pterygoid muscle

Lateral pterygoid plate

Levator veli palatini muscle

Pharyngeal recess

Longus capitis muscle

Rectus capitis anterior muscle

Superficial temporal artery

Sympathetic trunk

Styloglossus muscle

Stylohyoid muscle

Paranasal Sinuses

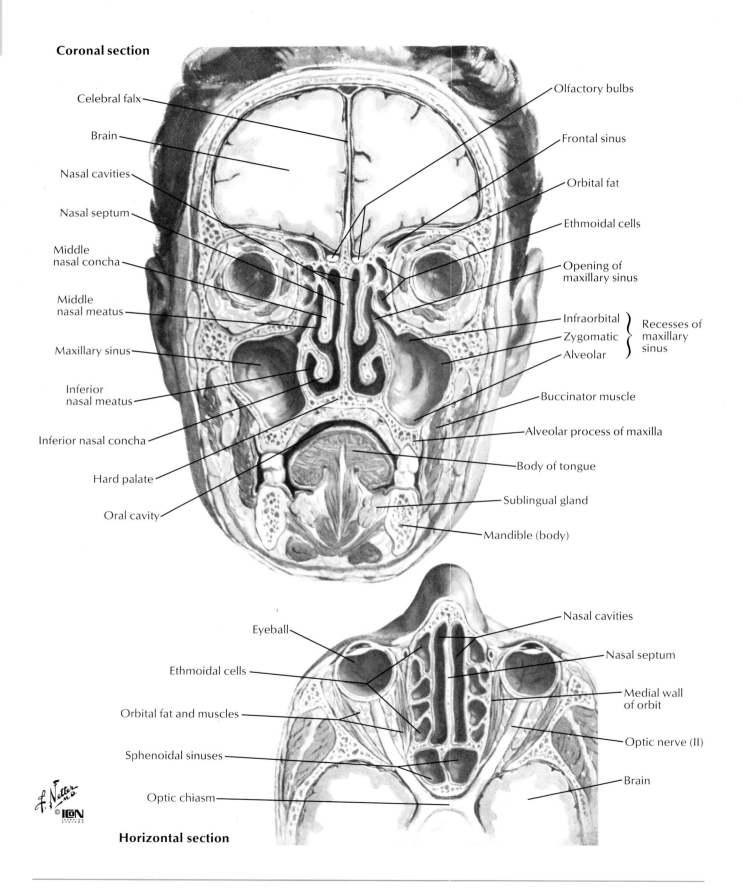

Coronal section

Celebral falx

Brain

Nasal cavities

Nasal septum

Middle nasal concha

Middle nasal meatus

Maxillary sinus

Inferior nasal meatus

Inferior nasal concha

Hard palate

Oral cavity

Olfactory bulbs

Frontal sinus

Orbital fat

Ethmoidal cells

Opening of maxillary sinus

Infraorbital ⎫
Zygomatic ⎬ Recesses of maxillary sinus
Alveolar   ⎭

Buccinator muscle

Alveolar process of maxilla

Body of tongue

Sublingual gland

Mandible (body)

Eyeball

Ethmoidal cells

Orbital fat and muscles

Sphenoidal sinuses

Optic chiasm

Nasal cavities

Nasal septum

Medial wall of orbit

Optic nerve (II)

Brain

Horizontal section

PLATE 44   **HEAD AND NECK**

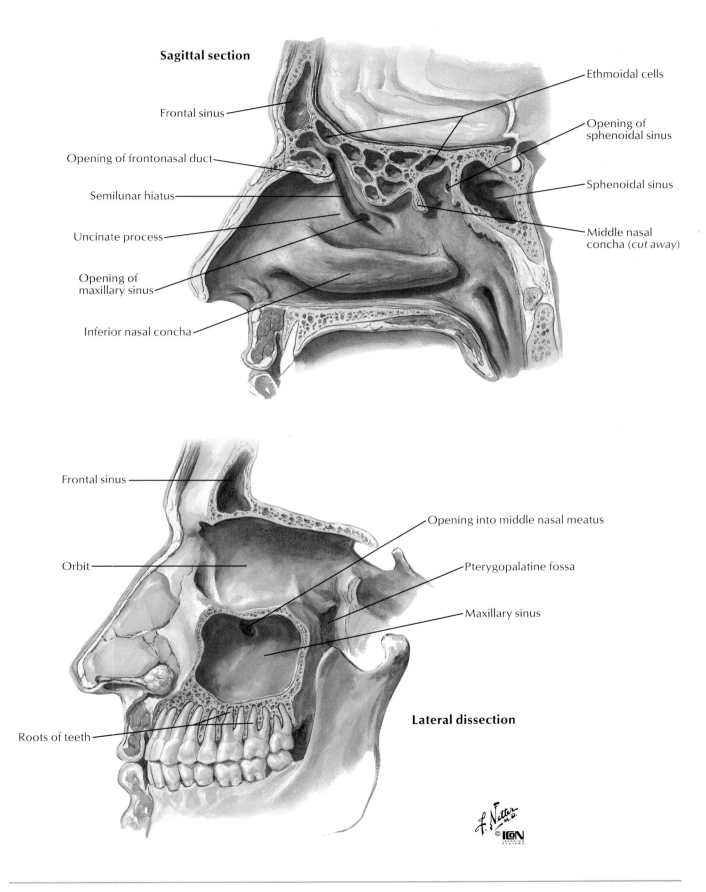

Sagittal section

Frontal sinus

Opening of frontonasal duct

Semilunar hiatus

Uncinate process

Opening of
maxillary sinus

Inferior nasal concha

Ethmoidal cells

Opening of
sphenoidal sinus

Sphenoidal sinus

Middle nasal
concha (*cut away*)

Frontal sinus

Orbit

Roots of teeth

Opening into middle nasal meatus

Pterygopalatine fossa

Maxillary sinus

Lateral dissection

Paranasal Sinuses: Changes With Age

Bones of nasal cavity and paranasal sinuses at birth

Sinus represents one or more anterior ethmoidal cells opening into semilunar hiatus of middle nasal meatus

Sinus represents one or more middle ethmoidal cells opening into middle nasal meatus

Sinuses represent two or more posterior ethmoidal cells opening into superior nasal meatus

Sphenoidal sinus within bony shell (sphenoidal concha) located anterior and lateral to body of sphenoid bone (broken line indicates sinus lateral to sphenoid body)

Part of nasolacrimal duct that formed in depths of nasooptic furrow

Nasal bone

Lacrimal bone

Nasolacrimal foramen (becomes bony canal)

Part of nasolacrimal duct within nasal cavity with slit-like opening in inferior nasal meatus

Maxilla

Uncinate process of ethmoid bone

Semilunar hiatus

Body of sphenoid bone

Hypophyseal fossa

Vestigial remnant of Rathke's pouch

Medial plate of pterygoid process

Lower border of highest nasal concha

Lower border of superior nasal concha

Superior nasal meatus

Middle nasal concha (*cut edge*) (inferior nasal concha completely removed)

Palatine bone

Pterygoid hamulus

Maxillary sinus with opening into semilunar hiatus (striped area represents membrane forming most of medial wall of sinus)

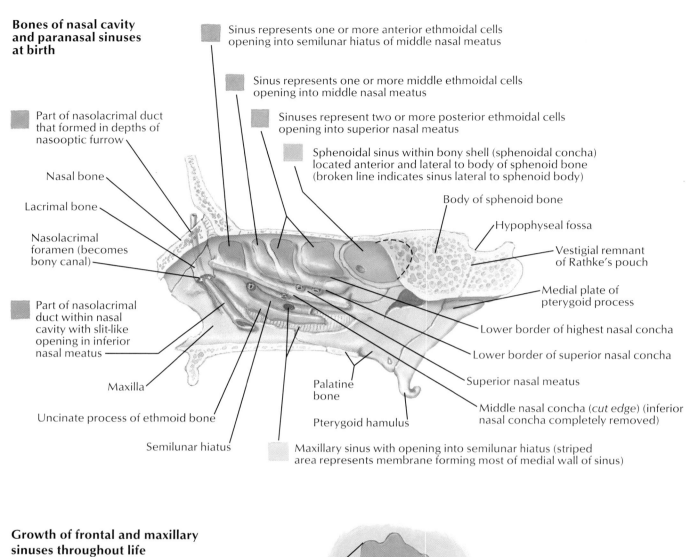

Growth of frontal and maxillary sinuses throughout life

Birth

1 year

4 years

7 years

12 years

Adult

Old age

Frontal sinus within frontal bone

Middle nasal concha

Nasal septum

Nasal cavity

Inferior nasal concha

Palate

Left orbit

Maxillary sinus within maxilla

Molar tooth

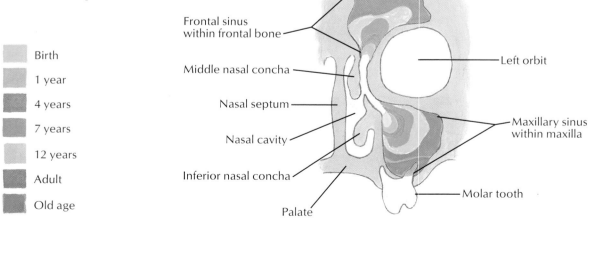

PLATE 46

HEAD AND NECK

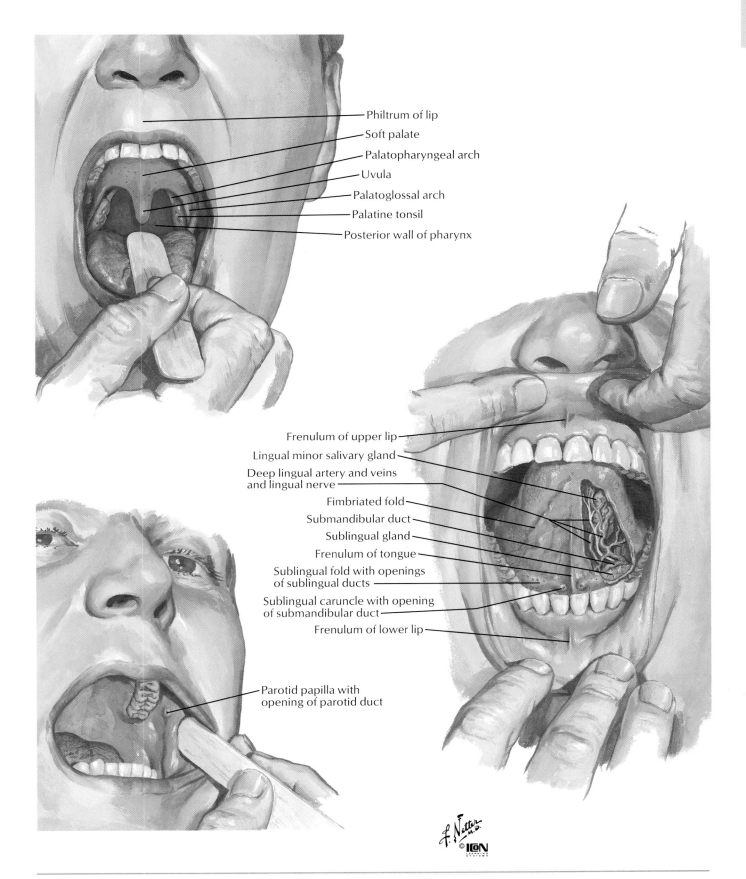

Philtrum of lip
Soft palate
Palatopharyngeal arch
Uvula
Palatoglossal arch
Palatine tonsil
Posterior wall of pharynx

Frenulum of upper lip
Lingual minor salivary gland
Deep lingual artery and veins and lingual nerve
Fimbriated fold
Submandibular duct
Sublingual gland
Frenulum of tongue
Sublingual fold with openings of sublingual ducts
Sublingual caruncle with opening of submandibular duct
Frenulum of lower lip

Parotid papilla with opening of parotid duct

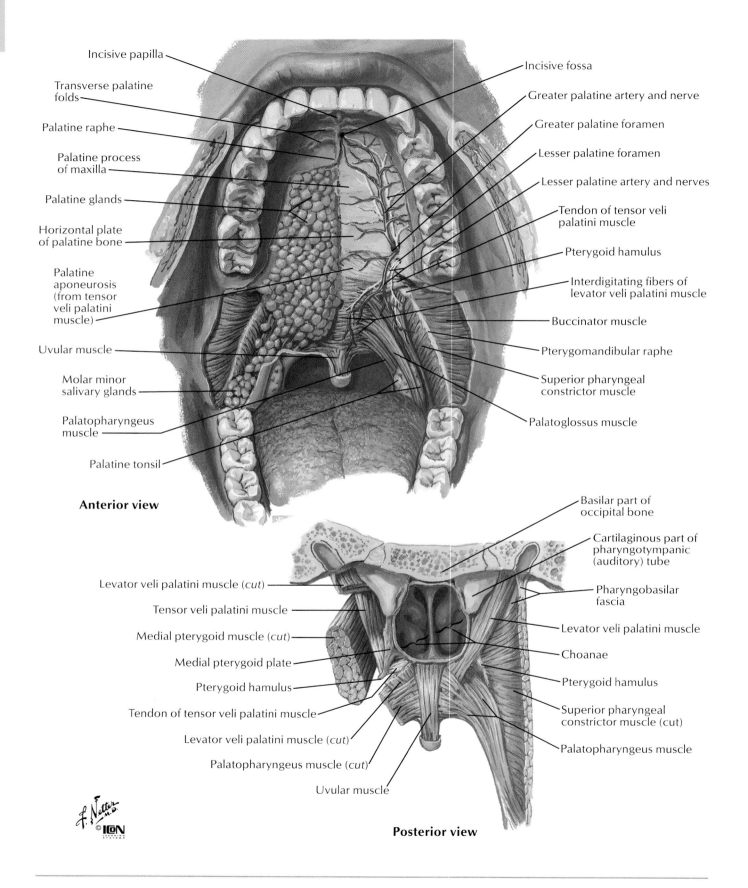

Incisive papilla

Transverse palatine folds

Palatine raphe

Palatine process of maxilla

Palatine glands

Horizontal plate of palatine bone

Palatine aponeurosis (from tensor veli palatini muscle)

Uvular muscle

Molar minor salivary glands

Palatopharyngeus muscle

Palatine tonsil

Incisive fossa

Greater palatine artery and nerve

Greater palatine foramen

Lesser palatine foramen

Lesser palatine artery and nerves

Tendon of tensor veli palatini muscle

Pterygoid hamulus

Interdigitating fibers of levator veli palatini muscle

Buccinator muscle

Pterygomandibular raphe

Superior pharyngeal constrictor muscle

Palatoglossus muscle

Anterior view

Levator veli palatini muscle (*cut*)

Tensor veli palatini muscle

Medial pterygoid muscle (*cut*)

Medial pterygoid plate

Pterygoid hamulus

Tendon of tensor veli palatini muscle

Levator veli palatini muscle (*cut*)

Palatopharyngeus muscle (*cut*)

Uvular muscle

Basilar part of occipital bone

Cartilaginous part of pharyngotympanic (auditory) tube

Pharyngobasilar fascia

Levator veli palatini muscle

Choanae

Pterygoid hamulus

Superior pharyngeal constrictor muscle (*cut*)

Palatopharyngeus muscle

Posterior view

PLATE 48

HEAD AND NECK

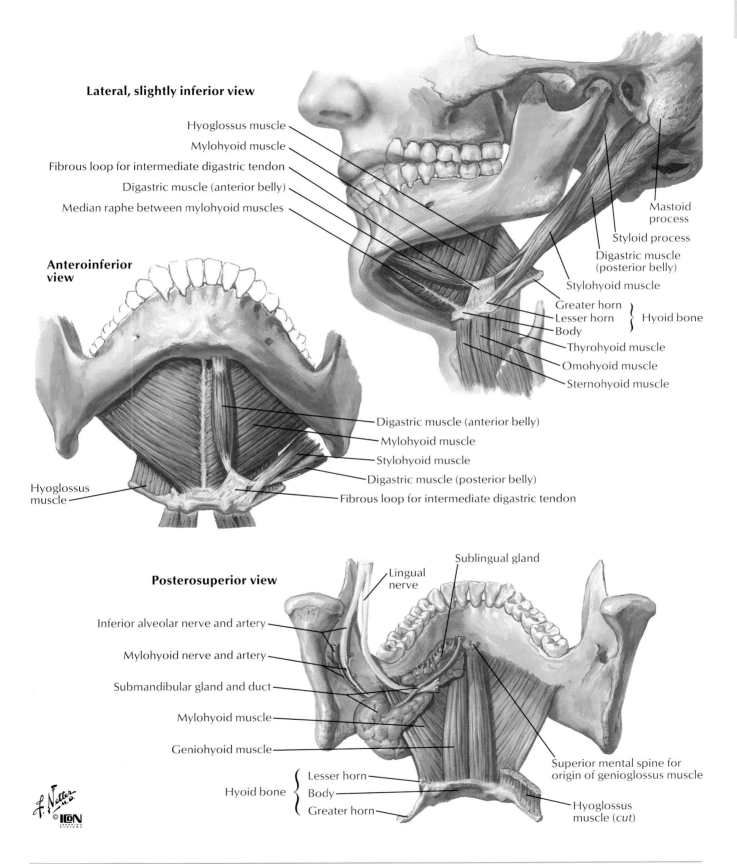

Lateral, slightly inferior view

Hyoglossus muscle

Mylohyoid muscle

Fibrous loop for intermediate digastric tendon

Digastric muscle (anterior belly)

Median raphe between mylohyoid muscles

Mastoid process

Styloid process

Digastric muscle (posterior belly)

Stylohyoid muscle

Greater horn

Lesser horn } Hyoid bone

Body

Thyrohyoid muscle

Omohyoid muscle

Sternohyoid muscle

Anteroinferior view

Digastric muscle (anterior belly)

Mylohyoid muscle

Stylohyoid muscle

Digastric muscle (posterior belly)

Fibrous loop for intermediate digastric tendon

Hyoglossus muscle

Posterosuperior view

Sublingual gland

Lingual nerve

Inferior alveolar nerve and artery

Mylohyoid nerve and artery

Submandibular gland and duct

Mylohyoid muscle

Geniohyoid muscle

Superior mental spine for origin of genioglossus muscle

Hyoid bone { Lesser horn

Body

Greater horn

Hyoglossus muscle (*cut*)

Muscles Involved in Mastication

FOR FACIAL MUSCLES SEE PLATE 22

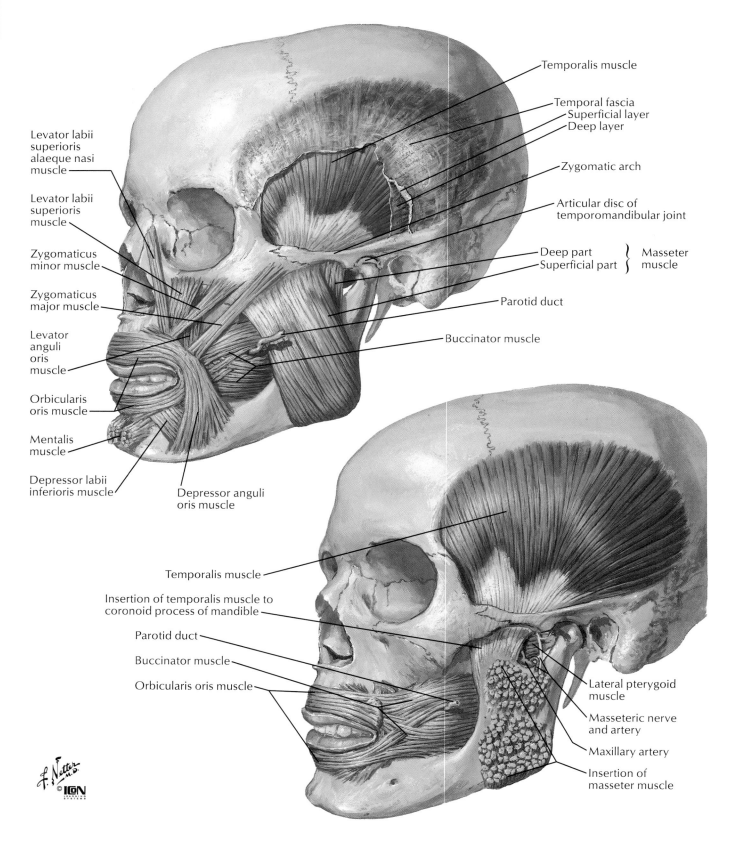

Temporalis muscle

Temporal fascia
Superficial layer
Deep layer

Zygomatic arch

Articular disc of
temporomandibular joint

Deep part
Superficial part } Masseter muscle

Parotid duct

Buccinator muscle

Levator labii
superioris
alaeque nasi
muscle

Levator labii
superioris
muscle

Zygomaticus
minor muscle

Zygomaticus
major muscle

Levator
anguli
oris
muscle

Orbicularis
oris muscle

Mentalis
muscle

Depressor labii
inferioris muscle

Depressor anguli
oris muscle

Temporalis muscle

Insertion of temporalis muscle to
coronoid process of mandible

Parotid duct

Buccinator muscle

Orbicularis oris muscle

Lateral pterygoid
muscle

Masseteric nerve
and artery

Maxillary artery

Insertion of
masseter muscle

PLATE 50

HEAD AND NECK

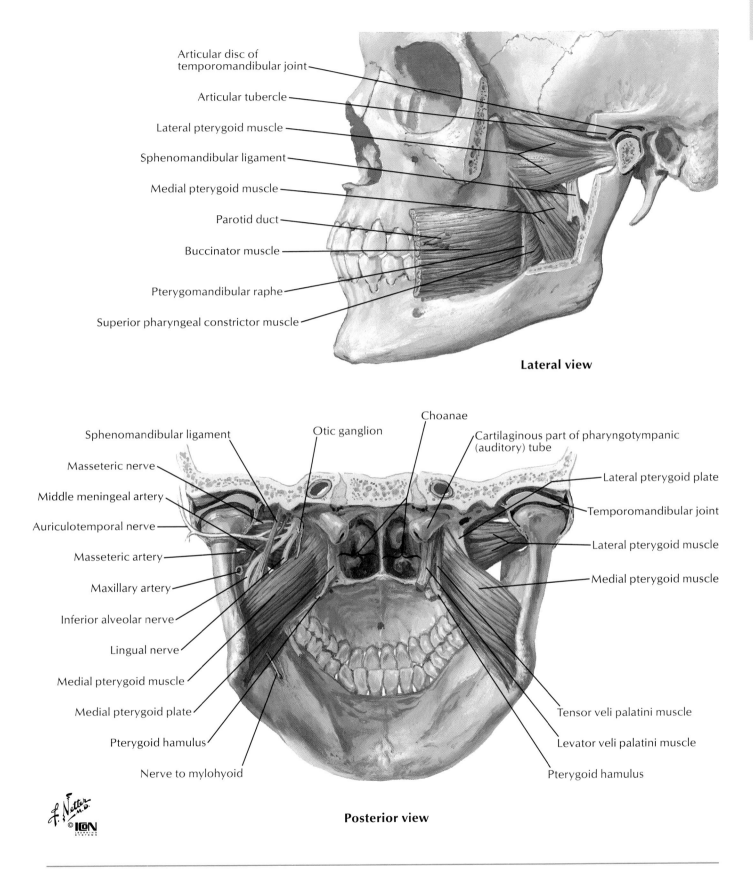

Articular disc of
temporomandibular joint

Articular tubercle

Lateral pterygoid muscle

Sphenomandibular ligament

Medial pterygoid muscle

Parotid duct

Buccinator muscle

Pterygomandibular raphe

Superior pharyngeal constrictor muscle

Lateral view

Sphenomandibular ligament

Otic ganglion

Choanae

Cartilaginous part of pharyngotympanic
(auditory) tube

Masseteric nerve

Middle meningeal artery

Auriculotemporal nerve

Masseteric artery

Maxillary artery

Inferior alveolar nerve

Lingual nerve

Medial pterygoid muscle

Medial pterygoid plate

Pterygoid hamulus

Nerve to mylohyoid

Lateral pterygoid plate

Temporomandibular joint

Lateral pterygoid muscle

Medial pterygoid muscle

Tensor veli palatini muscle

Levator veli palatini muscle

Pterygoid hamulus

Posterior view

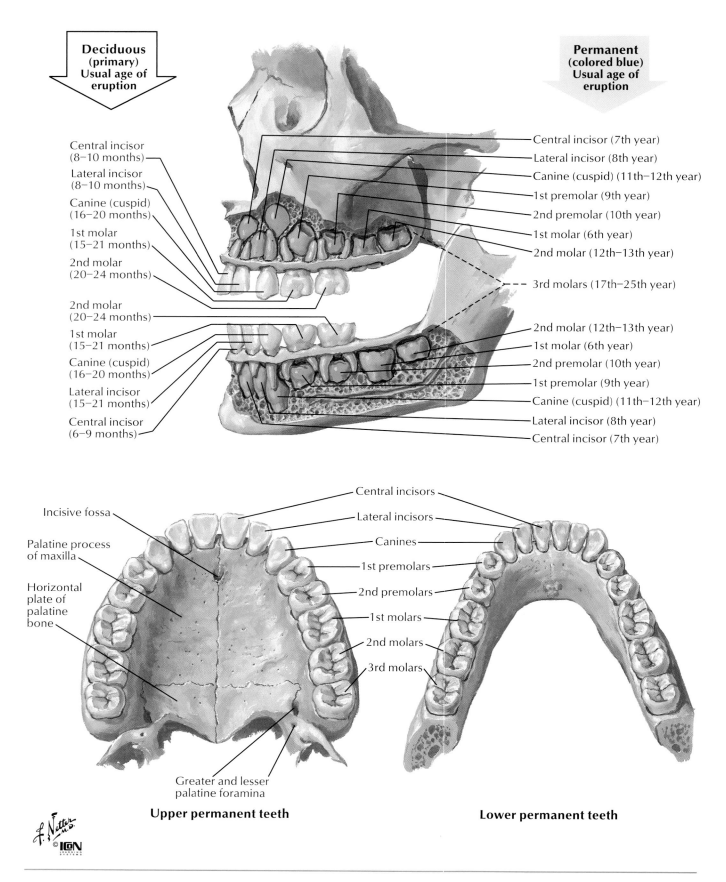

Deciduous (primary) Usual age of eruption

Central incisor (8–10 months)

Lateral incisor (8–10 months)

Canine (cuspid) (16–20 months)

1st molar (15–21 months)

2nd molar (20–24 months)

2nd molar (20–24 months)

1st molar (15–21 months)

Canine (cuspid) (16–20 months)

Lateral incisor (15–21 months)

Central incisor (6–9 months)

Permanent (colored blue) Usual age of eruption

Central incisor (7th year)

Lateral incisor (8th year)

Canine (cuspid) (11th–12th year)

1st premolar (9th year)

2nd premolar (10th year)

1st molar (6th year)

2nd molar (12th–13th year)

3rd molars (17th–25th year)

2nd molar (12th–13th year)

1st molar (6th year)

2nd premolar (10th year)

1st premolar (9th year)

Canine (cuspid) (11th–12th year)

Lateral incisor (8th year)

Central incisor (7th year)

Incisive fossa

Palatine process of maxilla

Horizontal plate of palatine bone

Central incisors

Lateral incisors

Canines

1st premolars

2nd premolars

1st molars

2nd molars

3rd molars

Greater and lesser palatine foramina

Upper permanent teeth

Lower permanent teeth

PLATE 52   **HEAD AND NECK**

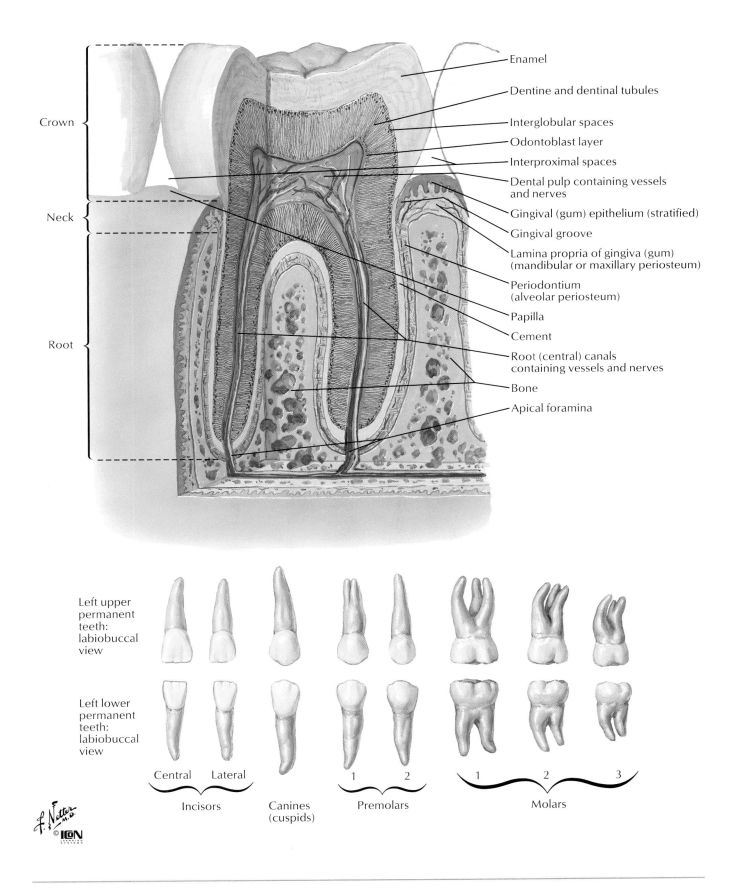

Crown

Neck

Root

Enamel

Dentine and dentinal tubules

Interglobular spaces

Odontoblast layer

Interproximal spaces

Dental pulp containing vessels and nerves

Gingival (gum) epithelium (stratified)

Gingival groove

Lamina propria of gingiva (gum) (mandibular or maxillary periosteum)

Periodontium (alveolar periosteum)

Papilla

Cement

Root (central) canals containing vessels and nerves

Bone

Apical foramina

Left upper permanent teeth: labiobuccal view

Left lower permanent teeth: labiobuccal view

Central   Lateral   1   2   1   2   3

Incisors   Canines   Premolars   Molars
                (cuspids)

Tongue

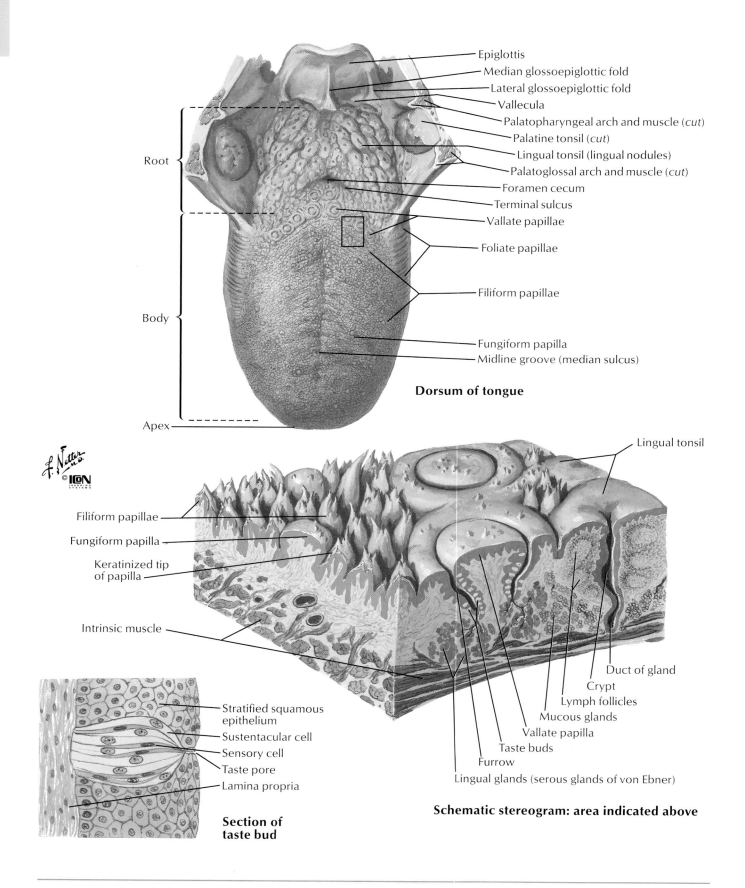

Epiglottis
Median glossoepiglottic fold
Lateral glossoepiglottic fold
Vallecula
Palatopharyngeal arch and muscle (*cut*)
Palatine tonsil (*cut*)
Lingual tonsil (lingual nodules)
Palatoglossal arch and muscle (*cut*)
Foramen cecum
Terminal sulcus
Vallate papillae
Foliate papillae
Filiform papillae
Fungiform papilla
Midline groove (median sulcus)

Root

Body

Apex

Dorsum of tongue

Lingual tonsil

Filiform papillae
Fungiform papilla
Keratinized tip of papilla

Intrinsic muscle

Duct of gland
Crypt
Lymph follicles
Mucous glands
Vallate papilla
Taste buds
Furrow
Lingual glands (serous glands of von Ebner)

Stratified squamous epithelium
Sustentacular cell
Sensory cell
Taste pore
Lamina propria

Section of taste bud

Schematic stereogram: area indicated above

PLATE 54

HEAD AND NECK

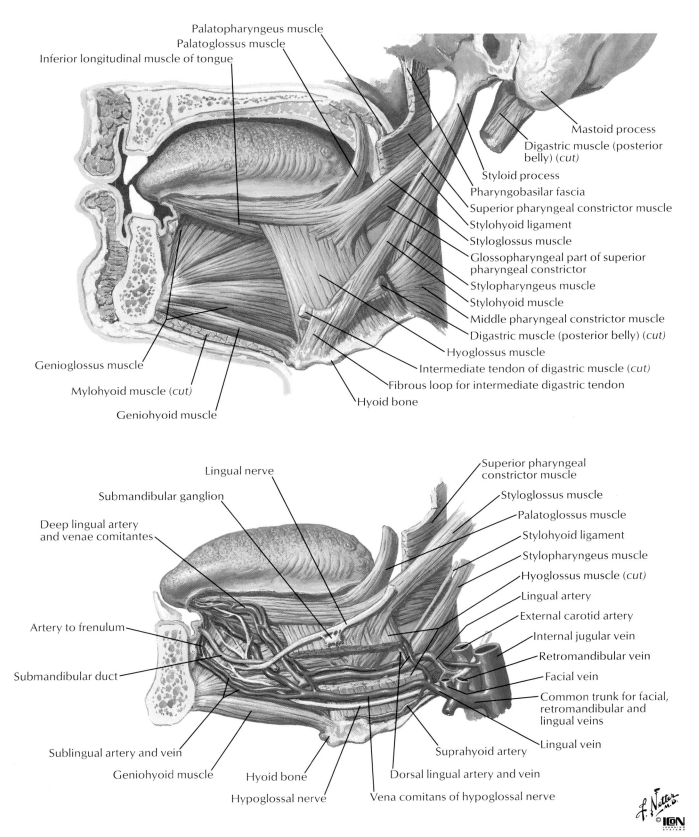

Palatopharyngeus muscle
Palatoglossus muscle
Inferior longitudinal muscle of tongue
Mastoid process
Digastric muscle (posterior belly) (cut)
Styloid process
Pharyngobasilar fascia
Superior pharyngeal constrictor muscle
Stylohyoid ligament
Styloglossus muscle
Glossopharyngeal part of superior pharyngeal constrictor
Stylopharyngeus muscle
Stylohyoid muscle
Middle pharyngeal constrictor muscle
Digastric muscle (posterior belly) (cut)
Hyoglossus muscle
Intermediate tendon of digastric muscle (cut)
Fibrous loop for intermediate digastric tendon
Hyoid bone
Genioglossus muscle
Mylohyoid muscle (cut)
Geniohyoid muscle

Lingual nerve
Submandibular ganglion
Deep lingual artery and venae comitantes
Artery to frenulum
Submandibular duct
Superior pharyngeal constrictor muscle
Styloglossus muscle
Palatoglossus muscle
Stylohyoid ligament
Stylopharyngeus muscle
Hyoglossus muscle (cut)
Lingual artery
External carotid artery
Internal jugular vein
Retromandibular vein
Facial vein
Common trunk for facial, retromandibular and lingual veins
Lingual vein
Sublingual artery and vein
Geniohyoid muscle
Hyoid bone
Hypoglossal nerve
Suprahyoid artery
Dorsal lingual artery and vein
Vena comitans of hypoglossal nerve

Tongue and Salivary Glands: Sections

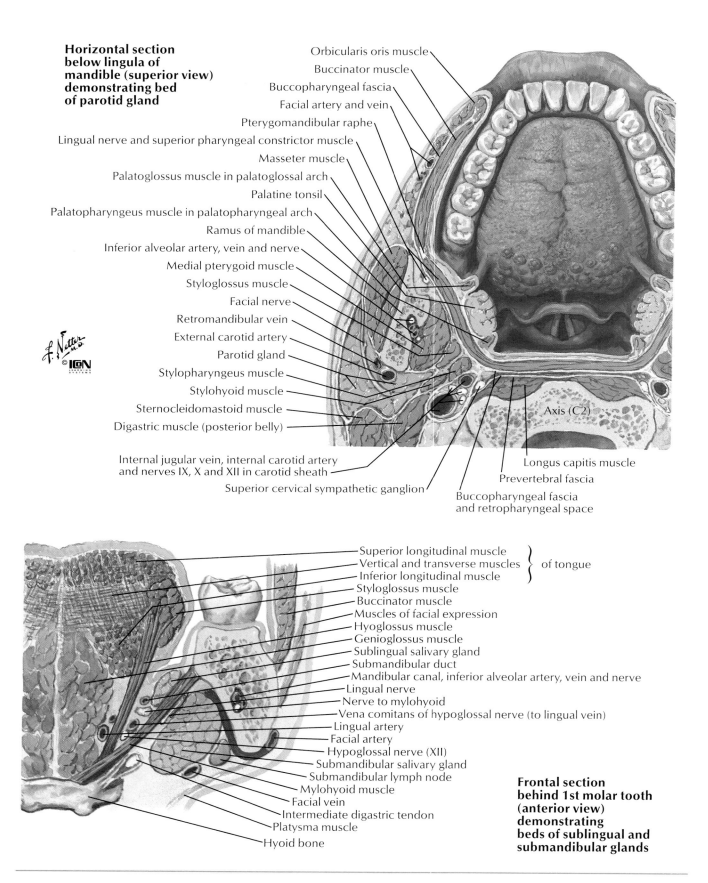

Horizontal section below lingula of mandible (superior view) demonstrating bed of parotid gland

Orbicularis oris muscle

Buccinator muscle

Buccopharyngeal fascia

Facial artery and vein

Pterygomandibular raphe

Lingual nerve and superior pharyngeal constrictor muscle

Masseter muscle

Palatoglossus muscle in palatoglossal arch

Palatine tonsil

Palatopharyngeus muscle in palatopharyngeal arch

Ramus of mandible

Inferior alveolar artery, vein and nerve

Medial pterygoid muscle

Styloglossus muscle

Facial nerve

Retromandibular vein

External carotid artery

Parotid gland

Stylopharyngeus muscle

Stylohyoid muscle

Sternocleidomastoid muscle

Digastric muscle (posterior belly)

Internal jugular vein, internal carotid artery and nerves IX, X and XII in carotid sheath

Superior cervical sympathetic ganglion

Axis (C2)

Longus capitis muscle

Prevertebral fascia

Buccopharyngeal fascia and retropharyngeal space

Superior longitudinal muscle

Vertical and transverse muscles } of tongue

Inferior longitudinal muscle

Styloglossus muscle

Buccinator muscle

Muscles of facial expression

Hyoglossus muscle

Genioglossus muscle

Sublingual salivary gland

Submandibular duct

Mandibular canal, inferior alveolar artery, vein and nerve

Lingual nerve

Nerve to mylohyoid

Vena comitans of hypoglossal nerve (to lingual vein)

Lingual artery

Facial artery

Hypoglossal nerve (XII)

Submandibular salivary gland

Submandibular lymph node

Mylohyoid muscle

Facial vein

Intermediate digastric tendon

Platysma muscle

Hyoid bone

Frontal section behind 1st molar tooth (anterior view) demonstrating beds of sublingual and submandibular glands

PLATE 56

HEAD AND NECK

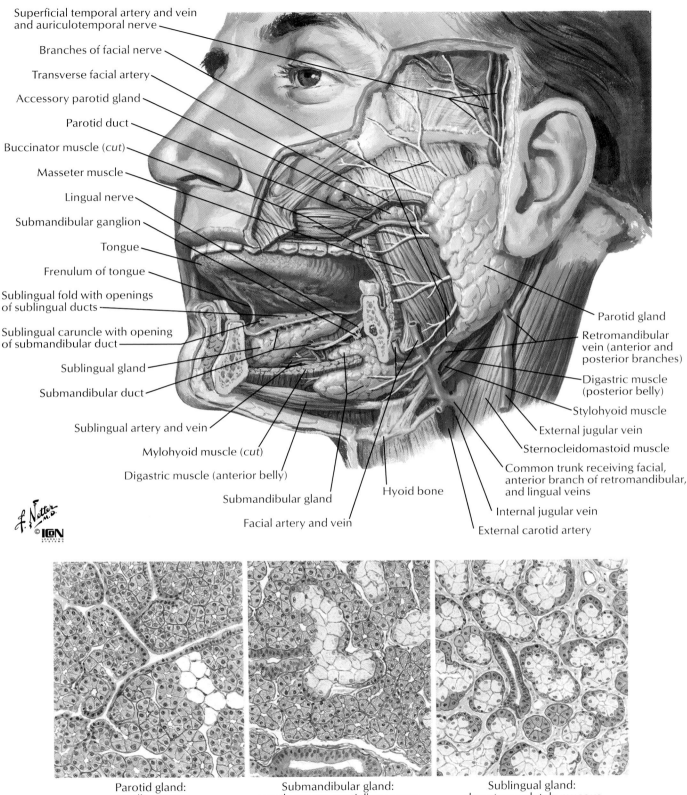

Superficial temporal artery and vein and auriculotemporal nerve

Branches of facial nerve

Transverse facial artery

Accessory parotid gland

Parotid duct

Buccinator muscle (*cut*)

Masseter muscle

Lingual nerve

Submandibular ganglion

Tongue

Frenulum of tongue

Sublingual fold with openings of sublingual ducts

Sublingual caruncle with opening of submandibular duct

Sublingual gland

Submandibular duct

Sublingual artery and vein

Mylohyoid muscle (*cut*)

Digastric muscle (anterior belly)

Submandibular gland

Facial artery and vein

Hyoid bone

Parotid gland

Retromandibular vein (anterior and posterior branches)

Digastric muscle (posterior belly)

Stylohyoid muscle

External jugular vein

Sternocleidomastoid muscle

Common trunk receiving facial, anterior branch of retromandibular, and lingual veins

Internal jugular vein

External carotid artery

Parotid gland: totally serous

Submandibular gland: mostly serous, partially mucous

Sublingual gland: almost completely mucous

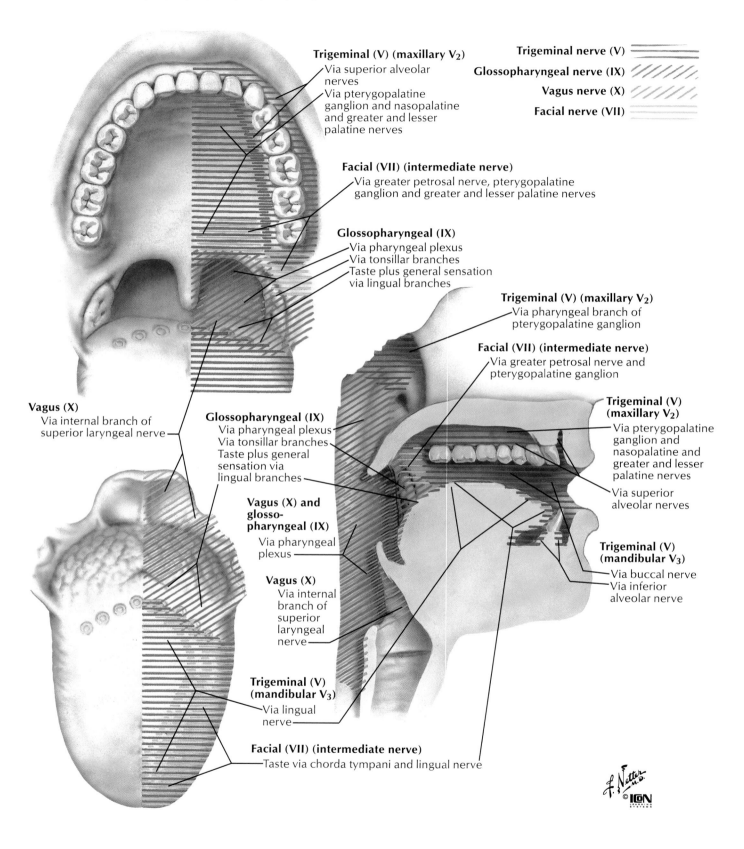

Trigeminal (V) (maxillary V₂)
Via superior alveolar nerves
Via pterygopalatine ganglion and nasopalatine and greater and lesser palatine nerves

Trigeminal nerve (V)
Glossopharyngeal nerve (IX)
Vagus nerve (X)
Facial nerve (VII)

Facial (VII) (intermediate nerve)
Via greater petrosal nerve, pterygopalatine ganglion and greater and lesser palatine nerves

Glossopharyngeal (IX)
Via pharyngeal plexus
Via tonsillar branches
Taste plus general sensation via lingual branches

Trigeminal (V) (maxillary V₂)
Via pharyngeal branch of pterygopalatine ganglion

Facial (VII) (intermediate nerve)
Via greater petrosal nerve and pterygopalatine ganglion

Trigeminal (V) (maxillary V₂)
Via pterygopalatine ganglion and nasopalatine and greater and lesser palatine nerves
Via superior alveolar nerves

Vagus (X)
Via internal branch of superior laryngeal nerve

Glossopharyngeal (IX)
Via pharyngeal plexus
Via tonsillar branches
Taste plus general sensation via lingual branches

Vagus (X) and glosso-pharyngeal (IX)
Via pharyngeal plexus

Vagus (X)
Via internal branch of superior laryngeal nerve

Trigeminal (V) (mandibular V₃)
Via buccal nerve
Via inferior alveolar nerve

Trigeminal (V) (mandibular V₃)
Via lingual nerve

Facial (VII) (intermediate nerve)
Taste via chorda tympani and lingual nerve

PLATE 58

HEAD AND NECK

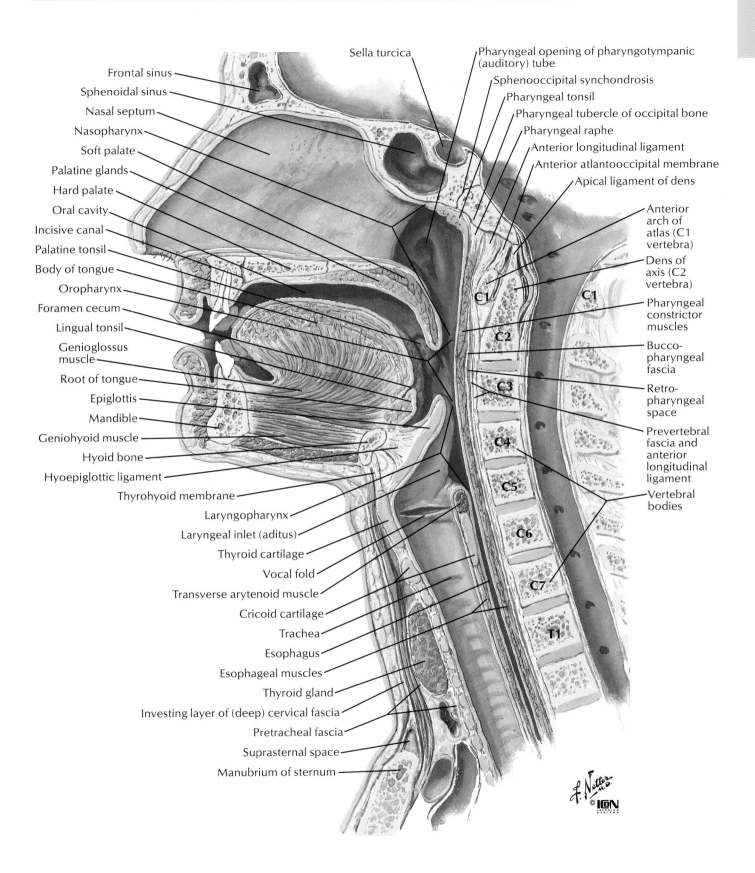

Frontal sinus

Sphenoidal sinus

Nasal septum

Nasopharynx

Soft palate

Palatine glands

Hard palate

Oral cavity

Incisive canal

Palatine tonsil

Body of tongue

Oropharynx

Foramen cecum

Lingual tonsil

Genioglossus muscle

Root of tongue

Epiglottis

Mandible

Geniohyoid muscle

Hyoid bone

Hyoepiglottic ligament

Thyrohyoid membrane

Laryngopharynx

Laryngeal inlet (aditus)

Thyroid cartilage

Vocal fold

Transverse arytenoid muscle

Cricoid cartilage

Trachea

Esophagus

Esophageal muscles

Thyroid gland

Investing layer of (deep) cervical fascia

Pretracheal fascia

Suprasternal space

Manubrium of sternum

Sella turcica

Pharyngeal opening of pharyngotympanic (auditory) tube

Sphenooccipital synchondrosis

Pharyngeal tonsil

Pharyngeal tubercle of occipital bone

Pharyngeal raphe

Anterior longitudinal ligament

Anterior atlantooccipital membrane

Apical ligament of dens

Anterior arch of atlas (C1 vertebra)

Dens of axis (C2 vertebra)

Pharyngeal constrictor muscles

Bucco-pharyngeal fascia

Retro-pharyngeal space

Prevertebral fascia and anterior longitudinal ligament

Vertebral bodies

C1

C2

C3

C4

C5

C6

C7

T1

C1

Fauces

**Medial view
Median (sagittal) section**

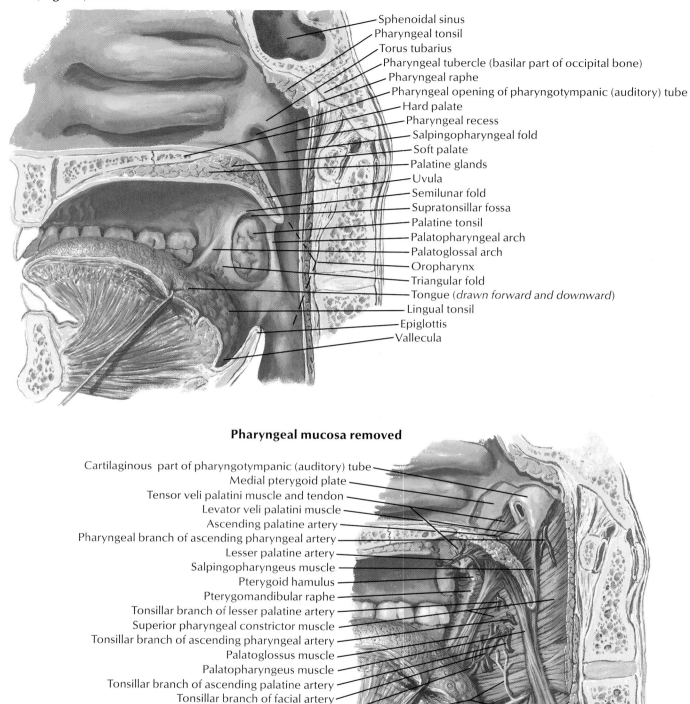

- Sphenoidal sinus
- Pharyngeal tonsil
- Torus tubarius
- Pharyngeal tubercle (basilar part of occipital bone)
- Pharyngeal raphe
- Pharyngeal opening of pharyngotympanic (auditory) tube
- Hard palate
- Pharyngeal recess
- Salpingopharyngeal fold
- Soft palate
- Palatine glands
- Uvula
- Semilunar fold
- Supratonsillar fossa
- Palatine tonsil
- Palatopharyngeal arch
- Palatoglossal arch
- Oropharynx
- Triangular fold
- Tongue (*drawn forward and downward*)
- Lingual tonsil
- Epiglottis
- Vallecula

Pharyngeal mucosa removed

- Cartilaginous part of pharyngotympanic (auditory) tube
- Medial pterygoid plate
- Tensor veli palatini muscle and tendon
- Levator veli palatini muscle
- Ascending palatine artery
- Pharyngeal branch of ascending pharyngeal artery
- Lesser palatine artery
- Salpingopharyngeus muscle
- Pterygoid hamulus
- Pterygomandibular raphe
- Tonsillar branch of lesser palatine artery
- Superior pharyngeal constrictor muscle
- Tonsillar branch of ascending pharyngeal artery
- Palatoglossus muscle
- Palatopharyngeus muscle
- Tonsillar branch of ascending palatine artery
- Tonsillar branch of facial artery
- Tonsillar branch of dorsal lingual artery
- Glossopharyngeal nerve (IX) and tonsillar branch
- Stylohyoid ligament
- Hyoglossus muscle
- Middle pharyngeal constrictor muscle
- Stylopharyngeus muscle

PLATE 60

HEAD AND NECK

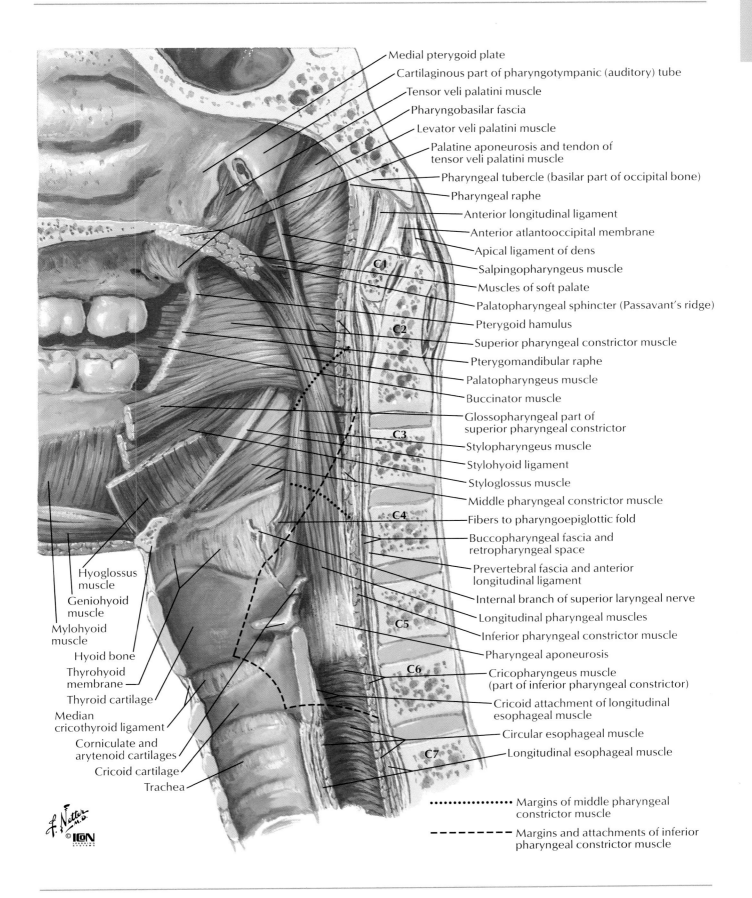

Medial pterygoid plate
Cartilaginous part of pharyngotympanic (auditory) tube
Tensor veli palatini muscle
Pharyngobasilar fascia
Levator veli palatini muscle
Palatine aponeurosis and tendon of tensor veli palatini muscle
Pharyngeal tubercle (basilar part of occipital bone)
Pharyngeal raphe
Anterior longitudinal ligament
Anterior atlantooccipital membrane
Apical ligament of dens
Salpingopharyngeus muscle
Muscles of soft palate
Palatopharyngeal sphincter (Passavant's ridge)
Pterygoid hamulus
Superior pharyngeal constrictor muscle
Pterygomandibular raphe
Palatopharyngeus muscle
Buccinator muscle
Glossopharyngeal part of superior pharyngeal constrictor
Stylopharyngeus muscle
Stylohyoid ligament
Styloglossus muscle
Middle pharyngeal constrictor muscle
Fibers to pharyngoepiglottic fold
Buccopharyngeal fascia and retropharyngeal space
Prevertebral fascia and anterior longitudinal ligament
Internal branch of superior laryngeal nerve
Longitudinal pharyngeal muscles
Inferior pharyngeal constrictor muscle
Pharyngeal aponeurosis
Cricopharyngeus muscle (part of inferior pharyngeal constrictor)
Cricoid attachment of longitudinal esophageal muscle
Circular esophageal muscle
Longitudinal esophageal muscle

C1
C2
C3
C4
C5
C6
C7

Hyoglossus muscle
Geniohyoid muscle
Mylohyoid muscle
Hyoid bone
Thyrohyoid membrane
Thyroid cartilage
Median cricothyroid ligament
Corniculate and arytenoid cartilages
Cricoid cartilage
Trachea

•••••••••••• Margins of middle pharyngeal constrictor muscle
– – – – – – – Margins and attachments of inferior pharyngeal constrictor muscle

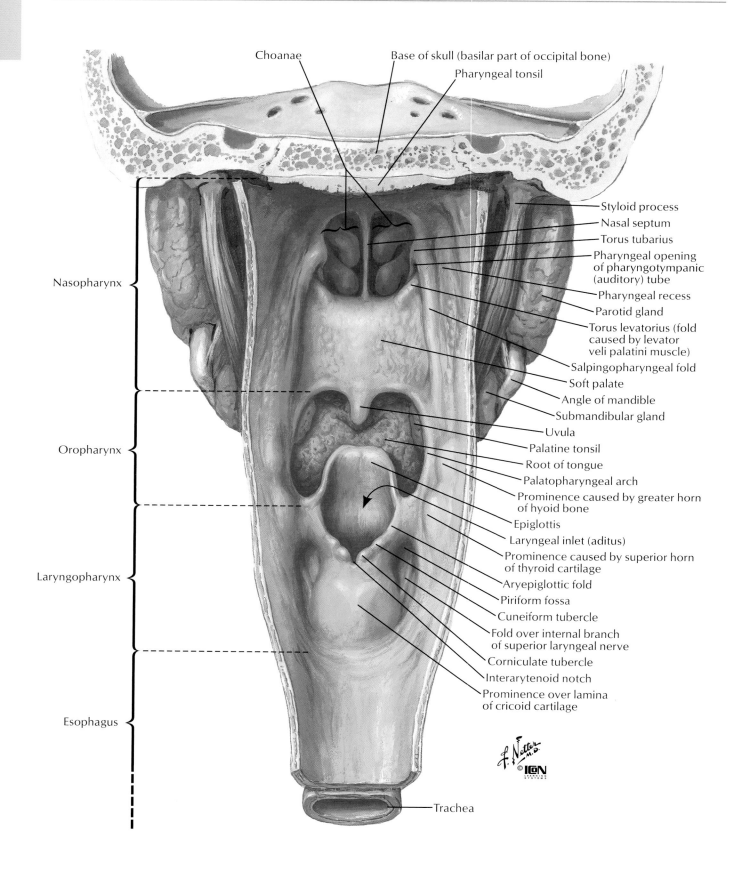

Choanae

Base of skull (basilar part of occipital bone)

Pharyngeal tonsil

Styloid process

Nasal septum

Torus tubarius

Pharyngeal opening
of pharyngotympanic
(auditory) tube

Pharyngeal recess

Parotid gland

Torus levatorius (fold
caused by levator
veli palatini muscle)

Salpingopharyngeal fold

Soft palate

Angle of mandible

Submandibular gland

Uvula

Palatine tonsil

Root of tongue

Palatopharyngeal arch

Prominence caused by greater horn
of hyoid bone

Epiglottis

Laryngeal inlet (aditus)

Prominence caused by superior horn
of thyroid cartilage

Aryepiglottic fold

Piriform fossa

Cuneiform tubercle

Fold over internal branch
of superior laryngeal nerve

Corniculate tubercle

Interarytenoid notch

Prominence over lamina
of cricoid cartilage

Nasopharynx

Oropharynx

Laryngopharynx

Esophagus

Trachea

PLATE 62

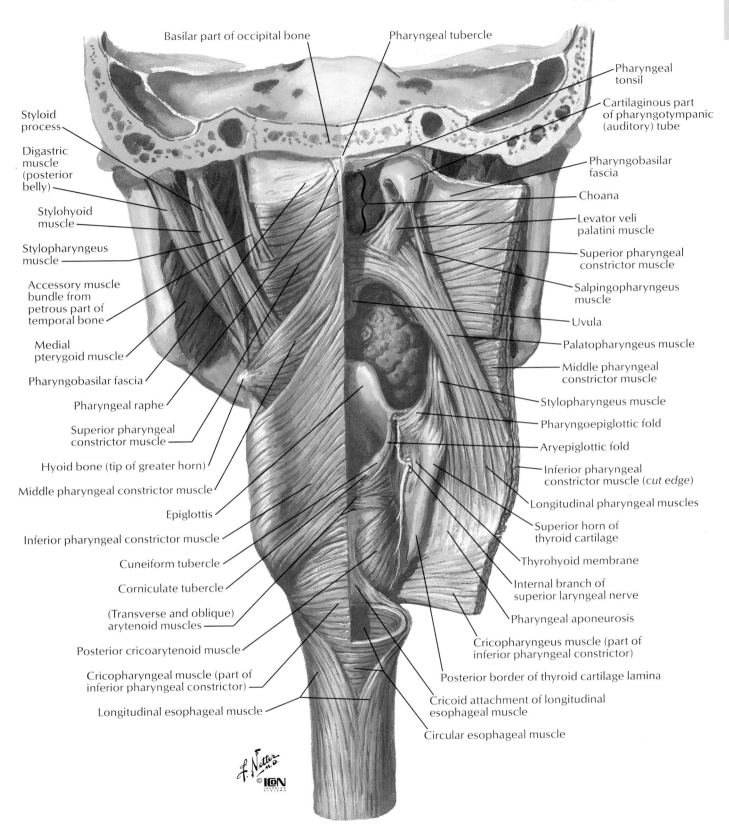

Basilar part of occipital bone

Pharyngeal tubercle

Pharyngeal tonsil

Cartilaginous part of pharyngotympanic (auditory) tube

Styloid process

Pharyngobasilar fascia

Digastric muscle (posterior belly)

Choana

Stylohyoid muscle

Levator veli palatini muscle

Stylopharyngeus muscle

Superior pharyngeal constrictor muscle

Accessory muscle bundle from petrous part of temporal bone

Salpingopharyngeus muscle

Uvula

Medial pterygoid muscle

Palatopharyngeus muscle

Pharyngobasilar fascia

Middle pharyngeal constrictor muscle

Pharyngeal raphe

Stylopharyngeus muscle

Superior pharyngeal constrictor muscle

Pharyngoepiglottic fold

Hyoid bone (tip of greater horn)

Aryepiglottic fold

Middle pharyngeal constrictor muscle

Inferior pharyngeal constrictor muscle (cut edge)

Epiglottis

Longitudinal pharyngeal muscles

Inferior pharyngeal constrictor muscle

Superior horn of thyroid cartilage

Cuneiform tubercle

Thyrohyoid membrane

Corniculate tubercle

Internal branch of superior laryngeal nerve

(Transverse and oblique) arytenoid muscles

Pharyngeal aponeurosis

Posterior cricoarytenoid muscle

Cricopharyngeus muscle (part of inferior pharyngeal constrictor)

Cricopharyngeal muscle (part of inferior pharyngeal constrictor)

Posterior border of thyroid cartilage lamina

Longitudinal esophageal muscle

Cricoid attachment of longitudinal esophageal muscle

Circular esophageal muscle

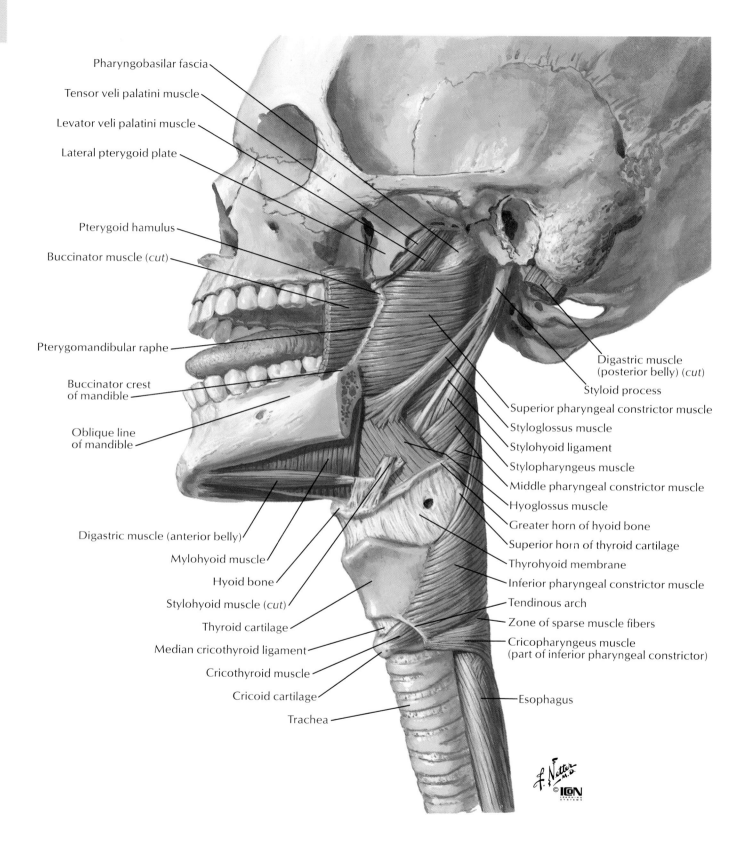

Pharyngobasilar fascia

Tensor veli palatini muscle

Levator veli palatini muscle

Lateral pterygoid plate

Pterygoid hamulus

Buccinator muscle (*cut*)

Pterygomandibular raphe

Buccinator crest of mandible

Oblique line of mandible

Digastric muscle (anterior belly)

Mylohyoid muscle

Hyoid bone

Stylohyoid muscle (*cut*)

Thyroid cartilage

Median cricothyroid ligament

Cricothyroid muscle

Cricoid cartilage

Trachea

Digastric muscle (posterior belly) (*cut*)

Styloid process

Superior pharyngeal constrictor muscle

Styloglossus muscle

Stylohyoid ligament

Stylopharyngeus muscle

Middle pharyngeal constrictor muscle

Hyoglossus muscle

Greater horn of hyoid bone

Superior horn of thyroid cartilage

Thyrohyoid membrane

Inferior pharyngeal constrictor muscle

Tendinous arch

Zone of sparse muscle fibers

Cricopharyngeus muscle (part of inferior pharyngeal constrictor)

Esophagus

PLATE 64

HEAD AND NECK

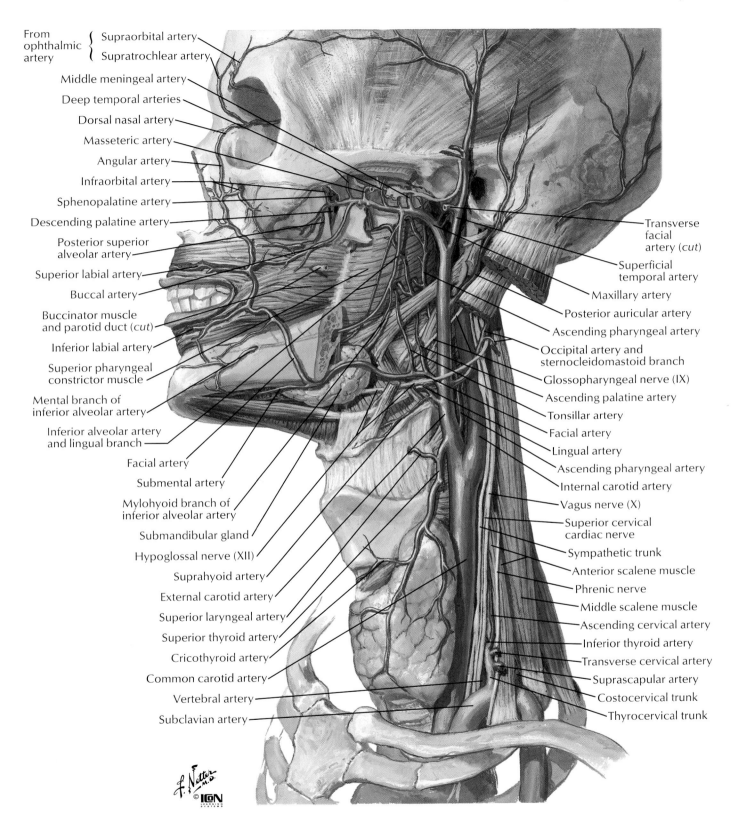

From ophthalmic artery { Supraorbital artery
Supratrochlear artery

Middle meningeal artery

Deep temporal arteries

Dorsal nasal artery

Masseteric artery

Angular artery

Infraorbital artery

Sphenopalatine artery

Descending palatine artery

Posterior superior alveolar artery

Superior labial artery

Buccal artery

Buccinator muscle and parotid duct (cut)

Inferior labial artery

Superior pharyngeal constrictor muscle

Mental branch of inferior alveolar artery

Inferior alveolar artery and lingual branch

Facial artery

Submental artery

Mylohyoid branch of inferior alveolar artery

Submandibular gland

Hypoglossal nerve (XII)

Suprahyoid artery

External carotid artery

Superior laryngeal artery

Superior thyroid artery

Cricothyroid artery

Common carotid artery

Vertebral artery

Subclavian artery

Transverse facial artery (cut)

Superficial temporal artery

Maxillary artery

Posterior auricular artery

Ascending pharyngeal artery

Occipital artery and sternocleidomastoid branch

Glossopharyngeal nerve (IX)

Ascending palatine artery

Tonsillar artery

Facial artery

Lingual artery

Ascending pharyngeal artery

Internal carotid artery

Vagus nerve (X)

Superior cervical cardiac nerve

Sympathetic trunk

Anterior scalene muscle

Phrenic nerve

Middle scalene muscle

Ascending cervical artery

Inferior thyroid artery

Transverse cervical artery

Suprascapular artery

Costocervical trunk

Thyrocervical trunk

Veins of Oral and Pharyngeal Regions

SEE ALSO PLATES 19, 27, 98

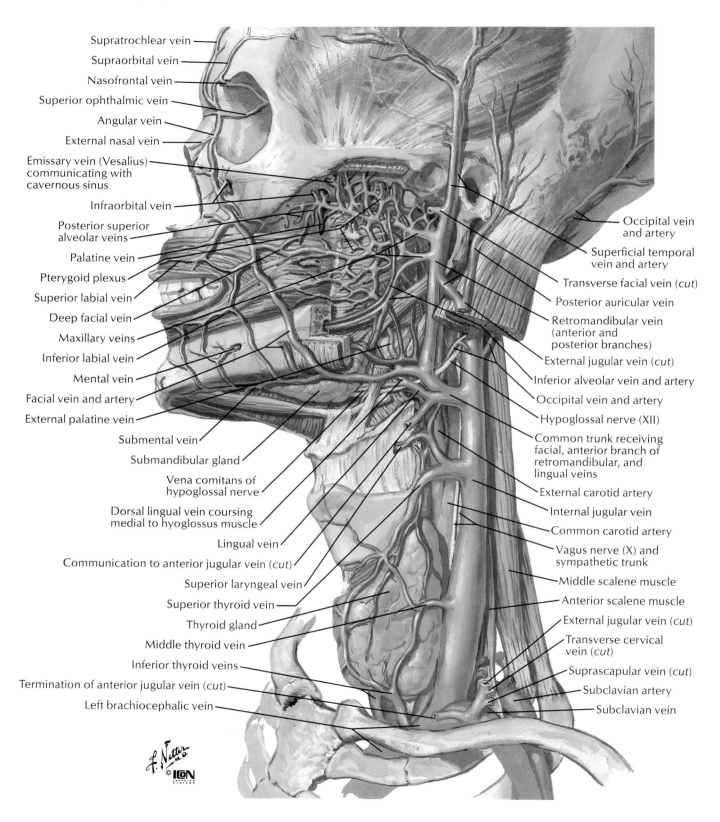

Supratrochlear vein

Supraorbital vein

Nasofrontal vein

Superior ophthalmic vein

Angular vein

External nasal vein

Emissary vein (Vesalius) communicating with cavernous sinus

Infraorbital vein

Posterior superior alveolar veins

Palatine vein

Pterygoid plexus

Superior labial vein

Deep facial vein

Maxillary veins

Inferior labial vein

Mental vein

Facial vein and artery

External palatine vein

Submental vein

Submandibular gland

Vena comitans of hypoglossal nerve

Dorsal lingual vein coursing medial to hyoglossus muscle

Lingual vein

Communication to anterior jugular vein (cut)

Superior laryngeal vein

Superior thyroid vein

Thyroid gland

Middle thyroid vein

Inferior thyroid veins

Termination of anterior jugular vein (cut)

Left brachiocephalic vein

Occipital vein and artery

Superficial temporal vein and artery

Transverse facial vein (cut)

Posterior auricular vein

Retromandibular vein (anterior and posterior branches)

External jugular vein (cut)

Inferior alveolar vein and artery

Occipital vein and artery

Hypoglossal nerve (XII)

Common trunk receiving facial, anterior branch of retromandibular, and lingual veins

External carotid artery

Internal jugular vein

Common carotid artery

Vagus nerve (X) and sympathetic trunk

Middle scalene muscle

Anterior scalene muscle

External jugular vein (cut)

Transverse cervical vein (cut)

Suprascapular vein (cut)

Subclavian artery

Subclavian vein

PLATE 66

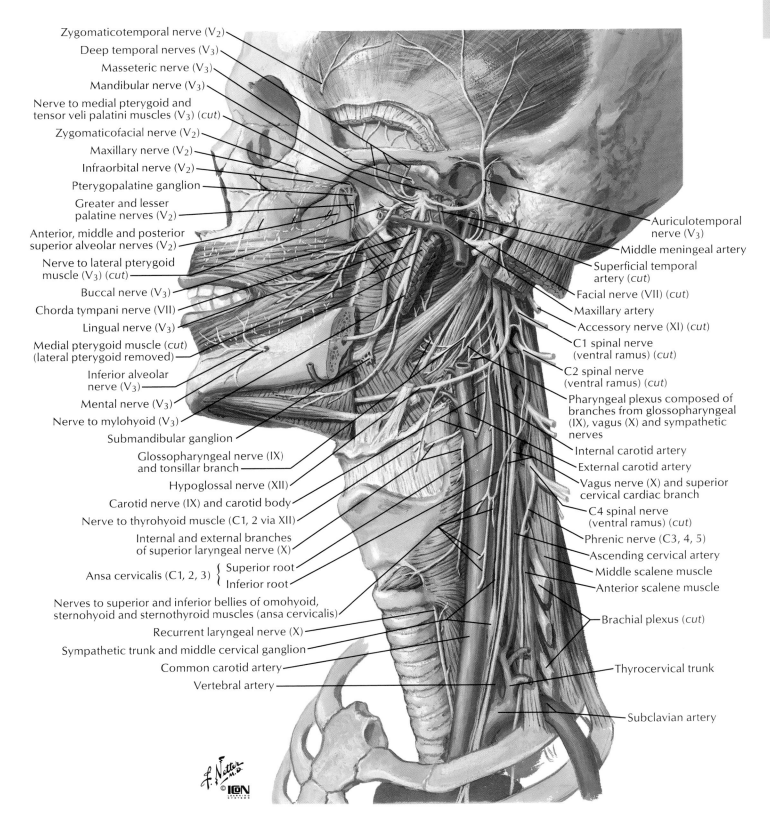

Zygomaticotemporal nerve (V₂)
Deep temporal nerves (V₃)
Masseteric nerve (V₃)
Mandibular nerve (V₃)
Nerve to medial pterygoid and tensor veli palatini muscles (V₃) (*cut*)
Zygomaticofacial nerve (V₂)
Maxillary nerve (V₂)
Infraorbital nerve (V₂)
Pterygopalatine ganglion
Greater and lesser palatine nerves (V₂)
Anterior, middle and posterior superior alveolar nerves (V₂)
Nerve to lateral pterygoid muscle (V₃) (*cut*)
Buccal nerve (V₃)
Chorda tympani nerve (VII)
Lingual nerve (V₃)
Medial pterygoid muscle (*cut*) (lateral pterygoid removed)
Inferior alveolar nerve (V₃)
Mental nerve (V₃)
Nerve to mylohyoid (V₃)
Submandibular ganglion
Glossopharyngeal nerve (IX) and tonsillar branch
Hypoglossal nerve (XII)
Carotid nerve (IX) and carotid body
Nerve to thyrohyoid muscle (C1, 2 via XII)
Internal and external branches of superior laryngeal nerve (X)
Ansa cervicalis (C1, 2, 3) { Superior root / Inferior root
Nerves to superior and inferior bellies of omohyoid, sternohyoid and sternothyroid muscles (ansa cervicalis)
Recurrent laryngeal nerve (X)
Sympathetic trunk and middle cervical ganglion
Common carotid artery
Vertebral artery

Auriculotemporal nerve (V₃)
Middle meningeal artery
Superficial temporal artery (*cut*)
Facial nerve (VII) (*cut*)
Maxillary artery
Accessory nerve (XI) (*cut*)
C1 spinal nerve (ventral ramus) (*cut*)
C2 spinal nerve (ventral ramus) (*cut*)
Pharyngeal plexus composed of branches from glossopharyngeal (IX), vagus (X) and sympathetic nerves
Internal carotid artery
External carotid artery
Vagus nerve (X) and superior cervical cardiac branch
C4 spinal nerve (ventral ramus) (*cut*)
Phrenic nerve (C3, 4, 5)
Ascending cervical artery
Middle scalene muscle
Anterior scalene muscle
Brachial plexus (*cut*)
Thyrocervical trunk
Subclavian artery

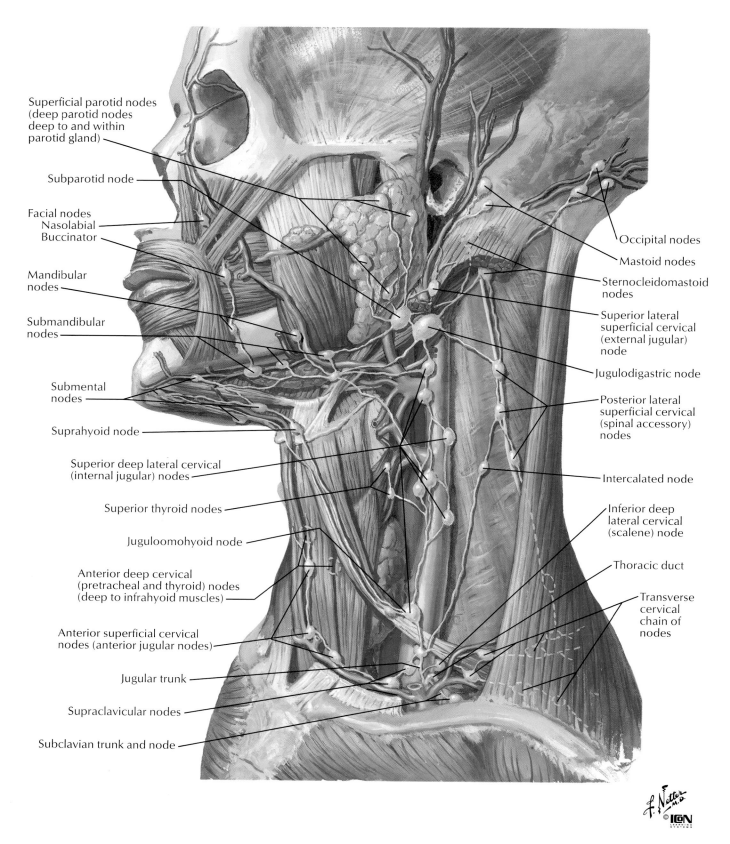

Superficial parotid nodes
(deep parotid nodes
deep to and within
parotid gland)

Subparotid node

Facial nodes
Nasolabial
Buccinator

Mandibular
nodes

Submandibular
nodes

Submental
nodes

Suprahyoid node

Superior deep lateral cervical
(internal jugular) nodes

Superior thyroid nodes

Juguloomohyoid node

Anterior deep cervical
(pretracheal and thyroid) nodes
(deep to infrahyoid muscles)

Anterior superficial cervical
nodes (anterior jugular nodes)

Jugular trunk

Supraclavicular nodes

Subclavian trunk and node

Occipital nodes

Mastoid nodes

Sternocleidomastoid
nodes

Superior lateral
superficial cervical
(external jugular)
node

Jugulodigastric node

Posterior lateral
superficial cervical
(spinal accessory)
nodes

Intercalated node

Inferior deep
lateral cervical
(scalene) node

Thoracic duct

Transverse
cervical
chain of
nodes

PLATE 68

HEAD AND NECK

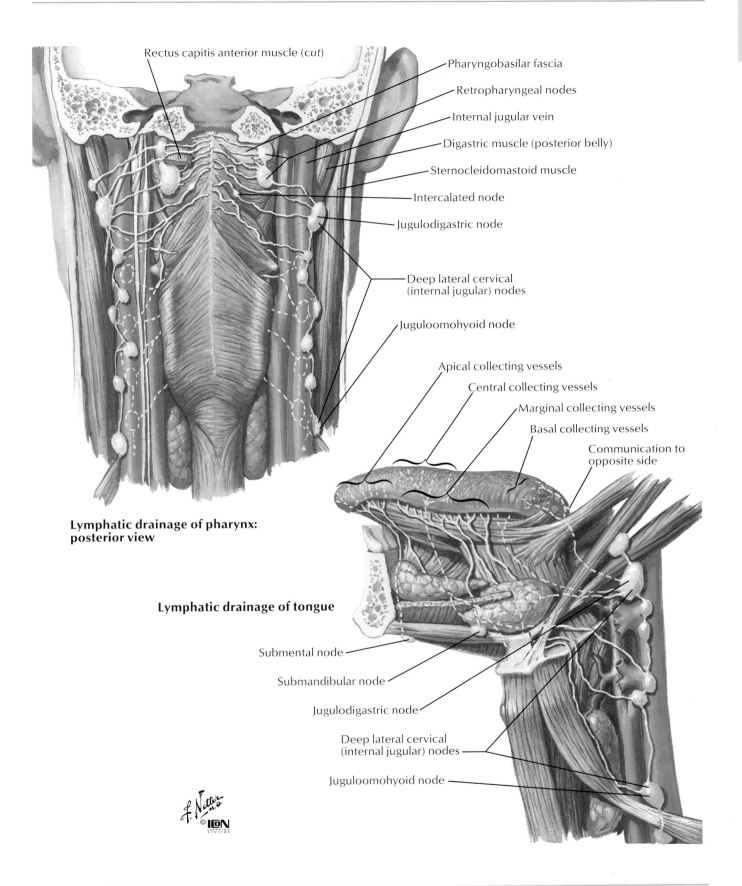

Rectus capitis anterior muscle (*cut*)

Pharyngobasilar fascia

Retropharyngeal nodes

Internal jugular vein

Digastric muscle (posterior belly)

Sternocleidomastoid muscle

Intercalated node

Jugulodigastric node

Deep lateral cervical
(internal jugular) nodes

Juguloomohyoid node

Apical collecting vessels

Central collecting vessels

Marginal collecting vessels

Basal collecting vessels

Communication to
opposite side

**Lymphatic drainage of pharynx:
posterior view**

Lymphatic drainage of tongue

Submental node

Submandibular node

Jugulodigastric node

Deep lateral cervical
(internal jugular) nodes

Juguloomohyoid node

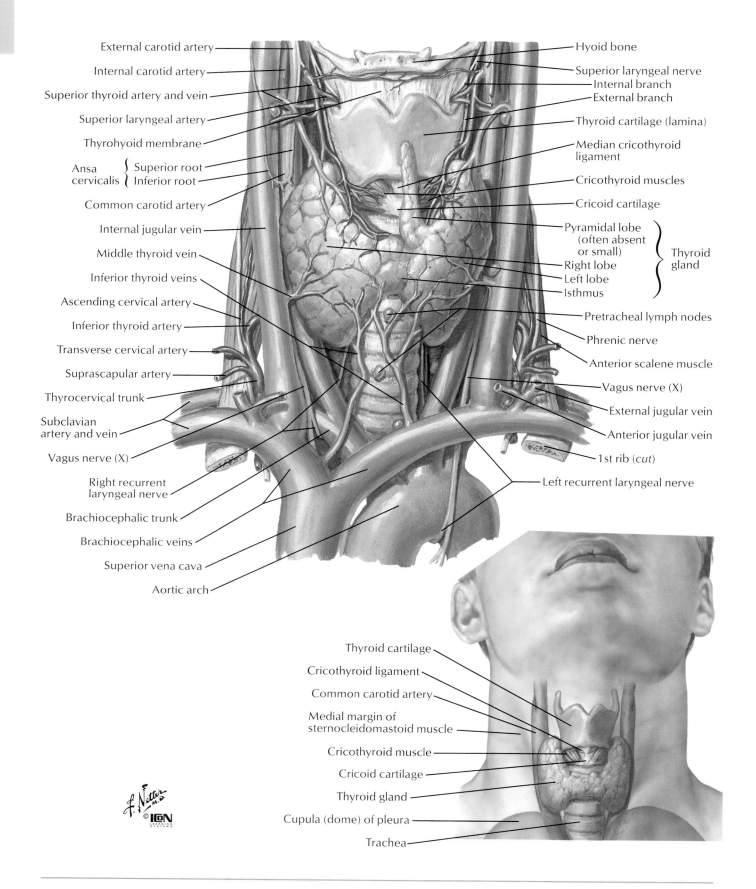

External carotid artery

Internal carotid artery

Superior thyroid artery and vein

Superior laryngeal artery

Thyrohyoid membrane

Ansa cervicalis
{ Superior root
{ Inferior root

Common carotid artery

Internal jugular vein

Middle thyroid vein

Inferior thyroid veins

Ascending cervical artery

Inferior thyroid artery

Transverse cervical artery

Suprascapular artery

Thyrocervical trunk

Subclavian artery and vein

Vagus nerve (X)

Right recurrent laryngeal nerve

Brachiocephalic trunk

Brachiocephalic veins

Superior vena cava

Aortic arch

Hyoid bone

Superior laryngeal nerve

Internal branch

External branch

Thyroid cartilage (lamina)

Median cricothyroid ligament

Cricothyroid muscles

Cricoid cartilage

Pyramidal lobe (often absent or small)

Right lobe

Left lobe   } Thyroid gland

Isthmus

Pretracheal lymph nodes

Phrenic nerve

Anterior scalene muscle

Vagus nerve (X)

External jugular vein

Anterior jugular vein

1st rib (*cut*)

Left recurrent laryngeal nerve

Thyroid cartilage

Cricothyroid ligament

Common carotid artery

Medial margin of sternocleidomastoid muscle

Cricothyroid muscle

Cricoid cartilage

Thyroid gland

Cupula (dome) of pleura

Trachea

PLATE 70   **HEAD AND NECK**

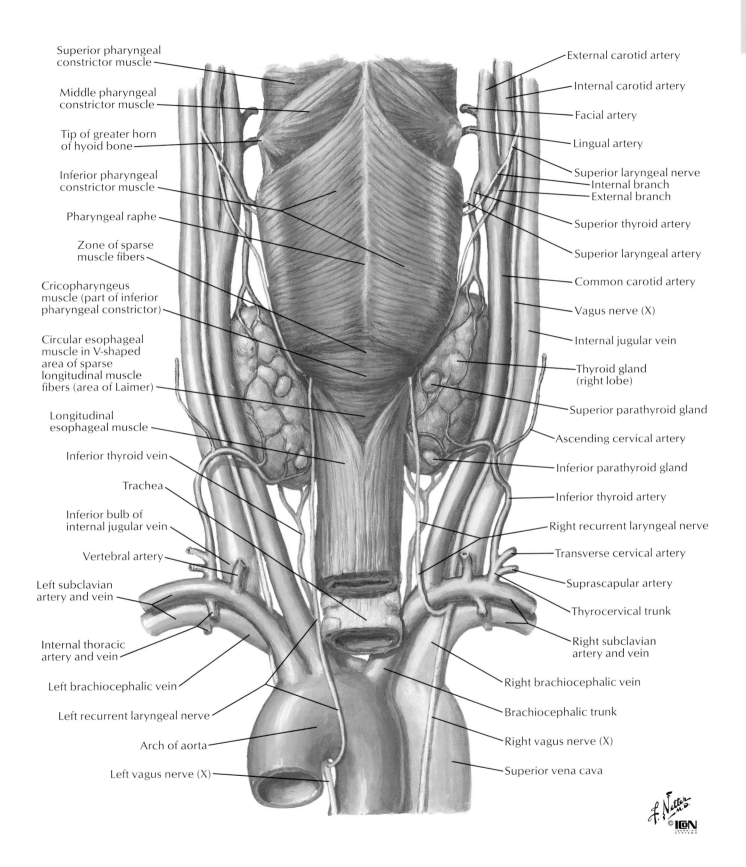

Superior pharyngeal constrictor muscle

Middle pharyngeal constrictor muscle

Tip of greater horn of hyoid bone

Inferior pharyngeal constrictor muscle

Pharyngeal raphe

Zone of sparse muscle fibers

Cricopharyngeus muscle (part of inferior pharyngeal constrictor)

Circular esophageal muscle in V-shaped area of sparse longitudinal muscle fibers (area of Laimer)

Longitudinal esophageal muscle

Inferior thyroid vein

Trachea

Inferior bulb of internal jugular vein

Vertebral artery

Left subclavian artery and vein

Internal thoracic artery and vein

Left brachiocephalic vein

Left recurrent laryngeal nerve

Arch of aorta

Left vagus nerve (X)

External carotid artery

Internal carotid artery

Facial artery

Lingual artery

Superior laryngeal nerve
Internal branch
External branch

Superior thyroid artery

Superior laryngeal artery

Common carotid artery

Vagus nerve (X)

Internal jugular vein

Thyroid gland (right lobe)

Superior parathyroid gland

Ascending cervical artery

Inferior parathyroid gland

Inferior thyroid artery

Right recurrent laryngeal nerve

Transverse cervical artery

Suprascapular artery

Thyrocervical trunk

Right subclavian artery and vein

Right brachiocephalic vein

Brachiocephalic trunk

Right vagus nerve (X)

Superior vena cava

Parathyroid Glands

SEE ALSO PLATE 76

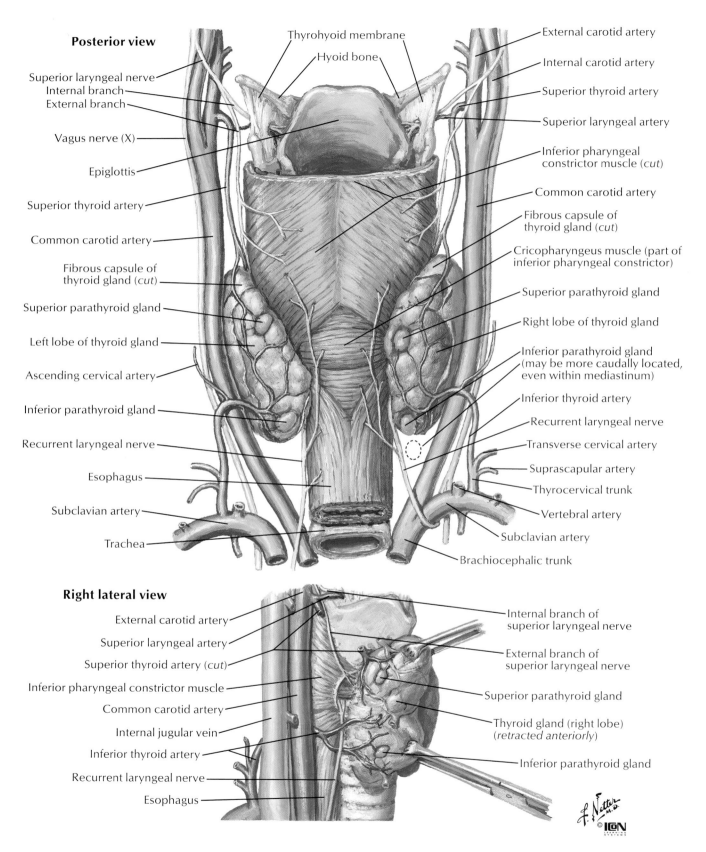

Posterior view

Thyrohyoid membrane

Hyoid bone

Superior laryngeal nerve
Internal branch
External branch

Vagus nerve (X)

Epiglottis

Superior thyroid artery

Common carotid artery

Fibrous capsule of
thyroid gland (*cut*)

Superior parathyroid gland

Left lobe of thyroid gland

Ascending cervical artery

Inferior parathyroid gland

Recurrent laryngeal nerve

Esophagus

Subclavian artery

Trachea

External carotid artery

Internal carotid artery

Superior thyroid artery

Superior laryngeal artery

Inferior pharyngeal
constrictor muscle (*cut*)

Common carotid artery

Fibrous capsule of
thyroid gland (*cut*)

Cricopharyngeus muscle (part of
inferior pharyngeal constrictor)

Superior parathyroid gland

Right lobe of thyroid gland

Inferior parathyroid gland
(may be more caudally located,
even within mediastinum)

Inferior thyroid artery

Recurrent laryngeal nerve

Transverse cervical artery

Suprascapular artery

Thyrocervical trunk

Vertebral artery

Subclavian artery

Brachiocephalic trunk

Right lateral view

External carotid artery

Superior laryngeal artery

Superior thyroid artery (*cut*)

Inferior pharyngeal constrictor muscle

Common carotid artery

Internal jugular vein

Inferior thyroid artery

Recurrent laryngeal nerve

Esophagus

Internal branch of
superior laryngeal nerve

External branch of
superior laryngeal nerve

Superior parathyroid gland

Thyroid gland (right lobe)
(*retracted anteriorly*)

Inferior parathyroid gland

F. Netter M.D.

©ICON

PLATE 72

HEAD AND NECK

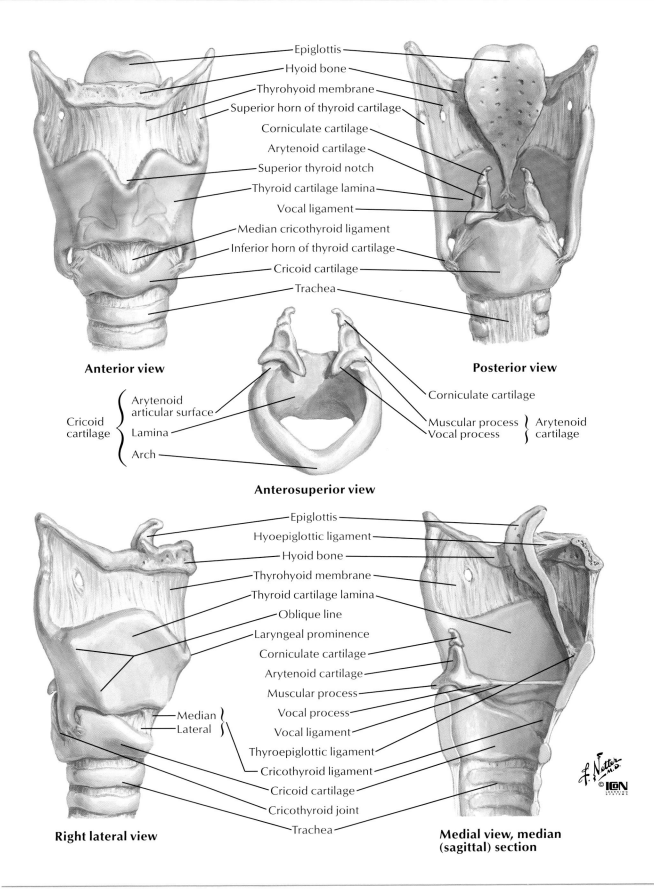

Epiglottis
Hyoid bone
Thyrohyoid membrane
Superior horn of thyroid cartilage
Corniculate cartilage
Arytenoid cartilage
Superior thyroid notch
Thyroid cartilage lamina
Vocal ligament
Median cricothyroid ligament
Inferior horn of thyroid cartilage
Cricoid cartilage
Trachea

Anterior view

Posterior view

Arytenoid articular surface
Cricoid cartilage
Lamina
Arch

Corniculate cartilage
Muscular process
Vocal process
Arytenoid cartilage

Anterosuperior view

Epiglottis
Hyoepiglottic ligament
Hyoid bone
Thyrohyoid membrane
Thyroid cartilage lamina
Oblique line
Laryngeal prominence
Corniculate cartilage
Arytenoid cartilage
Muscular process
Vocal process
Vocal ligament
Thyroepiglottic ligament
Median
Lateral
Cricothyroid ligament
Cricoid cartilage
Cricothyroid joint
Trachea

Right lateral view

Medial view, median (sagittal) section

Intrinsic Muscles of Larynx

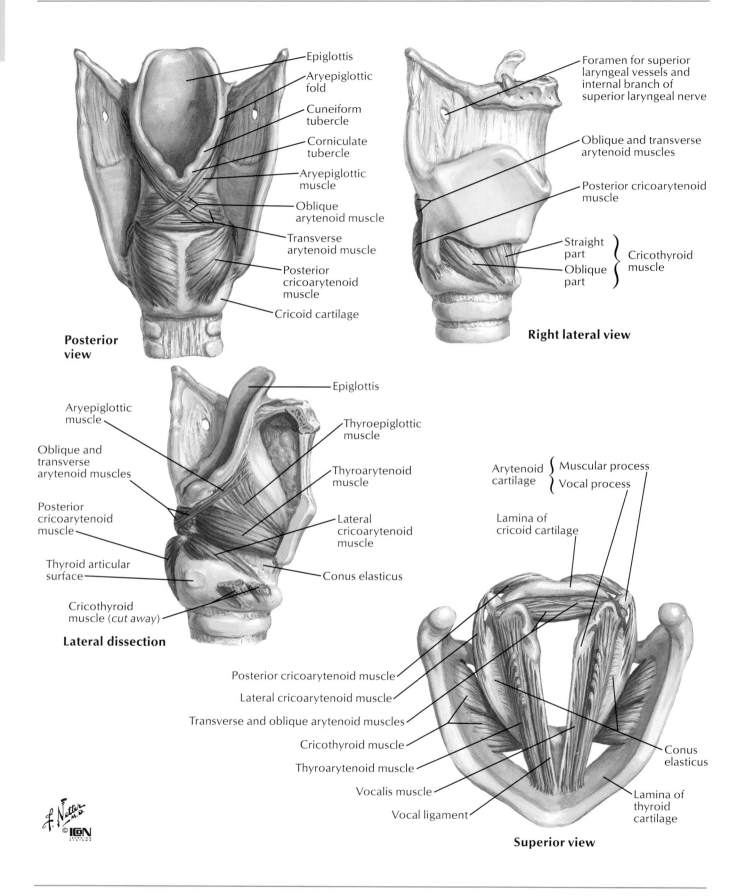

Epiglottis

Aryepiglottic fold

Cuneiform tubercle

Corniculate tubercle

Aryepiglottic muscle

Oblique arytenoid muscle

Transverse arytenoid muscle

Posterior cricoarytenoid muscle

Cricoid cartilage

Posterior view

Foramen for superior laryngeal vessels and internal branch of superior laryngeal nerve

Oblique and transverse arytenoid muscles

Posterior cricoarytenoid muscle

Straight part
Oblique part
} Cricothyroid muscle

Right lateral view

Aryepiglottic muscle

Oblique and transverse arytenoid muscles

Posterior cricoarytenoid muscle

Thyroid articular surface

Cricothyroid muscle (*cut away*)

Lateral dissection

Epiglottis

Thyroepiglottic muscle

Thyroarytenoid muscle

Lateral cricoarytenoid muscle

Conus elasticus

Arytenoid cartilage { Muscular process
Vocal process

Lamina of cricoid cartilage

Posterior cricoarytenoid muscle

Lateral cricoarytenoid muscle

Transverse and oblique arytenoid muscles

Cricothyroid muscle

Thyroarytenoid muscle

Vocalis muscle

Vocal ligament

Conus elasticus

Lamina of thyroid cartilage

Superior view

PLATE 74

HEAD AND NECK

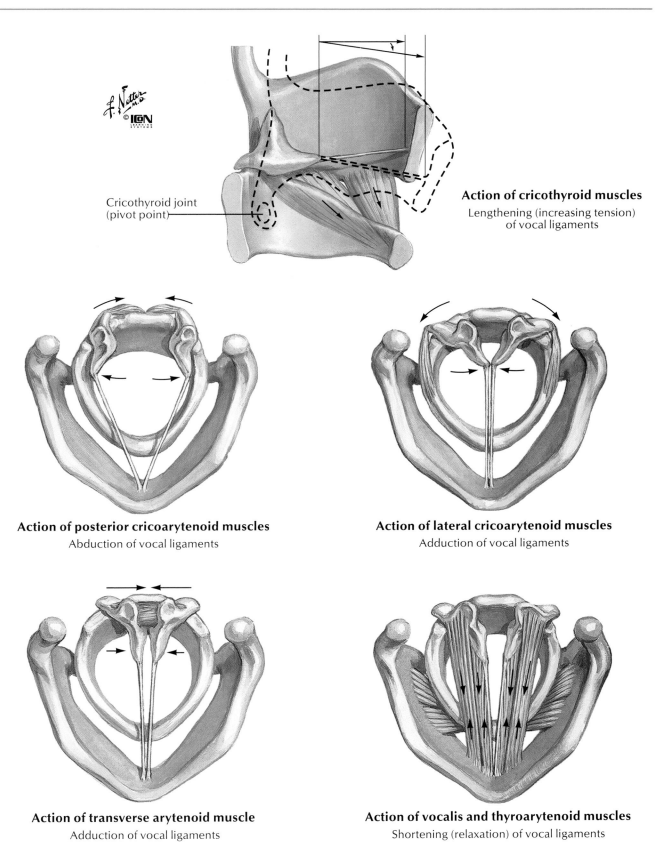

Action of cricothyroid muscles
Lengthening (increasing tension)
of vocal ligaments

Cricothyroid joint
(pivot point)

Action of posterior cricoarytenoid muscles
Abduction of vocal ligaments

Action of lateral cricoarytenoid muscles
Adduction of vocal ligaments

Action of transverse arytenoid muscle
Adduction of vocal ligaments

Action of vocalis and thyroarytenoid muscles
Shortening (relaxation) of vocal ligaments

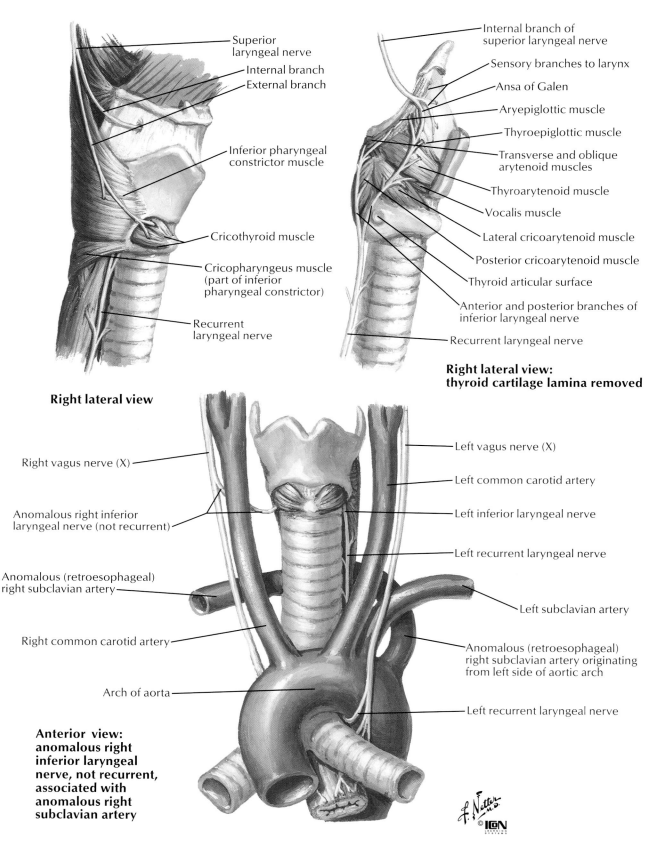

Superior laryngeal nerve

Internal branch

External branch

Inferior pharyngeal constrictor muscle

Cricothyroid muscle

Cricopharyngeus muscle (part of inferior pharyngeal constrictor)

Recurrent laryngeal nerve

Right lateral view

Internal branch of superior laryngeal nerve

Sensory branches to larynx

Ansa of Galen

Aryepiglottic muscle

Thyroepiglottic muscle

Transverse and oblique arytenoid muscles

Thyroarytenoid muscle

Vocalis muscle

Lateral cricoarytenoid muscle

Posterior cricoarytenoid muscle

Thyroid articular surface

Anterior and posterior branches of inferior laryngeal nerve

Recurrent laryngeal nerve

Right lateral view: thyroid cartilage lamina removed

Right vagus nerve (X)

Anomalous right inferior laryngeal nerve (not recurrent)

Anomalous (retroesophageal) right subclavian artery

Right common carotid artery

Arch of aorta

Left vagus nerve (X)

Left common carotid artery

Left inferior laryngeal nerve

Left recurrent laryngeal nerve

Left subclavian artery

Anomalous (retroesophageal) right subclavian artery originating from left side of aortic arch

Left recurrent laryngeal nerve

Anterior view: anomalous right inferior laryngeal nerve, not recurrent, associated with anomalous right subclavian artery

PLATE 76

HEAD AND NECK

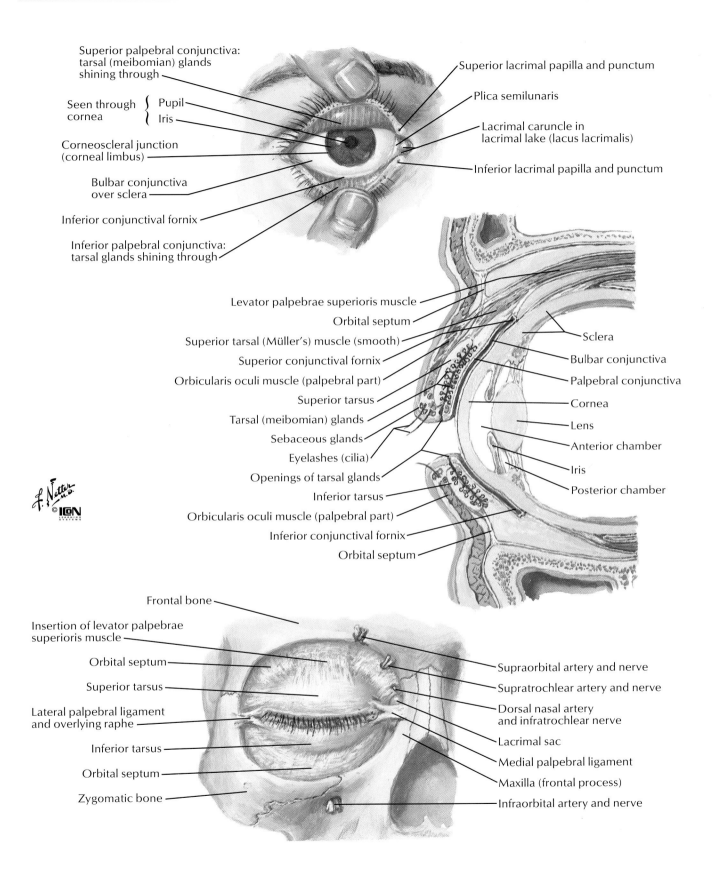

Superior palpebral conjunctiva: tarsal (meibomian) glands shining through

Seen through cornea { Pupil / Iris }

Corneoscleral junction (corneal limbus)

Bulbar conjunctiva over sclera

Inferior conjunctival fornix

Inferior palpebral conjunctiva: tarsal glands shining through

Superior lacrimal papilla and punctum

Plica semilunaris

Lacrimal caruncle in lacrimal lake (lacus lacrimalis)

Inferior lacrimal papilla and punctum

Levator palpebrae superioris muscle

Orbital septum

Superior tarsal (Müller's) muscle (smooth)

Superior conjunctival fornix

Orbicularis oculi muscle (palpebral part)

Superior tarsus

Tarsal (meibomian) glands

Sebaceous glands

Eyelashes (cilia)

Openings of tarsal glands

Inferior tarsus

Orbicularis oculi muscle (palpebral part)

Inferior conjunctival fornix

Orbital septum

Sclera

Bulbar conjunctiva

Palpebral conjunctiva

Cornea

Lens

Anterior chamber

Iris

Posterior chamber

Frontal bone

Insertion of levator palpebrae superioris muscle

Orbital septum

Superior tarsus

Lateral palpebral ligament and overlying raphe

Inferior tarsus

Orbital septum

Zygomatic bone

Supraorbital artery and nerve

Supratrochlear artery and nerve

Dorsal nasal artery and infratrochlear nerve

Lacrimal sac

Medial palpebral ligament

Maxilla (frontal process)

Infraorbital artery and nerve

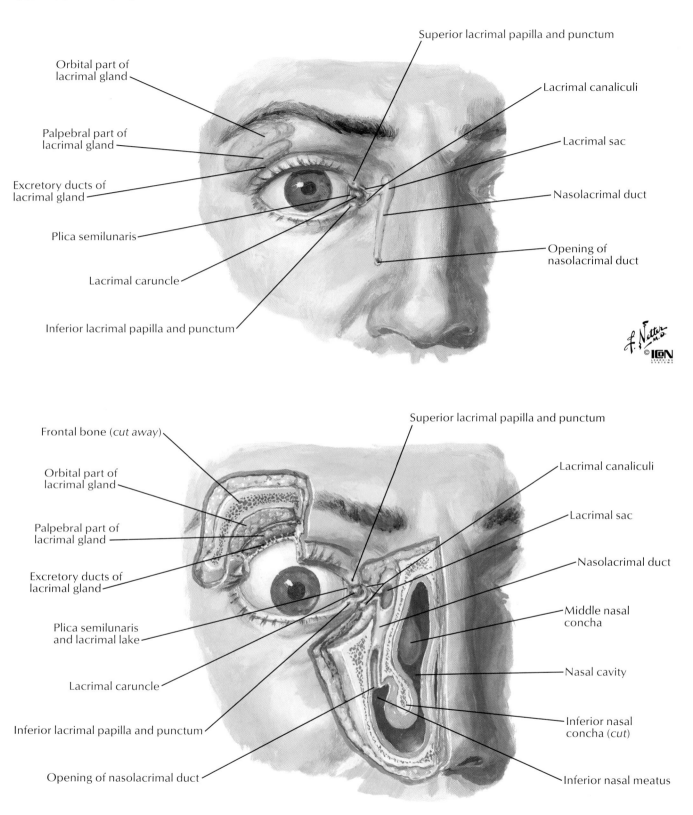

Superior lacrimal papilla and punctum

Orbital part of lacrimal gland

Palpebral part of lacrimal gland

Excretory ducts of lacrimal gland

Plica semilunaris

Lacrimal caruncle

Inferior lacrimal papilla and punctum

Lacrimal canaliculi

Lacrimal sac

Nasolacrimal duct

Opening of nasolacrimal duct

Frontal bone (*cut away*)

Orbital part of lacrimal gland

Palpebral part of lacrimal gland

Excretory ducts of lacrimal gland

Plica semilunaris and lacrimal lake

Lacrimal caruncle

Inferior lacrimal papilla and punctum

Opening of nasolacrimal duct

Superior lacrimal papilla and punctum

Lacrimal canaliculi

Lacrimal sac

Nasolacrimal duct

Middle nasal concha

Nasal cavity

Inferior nasal concha (*cut*)

Inferior nasal meatus

PLATE 78

HEAD AND NECK

Horizontal section

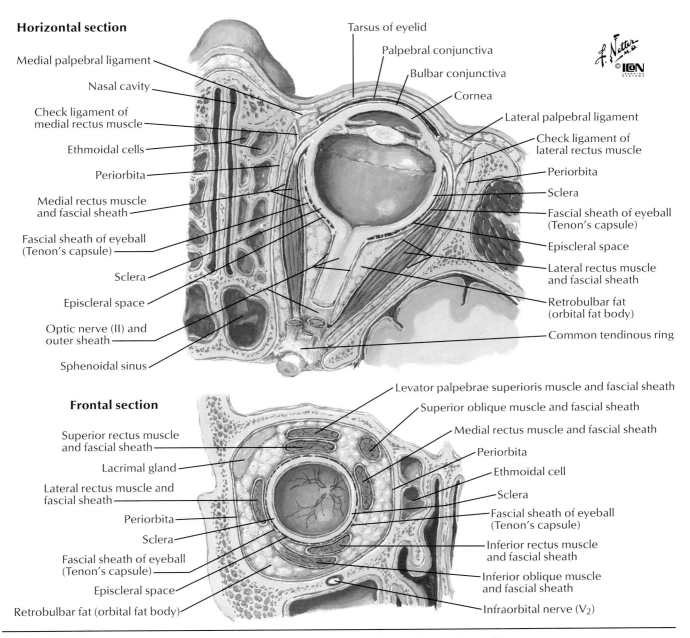

Medial palpebral ligament

Nasal cavity

Check ligament of medial rectus muscle

Ethmoidal cells

Periorbita

Medial rectus muscle and fascial sheath

Fascial sheath of eyeball (Tenon's capsule)

Sclera

Episcleral space

Optic nerve (II) and outer sheath

Sphenoidal sinus

Tarsus of eyelid

Palpebral conjunctiva

Bulbar conjunctiva

Cornea

Lateral palpebral ligament

Check ligament of lateral rectus muscle

Periorbita

Sclera

Fascial sheath of eyeball (Tenon's capsule)

Episcleral space

Lateral rectus muscle and fascial sheath

Retrobulbar fat (orbital fat body)

Common tendinous ring

Frontal section

Levator palpebrae superioris muscle and fascial sheath

Superior oblique muscle and fascial sheath

Medial rectus muscle and fascial sheath

Periorbita

Ethmoidal cell

Sclera

Fascial sheath of eyeball (Tenon's capsule)

Inferior rectus muscle and fascial sheath

Inferior oblique muscle and fascial sheath

Infraorbital nerve (V_2)

Superior rectus muscle and fascial sheath

Lacrimal gland

Lateral rectus muscle and fascial sheath

Periorbita

Sclera

Fascial sheath of eyeball (Tenon's capsule)

Episcleral space

Retrobulbar fat (orbital fat body)

Muscle attachments and nerves and vessels entering orbit

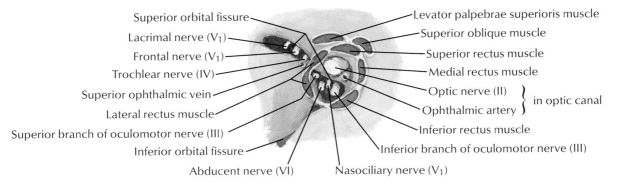

Superior orbital fissure

Lacrimal nerve (V_1)

Frontal nerve (V_1)

Trochlear nerve (IV)

Superior ophthalmic vein

Lateral rectus muscle

Superior branch of oculomotor nerve (III)

Inferior orbital fissure

Abducent nerve (VI)

Levator palpebrae superioris muscle

Superior oblique muscle

Superior rectus muscle

Medial rectus muscle

Optic nerve (II)

Ophthalmic artery

$\left.\begin{array}{c} \\ \end{array}\right\}$ in optic canal

Inferior rectus muscle

Inferior branch of oculomotor nerve (III)

Nasociliary nerve (V_1)

Extrinsic Eye Muscles

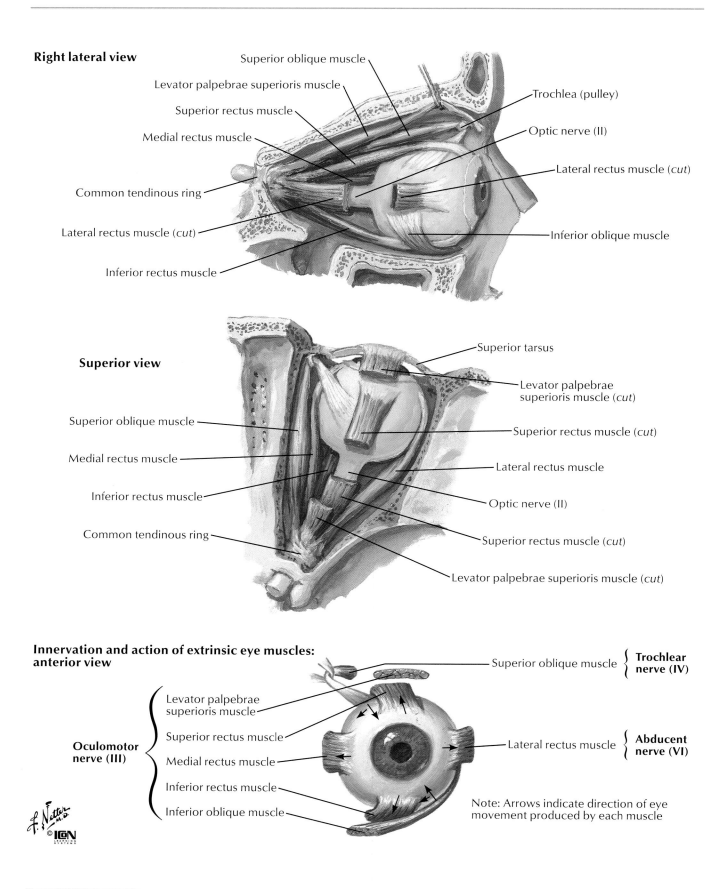

Right lateral view

Superior oblique muscle

Levator palpebrae superioris muscle

Superior rectus muscle

Medial rectus muscle

Common tendinous ring

Lateral rectus muscle (*cut*)

Inferior rectus muscle

Trochlea (pulley)

Optic nerve (II)

Lateral rectus muscle (*cut*)

Inferior oblique muscle

Superior view

Superior tarsus

Levator palpebrae superioris muscle (*cut*)

Superior rectus muscle (*cut*)

Superior oblique muscle

Medial rectus muscle

Lateral rectus muscle

Inferior rectus muscle

Optic nerve (II)

Common tendinous ring

Superior rectus muscle (*cut*)

Levator palpebrae superioris muscle (*cut*)

Innervation and action of extrinsic eye muscles: anterior view

Superior oblique muscle

Trochlear nerve (IV)

Levator palpebrae superioris muscle

Superior rectus muscle

Oculomotor nerve (III)

Medial rectus muscle

Lateral rectus muscle

Abducent nerve (VI)

Inferior rectus muscle

Inferior oblique muscle

Note: Arrows indicate direction of eye movement produced by each muscle

PLATE 80

HEAD AND NECK

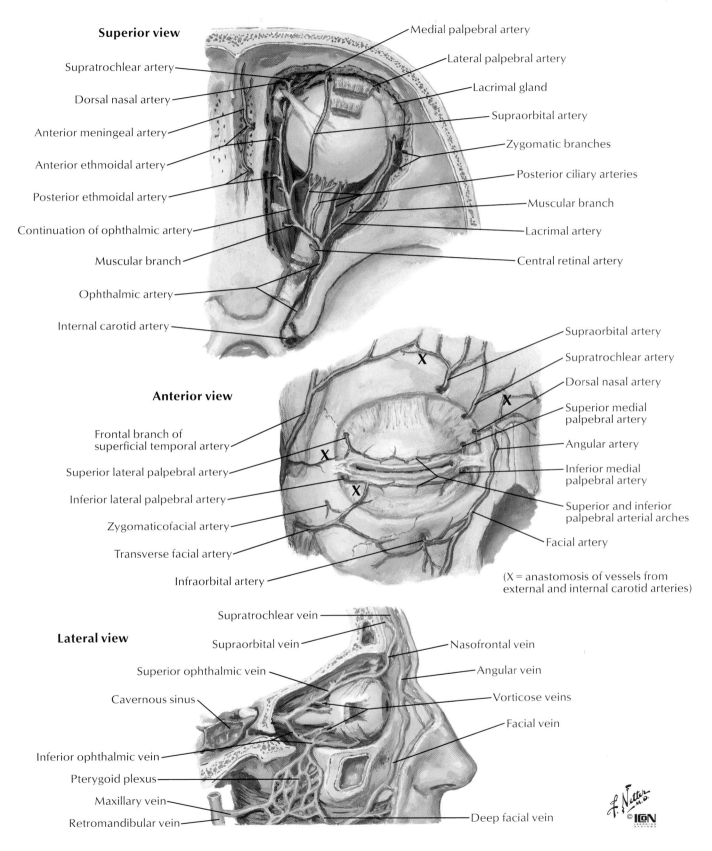

Superior view

Supratrochlear artery

Dorsal nasal artery

Anterior meningeal artery

Anterior ethmoidal artery

Posterior ethmoidal artery

Continuation of ophthalmic artery

Muscular branch

Ophthalmic artery

Internal carotid artery

Medial palpebral artery

Lateral palpebral artery

Lacrimal gland

Supraorbital artery

Zygomatic branches

Posterior ciliary arteries

Muscular branch

Lacrimal artery

Central retinal artery

Anterior view

Frontal branch of superficial temporal artery

Superior lateral palpebral artery

Inferior lateral palpebral artery

Zygomaticofacial artery

Transverse facial artery

Infraorbital artery

Supraorbital artery

Supratrochlear artery

Dorsal nasal artery

Superior medial palpebral artery

Angular artery

Inferior medial palpebral artery

Superior and inferior palpebral arterial arches

Facial artery

(X = anastomosis of vessels from external and internal carotid arteries)

Lateral view

Supratrochlear vein

Supraorbital vein

Superior ophthalmic vein

Cavernous sinus

Inferior ophthalmic vein

Pterygoid plexus

Maxillary vein

Retromandibular vein

Nasofrontal vein

Angular vein

Vorticose veins

Facial vein

Deep facial vein

Nerves of Orbit

SEE ALSO PLATES 41, 115, 126

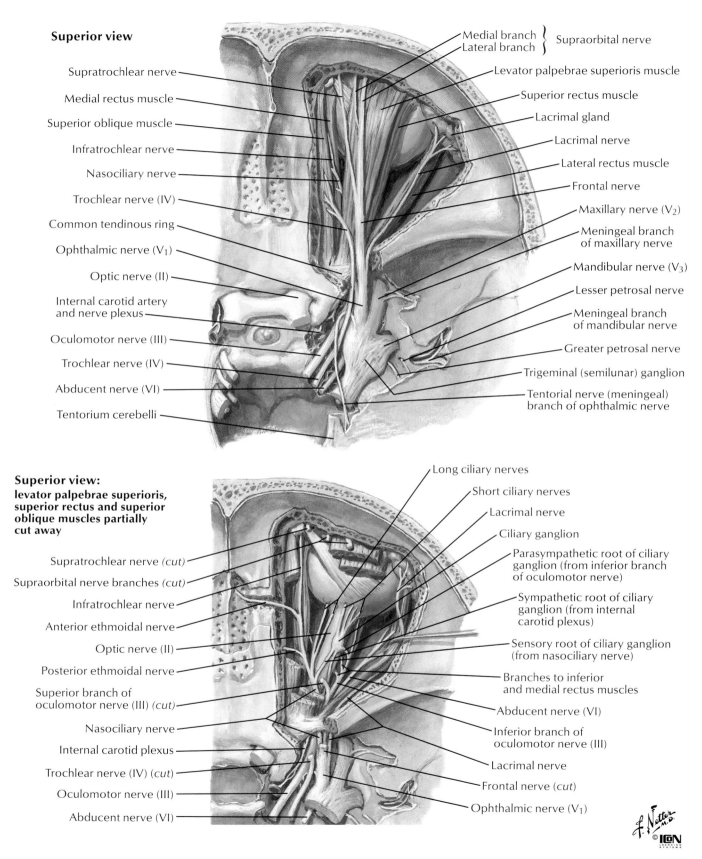

Superior view

Supratrochlear nerve

Medial rectus muscle

Superior oblique muscle

Infratrochlear nerve

Nasociliary nerve

Trochlear nerve (IV)

Common tendinous ring

Ophthalmic nerve (V₁)

Optic nerve (II)

Internal carotid artery and nerve plexus

Oculomotor nerve (III)

Trochlear nerve (IV)

Abducent nerve (VI)

Tentorium cerebelli

Medial branch } Supraorbital nerve
Lateral branch }

Levator palpebrae superioris muscle

Superior rectus muscle

Lacrimal gland

Lacrimal nerve

Lateral rectus muscle

Frontal nerve

Maxillary nerve (V₂)

Meningeal branch of maxillary nerve

Mandibular nerve (V₃)

Lesser petrosal nerve

Meningeal branch of mandibular nerve

Greater petrosal nerve

Trigeminal (semilunar) ganglion

Tentorial nerve (meningeal) branch of ophthalmic nerve

Superior view:
levator palpebrae superioris, superior rectus and superior oblique muscles partially cut away

Supratrochlear nerve *(cut)*

Supraorbital nerve branches *(cut)*

Infratrochlear nerve

Anterior ethmoidal nerve

Optic nerve (II)

Posterior ethmoidal nerve

Superior branch of oculomotor nerve (III) *(cut)*

Nasociliary nerve

Internal carotid plexus

Trochlear nerve (IV) *(cut)*

Oculomotor nerve (III)

Abducent nerve (VI)

Long ciliary nerves

Short ciliary nerves

Lacrimal nerve

Ciliary ganglion

Parasympathetic root of ciliary ganglion (from inferior branch of oculomotor nerve)

Sympathetic root of ciliary ganglion (from internal carotid plexus)

Sensory root of ciliary ganglion (from nasociliary nerve)

Branches to inferior and medial rectus muscles

Abducent nerve (VI)

Inferior branch of oculomotor nerve (III)

Lacrimal nerve

Frontal nerve *(cut)*

Ophthalmic nerve (V₁)

PLATE 82   **HEAD AND NECK**

Horizontal section

Zonular fibers
(suspensory ligament of lens)

Scleral venous sinus
(Schlemm's canal)

Scleral spur

Ciliary body and ciliary muscle

Ciliary part of retina

Tendon of
lateral rectus
muscle

Capsule of lens

Iris

Lens

Cornea

Anterior chamber

Posterior chamber

Iridocorneal angle

Ciliary processes

Bulbar conjunctiva

Ora serrata

Tendon of
medial rectus
muscle

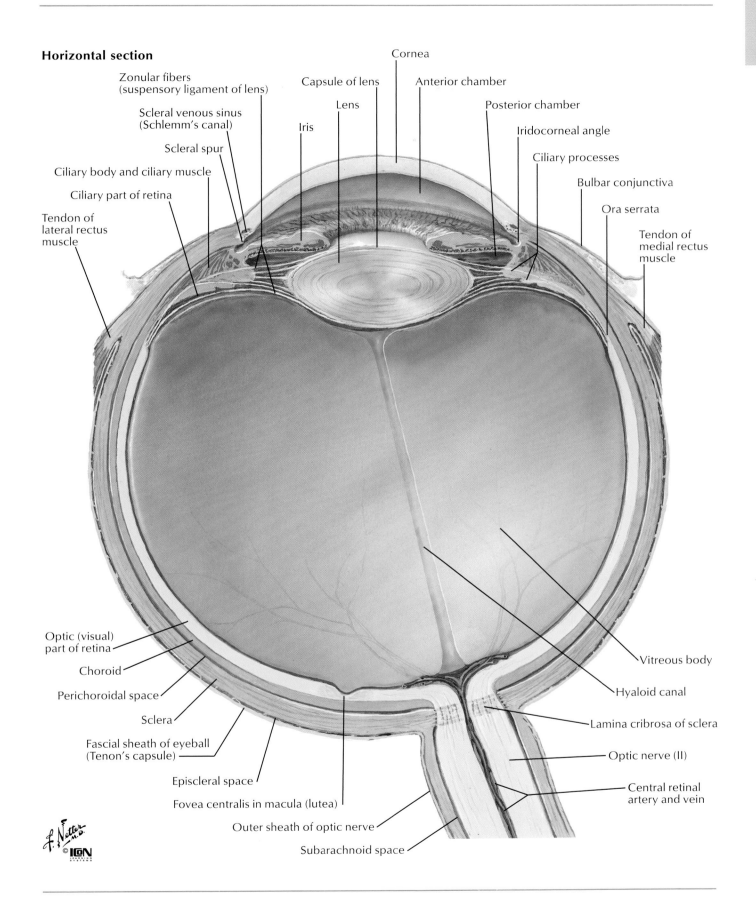

Optic (visual)
part of retina

Choroid

Perichoroidal space

Sclera

Fascial sheath of eyeball
(Tenon's capsule)

Episcleral space

Fovea centralis in macula (lutea)

Outer sheath of optic nerve

Subarachnoid space

Vitreous body

Hyaloid canal

Lamina cribrosa of sclera

Optic nerve (II)

Central retinal
artery and vein

Anterior and Posterior Chambers of Eye

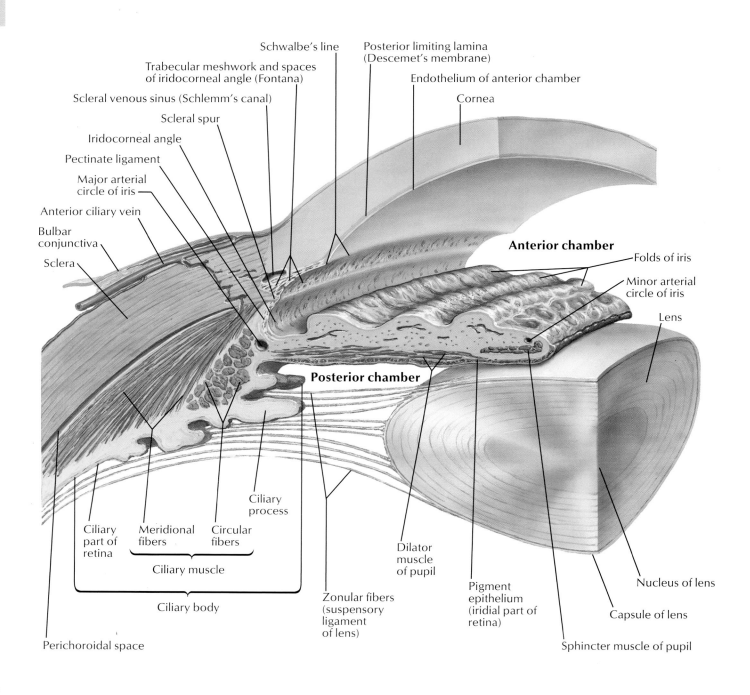

Schwalbe's line

Trabecular meshwork and spaces
of iridocorneal angle (Fontana)

Scleral venous sinus (Schlemm's canal)

Scleral spur

Iridocorneal angle

Pectinate ligament

Major arterial
circle of iris

Anterior ciliary vein

Bulbar
conjunctiva

Sclera

Posterior limiting lamina
(Descemet's membrane)

Endothelium of anterior chamber

Cornea

Anterior chamber

Folds of iris

Minor arterial
circle of iris

Lens

Posterior chamber

Ciliary
process

Ciliary
part of
retina

Meridional
fibers

Circular
fibers

Ciliary muscle

Ciliary body

Perichoroidal space

Zonular fibers
(suspensory
ligament
of lens)

Dilator
muscle
of pupil

Pigment
epithelium
(iridial part of
retina)

Sphincter muscle of pupil

Nucleus of lens

Capsule of lens

Note: For clarity, only single plane of zonular fibers shown;
actually, fibers surround entire circumference of lens

PLATE 84

HEAD AND NECK

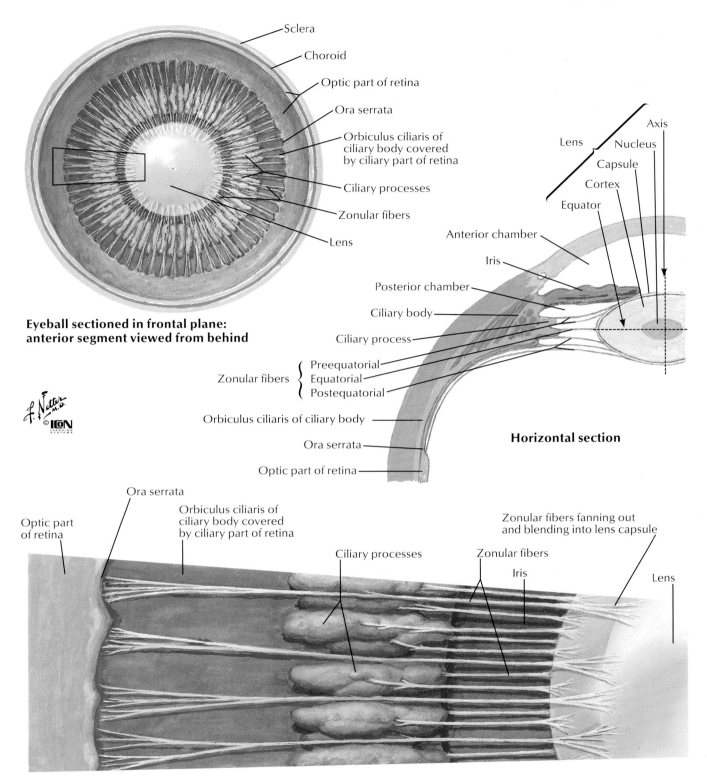

Sclera

Choroid

Optic part of retina

Ora serrata

Orbiculus ciliaris of ciliary body covered by ciliary part of retina

Ciliary processes

Zonular fibers

Lens

Eyeball sectioned in frontal plane: anterior segment viewed from behind

Axis

Lens

Nucleus

Capsule

Cortex

Equator

Anterior chamber

Iris

Posterior chamber

Ciliary body

Ciliary process

Zonular fibers { Preequatorial Equatorial Postequatorial

Orbiculus ciliaris of ciliary body

Ora serrata

Optic part of retina

Horizontal section

Ora serrata

Optic part of retina

Orbiculus ciliaris of ciliary body covered by ciliary part of retina

Ciliary processes

Zonular fibers fanning out and blending into lens capsule

Zonular fibers

Iris

Lens

Enlargement of segment outlined in top illustration (semischematic)

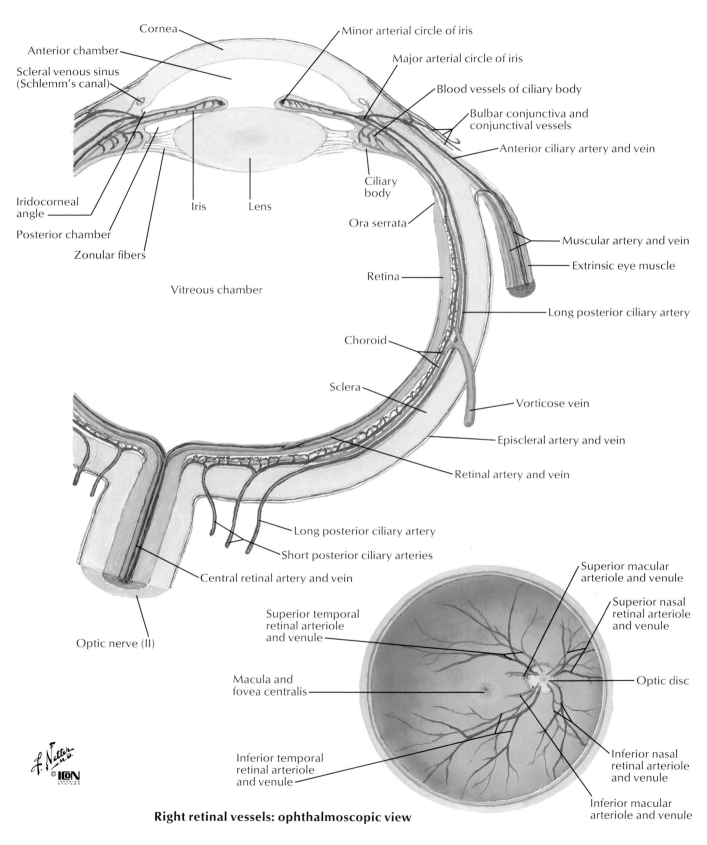

Cornea

Anterior chamber

Scleral venous sinus (Schlemm's canal)

Iridocorneal angle

Posterior chamber

Zonular fibers

Iris

Lens

Vitreous chamber

Minor arterial circle of iris

Major arterial circle of iris

Blood vessels of ciliary body

Bulbar conjunctiva and conjunctival vessels

Anterior ciliary artery and vein

Ciliary body

Ora serrata

Retina

Choroid

Sclera

Muscular artery and vein

Extrinsic eye muscle

Long posterior ciliary artery

Vorticose vein

Episcleral artery and vein

Retinal artery and vein

Long posterior ciliary artery

Short posterior ciliary arteries

Central retinal artery and vein

Optic nerve (II)

Superior temporal retinal arteriole and venule

Macula and fovea centralis

Inferior temporal retinal arteriole and venule

Superior macular arteriole and venule

Superior nasal retinal arteriole and venule

Optic disc

Inferior nasal retinal arteriole and venule

Inferior macular arteriole and venule

Right retinal vessels: ophthalmoscopic view

PLATE 86

HEAD AND NECK

Frontal section

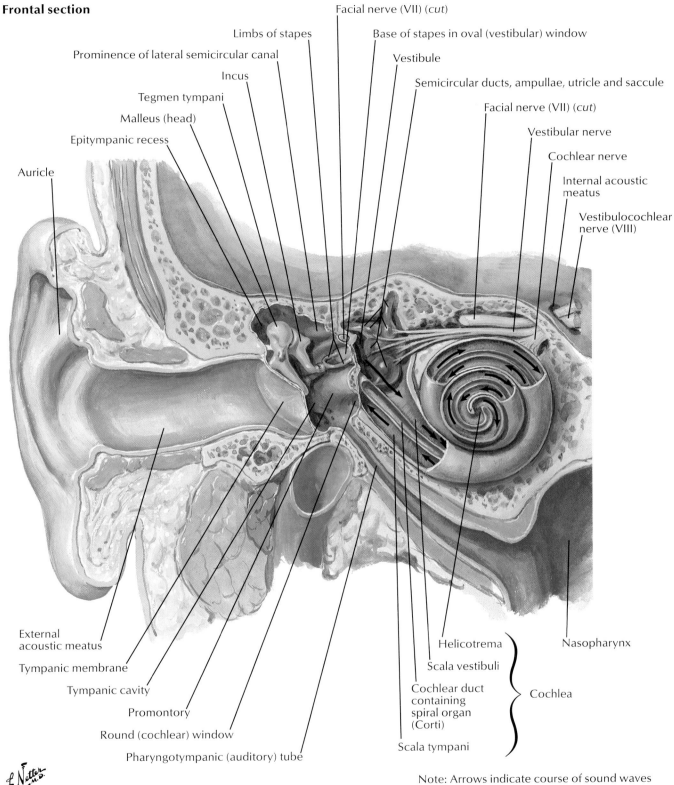

Facial nerve (VII) (*cut*)

Base of stapes in oval (vestibular) window

Limbs of stapes

Prominence of lateral semicircular canal

Vestibule

Incus

Semicircular ducts, ampullae, utricle and saccule

Tegmen tympani

Facial nerve (VII) (*cut*)

Malleus (head)

Vestibular nerve

Epitympanic recess

Cochlear nerve

Auricle

Internal acoustic meatus

Vestibulocochlear nerve (VIII)

External acoustic meatus

Tympanic membrane

Tympanic cavity

Promontory

Round (cochlear) window

Pharyngotympanic (auditory) tube

Helicotrema

Scala vestibuli

Cochlear duct containing spiral organ (Corti)

Scala tympani

Nasopharynx

Cochlea

Note: Arrows indicate course of sound waves

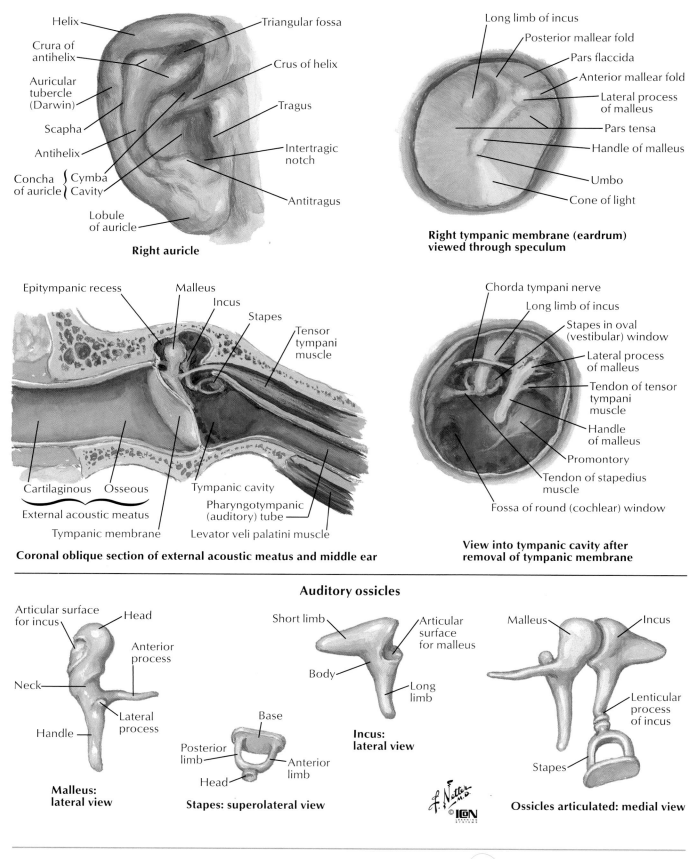

Right auricle

Helix

Crura of antihelix

Auricular tubercle (Darwin)

Scapha

Antihelix

Concha of auricle { Cymba / Cavity

Lobule of auricle

Triangular fossa

Crus of helix

Tragus

Intertragic notch

Antitragus

Right tympanic membrane (eardrum) viewed through speculum

Long limb of incus

Posterior mallear fold

Pars flaccida

Anterior mallear fold

Lateral process of malleus

Pars tensa

Handle of malleus

Umbo

Cone of light

Coronal oblique section of external acoustic meatus and middle ear

Epitympanic recess

Malleus

Incus

Stapes

Tensor tympani muscle

Cartilaginous   Osseous

External acoustic meatus

Tympanic membrane

Tympanic cavity

Pharyngotympanic (auditory) tube

Levator veli palatini muscle

View into tympanic cavity after removal of tympanic membrane

Chorda tympani nerve

Long limb of incus

Stapes in oval (vestibular) window

Lateral process of malleus

Tendon of tensor tympani muscle

Handle of malleus

Promontory

Tendon of stapedius muscle

Fossa of round (cochlear) window

Auditory ossicles

Articular surface for incus

Head

Anterior process

Neck

Lateral process

Handle

Malleus: lateral view

Base

Posterior limb

Head

Anterior limb

Stapes: superolateral view

Short limb

Articular surface for malleus

Body

Long limb

Incus: lateral view

Malleus

Incus

Lenticular process of incus

Stapes

Ossicles articulated: medial view

PLATE 88

HEAD AND NECK

Lateral wall of tympanic cavity: medial (internal) view

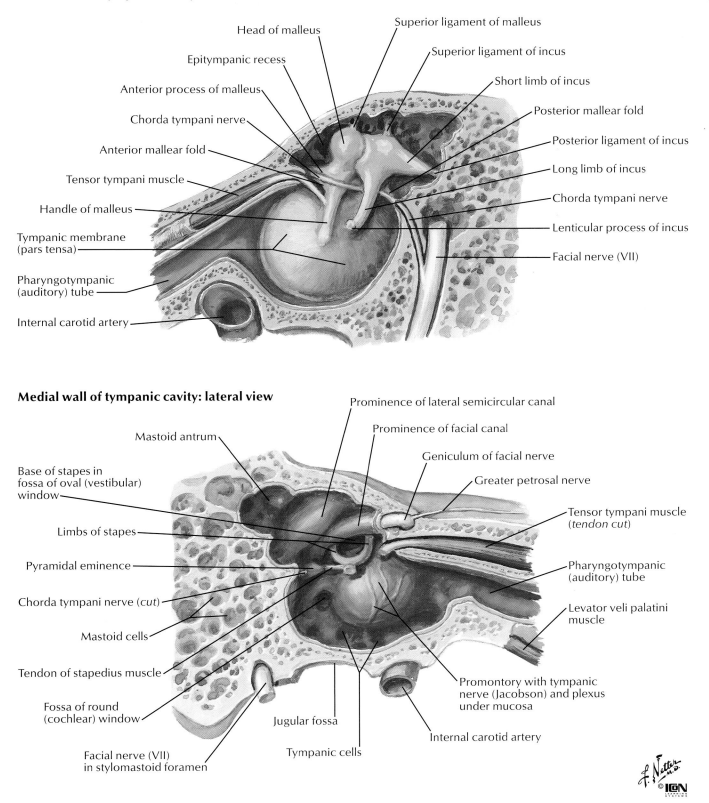

Head of malleus

Superior ligament of malleus

Epitympanic recess

Superior ligament of incus

Anterior process of malleus

Short limb of incus

Chorda tympani nerve

Posterior mallear fold

Anterior mallear fold

Posterior ligament of incus

Tensor tympani muscle

Long limb of incus

Handle of malleus

Chorda tympani nerve

Tympanic membrane
(pars tensa)

Lenticular process of incus

Pharyngotympanic
(auditory) tube

Facial nerve (VII)

Internal carotid artery

Medial wall of tympanic cavity: lateral view

Prominence of lateral semicircular canal

Mastoid antrum

Prominence of facial canal

Geniculum of facial nerve

Base of stapes in
fossa of oval (vestibular)
window

Greater petrosal nerve

Tensor tympani muscle
(*tendon cut*)

Limbs of stapes

Pyramidal eminence

Pharyngotympanic
(auditory) tube

Chorda tympani nerve (*cut*)

Levator veli palatini
muscle

Mastoid cells

Tendon of stapedius muscle

Promontory with tympanic
nerve (Jacobson) and plexus
under mucosa

Fossa of round
(cochlear) window

Jugular fossa

Internal carotid artery

Facial nerve (VII)
in stylomastoid foramen

Tympanic cells

Bony and Membranous Labyrinths

SEE ALSO PLATE 118

Right bony labyrinth (otic capsule), anterolateral view: surrounding cancellous bone removed

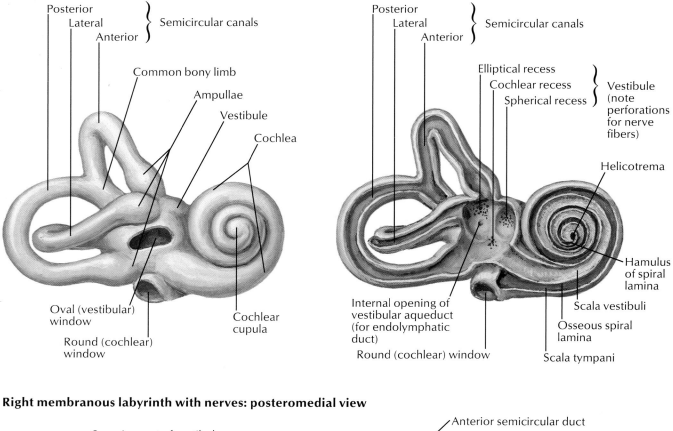

Posterior
Lateral
Anterior
} Semicircular canals

Common bony limb

Ampullae

Vestibule

Cochlea

Oval (vestibular) window

Round (cochlear) window

Cochlear cupula

Dissected right bony labyrinth (otic capsule): membranous labyrinth removed

Posterior
Lateral
Anterior
} Semicircular canals

Elliptical recess
Cochlear recess
Spherical recess
} Vestibule (note perforations for nerve fibers)

Helicotrema

Hamulus of spiral lamina

Scala vestibuli

Osseous spiral lamina

Scala tympani

Internal opening of vestibular aqueduct (for endolymphatic duct)

Round (cochlear) window

Right membranous labyrinth with nerves: posteromedial view

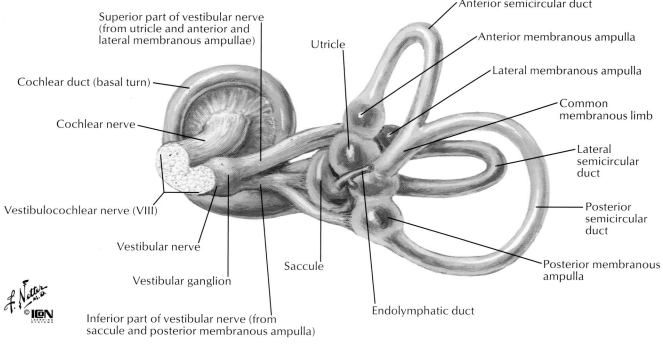

Superior part of vestibular nerve (from utricle and anterior and lateral membranous ampullae)

Utricle

Anterior semicircular duct

Anterior membranous ampulla

Lateral membranous ampulla

Cochlear duct (basal turn)

Cochlear nerve

Common membranous limb

Lateral semicircular duct

Posterior semicircular duct

Vestibulocochlear nerve (VIII)

Vestibular nerve

Vestibular ganglion

Saccule

Endolymphatic duct

Posterior membranous ampulla

Inferior part of vestibular nerve (from saccule and posterior membranous ampulla)

PLATE 90

Bony and membranous labyrinths: schema

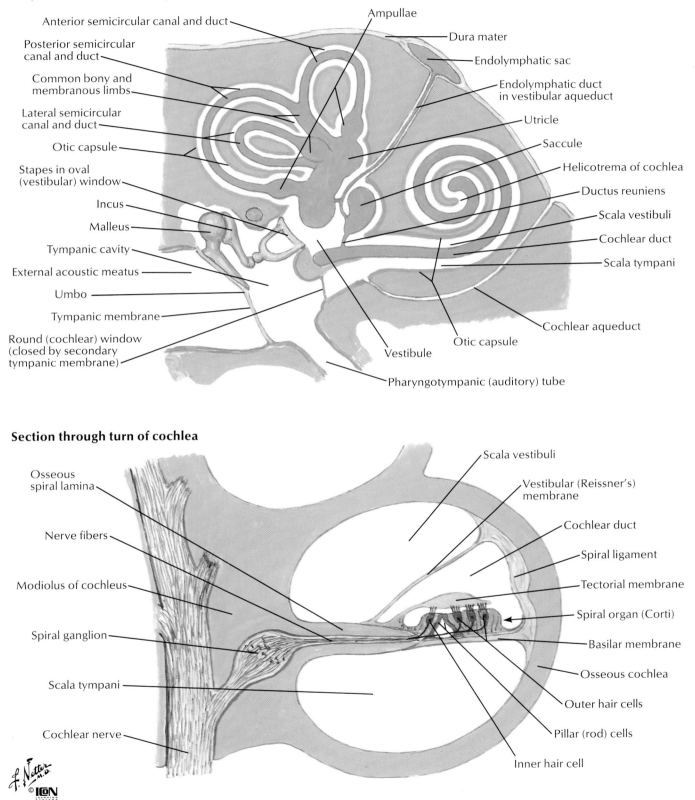

Anterior semicircular canal and duct

Posterior semicircular canal and duct

Common bony and membranous limbs

Lateral semicircular canal and duct

Otic capsule

Stapes in oval (vestibular) window

Incus

Malleus

Tympanic cavity

External acoustic meatus

Umbo

Tympanic membrane

Round (cochlear) window (closed by secondary tympanic membrane)

Ampullae

Dura mater

Endolymphatic sac

Endolymphatic duct in vestibular aqueduct

Utricle

Saccule

Helicotrema of cochlea

Ductus reuniens

Scala vestibuli

Cochlear duct

Scala tympani

Cochlear aqueduct

Otic capsule

Vestibule

Pharyngotympanic (auditory) tube

Section through turn of cochlea

Osseous spiral lamina

Nerve fibers

Modiolus of cochleus

Spiral ganglion

Scala tympani

Cochlear nerve

Scala vestibuli

Vestibular (Reissner's) membrane

Cochlear duct

Spiral ligament

Tectorial membrane

Spiral organ (Corti)

Basilar membrane

Osseous cochlea

Outer hair cells

Pillar (rod) cells

Inner hair cell

Orientation of Labyrinth in Skull

Superior projection of right bony labyrinth on floor of skull

Cochlea

Cochlear nerve

Facial nerve (VII)

Internal acoustic opening

Vestibulocochlear nerve (VIII)

Vestibular nerve

Petrous part of temporal bone

External opening of vestibular aqueduct (for endolymphatic duct)

Groove for greater petrosal nerve

Geniculum of facial nerve

Plane of anterior semicircular canal

Lateral semicircular canal

Plane of posterior semicircular canal

Lateral projection of right membranous labyrinth

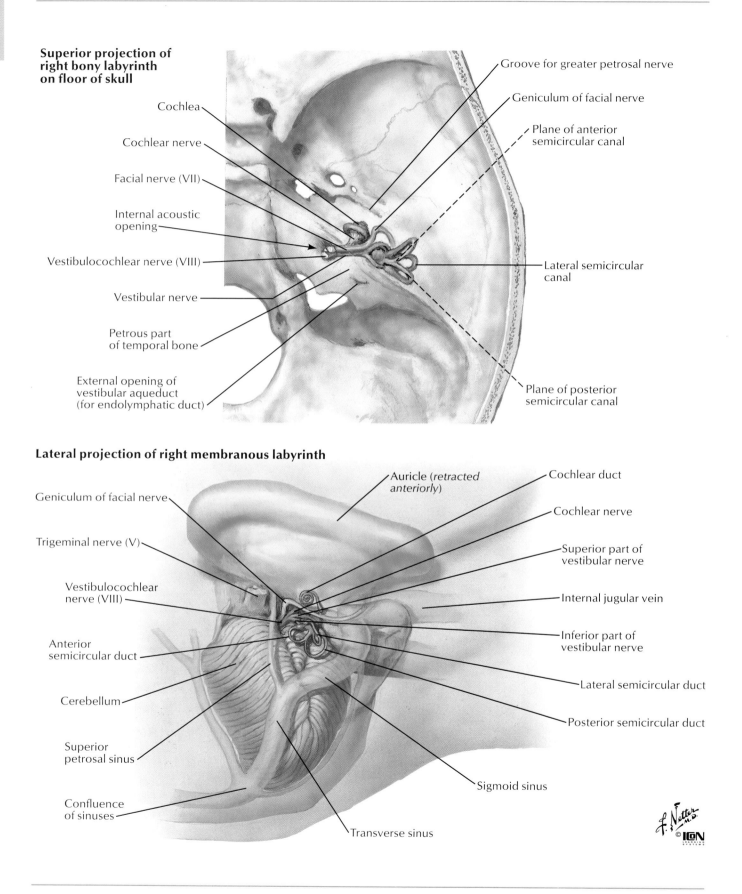

Geniculum of facial nerve

Trigeminal nerve (V)

Vestibulocochlear nerve (VIII)

Anterior semicircular duct

Cerebellum

Superior petrosal sinus

Confluence of sinuses

Auricle (*retracted anteriorly*)

Transverse sinus

Cochlear duct

Cochlear nerve

Superior part of vestibular nerve

Internal jugular vein

Inferior part of vestibular nerve

Lateral semicircular duct

Posterior semicircular duct

Sigmoid sinus

PLATE 92

HEAD AND NECK

Cartilaginous part of pharyngotympanic (auditory) tube at base of skull: inferior view

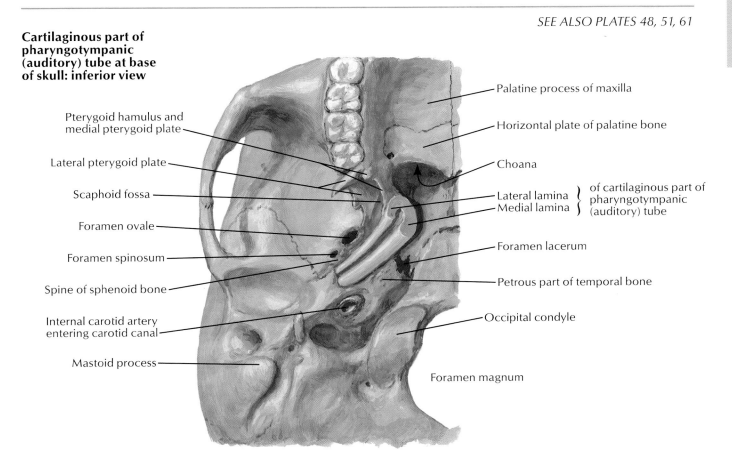

Pterygoid hamulus and medial pterygoid plate

Lateral pterygoid plate

Scaphoid fossa

Foramen ovale

Foramen spinosum

Spine of sphenoid bone

Internal carotid artery entering carotid canal

Mastoid process

Palatine process of maxilla

Horizontal plate of palatine bone

Choana

Lateral lamina ⎫ of cartilaginous part of
Medial lamina ⎬ pharyngotympanic
⎭ (auditory) tube

Foramen lacerum

Petrous part of temporal bone

Occipital condyle

Foramen magnum

Section through cartilaginous part of pharyngotympanic (auditory) tube, with tube closed

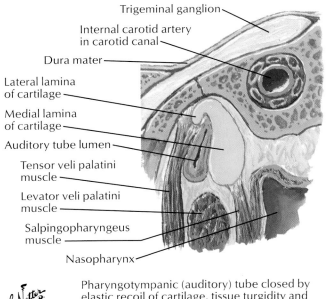

Trigeminal ganglion

Internal carotid artery in carotid canal

Dura mater

Lateral lamina of cartilage

Medial lamina of cartilage

Auditory tube lumen

Tensor veli palatini muscle

Levator veli palatini muscle

Salpingopharyngeus muscle

Nasopharynx

Pharyngotympanic (auditory) tube closed by elastic recoil of cartilage, tissue turgidity and tension of salpingopharyngeus muscles

Section through cartilaginous part of pharyngotympanic (auditory) tube, with tube open

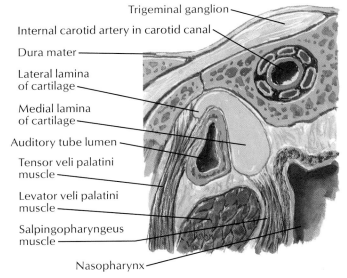

Trigeminal ganglion

Internal carotid artery in carotid canal

Dura mater

Lateral lamina of cartilage

Medial lamina of cartilage

Auditory tube lumen

Tensor veli palatini muscle

Levator veli palatini muscle

Salpingopharyngeus muscle

Nasopharynx

Lumen opened chiefly when attachment of tensor veli palatini muscle pulls wall of tube laterally during swallowing

Meninges and Diploic Veins

SEE ALSO PLATE 19

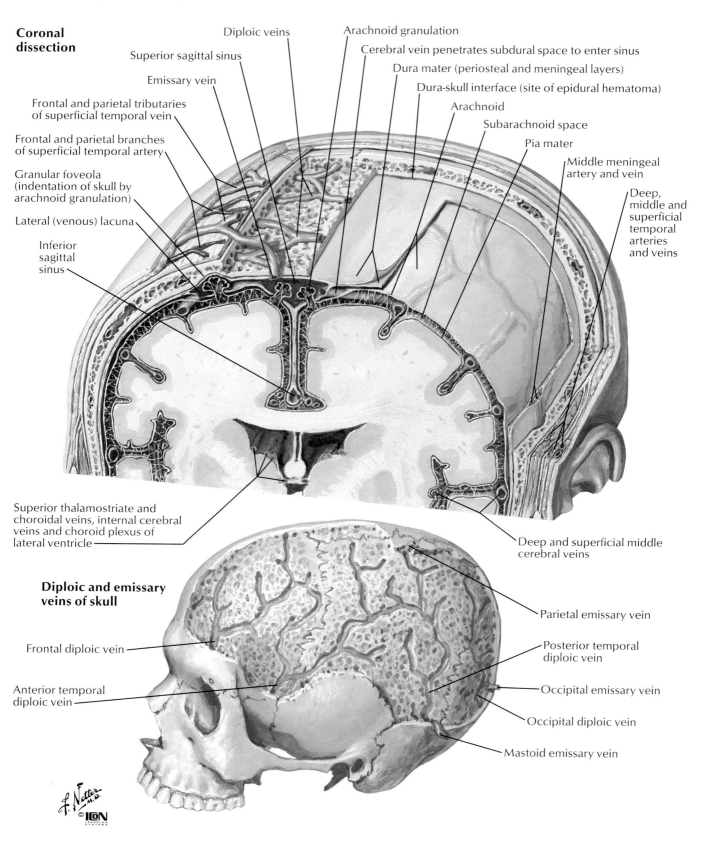

Coronal dissection

Diploic veins

Superior sagittal sinus

Emissary vein

Arachnoid granulation

Cerebral vein penetrates subdural space to enter sinus

Dura mater (periosteal and meningeal layers)

Dura-skull interface (site of epidural hematoma)

Arachnoid

Subarachnoid space

Pia mater

Frontal and parietal tributaries of superficial temporal vein

Frontal and parietal branches of superficial temporal artery

Granular foveola (indentation of skull by arachnoid granulation)

Lateral (venous) lacuna

Inferior sagittal sinus

Middle meningeal artery and vein

Deep, middle and superficial temporal arteries and veins

Superior thalamostriate and choroidal veins, internal cerebral veins and choroid plexus of lateral ventricle

Deep and superficial middle cerebral veins

Diploic and emissary veins of skull

Parietal emissary vein

Frontal diploic vein

Posterior temporal diploic vein

Anterior temporal diploic vein

Occipital emissary vein

Occipital diploic vein

Mastoid emissary vein

PLATE 94   **HEAD AND NECK**

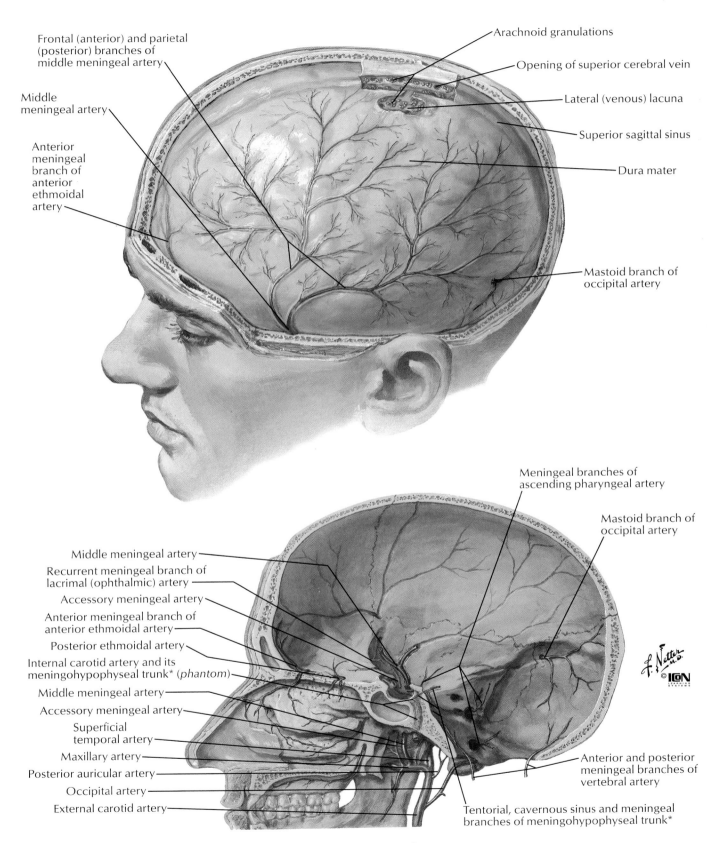

Frontal (anterior) and parietal (posterior) branches of middle meningeal artery

Middle meningeal artery

Anterior meningeal branch of anterior ethmoidal artery

Arachnoid granulations

Opening of superior cerebral vein

Lateral (venous) lacuna

Superior sagittal sinus

Dura mater

Mastoid branch of occipital artery

Meningeal branches of ascending pharyngeal artery

Mastoid branch of occipital artery

Middle meningeal artery

Recurrent meningeal branch of lacrimal (ophthalmic) artery

Accessory meningeal artery

Anterior meningeal branch of anterior ethmoidal artery

Posterior ethmoidal artery

Internal carotid artery and its meningohypophyseal trunk* (phantom)

Middle meningeal artery

Accessory meningeal artery

Superficial temporal artery

Maxillary artery

Posterior auricular artery

Occipital artery

External carotid artery

Anterior and posterior meningeal branches of vertebral artery

Tentorial, cavernous sinus and meningeal branches of meningohypophyseal trunk*

*Variant; most commonly, these branches arise directly from internal carotid artery

FOR DEEP VEINS OF BRAIN SEE PLATE 138

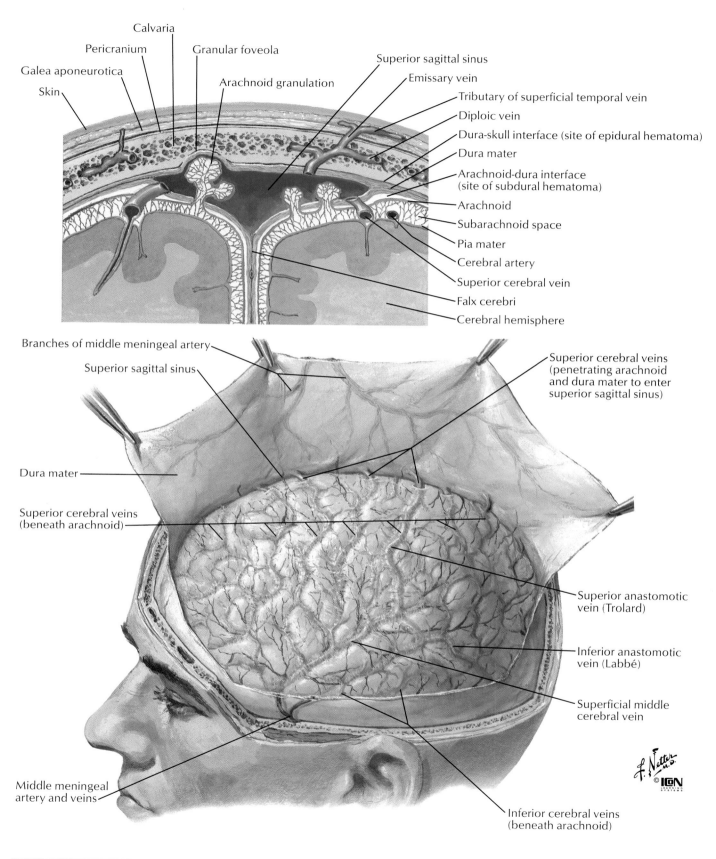

Calvaria

Pericranium

Granular foveola

Galea aponeurotica

Arachnoid granulation

Skin

Superior sagittal sinus

Emissary vein

Tributary of superficial temporal vein

Diploic vein

Dura-skull interface (site of epidural hematoma)

Dura mater

Arachnoid-dura interface (site of subdural hematoma)

Arachnoid

Subarachnoid space

Pia mater

Cerebral artery

Superior cerebral vein

Falx cerebri

Cerebral hemisphere

Branches of middle meningeal artery

Superior sagittal sinus

Dura mater

Superior cerebral veins (beneath arachnoid)

Superior cerebral veins (penetrating arachnoid and dura mater to enter superior sagittal sinus)

Superior anastomotic vein (Trolard)

Inferior anastomotic vein (Labbé)

Superficial middle cerebral vein

Middle meningeal artery and veins

Inferior cerebral veins (beneath arachnoid)

PLATE 96

HEAD AND NECK

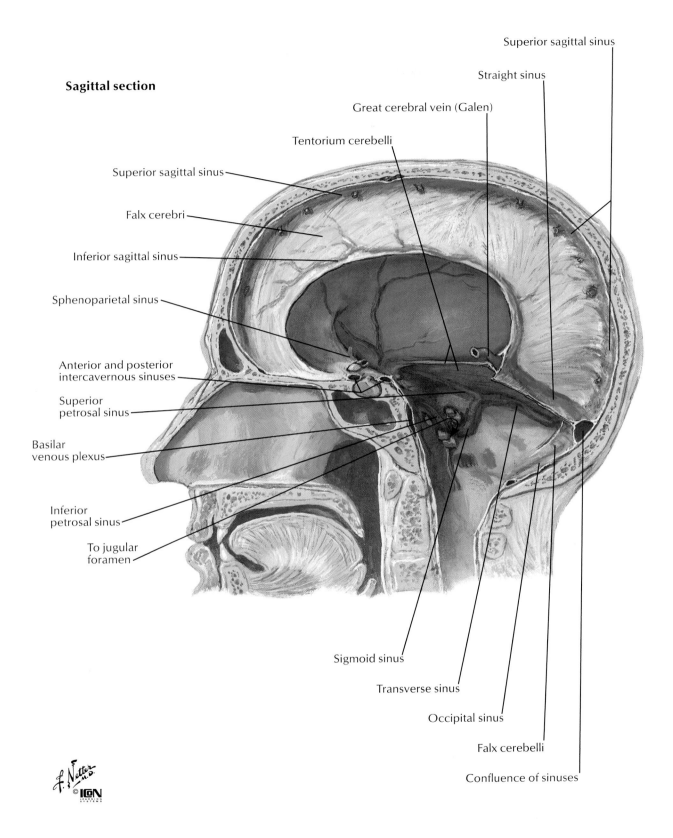

Sagittal section

Superior sagittal sinus

Straight sinus

Great cerebral vein (Galen)

Tentorium cerebelli

Superior sagittal sinus

Falx cerebri

Inferior sagittal sinus

Sphenoparietal sinus

Anterior and posterior intercavernous sinuses

Superior petrosal sinus

Basilar venous plexus

Inferior petrosal sinus

To jugular foramen

Sigmoid sinus

Transverse sinus

Occipital sinus

Falx cerebelli

Confluence of sinuses

Dural Venous Sinuses (continued)

SEE ALSO PLATE 81

Skull sectioned horizontally: superior view

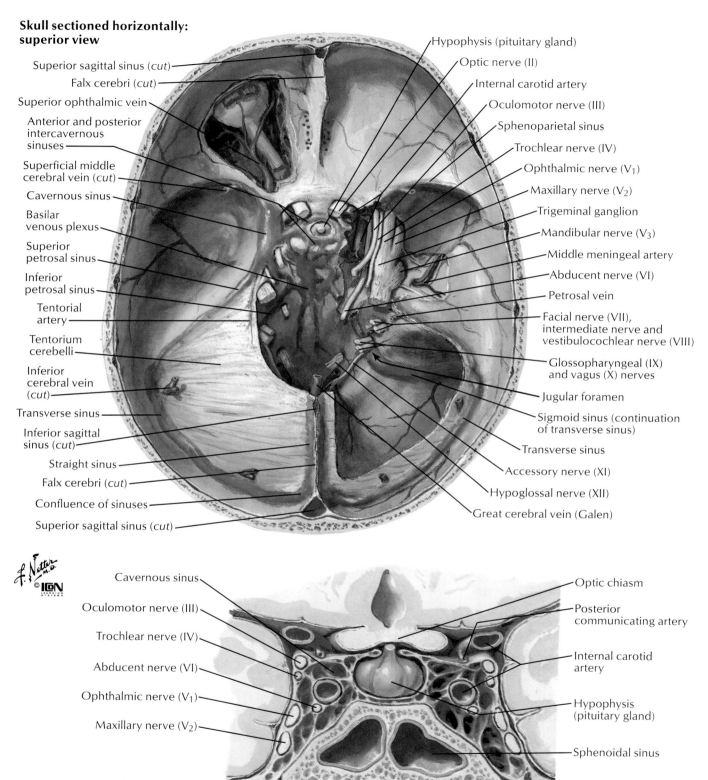

Superior sagittal sinus (*cut*)

Falx cerebri (*cut*)

Superior ophthalmic vein

Anterior and posterior intercavernous sinuses

Superficial middle cerebral vein (*cut*)

Cavernous sinus

Basilar venous plexus

Superior petrosal sinus

Inferior petrosal sinus

Tentorial artery

Tentorium cerebelli

Inferior cerebral vein (*cut*)

Transverse sinus

Inferior sagittal sinus (*cut*)

Straight sinus

Falx cerebri (*cut*)

Confluence of sinuses

Superior sagittal sinus (*cut*)

Hypophysis (pituitary gland)

Optic nerve (II)

Internal carotid artery

Oculomotor nerve (III)

Sphenoparietal sinus

Trochlear nerve (IV)

Ophthalmic nerve (V₁)

Maxillary nerve (V₂)

Trigeminal ganglion

Mandibular nerve (V₃)

Middle meningeal artery

Abducent nerve (VI)

Petrosal vein

Facial nerve (VII), intermediate nerve and vestibulocochlear nerve (VIII)

Glossopharyngeal (IX) and vagus (X) nerves

Jugular foramen

Sigmoid sinus (continuation of transverse sinus)

Transverse sinus

Accessory nerve (XI)

Hypoglossal nerve (XII)

Great cerebral vein (Galen)

Cavernous sinus

Oculomotor nerve (III)

Trochlear nerve (IV)

Abducent nerve (VI)

Ophthalmic nerve (V₁)

Maxillary nerve (V₂)

Coronal section through cavernous sinus

Optic chiasm

Posterior communicating artery

Internal carotid artery

Hypophysis (pituitary gland)

Sphenoidal sinus

Nasopharynx

PLATE 98

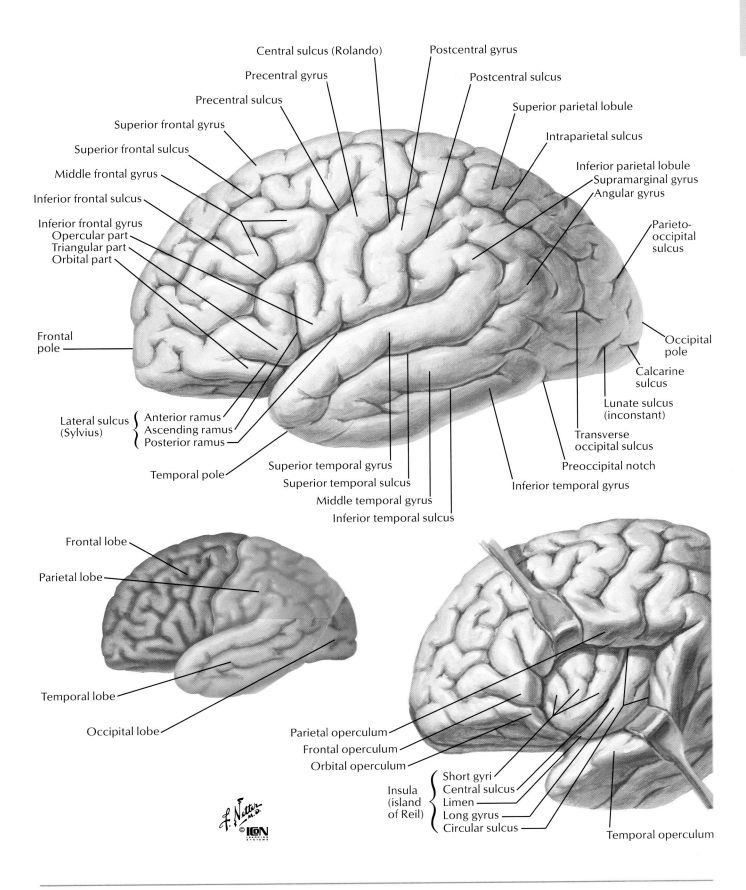

Central sulcus (Rolando)
Postcentral gyrus
Precentral gyrus
Postcentral sulcus
Precentral sulcus
Superior parietal lobule
Superior frontal gyrus
Intraparietal sulcus
Superior frontal sulcus
Inferior parietal lobule
Middle frontal gyrus
Supramarginal gyrus
Inferior frontal sulcus
Angular gyrus
Inferior frontal gyrus
Parieto-occipital sulcus
Opercular part
Triangular part
Orbital part
Frontal pole
Occipital pole
Calcarine sulcus
Lunate sulcus (inconstant)
Lateral sulcus (Sylvius) { Anterior ramus
Ascending ramus
Posterior ramus
Transverse occipital sulcus
Temporal pole
Preoccipital notch
Superior temporal gyrus
Inferior temporal gyrus
Superior temporal sulcus
Middle temporal gyrus
Inferior temporal sulcus

Frontal lobe
Parietal lobe
Temporal lobe
Occipital lobe

Parietal operculum
Frontal operculum
Orbital operculum
Insula (island of Reil) { Short gyri
Central sulcus
Limen
Long gyrus
Circular sulcus
Temporal operculum

Cerebrum: Medial Views

FOR HYPOPHYSIS SEE PLATE 140

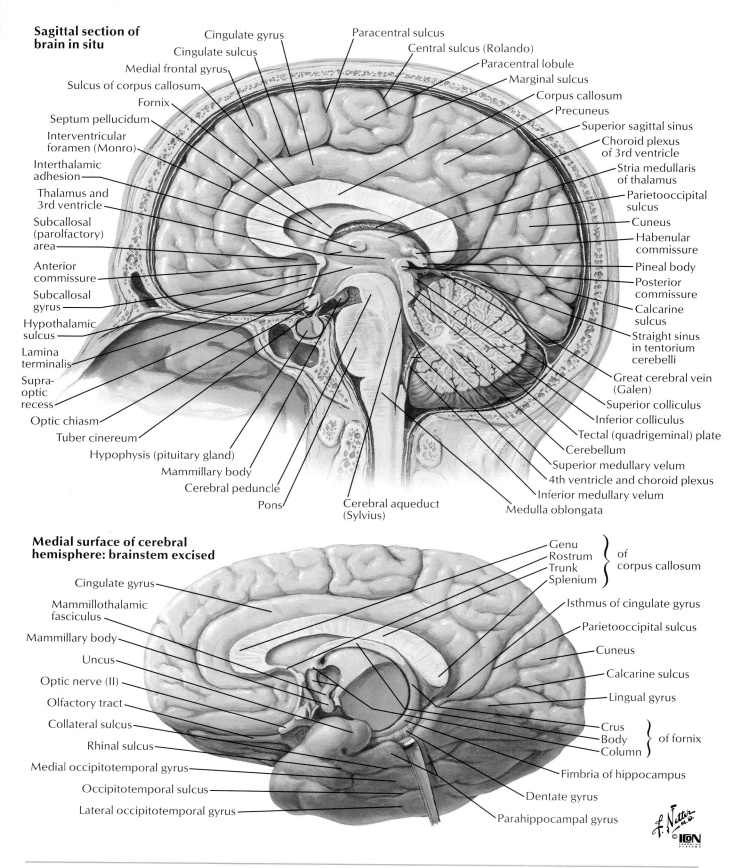

Sagittal section of brain in situ

Cingulate gyrus
Cingulate sulcus
Medial frontal gyrus
Sulcus of corpus callosum
Fornix
Septum pellucidum
Interventricular foramen (Monro)
Interthalamic adhesion
Thalamus and 3rd ventricle
Subcallosal (parolfactory) area
Anterior commissure
Subcallosal gyrus
Hypothalamic sulcus
Lamina terminalis
Supra-optic recess
Optic chiasm
Tuber cinereum
Hypophysis (pituitary gland)
Mammillary body
Cerebral peduncle
Pons

Paracentral sulcus
Central sulcus (Rolando)
Paracentral lobule
Marginal sulcus
Corpus callosum
Precuneus
Superior sagittal sinus
Choroid plexus of 3rd ventricle
Stria medullaris of thalamus
Parietooccipital sulcus
Cuneus
Habenular commissure
Pineal body
Posterior commissure
Calcarine sulcus
Straight sinus in tentorium cerebelli
Great cerebral vein (Galen)
Superior colliculus
Inferior colliculus
Tectal (quadrigeminal) plate
Cerebellum
Superior medullary velum
4th ventricle and choroid plexus
Inferior medullary velum
Medulla oblongata

Cerebral aqueduct (Sylvius)

Medial surface of cerebral hemisphere: brainstem excised

Cingulate gyrus
Mammillothalamic fasciculus
Mammillary body
Uncus
Optic nerve (II)
Olfactory tract
Collateral sulcus
Rhinal sulcus
Medial occipitotemporal gyrus
Occipitotemporal sulcus
Lateral occipitotemporal gyrus

Genu
Rostrum
Trunk
Splenium
} of corpus callosum

Isthmus of cingulate gyrus
Parietooccipital sulcus
Cuneus
Calcarine sulcus
Lingual gyrus
Crus
Body
Column
} of fornix
Fimbria of hippocampus
Dentate gyrus
Parahippocampal gyrus

PLATE 100

HEAD AND NECK

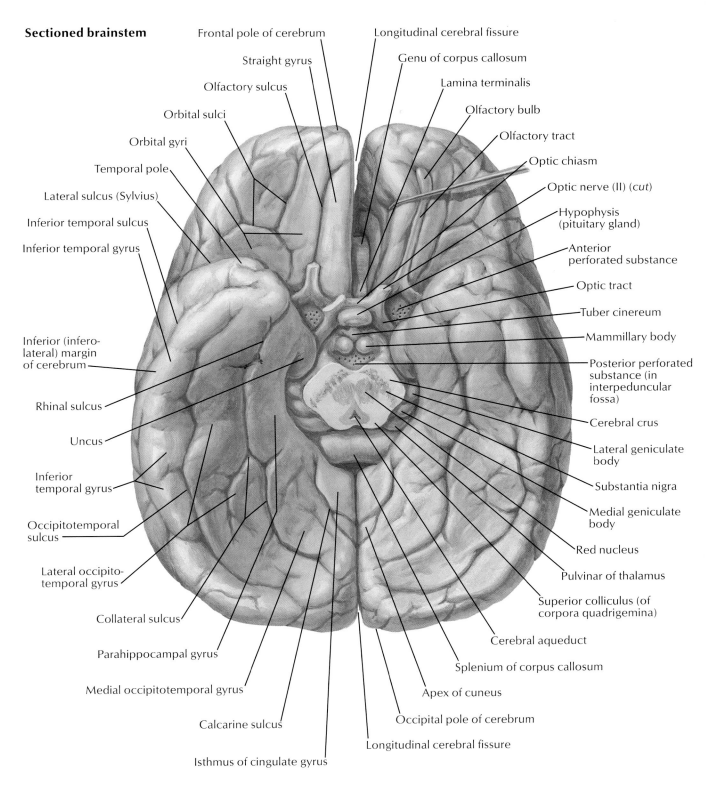

Sectioned brainstem

Frontal pole of cerebrum

Straight gyrus

Olfactory sulcus

Orbital sulci

Orbital gyri

Temporal pole

Lateral sulcus (Sylvius)

Inferior temporal sulcus

Inferior temporal gyrus

Inferior (infero-lateral) margin of cerebrum

Rhinal sulcus

Uncus

Inferior temporal gyrus

Occipitotemporal sulcus

Lateral occipito-temporal gyrus

Collateral sulcus

Parahippocampal gyrus

Medial occipitotemporal gyrus

Calcarine sulcus

Isthmus of cingulate gyrus

Longitudinal cerebral fissure

Genu of corpus callosum

Lamina terminalis

Olfactory bulb

Olfactory tract

Optic chiasm

Optic nerve (II) (cut)

Hypophysis (pituitary gland)

Anterior perforated substance

Optic tract

Tuber cinereum

Mammillary body

Posterior perforated substance (in interpeduncular fossa)

Cerebral crus

Lateral geniculate body

Substantia nigra

Medial geniculate body

Red nucleus

Pulvinar of thalamus

Superior colliculus (of corpora quadrigemina)

Cerebral aqueduct

Splenium of corpus callosum

Apex of cuneus

Occipital pole of cerebrum

Longitudinal cerebral fissure

Ventricles of Brain

Left lateral phantom view

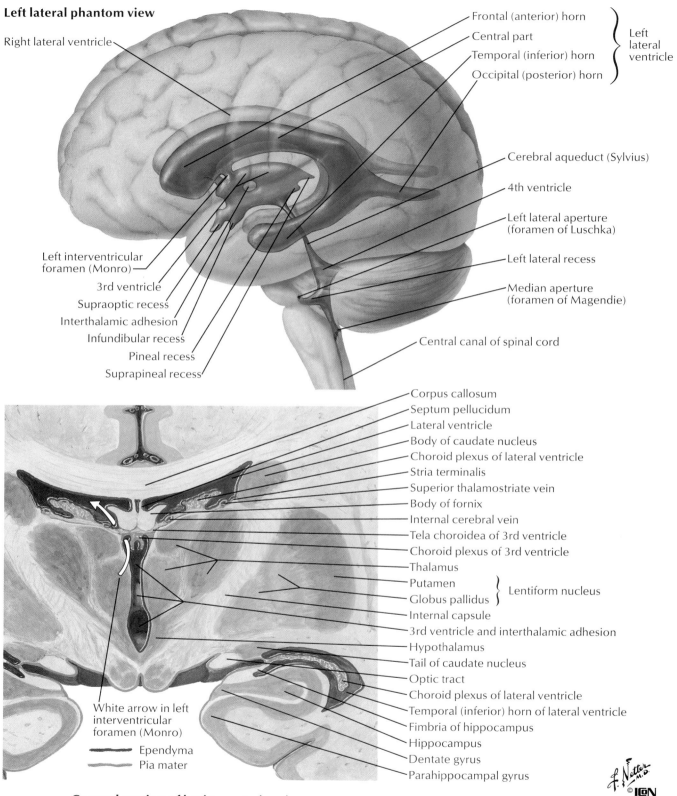

Right lateral ventricle

Frontal (anterior) horn
Central part
Temporal (inferior) horn
Occipital (posterior) horn

Left lateral ventricle

Cerebral aqueduct (Sylvius)

4th ventricle

Left lateral aperture (foramen of Luschka)

Left lateral recess

Median aperture (foramen of Magendie)

Left interventricular foramen (Monro)
3rd ventricle
Supraoptic recess
Interthalamic adhesion
Infundibular recess
Pineal recess
Suprapineal recess

Central canal of spinal cord

Corpus callosum
Septum pellucidum
Lateral ventricle
Body of caudate nucleus
Choroid plexus of lateral ventricle
Stria terminalis
Superior thalamostriate vein
Body of fornix
Internal cerebral vein
Tela choroidea of 3rd ventricle
Choroid plexus of 3rd ventricle
Thalamus
Putamen
Globus pallidus
Internal capsule
3rd ventricle and interthalamic adhesion
Hypothalamus
Tail of caudate nucleus
Optic tract
Choroid plexus of lateral ventricle
Temporal (inferior) horn of lateral ventricle
Fimbria of hippocampus
Hippocampus
Dentate gyrus
Parahippocampal gyrus

Lentiform nucleus

White arrow in left interventricular foramen (Monro)
Ependyma
Pia mater

Coronal section of brain: posterior view

PLATE 102

HEAD AND NECK

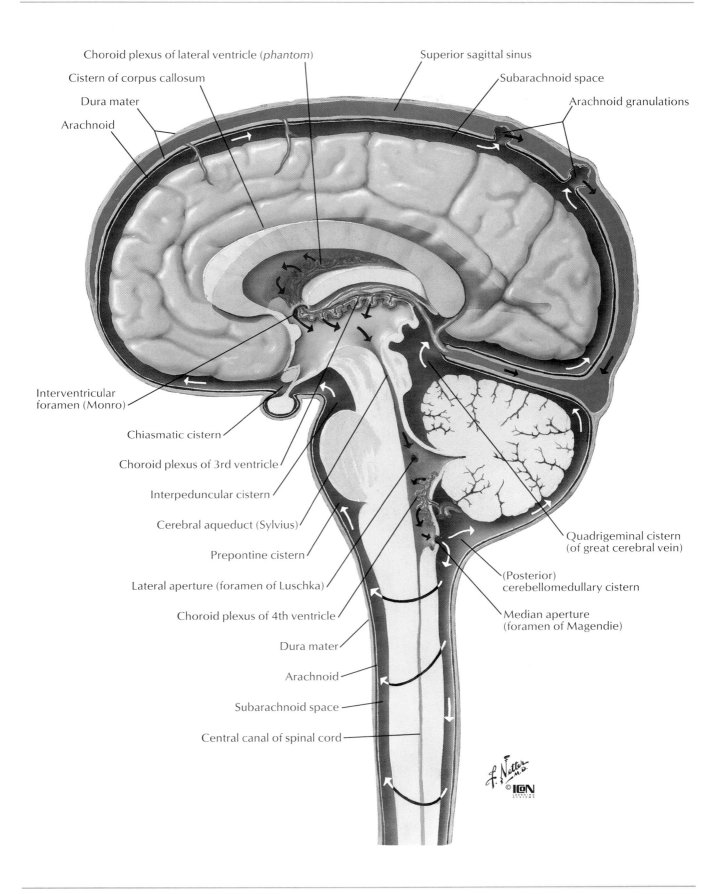

Choroid plexus of lateral ventricle (*phantom*)

Cistern of corpus callosum

Dura mater

Arachnoid

Superior sagittal sinus

Subarachnoid space

Arachnoid granulations

Interventricular foramen (Monro)

Chiasmatic cistern

Choroid plexus of 3rd ventricle

Interpeduncular cistern

Cerebral aqueduct (Sylvius)

Prepontine cistern

Lateral aperture (foramen of Luschka)

Choroid plexus of 4th ventricle

Dura mater

Arachnoid

Subarachnoid space

Central canal of spinal cord

Quadrigeminal cistern (of great cerebral vein)

(Posterior) cerebellomedullary cistern

Median aperture (foramen of Magendie)

Basal Nuclei (Ganglia)

Horizontal sections through cerebrum

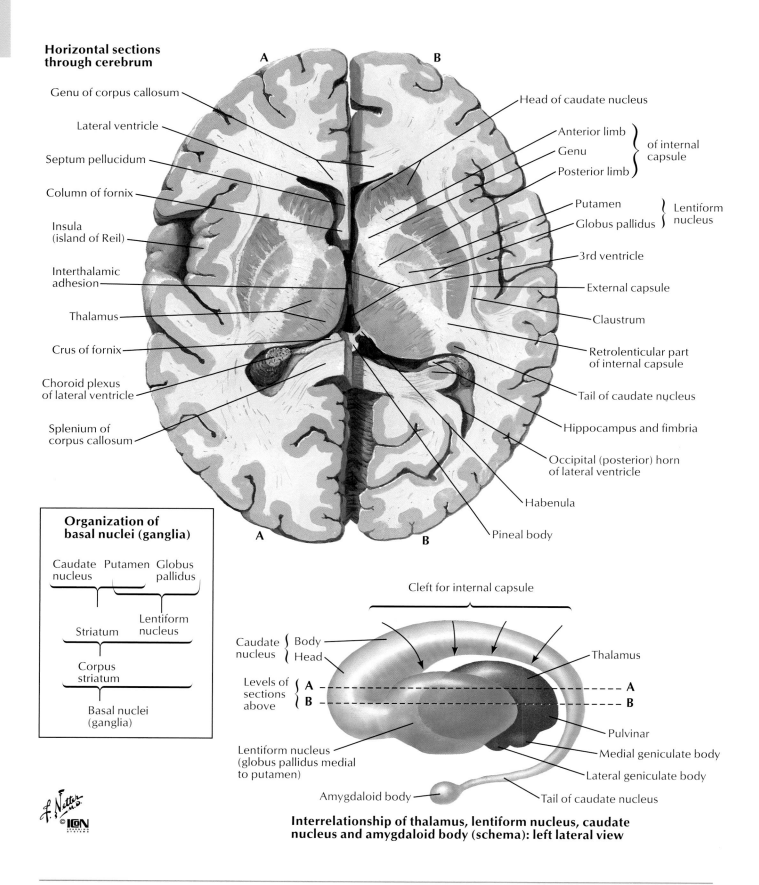

Genu of corpus callosum

Lateral ventricle

Septum pellucidum

Column of fornix

Insula (island of Reil)

Interthalamic adhesion

Thalamus

Crus of fornix

Choroid plexus of lateral ventricle

Splenium of corpus callosum

A

B

Head of caudate nucleus

Anterior limb
Genu } of internal capsule
Posterior limb

Putamen } Lentiform nucleus
Globus pallidus

3rd ventricle

External capsule

Claustrum

Retrolenticular part of internal capsule

Tail of caudate nucleus

Hippocampus and fimbria

Occipital (posterior) horn of lateral ventricle

Habenula

Pineal body

A   B

Organization of basal nuclei (ganglia)

Caudate nucleus   Putamen   Globus pallidus

Lentiform nucleus

Striatum

Corpus striatum

Basal nuclei (ganglia)

Cleft for internal capsule

Caudate { Body
nucleus { Head

Levels of sections above { A
{ B

Lentiform nucleus (globus pallidus medial to putamen)

Amygdaloid body

Thalamus

A

B

Pulvinar

Medial geniculate body

Lateral geniculate body

Tail of caudate nucleus

Interrelationship of thalamus, lentiform nucleus, caudate nucleus and amygdaloid body (schema): left lateral view

PLATE 104

HEAD AND NECK

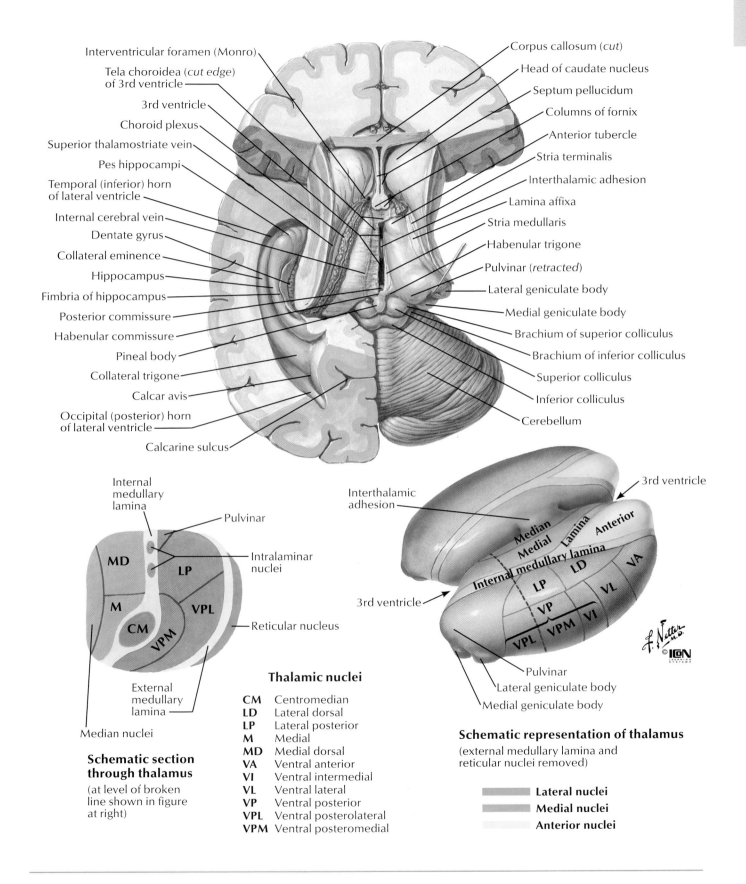

Interventricular foramen (Monro)

Tela choroidea (*cut edge*) of 3rd ventricle

3rd ventricle

Choroid plexus

Superior thalamostriate vein

Pes hippocampi

Temporal (inferior) horn of lateral ventricle

Internal cerebral vein

Dentate gyrus

Collateral eminence

Hippocampus

Fimbria of hippocampus

Posterior commissure

Habenular commissure

Pineal body

Collateral trigone

Calcar avis

Occipital (posterior) horn of lateral ventricle

Calcarine sulcus

Corpus callosum (*cut*)

Head of caudate nucleus

Septum pellucidum

Columns of fornix

Anterior tubercle

Stria terminalis

Interthalamic adhesion

Lamina affixa

Stria medullaris

Habenular trigone

Pulvinar (*retracted*)

Lateral geniculate body

Medial geniculate body

Brachium of superior colliculus

Brachium of inferior colliculus

Superior colliculus

Inferior colliculus

Cerebellum

Internal medullary lamina

Pulvinar

Intralaminar nuclei

MD

LP

M

VPL

CM

VPM

Reticular nucleus

External medullary lamina

Median nuclei

Schematic section through thalamus

(at level of broken line shown in figure at right)

Thalamic nuclei

CM	Centromedian
LD	Lateral dorsal
LP	Lateral posterior
M	Medial
MD	Medial dorsal
VA	Ventral anterior
VI	Ventral intermedial
VL	Ventral lateral
VP	Ventral posterior
VPL	Ventral posterolateral
VPM	Ventral posteromedial

Interthalamic adhesion

3rd ventricle

Median
Medial
Lamina
Anterior
Internal medullary lamina
LP
LD
VA
VP
VL
VPL
VPM
VI
3rd ventricle

Pulvinar

Lateral geniculate body

Medial geniculate body

Schematic representation of thalamus

(external medullary lamina and reticular nuclei removed)

Lateral nuclei
Medial nuclei
Anterior nuclei

Hippocampus and Fornix

Superior dissection

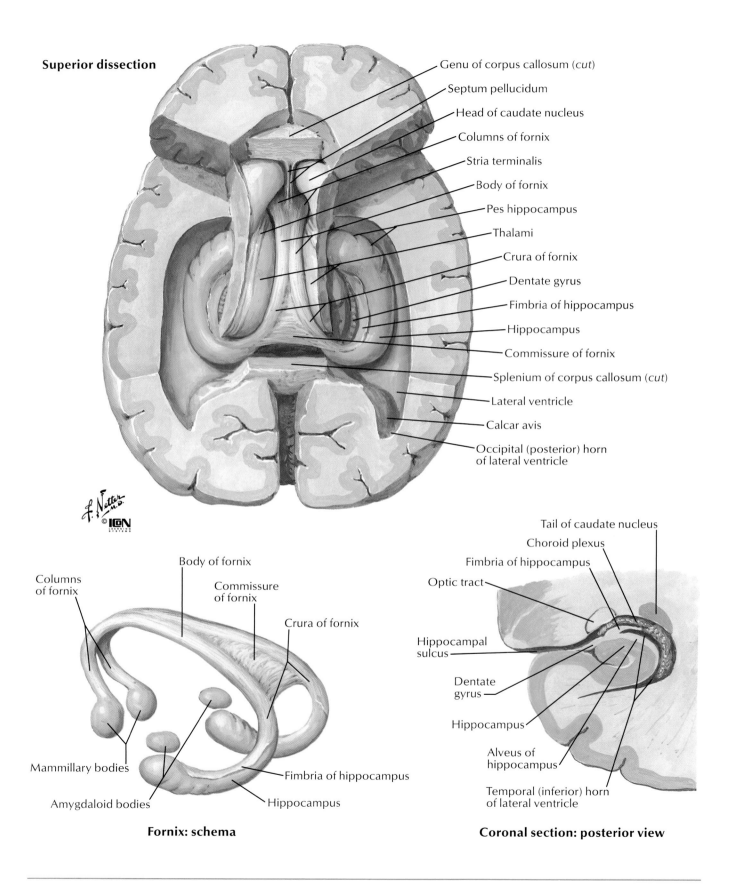

Genu of corpus callosum (*cut*)

Septum pellucidum

Head of caudate nucleus

Columns of fornix

Stria terminalis

Body of fornix

Pes hippocampus

Thalami

Crura of fornix

Dentate gyrus

Fimbria of hippocampus

Hippocampus

Commissure of fornix

Splenium of corpus callosum (*cut*)

Lateral ventricle

Calcar avis

Occipital (posterior) horn of lateral ventricle

Columns of fornix

Body of fornix

Commissure of fornix

Crura of fornix

Mammillary bodies

Amygdaloid bodies

Fimbria of hippocampus

Hippocampus

Fornix: schema

Tail of caudate nucleus

Choroid plexus

Fimbria of hippocampus

Optic tract

Hippocampal sulcus

Dentate gyrus

Hippocampus

Alveus of hippocampus

Temporal (inferior) horn of lateral ventricle

Coronal section: posterior view

PLATE 106

HEAD AND NECK

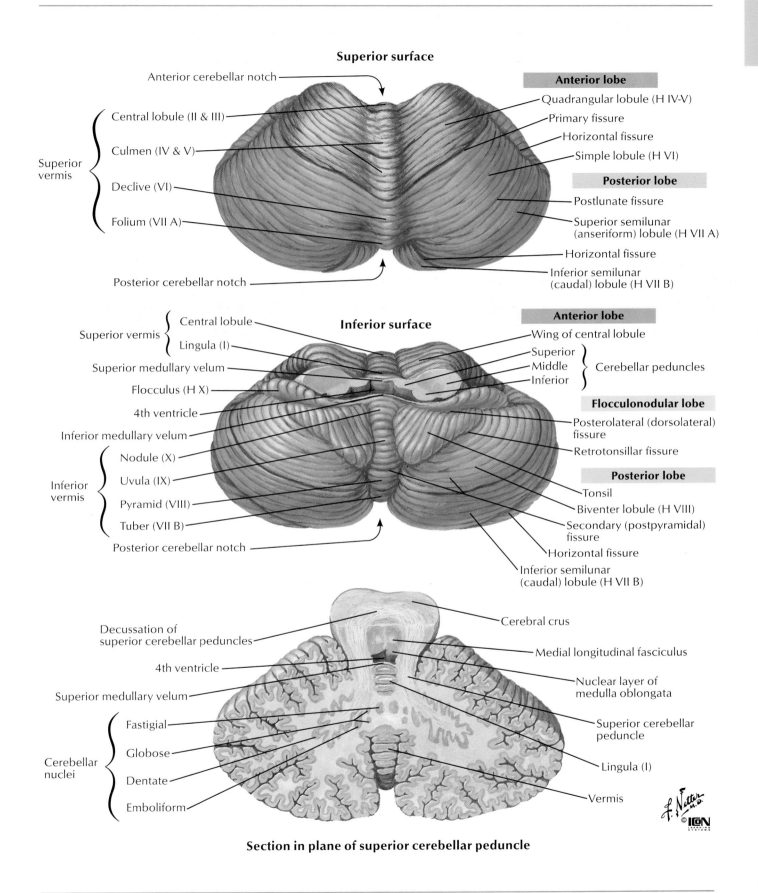

Superior surface

Anterior cerebellar notch

Anterior lobe

Central lobule (II & III)

Culmen (IV & V)

Superior vermis

Declive (VI)

Folium (VII A)

Quadrangular lobule (H IV-V)

Primary fissure

Horizontal fissure

Simple lobule (H VI)

Posterior lobe

Postlunate fissure

Superior semilunar (anseriform) lobule (H VII A)

Horizontal fissure

Inferior semilunar (caudal) lobule (H VII B)

Posterior cerebellar notch

Inferior surface

Superior vermis — Central lobule / Lingula (I)

Superior medullary velum

Flocculus (H X)

4th ventricle

Inferior medullary velum

Nodule (X)

Uvula (IX)

Inferior vermis

Pyramid (VIII)

Tuber (VII B)

Posterior cerebellar notch

Anterior lobe

Wing of central lobule

Superior
Middle — Cerebellar peduncles
Inferior

Flocculonodular lobe

Posterolateral (dorsolateral) fissure

Retrotonsillar fissure

Posterior lobe

Tonsil

Biventer lobule (H VIII)

Secondary (postpyramidal) fissure

Horizontal fissure

Inferior semilunar (caudal) lobule (H VII B)

Decussation of superior cerebellar peduncles

4th ventricle

Superior medullary velum

Fastigial

Globose

Cerebellar nuclei

Dentate

Emboliform

Cerebral crus

Medial longitudinal fasciculus

Nuclear layer of medulla oblongata

Superior cerebellar peduncle

Lingula (I)

Vermis

Section in plane of superior cerebellar peduncle

Brainstem

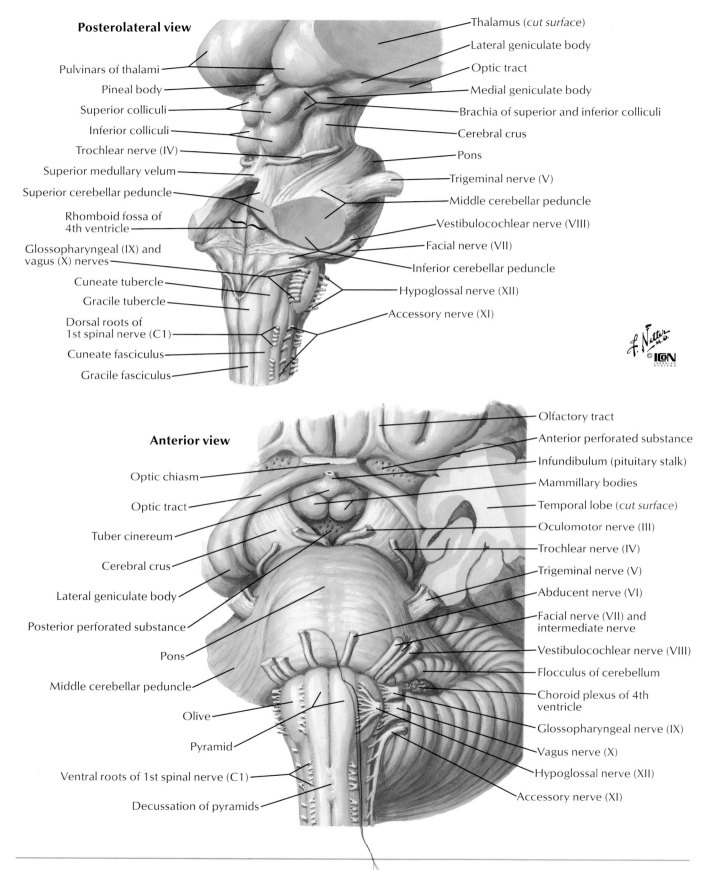

Posterolateral view

Pulvinars of thalami

Pineal body

Superior colliculi

Inferior colliculi

Trochlear nerve (IV)

Superior medullary velum

Superior cerebellar peduncle

Rhomboid fossa of 4th ventricle

Glossopharyngeal (IX) and vagus (X) nerves

Cuneate tubercle

Gracile tubercle

Dorsal roots of 1st spinal nerve (C1)

Cuneate fasciculus

Gracile fasciculus

Thalamus (*cut surface*)

Lateral geniculate body

Optic tract

Medial geniculate body

Brachia of superior and inferior colliculi

Cerebral crus

Pons

Trigeminal nerve (V)

Middle cerebellar peduncle

Vestibulocochlear nerve (VIII)

Facial nerve (VII)

Inferior cerebellar peduncle

Hypoglossal nerve (XII)

Accessory nerve (XI)

Anterior view

Optic chiasm

Optic tract

Tuber cinereum

Cerebral crus

Lateral geniculate body

Posterior perforated substance

Pons

Middle cerebellar peduncle

Olive

Pyramid

Ventral roots of 1st spinal nerve (C1)

Decussation of pyramids

Olfactory tract

Anterior perforated substance

Infundibulum (pituitary stalk)

Mammillary bodies

Temporal lobe (*cut surface*)

Oculomotor nerve (III)

Trochlear nerve (IV)

Trigeminal nerve (V)

Abducent nerve (VI)

Facial nerve (VII) and intermediate nerve

Vestibulocochlear nerve (VIII)

Flocculus of cerebellum

Choroid plexus of 4th ventricle

Glossopharyngeal nerve (IX)

Vagus nerve (X)

Hypoglossal nerve (XII)

Accessory nerve (XI)

PLATE 108

HEAD AND NECK

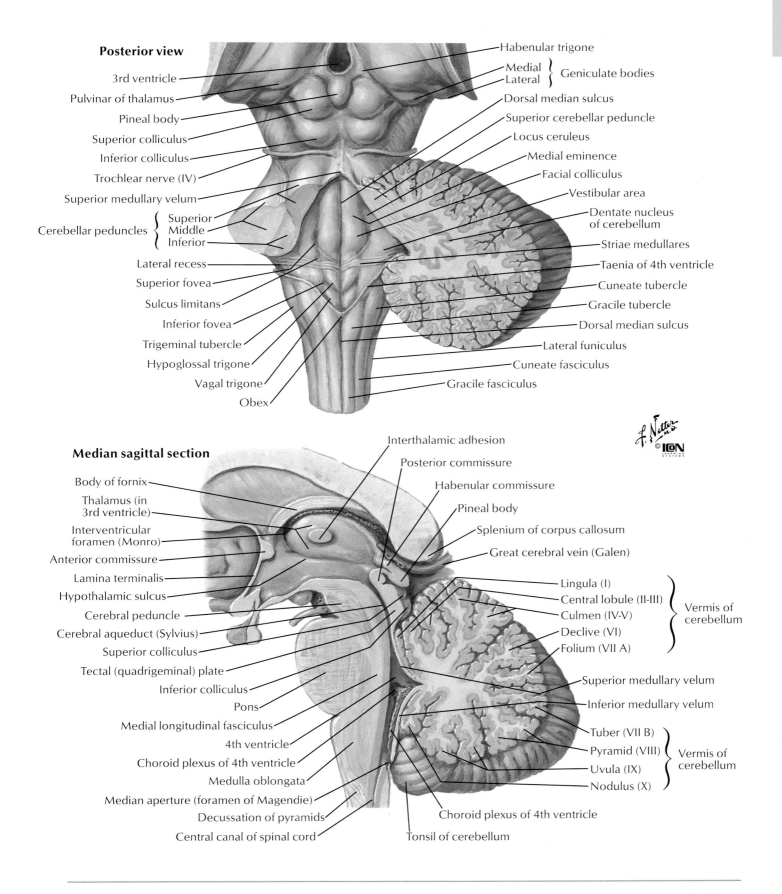

Posterior view

3rd ventricle
Pulvinar of thalamus
Pineal body
Superior colliculus
Inferior colliculus
Trochlear nerve (IV)
Superior medullary velum
Cerebellar peduncles { Superior / Middle / Inferior }
Lateral recess
Superior fovea
Sulcus limitans
Inferior fovea
Trigeminal tubercle
Hypoglossal trigone
Vagal trigone
Obex

Habenular trigone
Medial } Lateral } Geniculate bodies
Dorsal median sulcus
Superior cerebellar peduncle
Locus ceruleus
Medial eminence
Facial colliculus
Vestibular area
Dentate nucleus of cerebellum
Striae medullares
Taenia of 4th ventricle
Cuneate tubercle
Gracile tubercle
Dorsal median sulcus
Lateral funiculus
Cuneate fasciculus
Gracile fasciculus

Median sagittal section

Body of fornix
Thalamus (in 3rd ventricle)
Interventricular foramen (Monro)
Anterior commissure
Lamina terminalis
Hypothalamic sulcus
Cerebral peduncle
Cerebral aqueduct (Sylvius)
Superior colliculus
Tectal (quadrigeminal) plate
Inferior colliculus
Pons
Medial longitudinal fasciculus
4th ventricle
Choroid plexus of 4th ventricle
Medulla oblongata
Median aperture (foramen of Magendie)
Decussation of pyramids
Central canal of spinal cord

Interthalamic adhesion
Posterior commissure
Habenular commissure
Pineal body
Splenium of corpus callosum
Great cerebral vein (Galen)
Lingula (I)
Central lobule (II-III)
Culmen (IV-V)
Declive (VI)
Folium (VII A)
} Vermis of cerebellum
Superior medullary velum
Inferior medullary velum
Tuber (VII B)
Pyramid (VIII)
Uvula (IX)
Nodulus (X)
} Vermis of cerebellum
Choroid plexus of 4th ventricle
Tonsil of cerebellum

Cranial Nerve Nuclei in Brainstem: Schema

Posterior phantom view

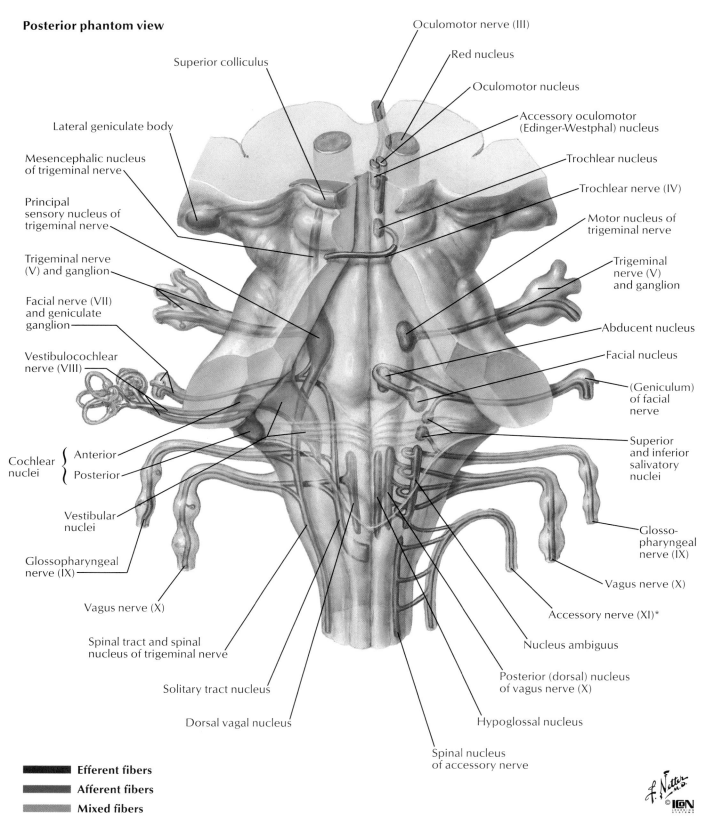

Oculomotor nerve (III)

Superior colliculus

Red nucleus

Oculomotor nucleus

Lateral geniculate body

Accessory oculomotor
(Edinger-Westphal) nucleus

Mesencephalic nucleus
of trigeminal nerve

Trochlear nucleus

Principal
sensory nucleus of
trigeminal nerve

Trochlear nerve (IV)

Motor nucleus of
trigeminal nerve

Trigeminal nerve
(V) and ganglion

Trigeminal
nerve (V)
and ganglion

Facial nerve (VII)
and geniculate
ganglion

Abducent nucleus

Facial nucleus

Vestibulocochlear
nerve (VIII)

(Geniculum)
of facial
nerve

Cochlear nuclei { Anterior
                  Posterior

Superior
and inferior
salivatory
nuclei

Vestibular
nuclei

Glosso-
pharyngeal
nerve (IX)

Glossopharyngeal
nerve (IX)

Vagus nerve (X)

Vagus nerve (X)

Accessory nerve (XI)*

Spinal tract and spinal
nucleus of trigeminal nerve

Nucleus ambiguus

Solitary tract nucleus

Posterior (dorsal) nucleus
of vagus nerve (X)

Dorsal vagal nucleus

Hypoglossal nucleus

Spinal nucleus
of accessory nerve

■■■ Efferent fibers
■■■ Afferent fibers
■■■ Mixed fibers

*Recent evidence suggests that the accessory nerve lacks a cranial root and has no connection to the vagus nerve.
Verification of this finding awaits further investigation

PLATE 110   **HEAD AND NECK**

Medial dissection

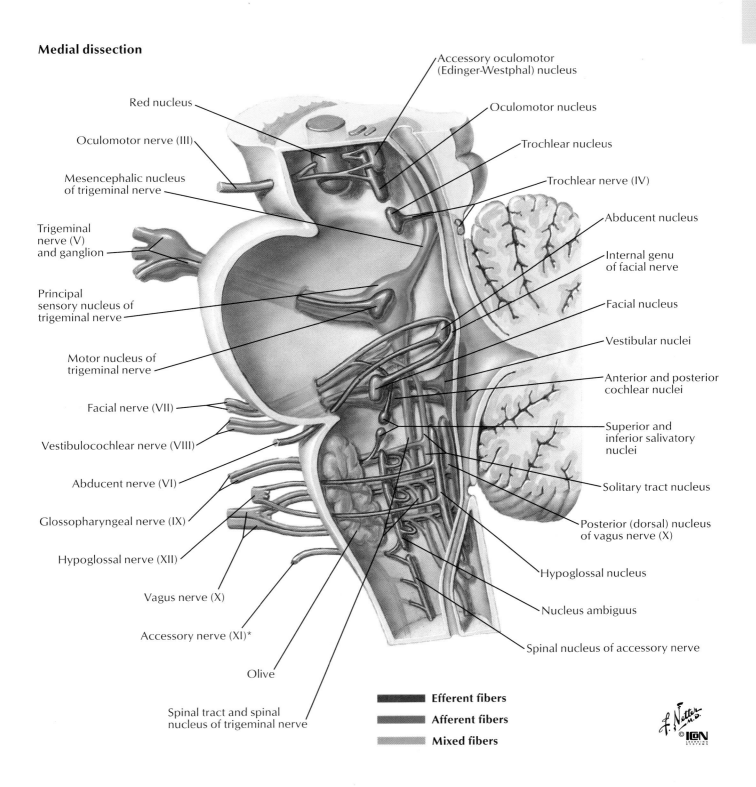

Accessory oculomotor (Edinger-Westphal) nucleus

Red nucleus

Oculomotor nerve (III)

Oculomotor nucleus

Trochlear nucleus

Mesencephalic nucleus of trigeminal nerve

Trochlear nerve (IV)

Trigeminal nerve (V) and ganglion

Abducent nucleus

Principal sensory nucleus of trigeminal nerve

Internal genu of facial nerve

Facial nucleus

Motor nucleus of trigeminal nerve

Vestibular nuclei

Anterior and posterior cochlear nuclei

Facial nerve (VII)

Vestibulocochlear nerve (VIII)

Superior and inferior salivatory nuclei

Abducent nerve (VI)

Solitary tract nucleus

Glossopharyngeal nerve (IX)

Posterior (dorsal) nucleus of vagus nerve (X)

Hypoglossal nerve (XII)

Hypoglossal nucleus

Vagus nerve (X)

Nucleus ambiguus

Accessory nerve (XI)*

Spinal nucleus of accessory nerve

Olive

Efferent fibers

Afferent fibers

Mixed fibers

Spinal tract and spinal nucleus of trigeminal nerve

*Recent evidence suggests that the accessory nerve lacks a cranial root and has no connection to the vagus nerve. Verification of this finding awaits further investigation

CRANIAL AND CERVICAL NERVES

PLATE 111

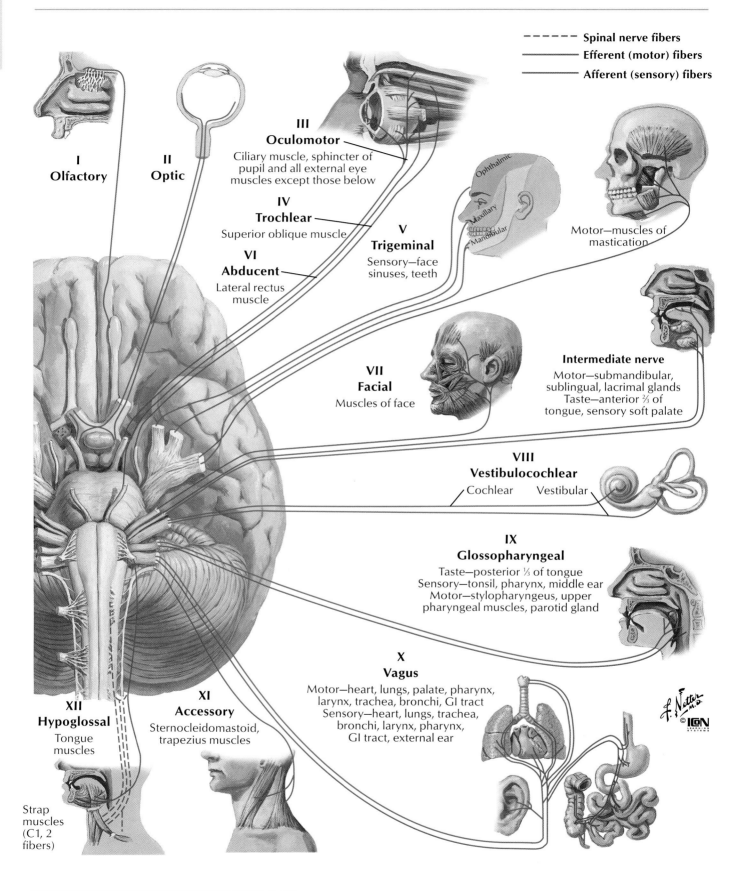

------ Spinal nerve fibers
———— Efferent (motor) fibers
———— Afferent (sensory) fibers

I
Olfactory

II
Optic

III
Oculomotor
Ciliary muscle, sphincter of
pupil and all external eye
muscles except those below

IV
Trochlear
Superior oblique muscle

VI
Abducent
Lateral rectus
muscle

V
Trigeminal
Sensory—face
sinuses, teeth

Ophthalmic
Maxillary
Mandibular

Motor—muscles of
mastication

VII
Facial
Muscles of face

Intermediate nerve
Motor—submandibular,
sublingual, lacrimal glands
Taste—anterior ⅔ of
tongue, sensory soft palate

VIII
Vestibulocochlear
Cochlear   Vestibular

IX
Glossopharyngeal
Taste—posterior ⅓ of tongue
Sensory—tonsil, pharynx, middle ear
Motor—stylopharyngeus, upper
pharyngeal muscles, parotid gland

X
Vagus
Motor—heart, lungs, palate, pharynx,
larynx, trachea, bronchi, GI tract
Sensory—heart, lungs, trachea,
bronchi, larynx, pharynx,
GI tract, external ear

XII
Hypoglossal
Tongue
muscles

Strap
muscles
(C1, 2
fibers)

XI
Accessory
Sternocleidomastoid,
trapezius muscles

PLATE 112   **HEAD AND NECK**

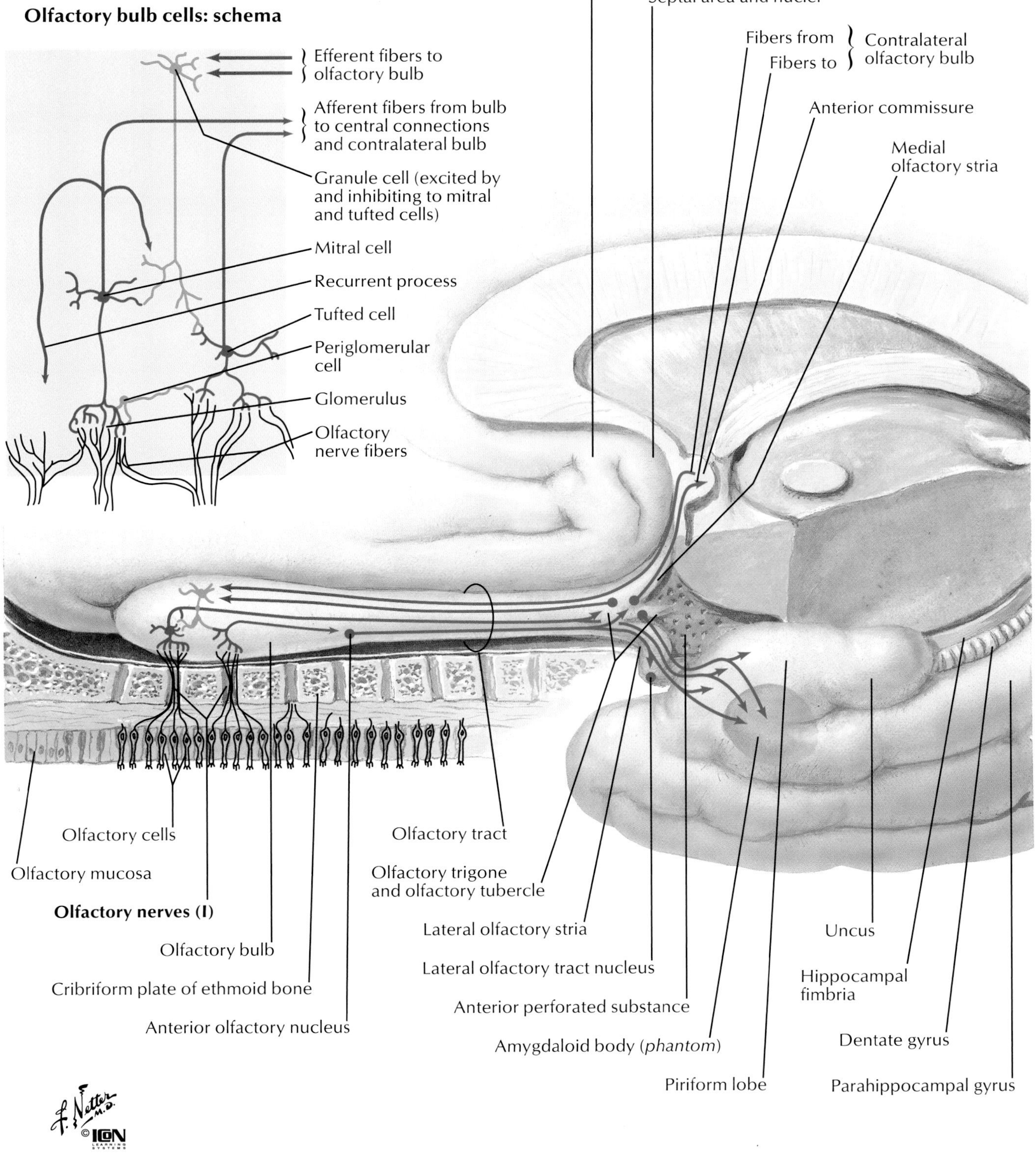

Olfactory bulb cells: schema

Efferent fibers to olfactory bulb

Afferent fibers from bulb to central connections and contralateral bulb

Granule cell (excited by and inhibiting to mitral and tufted cells)

Mitral cell

Recurrent process

Tufted cell

Periglomerular cell

Glomerulus

Olfactory nerve fibers

Subcallosal (parolfactory) area

Septal area and nuclei

Fibers from } Contralateral
Fibers to } olfactory bulb

Anterior commissure

Medial olfactory stria

Olfactory cells

Olfactory mucosa

Olfactory nerves (I)

Olfactory bulb

Cribriform plate of ethmoid bone

Anterior olfactory nucleus

Olfactory tract

Olfactory trigone and olfactory tubercle

Lateral olfactory stria

Lateral olfactory tract nucleus

Anterior perforated substance

Amygdaloid body (*phantom*)

Piriform lobe

Uncus

Hippocampal fimbria

Dentate gyrus

Parahippocampal gyrus

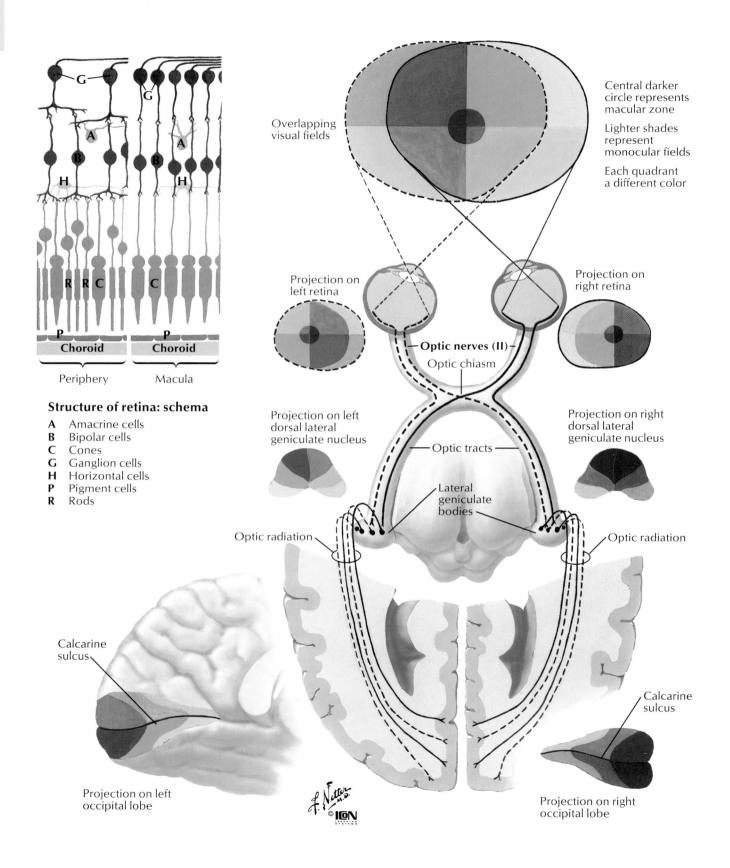

Overlapping visual fields

Central darker circle represents macular zone

Lighter shades represent monocular fields

Each quadrant a different color

R R C

C

Choroid

Choroid

Periphery

Macula

Structure of retina: schema

A Amacrine cells
B Bipolar cells
C Cones
G Ganglion cells
H Horizontal cells
P Pigment cells
R Rods

Projection on left retina

Projection on right retina

Optic nerves (II)

Optic chiasm

Projection on left dorsal lateral geniculate nucleus

Projection on right dorsal lateral geniculate nucleus

Optic tracts

Lateral geniculate bodies

Optic radiation

Optic radiation

Calcarine sulcus

Calcarine sulcus

Projection on left occipital lobe

Projection on right occipital lobe

PLATE 114

HEAD AND NECK

Oculomotor (III), Trochlear (IV) and Abducent (VI) Nerves: Schema

SEE ALSO PLATES 82, 126, 160

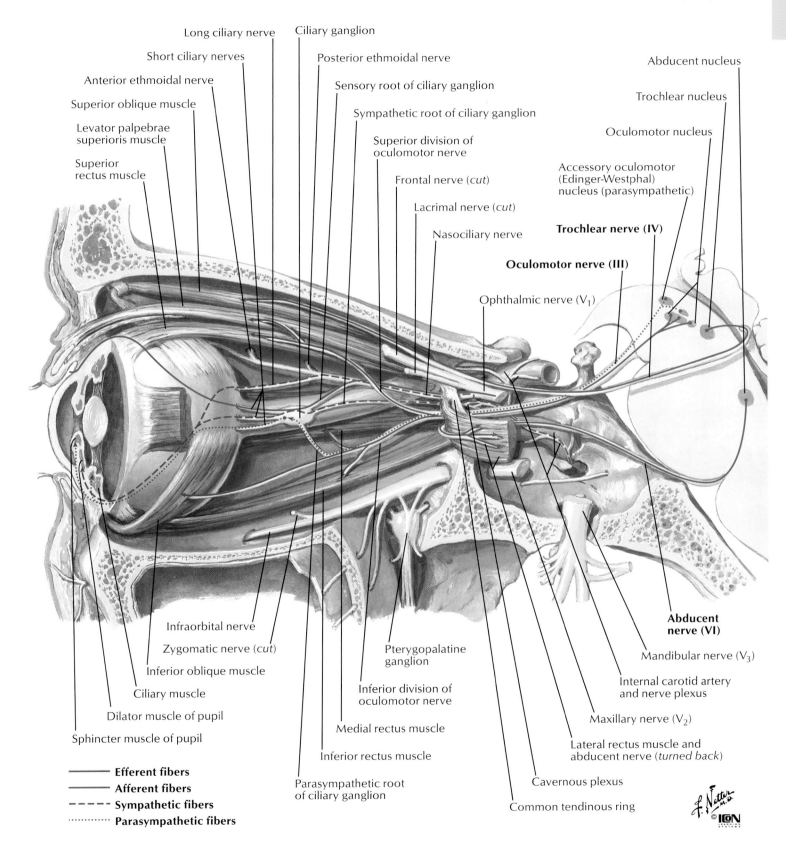

Long ciliary nerve

Short ciliary nerves

Anterior ethmoidal nerve

Superior oblique muscle

Levator palpebrae superioris muscle

Superior rectus muscle

Ciliary ganglion

Posterior ethmoidal nerve

Sensory root of ciliary ganglion

Sympathetic root of ciliary ganglion

Superior division of oculomotor nerve

Frontal nerve (*cut*)

Lacrimal nerve (*cut*)

Nasociliary nerve

Abducent nucleus

Trochlear nucleus

Oculomotor nucleus

Accessory oculomotor (Edinger-Westphal) nucleus (parasympathetic)

Trochlear nerve (IV)

Oculomotor nerve (III)

Ophthalmic nerve (V_1)

Infraorbital nerve

Zygomatic nerve (*cut*)

Inferior oblique muscle

Ciliary muscle

Dilator muscle of pupil

Sphincter muscle of pupil

Pterygopalatine ganglion

Inferior division of oculomotor nerve

Medial rectus muscle

Inferior rectus muscle

Parasympathetic root of ciliary ganglion

Abducent nerve (VI)

Mandibular nerve (V_3)

Internal carotid artery and nerve plexus

Maxillary nerve (V_2)

Lateral rectus muscle and abducent nerve (*turned back*)

Cavernous plexus

Common tendinous ring

——— **Efferent fibers**
——— **Afferent fibers**
- - - **Sympathetic fibers**
········ **Parasympathetic fibers**

f. Netter
M.D.

Trigeminal Nerve (V): Schema

SEE ALSO PLATES 20, 38, 39, 41, 42, 160

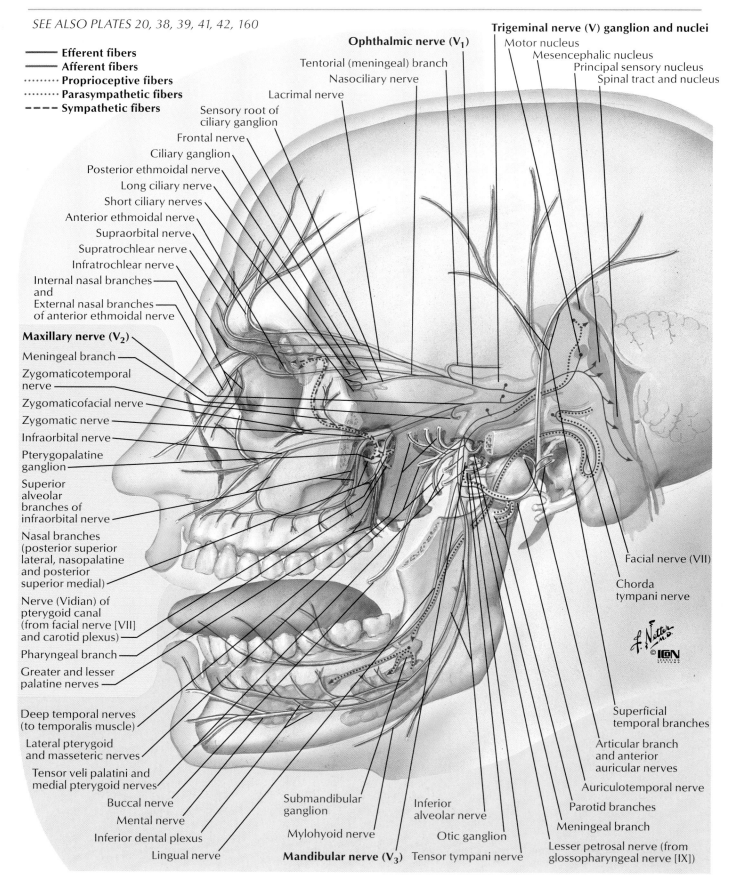

—— Efferent fibers
—— Afferent fibers
·········· Proprioceptive fibers
·········· Parasympathetic fibers
– – – – Sympathetic fibers

Ophthalmic nerve (V₁)
Tentorial (meningeal) branch
Nasociliary nerve
Lacrimal nerve
Sensory root of ciliary ganglion
Frontal nerve
Ciliary ganglion
Posterior ethmoidal nerve
Long ciliary nerve
Short ciliary nerves
Anterior ethmoidal nerve
Supraorbital nerve
Supratrochlear nerve
Infratrochlear nerve
Internal nasal branches and
External nasal branches of anterior ethmoidal nerve

Trigeminal nerve (V) ganglion and nuclei
Motor nucleus
Mesencephalic nucleus
Principal sensory nucleus
Spinal tract and nucleus

Maxillary nerve (V₂)
Meningeal branch
Zygomaticotemporal nerve
Zygomaticofacial nerve
Zygomatic nerve
Infraorbital nerve
Pterygopalatine ganglion
Superior alveolar branches of infraorbital nerve
Nasal branches (posterior superior lateral, nasopalatine and posterior superior medial)
Nerve (Vidian) of pterygoid canal (from facial nerve [VII] and carotid plexus)
Pharyngeal branch
Greater and lesser palatine nerves
Deep temporal nerves (to temporalis muscle)
Lateral pterygoid and masseteric nerves
Tensor veli palatini and medial pterygoid nerves
Buccal nerve
Mental nerve
Inferior dental plexus
Lingual nerve

Facial nerve (VII)
Chorda tympani nerve

Superficial temporal branches
Articular branch and anterior auricular nerves
Auriculotemporal nerve
Parotid branches
Meningeal branch
Lesser petrosal nerve (from glossopharyngeal nerve [IX])

Submandibular ganglion
Mylohyoid nerve
Mandibular nerve (V₃)
Inferior alveolar nerve
Otic ganglion
Tensor tympani nerve

f. Netter M.D.

PLATE 116

HEAD AND NECK

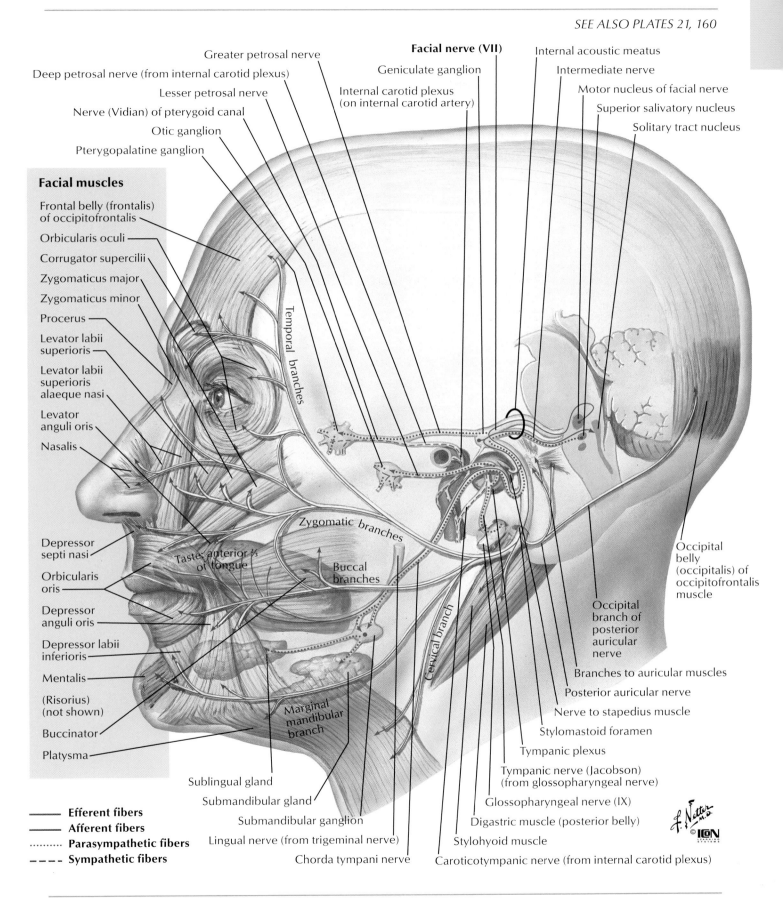

Greater petrosal nerve

Deep petrosal nerve (from internal carotid plexus)

Lesser petrosal nerve

Nerve (Vidian) of pterygoid canal

Otic ganglion

Pterygopalatine ganglion

Facial nerve (VII)

Geniculate ganglion

Internal carotid plexus (on internal carotid artery)

Internal acoustic meatus

Intermediate nerve

Motor nucleus of facial nerve

Superior salivatory nucleus

Solitary tract nucleus

Facial muscles

Frontal belly (frontalis) of occipitofrontalis

Orbicularis oculi

Corrugator supercilii

Zygomaticus major

Zygomaticus minor

Procerus

Levator labii superioris

Levator labii superioris alaeque nasi

Levator anguli oris

Nasalis

Depressor septi nasi

Orbicularis oris

Depressor anguli oris

Depressor labii inferioris

Mentalis

(Risorius) (not shown)

Buccinator

Platysma

Temporal branches

Zygomatic branches

Taste: anterior ⅔ of tongue

Buccal branches

Marginal mandibular branch

Cervical branch

Sublingual gland

Submandibular gland

Submandibular ganglion

Lingual nerve (from trigeminal nerve)

Chorda tympani nerve

Occipital belly (occipitalis) of occipitofrontalis muscle

Occipital branch of posterior auricular nerve

Branches to auricular muscles

Posterior auricular nerve

Nerve to stapedius muscle

Stylomastoid foramen

Tympanic plexus

Tympanic nerve (Jacobson) (from glossopharyngeal nerve)

Glossopharyngeal nerve (IX)

Digastric muscle (posterior belly)

Stylohyoid muscle

Caroticotympanic nerve (from internal carotid plexus)

——— **Efferent fibers**

——— **Afferent fibers**

·········· **Parasympathetic fibers**

‑ ‑ ‑ ‑ **Sympathetic fibers**

F. Netter M.D.
© ICN LEARNING SYSTEMS

Vestibulocochlear Nerve (VIII): Schema

Afferent fibers

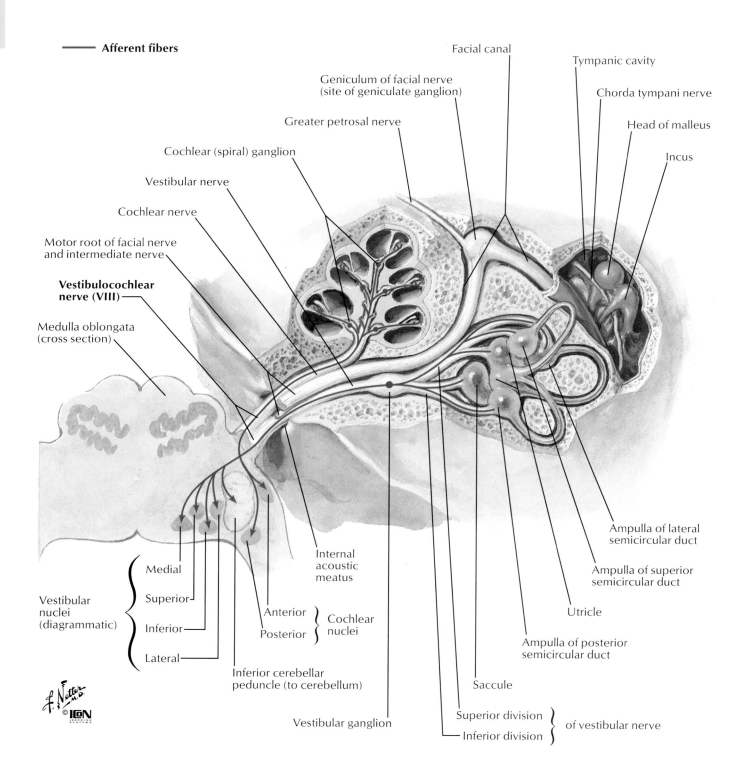

Facial canal

Geniculum of facial nerve
(site of geniculate ganglion)

Greater petrosal nerve

Tympanic cavity

Chorda tympani nerve

Head of malleus

Incus

Cochlear (spiral) ganglion

Vestibular nerve

Cochlear nerve

Motor root of facial nerve
and intermediate nerve

**Vestibulocochlear
nerve (VIII)**

Medulla oblongata
(cross section)

Internal
acoustic
meatus

Medial

Superior

Inferior

Lateral

Vestibular
nuclei
(diagrammatic)

Anterior

Posterior

Cochlear
nuclei

Inferior cerebellar
peduncle (to cerebellum)

Vestibular ganglion

Saccule

Superior division

Inferior division

of vestibular nerve

Ampulla of lateral
semicircular duct

Ampulla of superior
semicircular duct

Utricle

Ampulla of posterior
semicircular duct

PLATE 118

HEAD AND NECK

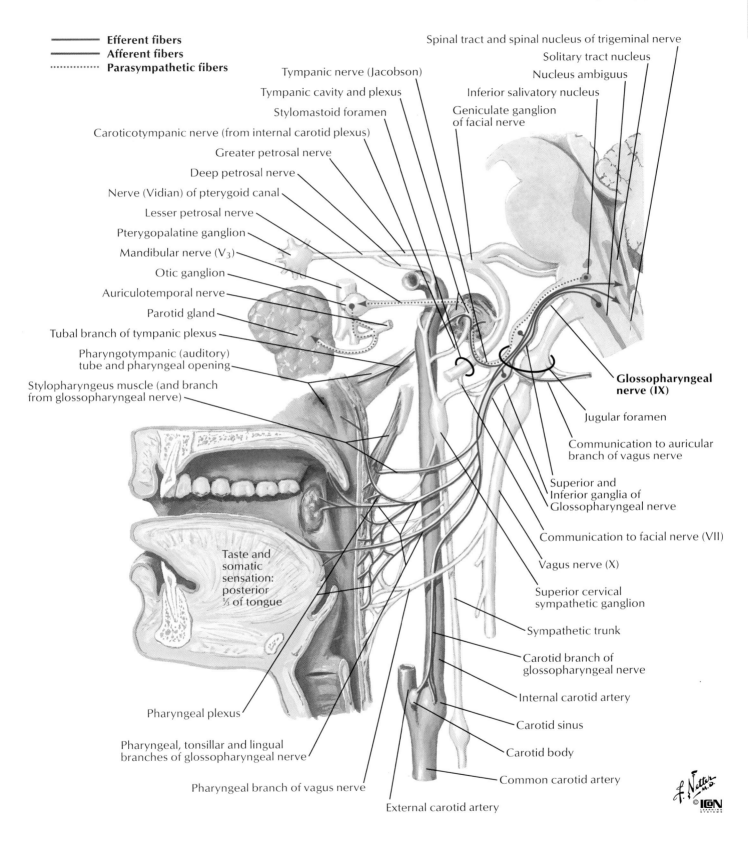

Efferent fibers
Afferent fibers
Parasympathetic fibers

Spinal tract and spinal nucleus of trigeminal nerve

Solitary tract nucleus

Tympanic nerve (Jacobson)

Nucleus ambiguus

Tympanic cavity and plexus

Inferior salivatory nucleus

Stylomastoid foramen

Geniculate ganglion of facial nerve

Caroticotympanic nerve (from internal carotid plexus)

Greater petrosal nerve

Deep petrosal nerve

Nerve (Vidian) of pterygoid canal

Lesser petrosal nerve

Pterygopalatine ganglion

Mandibular nerve (V₃)

Otic ganglion

Auriculotemporal nerve

Parotid gland

Tubal branch of tympanic plexus

Pharyngotympanic (auditory) tube and pharyngeal opening

Stylopharyngeus muscle (and branch from glossopharyngeal nerve)

Glossopharyngeal nerve (IX)

Jugular foramen

Communication to auricular branch of vagus nerve

Superior and Inferior ganglia of Glossopharyngeal nerve

Communication to facial nerve (VII)

Vagus nerve (X)

Superior cervical sympathetic ganglion

Taste and somatic sensation: posterior ⅓ of tongue

Sympathetic trunk

Carotid branch of glossopharyngeal nerve

Internal carotid artery

Carotid sinus

Pharyngeal plexus

Carotid body

Pharyngeal, tonsillar and lingual branches of glossopharyngeal nerve

Common carotid artery

Pharyngeal branch of vagus nerve

External carotid artery

Vagus Nerve (X): Schema

SEE ALSO PLATE 160

Glossopharyngeal nerve (IX)

Meningeal branch of vagus nerve

Auricular branch of vagus nerve

Pharyngotympanic (auditory) tube

Levator veli palatini muscle

Salpingopharyngeus muscle

Palatoglossus muscle

Palatopharyngeus muscle

Superior pharyngeal constrictor muscle

Stylopharyngeus muscle

Middle pharyngeal constrictor muscle

Inferior pharyngeal constrictor muscle

Cricothyroid muscle

Trachea

Esophagus

Right subclavian artery

Right recurrent laryngeal nerve

Heart

Hepatic branch of anterior vagal trunk (in lesser omentum)

Celiac branches from anterior and posterior vagal trunks to celiac plexus

Celiac and superior mesenteric ganglia and celiac plexus

Hepatic plexus

Gallbladder and bile ducts

Liver

Pyloric branch from hepatic plexus

Pancreas

Duodenum

Ascending colon

Cecum

Appendix

Posterior nucleus of vagus nerve (parasympathetic and visceral afferent)

Solitary tract nucleus (visceral afferents including taste)

Spinal tract and spinal nucleus of trigeminal nerve (somatic afferent)

Nucleus ambiguus (motor to pharyngeal and laryngeal muscles)

Cranial root of accessory nerve* (see next plate)

Vagus nerve (X)

Jugular foramen

Superior ganglion of vagus nerve

Inferior ganglion of vagus nerve

Pharyngeal branch of vagus nerve (motor to muscles of palate and lower pharynx; sensory to lower pharynx)

Communicating branch of vagus nerve to carotid branch of glossopharyngeal nerve

Pharyngeal plexus

Superior laryngeal nerve:
Internal branch (sensory and parasympathetic)
External branch (motor to cricothyroid muscle)

Superior cervical cardiac branch of vagus nerve

Inferior cervical cardiac branch of vagus nerve

Thoracic cardiac branch of vagus nerve

Left recurrent laryngeal nerve (motor to muscles of larynx except cricothyroid; sensory and parasympathetic to larynx below vocal folds; parasympathetic, efferent and afferent to upper esophagus and trachea)

Pulmonary plexus

Cardiac plexus

Esophageal plexus

Anterior vagal trunk

Gastric branches of anterior vagal trunk (branches from posterior trunk behind stomach)

Vagal branches (parasympathetic motor, secretomotor and afferent fibers) accompany superior mesenteric artery and its branches usually as far as left colic (splenic) flexure

Small intestine

Efferent fibers
Afferent fibers
Parasympathetic fibers

PLATE 120

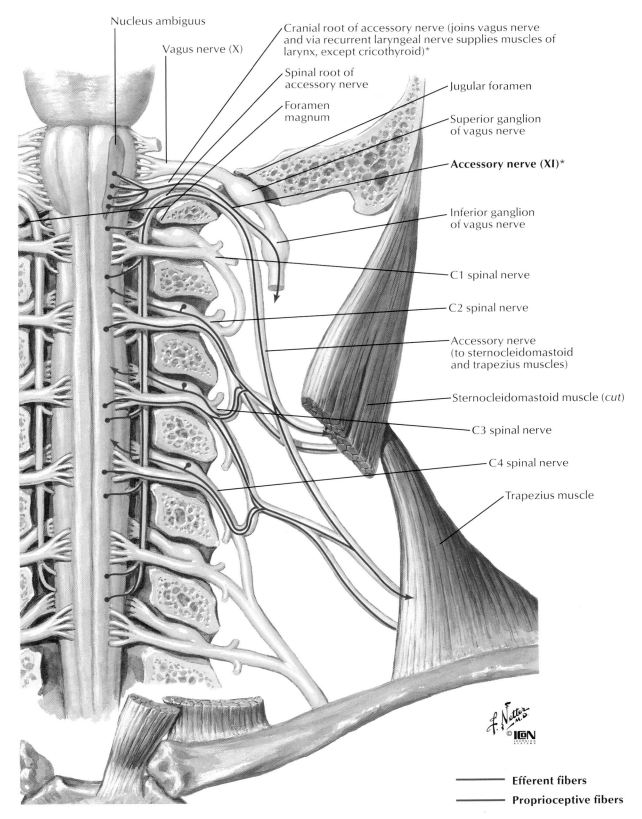

Nucleus ambiguus

Vagus nerve (X)

Cranial root of accessory nerve (joins vagus nerve and via recurrent laryngeal nerve supplies muscles of larynx, except cricothyroid)*

Spinal root of accessory nerve

Foramen magnum

Jugular foramen

Superior ganglion of vagus nerve

Accessory nerve (XI)*

Inferior ganglion of vagus nerve

C1 spinal nerve

C2 spinal nerve

Accessory nerve (to sternocleidomastoid and trapezius muscles)

Sternocleidomastoid muscle (*cut*)

C3 spinal nerve

C4 spinal nerve

Trapezius muscle

—— Efferent fibers
—— Proprioceptive fibers

*Recent evidence suggests that the accessory nerve lacks a cranial root and has no connection to the vagus nerve. Verification of this finding awaits further investigation.

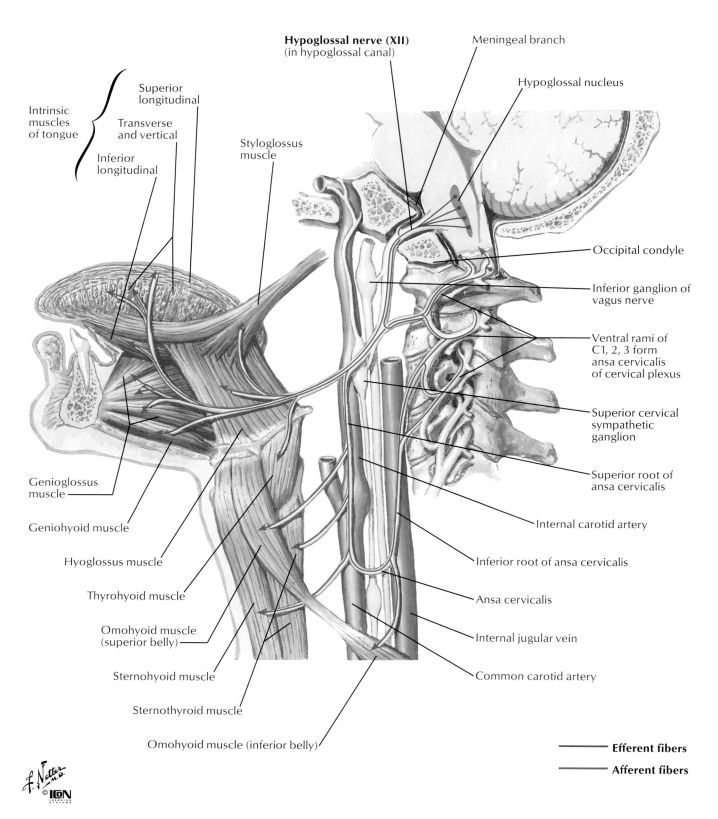

Hypoglossal nerve (XII)
(in hypoglossal canal)

Meningeal branch

Hypoglossal nucleus

Intrinsic muscles of tongue

Superior longitudinal

Transverse and vertical

Inferior longitudinal

Styloglossus muscle

Occipital condyle

Inferior ganglion of vagus nerve

Ventral rami of C1, 2, 3 form ansa cervicalis of cervical plexus

Superior cervical sympathetic ganglion

Superior root of ansa cervicalis

Internal carotid artery

Inferior root of ansa cervicalis

Ansa cervicalis

Internal jugular vein

Common carotid artery

Genioglossus muscle

Geniohyoid muscle

Hyoglossus muscle

Thyrohyoid muscle

Omohyoid muscle (superior belly)

Sternohyoid muscle

Sternothyroid muscle

Omohyoid muscle (inferior belly)

——— **Efferent fibers**
——— **Afferent fibers**

PLATE 122

HEAD AND NECK

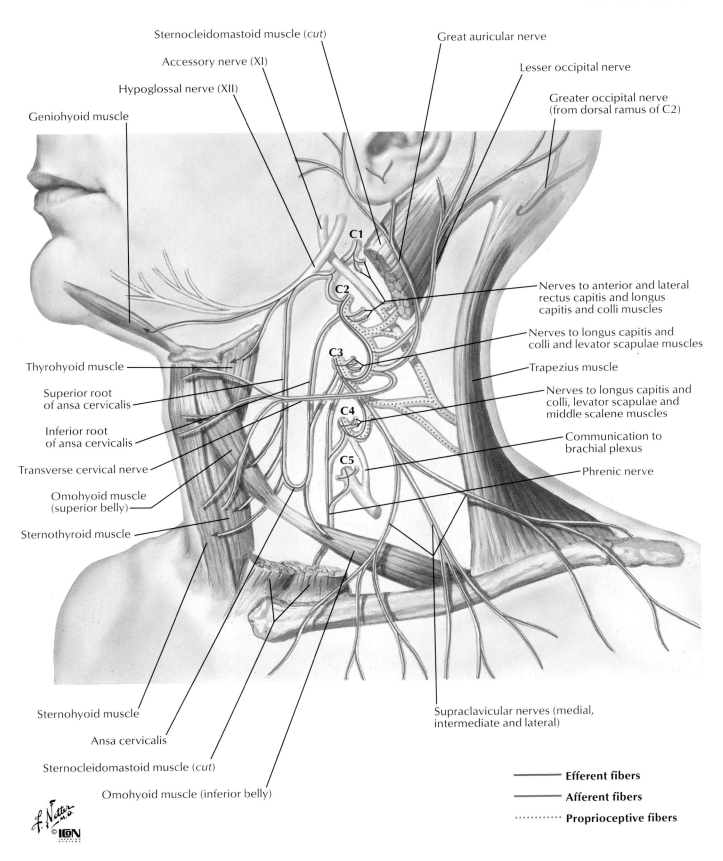

Sternocleidomastoid muscle (*cut*)

Accessory nerve (XI)

Hypoglossal nerve (XII)

Geniohyoid muscle

Great auricular nerve

Lesser occipital nerve

Greater occipital nerve
(from dorsal ramus of C2)

C1

C2

Nerves to anterior and lateral
rectus capitis and longus
capitis and colli muscles

Nerves to longus capitis and
colli and levator scapulae muscles

C3

Thyrohyoid muscle

Trapezius muscle

Superior root
of ansa cervicalis

Nerves to longus capitis and
colli, levator scapulae and
middle scalene muscles

C4

Inferior root
of ansa cervicalis

Communication to
brachial plexus

Transverse cervical nerve

C5

Phrenic nerve

Omohyoid muscle
(superior belly)

Sternothyroid muscle

Sternohyoid muscle

Supraclavicular nerves (medial,
intermediate and lateral)

Ansa cervicalis

Sternocleidomastoid muscle (*cut*)

Omohyoid muscle (inferior belly)

—— **Efferent fibers**

—— **Afferent fibers**

·········· **Proprioceptive fibers**

SEE ALSO PLATES 67, 119, 120, 159, 205, 222, 236, 308

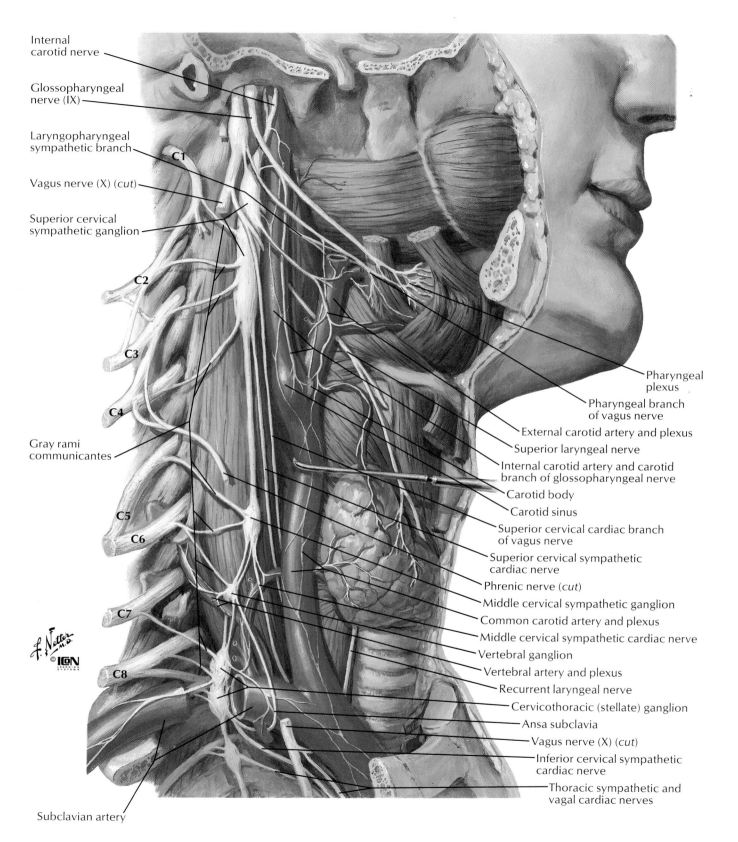

Internal
carotid nerve

Glossopharyngeal
nerve (IX)

Laryngopharyngeal
sympathetic branch

Vagus nerve (X) (*cut*)

Superior cervical
sympathetic ganglion

C1

C2

C3

C4

Gray rami
communicantes

C5

C6

C7

C8

Subclavian artery

Pharyngeal
plexus

Pharyngeal branch
of vagus nerve

External carotid artery and plexus

Superior laryngeal nerve

Internal carotid artery and carotid
branch of glossopharyngeal nerve

Carotid body

Carotid sinus

Superior cervical cardiac branch
of vagus nerve

Superior cervical sympathetic
cardiac nerve

Phrenic nerve (*cut*)

Middle cervical sympathetic ganglion

Common carotid artery and plexus

Middle cervical sympathetic cardiac nerve

Vertebral ganglion

Vertebral artery and plexus

Recurrent laryngeal nerve

Cervicothoracic (stellate) ganglion

Ansa subclavia

Vagus nerve (X) (*cut*)

Inferior cervical sympathetic
cardiac nerve

Thoracic sympathetic and
vagal cardiac nerves

PLATE 124

HEAD AND NECK

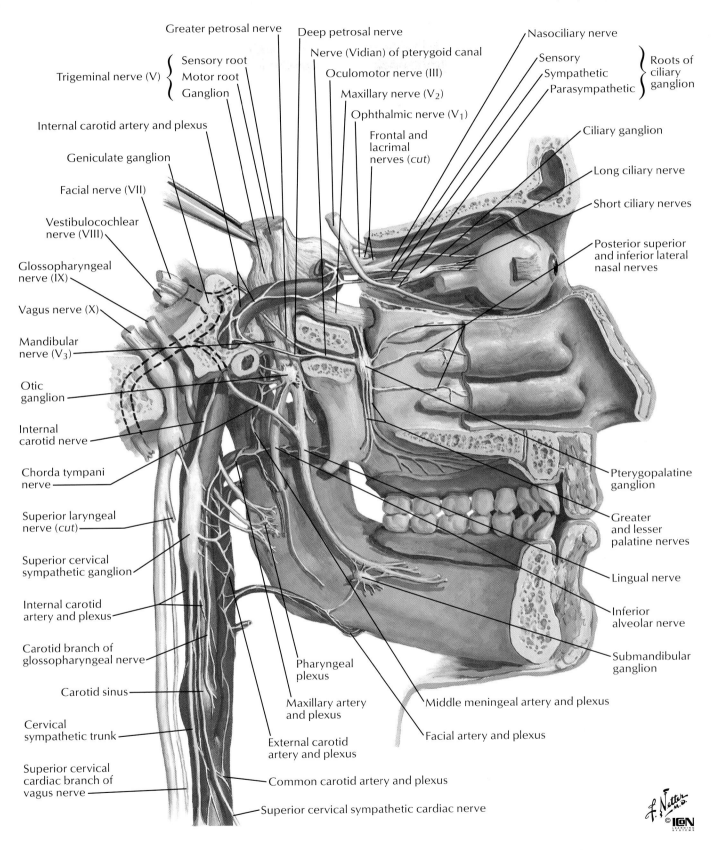

Greater petrosal nerve

Deep petrosal nerve

Nasociliary nerve

Nerve (Vidian) of pterygoid canal

Trigeminal nerve (V) { Sensory root / Motor root / Ganglion

Sensory
Sympathetic
Parasympathetic } Roots of ciliary ganglion

Oculomotor nerve (III)

Internal carotid artery and plexus

Maxillary nerve (V₂)

Ciliary ganglion

Geniculate ganglion

Ophthalmic nerve (V₁)

Long ciliary nerve

Facial nerve (VII)

Frontal and lacrimal nerves (*cut*)

Short ciliary nerves

Vestibulocochlear nerve (VIII)

Posterior superior and inferior lateral nasal nerves

Glossopharyngeal nerve (IX)

Vagus nerve (X)

Mandibular nerve (V₃)

Otic ganglion

Internal carotid nerve

Pterygopalatine ganglion

Chorda tympani nerve

Superior laryngeal nerve (*cut*)

Superior cervical sympathetic ganglion

Greater and lesser palatine nerves

Internal carotid artery and plexus

Lingual nerve

Carotid branch of glossopharyngeal nerve

Inferior alveolar nerve

Carotid sinus

Submandibular ganglion

Cervical sympathetic trunk

Pharyngeal plexus

Middle meningeal artery and plexus

Maxillary artery and plexus

Superior cervical cardiac branch of vagus nerve

External carotid artery and plexus

Facial artery and plexus

Common carotid artery and plexus

Superior cervical sympathetic cardiac nerve

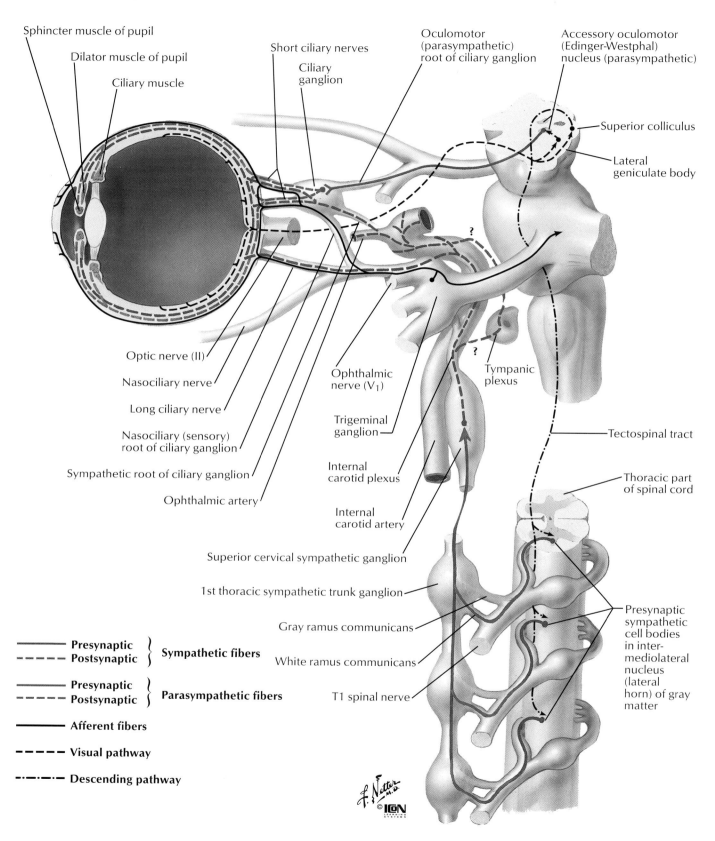

Sphincter muscle of pupil

Dilator muscle of pupil

Ciliary muscle

Short ciliary nerves

Ciliary ganglion

Oculomotor (parasympathetic) root of ciliary ganglion

Accessory oculomotor (Edinger-Westphal) nucleus (parasympathetic)

Superior colliculus

Lateral geniculate body

Optic nerve (II)

Nasociliary nerve

Long ciliary nerve

Nasociliary (sensory) root of ciliary ganglion

Sympathetic root of ciliary ganglion

Ophthalmic artery

Ophthalmic nerve (V₁)

Trigeminal ganglion

Internal carotid plexus

Internal carotid artery

Tympanic plexus

Tectospinal tract

Thoracic part of spinal cord

Superior cervical sympathetic ganglion

1st thoracic sympathetic trunk ganglion

Gray ramus communicans

White ramus communicans

T1 spinal nerve

Presynaptic sympathetic cell bodies in inter-mediolateral nucleus (lateral horn) of gray matter

—————— **Presynaptic**	} **Sympathetic fibers**
- - - - - **Postsynaptic**	
—————— **Presynaptic**	} **Parasympathetic fibers**
- - - - - **Postsynaptic**	
—————— **Afferent fibers**	
- - - - - **Visual pathway**	
-··-··- **Descending pathway**	

PLATE 126

HEAD AND NECK

Pterygopalatine and Submandibular Ganglia: Schema

Ophthalmic nerve (V$_1$)

Mandibular nerve (V$_3$)

Otic ganglion

Lingual nerve

Maxillary nerve (V$_2$)

Nerve (Vidian) of pterygoid canal

Pterygopalatine ganglion

Lacrimal gland

Trigeminal ganglion

Deep petrosal nerve

Greater petrosal nerve

Chorda tympani nerve

Trigeminal nerve (V)

Facial nerve (VII) (intermediate nerve)

Superior salivatory nucleus

Descending palatine nerves

Posterior nasal nerves

Pharyngeal nerve

Maxillary artery

Internal carotid nerve

Glossopharyngeal nerve (IX)

Superior cervical sympathetic ganglion

Palatine nerves { Greater Lesser

Sympathetic trunk

T1 and T2 spinal nerves

Submandibular ganglion

Thoracic spinal cord

Dorsal root

Sublingual gland

Submandibular gland

Facial artery

Lingual artery

External carotid artery and plexus

Common carotid artery

White   Gray

Rami communicantes

Internal carotid artery

Ventral root

Sympathetic presynaptic cell bodies in intermediolateral nucleus (lateral horn) of gray matter

——— Sympathetic presynaptic fibers

– – – Sympathetic postsynaptic fibers

——— Parasympathetic presynaptic fibers

– – – Parasympathetic postsynaptic fibers

Otic Ganglion: Schema

SEE ALSO PLATE 160

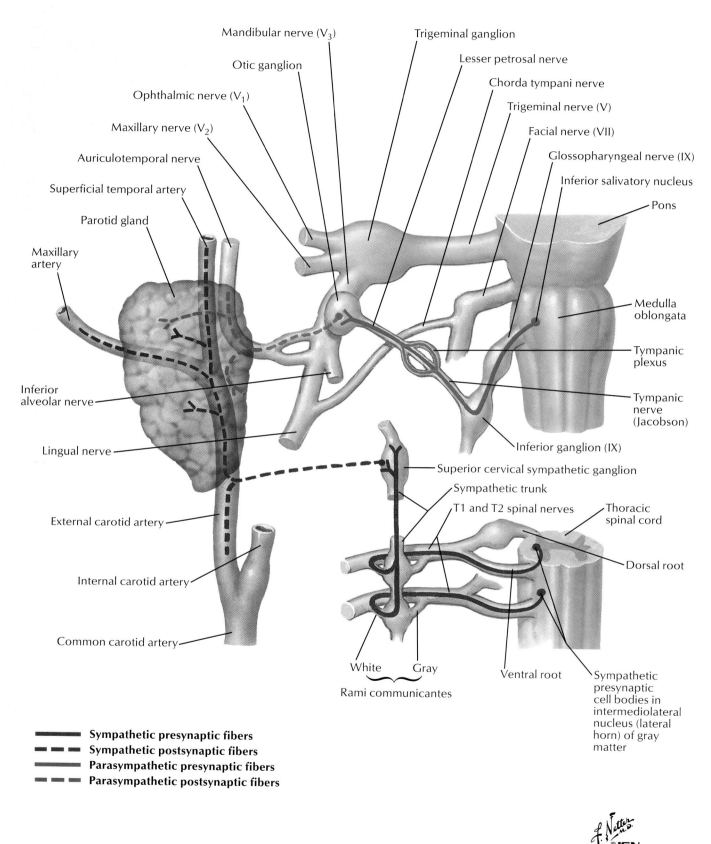

Mandibular nerve (V₃)

Otic ganglion

Ophthalmic nerve (V₁)

Maxillary nerve (V₂)

Auriculotemporal nerve

Superficial temporal artery

Parotid gland

Maxillary artery

Inferior alveolar nerve

Lingual nerve

External carotid artery

Internal carotid artery

Common carotid artery

Trigeminal ganglion

Lesser petrosal nerve

Chorda tympani nerve

Trigeminal nerve (V)

Facial nerve (VII)

Glossopharyngeal nerve (IX)

Inferior salivatory nucleus

Pons

Medulla oblongata

Tympanic plexus

Tympanic nerve (Jacobson)

Inferior ganglion (IX)

Superior cervical sympathetic ganglion

Sympathetic trunk

T1 and T2 spinal nerves

Thoracic spinal cord

Dorsal root

Ventral root

Sympathetic presynaptic cell bodies in intermediolateral nucleus (lateral horn) of gray matter

White   Gray

Rami communicantes

━━━━━ Sympathetic presynaptic fibers
━ ━ ━ Sympathetic postsynaptic fibers
━━━━━ Parasympathetic presynaptic fibers
━ ━ ━ Parasympathetic postsynaptic fibers

PLATE 128

HEAD AND NECK

——————— **Usual pathway**

- - - - - - - **Accessory pathway**

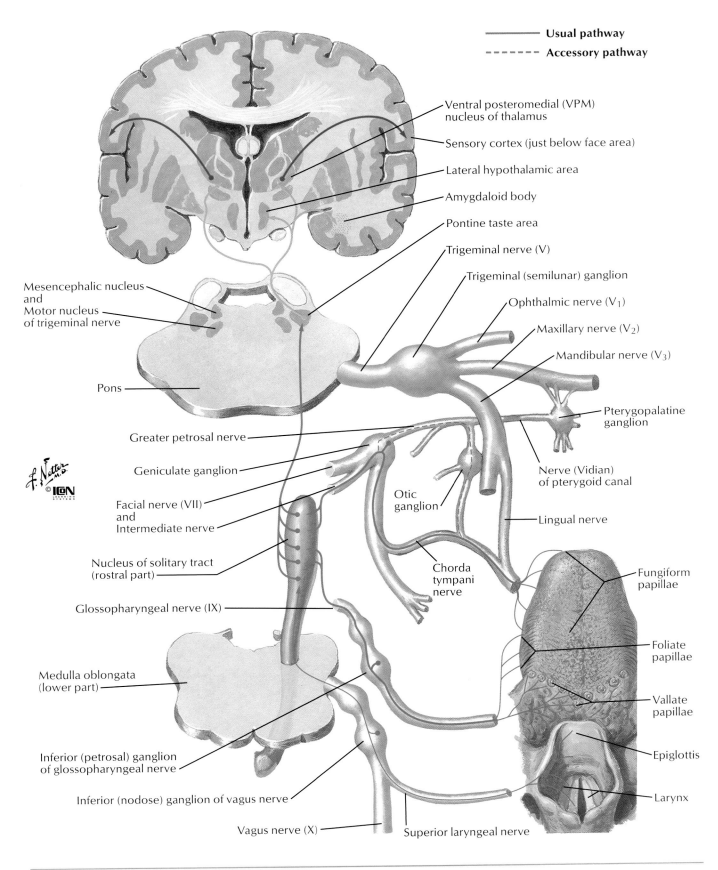

Ventral posteromedial (VPM) nucleus of thalamus

Sensory cortex (just below face area)

Lateral hypothalamic area

Amygdaloid body

Pontine taste area

Trigeminal nerve (V)

Trigeminal (semilunar) ganglion

Ophthalmic nerve (V₁)

Maxillary nerve (V₂)

Mandibular nerve (V₃)

Pterygopalatine ganglion

Nerve (Vidian) of pterygoid canal

Lingual nerve

Fungiform papillae

Foliate papillae

Vallate papillae

Epiglottis

Larynx

Mesencephalic nucleus and Motor nucleus of trigeminal nerve

Pons

Greater petrosal nerve

Geniculate ganglion

Facial nerve (VII) and Intermediate nerve

Nucleus of solitary tract (rostral part)

Glossopharyngeal nerve (IX)

Medulla oblongata (lower part)

Inferior (petrosal) ganglion of glossopharyngeal nerve

Inferior (nodose) ganglion of vagus nerve

Vagus nerve (X)

Superior laryngeal nerve

Otic ganglion

Chorda tympani nerve

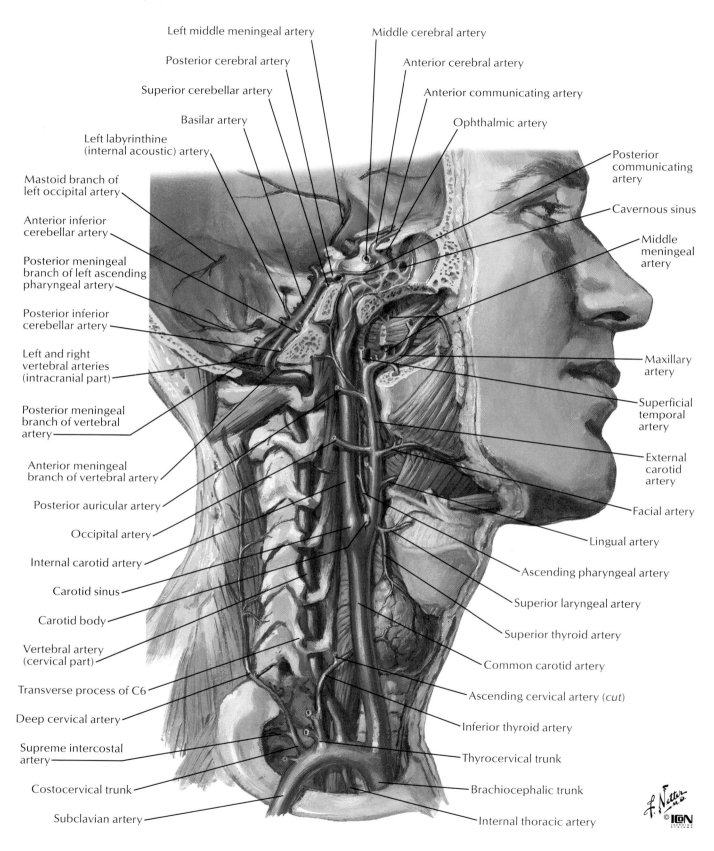

Left middle meningeal artery

Middle cerebral artery

Posterior cerebral artery

Anterior cerebral artery

Superior cerebellar artery

Anterior communicating artery

Basilar artery

Ophthalmic artery

Left labyrinthine (internal acoustic) artery

Posterior communicating artery

Mastoid branch of left occipital artery

Cavernous sinus

Anterior inferior cerebellar artery

Middle meningeal artery

Posterior meningeal branch of left ascending pharyngeal artery

Posterior inferior cerebellar artery

Left and right vertebral arteries (intracranial part)

Maxillary artery

Posterior meningeal branch of vertebral artery

Superficial temporal artery

Anterior meningeal branch of vertebral artery

External carotid artery

Posterior auricular artery

Facial artery

Occipital artery

Lingual artery

Internal carotid artery

Ascending pharyngeal artery

Carotid sinus

Superior laryngeal artery

Carotid body

Superior thyroid artery

Vertebral artery (cervical part)

Common carotid artery

Transverse process of C6

Ascending cervical artery (cut)

Deep cervical artery

Inferior thyroid artery

Supreme intercostal artery

Thyrocervical trunk

Costocervical trunk

Brachiocephalic trunk

Subclavian artery

Internal thoracic artery

PLATE 130

HEAD AND NECK

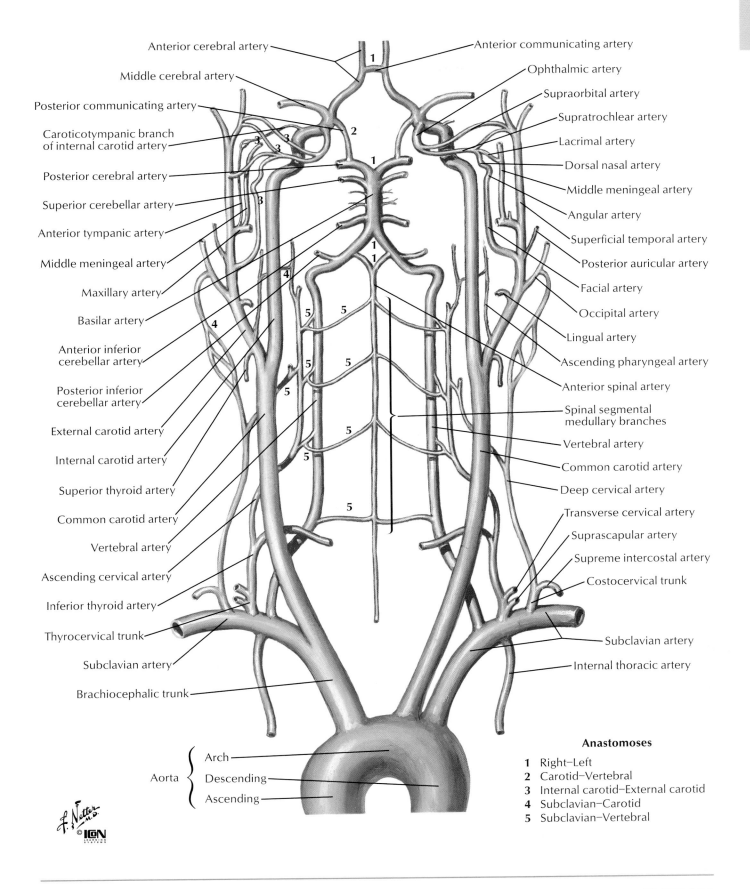

Anterior cerebral artery

Middle cerebral artery

Posterior communicating artery

Caroticotympanic branch of internal carotid artery

Posterior cerebral artery

Superior cerebellar artery

Anterior tympanic artery

Middle meningeal artery

Maxillary artery

Basilar artery

Anterior inferior cerebellar artery

Posterior inferior cerebellar artery

External carotid artery

Internal carotid artery

Superior thyroid artery

Common carotid artery

Vertebral artery

Ascending cervical artery

Inferior thyroid artery

Thyrocervical trunk

Subclavian artery

Brachiocephalic trunk

Anterior communicating artery

Ophthalmic artery

Supraorbital artery

Supratrochlear artery

Lacrimal artery

Dorsal nasal artery

Middle meningeal artery

Angular artery

Superficial temporal artery

Posterior auricular artery

Facial artery

Occipital artery

Lingual artery

Ascending pharyngeal artery

Anterior spinal artery

Spinal segmental medullary branches

Vertebral artery

Common carotid artery

Deep cervical artery

Transverse cervical artery

Suprascapular artery

Supreme intercostal artery

Costocervical trunk

Subclavian artery

Internal thoracic artery

Aorta { Arch / Descending / Ascending

Anastomoses

1 Right–Left
2 Carotid–Vertebral
3 Internal carotid–External carotid
4 Subclavian–Carotid
5 Subclavian–Vertebral

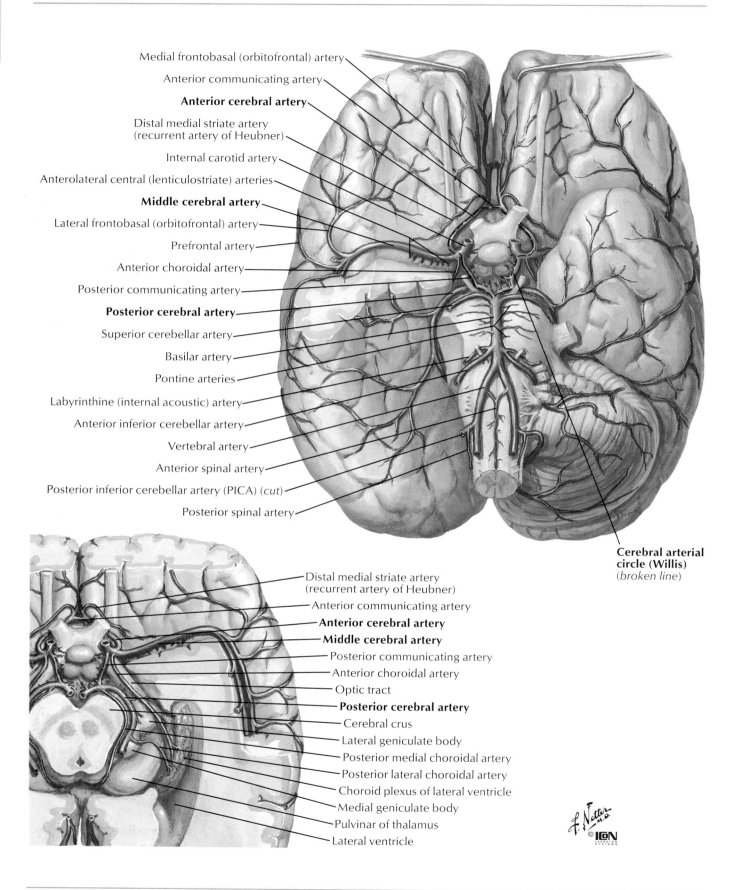

Medial frontobasal (orbitofrontal) artery

Anterior communicating artery

Anterior cerebral artery

Distal medial striate artery
(recurrent artery of Heubner)

Internal carotid artery

Anterolateral central (lenticulostriate) arteries

Middle cerebral artery

Lateral frontobasal (orbitofrontal) artery

Prefrontal artery

Anterior choroidal artery

Posterior communicating artery

Posterior cerebral artery

Superior cerebellar artery

Basilar artery

Pontine arteries

Labyrinthine (internal acoustic) artery

Anterior inferior cerebellar artery

Vertebral artery

Anterior spinal artery

Posterior inferior cerebellar artery (PICA) (*cut*)

Posterior spinal artery

**Cerebral arterial
circle (Willis)**
(*broken line*)

Distal medial striate artery
(recurrent artery of Heubner)

Anterior communicating artery

Anterior cerebral artery

Middle cerebral artery

Posterior communicating artery

Anterior choroidal artery

Optic tract

Posterior cerebral artery

Cerebral crus

Lateral geniculate body

Posterior medial choroidal artery

Posterior lateral choroidal artery

Choroid plexus of lateral ventricle

Medial geniculate body

Pulvinar of thalamus

Lateral ventricle

PLATE 132

HEAD AND NECK

Vessels dissected out: inferior view

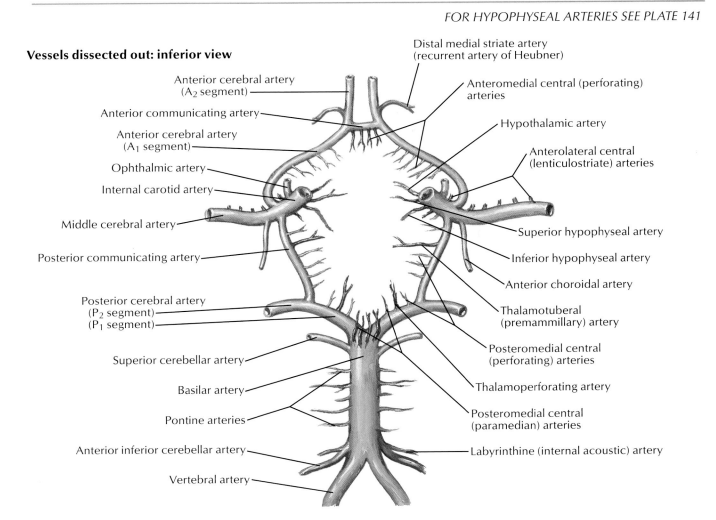

- Anterior cerebral artery (A_2 segment)
- Anterior communicating artery
- Anterior cerebral artery (A_1 segment)
- Ophthalmic artery
- Internal carotid artery
- Middle cerebral artery
- Posterior communicating artery
- Posterior cerebral artery (P_2 segment) (P_1 segment)
- Superior cerebellar artery
- Basilar artery
- Pontine arteries
- Anterior inferior cerebellar artery
- Vertebral artery

- Distal medial striate artery (recurrent artery of Heubner)
- Anteromedial central (perforating) arteries
- Hypothalamic artery
- Anterolateral central (lenticulostriate) arteries
- Superior hypophyseal artery
- Inferior hypophyseal artery
- Anterior choroidal artery
- Thalamotuberal (premammillary) artery
- Posteromedial central (perforating) arteries
- Thalamoperforating artery
- Posteromedial central (paramedian) arteries
- Labyrinthine (internal acoustic) artery

Vessels in situ: inferior view

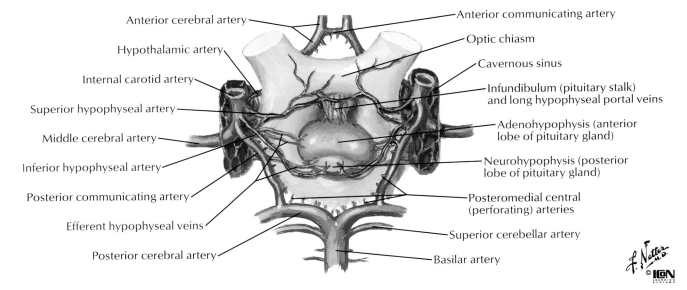

- Anterior cerebral artery
- Hypothalamic artery
- Internal carotid artery
- Superior hypophyseal artery
- Middle cerebral artery
- Inferior hypophyseal artery
- Posterior communicating artery
- Efferent hypophyseal veins
- Posterior cerebral artery

- Anterior communicating artery
- Optic chiasm
- Cavernous sinus
- Infundibulum (pituitary stalk) and long hypophyseal portal veins
- Adenohypophysis (anterior lobe of pituitary gland)
- Neurohypophysis (posterior lobe of pituitary gland)
- Posteromedial central (perforating) arteries
- Superior cerebellar artery
- Basilar artery

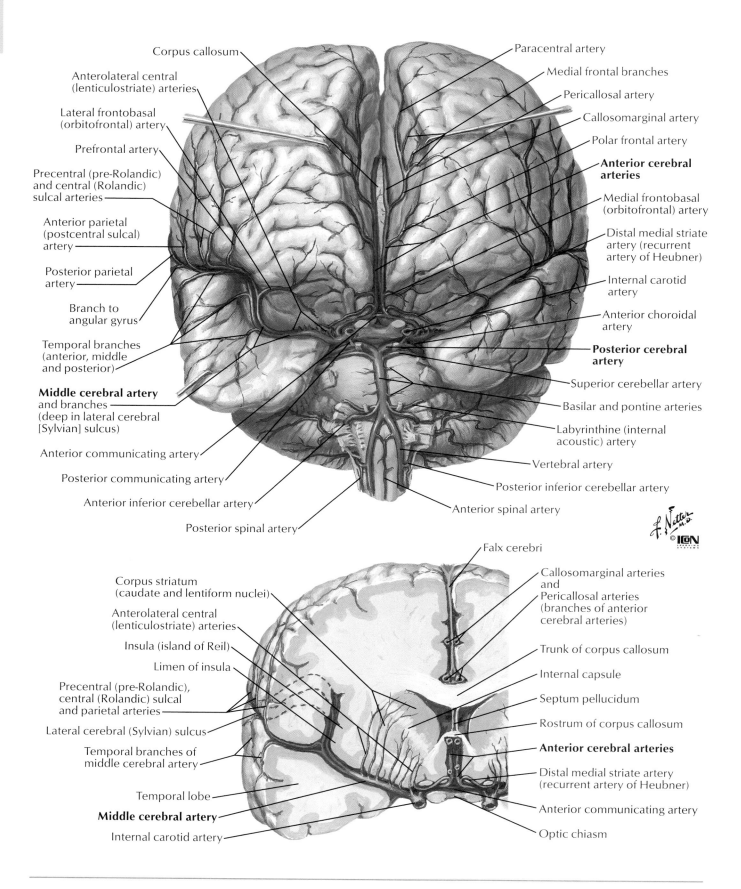

Corpus callosum

Anterolateral central (lenticulostriate) arteries

Lateral frontobasal (orbitofrontal) artery

Prefrontal artery

Precentral (pre-Rolandic) and central (Rolandic) sulcal arteries

Anterior parietal (postcentral sulcal) artery

Posterior parietal artery

Branch to angular gyrus

Temporal branches (anterior, middle and posterior)

Middle cerebral artery and branches (deep in lateral cerebral [Sylvian] sulcus)

Anterior communicating artery

Posterior communicating artery

Anterior inferior cerebellar artery

Posterior spinal artery

Paracentral artery

Medial frontal branches

Pericallosal artery

Callosomarginal artery

Polar frontal artery

Anterior cerebral arteries

Medial frontobasal (orbitofrontal) artery

Distal medial striate artery (recurrent artery of Heubner)

Internal carotid artery

Anterior choroidal artery

Posterior cerebral artery

Superior cerebellar artery

Basilar and pontine arteries

Labyrinthine (internal acoustic) artery

Vertebral artery

Posterior inferior cerebellar artery

Anterior spinal artery

Corpus striatum (caudate and lentiform nuclei)

Anterolateral central (lenticulostriate) arteries

Insula (island of Reil)

Limen of insula

Precentral (pre-Rolandic), central (Rolandic) sulcal and parietal arteries

Lateral cerebral (Sylvian) sulcus

Temporal branches of middle cerebral artery

Temporal lobe

Middle cerebral artery

Internal carotid artery

Falx cerebri

Callosomarginal arteries and Pericallosal arteries (branches of anterior cerebral arteries)

Trunk of corpus callosum

Internal capsule

Septum pellucidum

Rostrum of corpus callosum

Anterior cerebral arteries

Distal medial striate artery (recurrent artery of Heubner)

Anterior communicating artery

Optic chiasm

PLATE 134

HEAD AND NECK

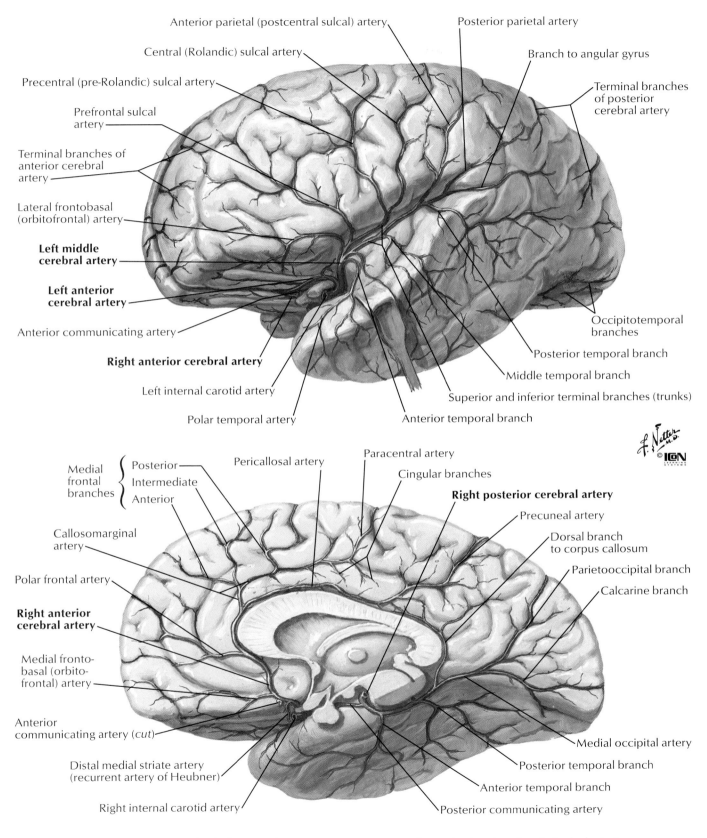

Anterior parietal (postcentral sulcal) artery

Central (Rolandic) sulcal artery

Precentral (pre-Rolandic) sulcal artery

Prefrontal sulcal artery

Terminal branches of anterior cerebral artery

Lateral frontobasal (orbitofrontal) artery

Left middle cerebral artery

Left anterior cerebral artery

Anterior communicating artery

Right anterior cerebral artery

Left internal carotid artery

Polar temporal artery

Posterior parietal artery

Branch to angular gyrus

Terminal branches of posterior cerebral artery

Occipitotemporal branches

Posterior temporal branch

Middle temporal branch

Superior and inferior terminal branches (trunks)

Anterior temporal branch

Medial frontal branches { Posterior, Intermediate, Anterior

Pericallosal artery

Paracentral artery

Cingular branches

Right posterior cerebral artery

Precuneal artery

Callosomarginal artery

Polar frontal artery

Right anterior cerebral artery

Medial fronto-basal (orbito-frontal) artery

Anterior communicating artery (*cut*)

Distal medial striate artery (recurrent artery of Heubner)

Right internal carotid artery

Dorsal branch to corpus callosum

Parietooccipital branch

Calcarine branch

Medial occipital artery

Posterior temporal branch

Anterior temporal branch

Posterior communicating artery

Note: Anterior parietal (postcentral sulcal) artery also occurs as separate anterior parietal and postcentral sulcal arteries

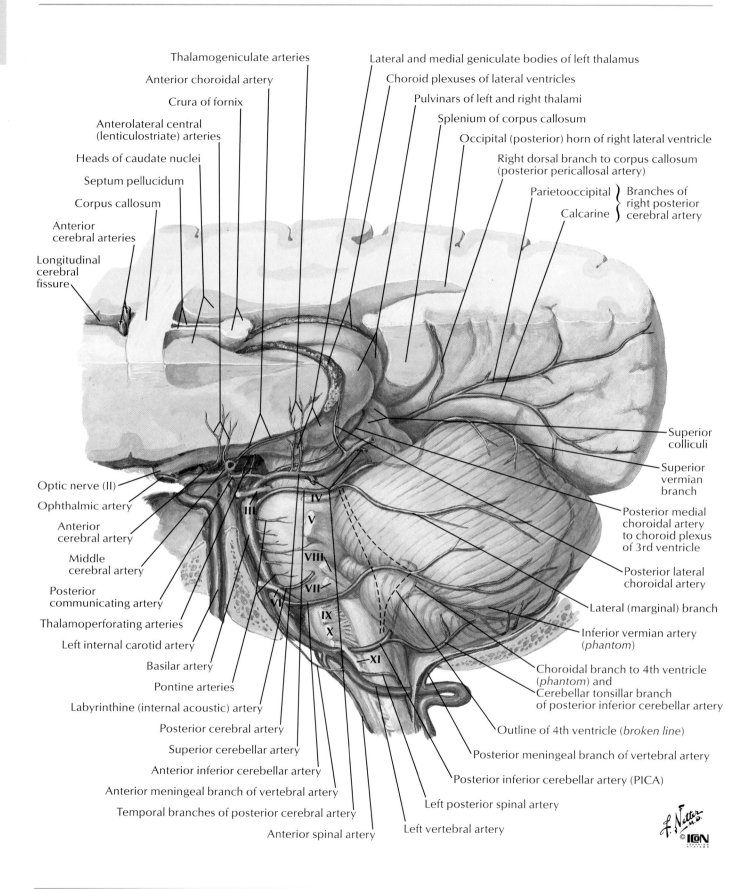

Thalamogeniculate arteries

Anterior choroidal artery

Crura of fornix

Anterolateral central
(lenticulostriate) arteries

Heads of caudate nuclei

Septum pellucidum

Corpus callosum

Anterior
cerebral arteries

Longitudinal
cerebral
fissure

Lateral and medial geniculate bodies of left thalamus

Choroid plexuses of lateral ventricles

Pulvinars of left and right thalami

Splenium of corpus callosum

Occipital (posterior) horn of right lateral ventricle

Right dorsal branch to corpus callosum
(posterior pericallosal artery)

Parietooccipital ⎫ Branches of
⎬ right posterior
Calcarine ⎭ cerebral artery

Optic nerve (II)

Ophthalmic artery

Anterior
cerebral artery

Middle
cerebral artery

Posterior
communicating artery

Thalamoperforating arteries

Left internal carotid artery

Basilar artery

Pontine arteries

Labyrinthine (internal acoustic) artery

Posterior cerebral artery

Superior cerebellar artery

Anterior inferior cerebellar artery

Anterior meningeal branch of vertebral artery

Temporal branches of posterior cerebral artery

Anterior spinal artery

Superior
colliculi

Superior
vermian
branch

Posterior medial
choroidal artery
to choroid plexus
of 3rd ventricle

Posterior lateral
choroidal artery

Lateral (marginal) branch

Inferior vermian artery
(phantom)

Choroidal branch to 4th ventricle
(phantom) and
Cerebellar tonsillar branch
of posterior inferior cerebellar artery

Outline of 4th ventricle (broken line)

Posterior meningeal branch of vertebral artery

Posterior inferior cerebellar artery (PICA)

Left posterior spinal artery

Left vertebral artery

III

IV

V

VIII

VII

VI

IX

X

XI

PLATE 136

HEAD AND NECK

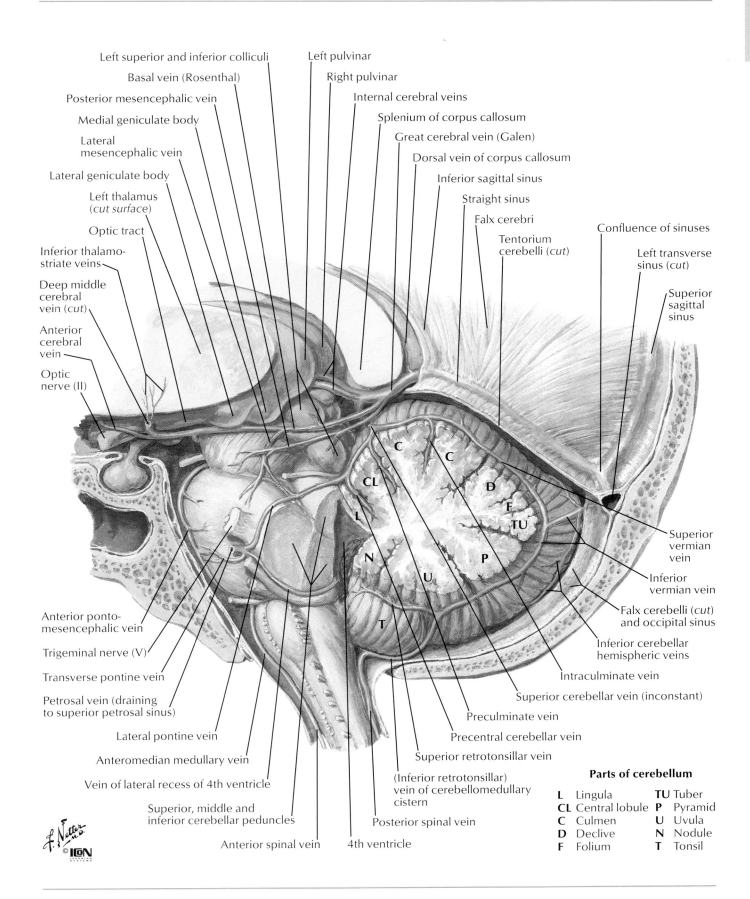

Left superior and inferior colliculi

Basal vein (Rosenthal)

Posterior mesencephalic vein

Medial geniculate body

Lateral mesencephalic vein

Lateral geniculate body

Left thalamus (*cut surface*)

Optic tract

Inferior thalamo-striate veins

Deep middle cerebral vein (*cut*)

Anterior cerebral vein

Optic nerve (II)

Left pulvinar

Right pulvinar

Internal cerebral veins

Splenium of corpus callosum

Great cerebral vein (Galen)

Dorsal vein of corpus callosum

Inferior sagittal sinus

Straight sinus

Falx cerebri

Tentorium cerebelli (*cut*)

Confluence of sinuses

Left transverse sinus (*cut*)

Superior sagittal sinus

Superior vermian vein

Inferior vermian vein

Falx cerebelli (*cut*) and occipital sinus

Inferior cerebellar hemispheric veins

Intraculminate vein

Superior cerebellar vein (inconstant)

Preculminate vein

Precentral cerebellar vein

Superior retrotonsillar vein

(Inferior retrotonsillar) vein of cerebellomedullary cistern

Posterior spinal vein

4th ventricle

Anterior spinal vein

Superior, middle and inferior cerebellar peduncles

Vein of lateral recess of 4th ventricle

Anteromedian medullary vein

Lateral pontine vein

Petrosal vein (draining to superior petrosal sinus)

Transverse pontine vein

Trigeminal nerve (V)

Anterior ponto-mesencephalic vein

Parts of cerebellum

L	Lingula	**TU**	Tuber
CL	Central lobule	**P**	Pyramid
C	Culmen	**U**	Uvula
D	Declive	**N**	Nodule
F	Folium	**T**	Tonsil

Deep Veins of Brain

FOR SUPERFICIAL VEINS OF BRAIN SEE PLATE 96

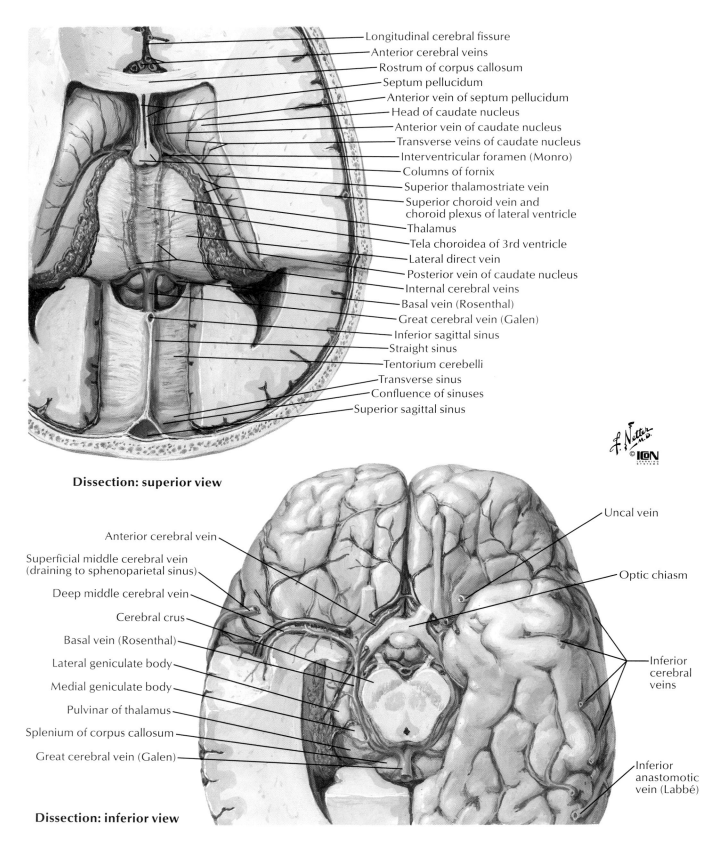

Longitudinal cerebral fissure
Anterior cerebral veins
Rostrum of corpus callosum
Septum pellucidum
Anterior vein of septum pellucidum
Head of caudate nucleus
Anterior vein of caudate nucleus
Transverse veins of caudate nucleus
Interventricular foramen (Monro)
Columns of fornix
Superior thalamostriate vein
Superior choroid vein and choroid plexus of lateral ventricle
Thalamus
Tela choroidea of 3rd ventricle
Lateral direct vein
Posterior vein of caudate nucleus
Internal cerebral veins
Basal vein (Rosenthal)
Great cerebral vein (Galen)
Inferior sagittal sinus
Straight sinus
Tentorium cerebelli
Transverse sinus
Confluence of sinuses
Superior sagittal sinus

Dissection: superior view

Anterior cerebral vein
Superficial middle cerebral vein (draining to sphenoparietal sinus)
Deep middle cerebral vein
Cerebral crus
Basal vein (Rosenthal)
Lateral geniculate body
Medial geniculate body
Pulvinar of thalamus
Splenium of corpus callosum
Great cerebral vein (Galen)

Uncal vein
Optic chiasm
Inferior cerebral veins
Inferior anastomotic vein (Labbé)

Dissection: inferior view

PLATE 138

HEAD AND NECK

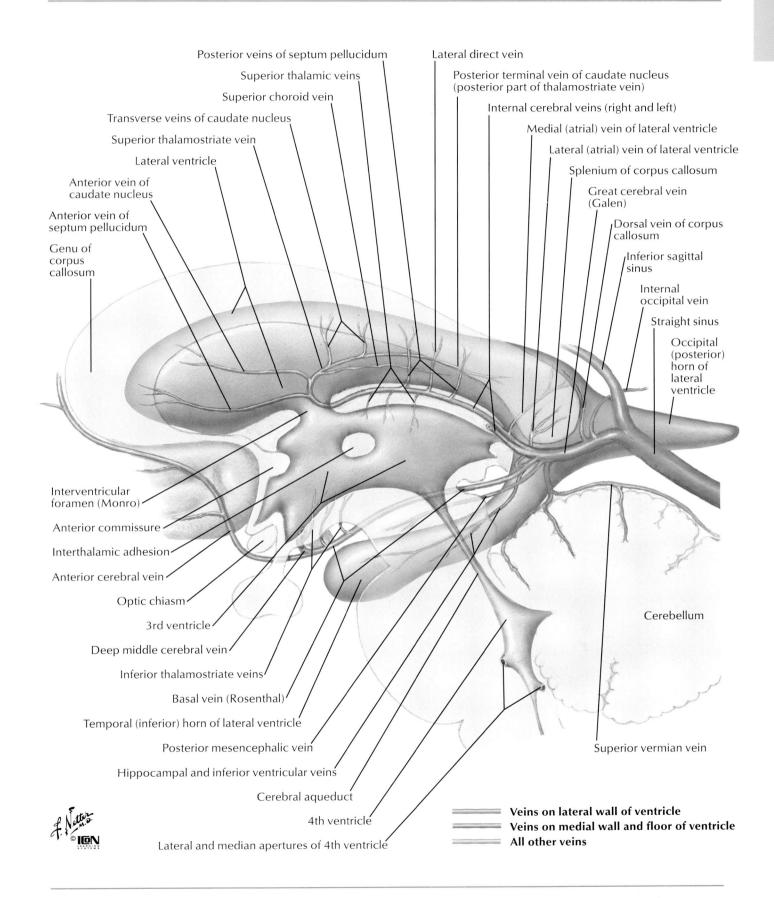

Posterior veins of septum pellucidum

Superior thalamic veins

Superior choroid vein

Transverse veins of caudate nucleus

Superior thalamostriate vein

Lateral ventricle

Anterior vein of caudate nucleus

Anterior vein of septum pellucidum

Genu of corpus callosum

Lateral direct vein

Posterior terminal vein of caudate nucleus (posterior part of thalamostriate vein)

Internal cerebral veins (right and left)

Medial (atrial) vein of lateral ventricle

Lateral (atrial) vein of lateral ventricle

Splenium of corpus callosum

Great cerebral vein (Galen)

Dorsal vein of corpus callosum

Inferior sagittal sinus

Internal occipital vein

Straight sinus

Occipital (posterior) horn of lateral ventricle

Interventricular foramen (Monro)

Anterior commissure

Interthalamic adhesion

Anterior cerebral vein

Optic chiasm

3rd ventricle

Deep middle cerebral vein

Inferior thalamostriate veins

Basal vein (Rosenthal)

Temporal (inferior) horn of lateral ventricle

Posterior mesencephalic vein

Hippocampal and inferior ventricular veins

Cerebral aqueduct

4th ventricle

Lateral and median apertures of 4th ventricle

Cerebellum

Superior vermian vein

Veins on lateral wall of ventricle
Veins on medial wall and floor of ventricle
All other veins

F. Netter M.D.
©ICN LEARNING SYSTEMS

Hypothalamus and Hypophysis

SEE ALSO PLATES 100, 101

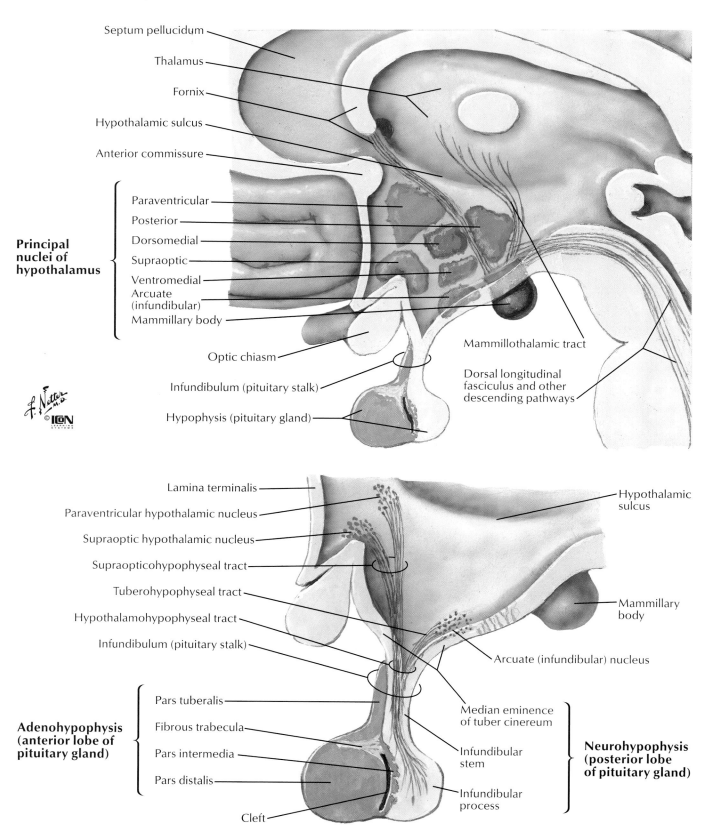

Septum pellucidum

Thalamus

Fornix

Hypothalamic sulcus

Anterior commissure

Principal nuclei of hypothalamus

Paraventricular

Posterior

Dorsomedial

Supraoptic

Ventromedial

Arcuate (infundibular)

Mammillary body

Optic chiasm

Infundibulum (pituitary stalk)

Hypophysis (pituitary gland)

Mammillothalamic tract

Dorsal longitudinal fasciculus and other descending pathways

Lamina terminalis

Paraventricular hypothalamic nucleus

Supraoptic hypothalamic nucleus

Supraopticohypophyseal tract

Tuberohypophyseal tract

Hypothalamohypophyseal tract

Infundibulum (pituitary stalk)

Hypothalamic sulcus

Mammillary body

Arcuate (infundibular) nucleus

Adenohypophysis (anterior lobe of pituitary gland)

Pars tuberalis

Fibrous trabecula

Pars intermedia

Pars distalis

Cleft

Median eminence of tuber cinereum

Infundibular stem

Infundibular process

Neurohypophysis (posterior lobe of pituitary gland)

PLATE 140

HEAD AND NECK

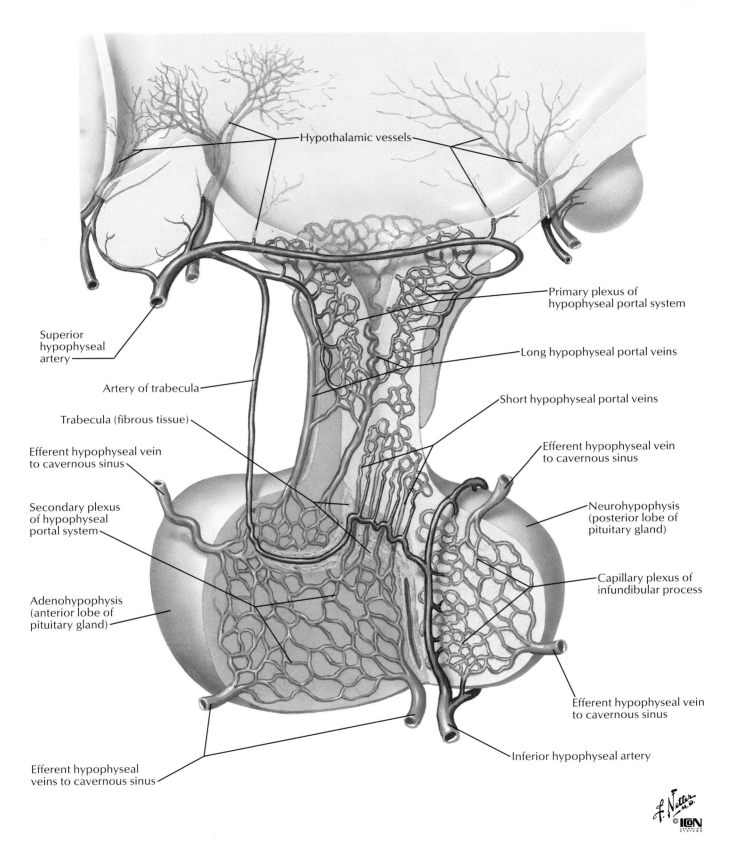

Hypothalamic vessels

Primary plexus of
hypophyseal portal system

Superior
hypophyseal
artery

Long hypophyseal portal veins

Artery of trabecula

Short hypophyseal portal veins

Trabecula (fibrous tissue)

Efferent hypophyseal vein
to cavernous sinus

Efferent hypophyseal vein
to cavernous sinus

Secondary plexus
of hypophyseal
portal system

Neurohypophysis
(posterior lobe of
pituitary gland)

Capillary plexus of
infundibular process

Adenohypophysis
(anterior lobe of
pituitary gland)

Efferent hypophyseal vein
to cavernous sinus

Efferent hypophyseal
veins to cavernous sinus

Inferior hypophyseal artery

Head Scans: Sagittal MR Images

SEE ALSO PLATE 100

Median (A) and paramedian (B,C) sagittal MR images

A

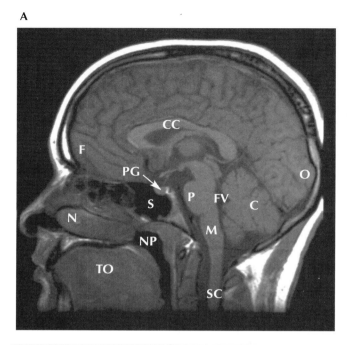

C	Cerebellum	**N**	Inferior nasal concha
CC	Corpus callosum	**NP**	Nasopharynx
E	Extraocular muscles	**O**	Occipital pole
		ON	Optic nerve
F	Frontal pole	**P**	Pons
FV	Fourth ventricle	**PG**	Pituitary gland
		S	Sphenoid sinus
L	Lateral ventricle	**SC**	Spinal cord
M	Medulla oblongata	**T**	Thalamus
		TC	Tentorium cerebelli
MB	Midbrain		
MS	Maxillary sinus	**TO**	Tongue

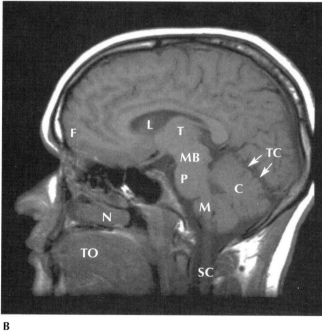

B

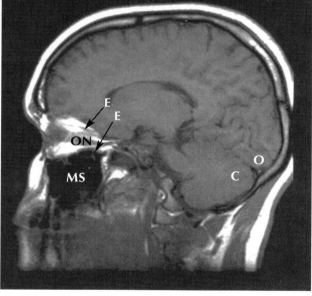

C

PLATE 142

HEAD AND NECK

Axial MR images of the head from inferior (A) to superior (C)

A

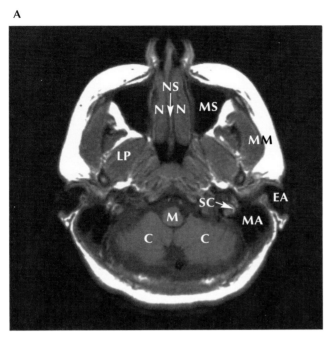

B	Basilar artery	**M**	Medulla oblongata
C	Cerebellum	**MA**	Mastoid air cells
CH	Cerebral hemisphere	**MB**	Midbrain
CS	Confluence of sinuses	**MM**	Masseter muscle
E	Eye	**MR**	Medial rectus muscle
EA	External acoustic meatus	**MS**	Maxillary sinus
ES	Ethmoid sinus	**N**	Nasal concha
F	Fat in orbit	**NS**	Nasal septum
FV	Fourth ventricle	**P**	Pons
L	Lens	**S**	Sphenoid sinus
LP	Lateral pterygoid muscle	**SC**	Semicircular canals
LR	Lateral rectus muscle	**SS**	Superior sagittal sinus
		T	Temporalis muscle
		TL	Temporal lobe

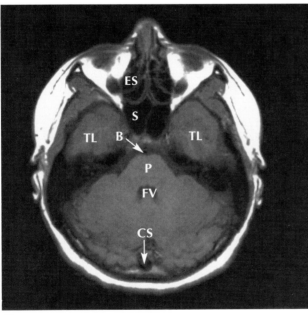

B

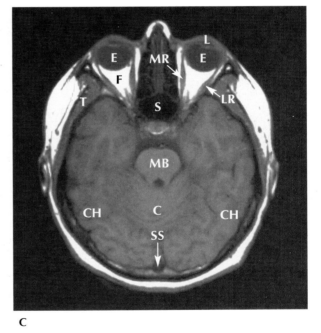

C

Head Scans: Coronal CT Images

SEE ALSO PLATES 44, 79

Coronal CT images of the head from anterior (A) to posterior (C)

A

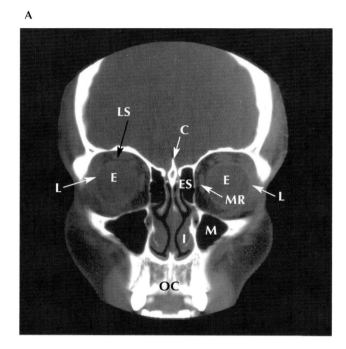

A	Anterior clinoid process	**LS**	Levator palpebrae superioris and superior rectus muscles
C	Crista galli		
E	Eye (vitreous chamber)	**M**	Maxillary sinus
ES	Ethmoid sinus	**MR**	Medial rectus muscle
I	Inferior nasal concha	**N**	Nasal septum
IR	Inferior rectus muscle	**O**	Optic nerve
		OC	Oral cavity
L	Lateral rectus muscle	**S**	Sphenoid sinus

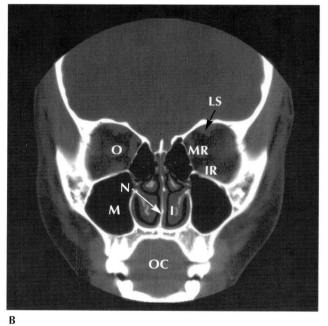

B

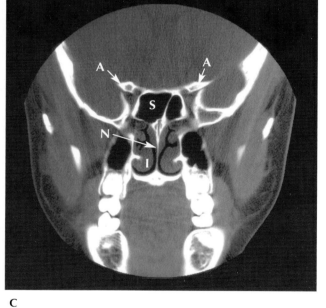

C

PLATE 144

HEAD AND NECK

Section II
BACK AND SPINAL CORD

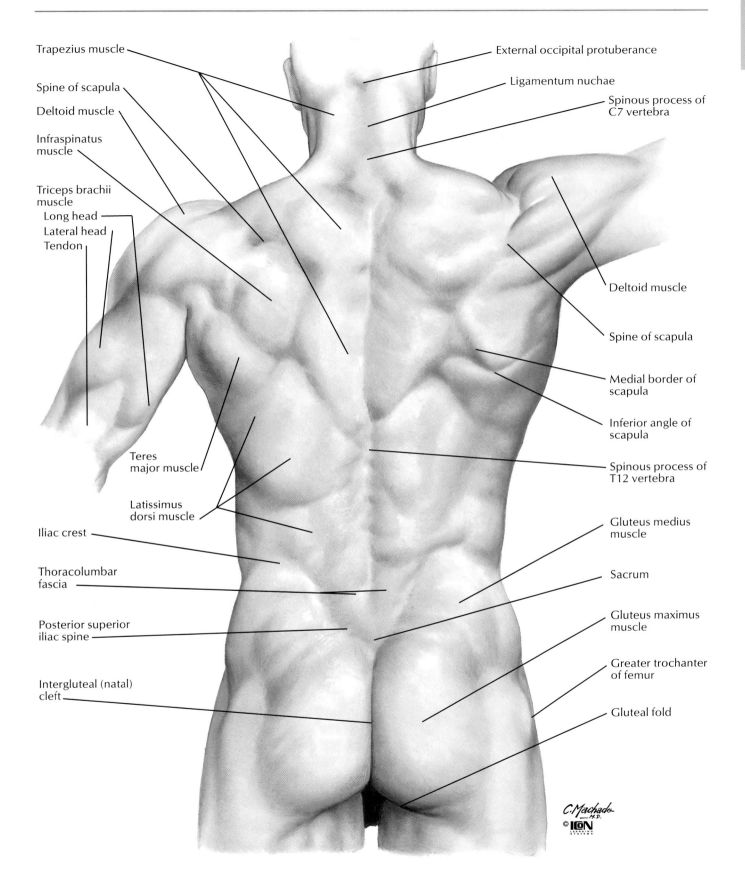

Trapezius muscle

Spine of scapula

Deltoid muscle

Infraspinatus
muscle

Triceps brachii
muscle
  Long head
  Lateral head
  Tendon

Teres
major muscle

Latissimus
dorsi muscle

Iliac crest

Thoracolumbar
fascia

Posterior superior
iliac spine

Intergluteal (natal)
cleft

External occipital protuberance

Ligamentum nuchae

Spinous process of
C7 vertebra

Deltoid muscle

Spine of scapula

Medial border of
scapula

Inferior angle of
scapula

Spinous process of
T12 vertebra

Gluteus medius
muscle

Sacrum

Gluteus maximus
muscle

Greater trochanter
of femur

Gluteal fold

SURFACE ANATOMY

PLATE 145

Vertebral Column

SEE ALSO PLATES 12, 15, 16, 147, 148, 150, 178, 240

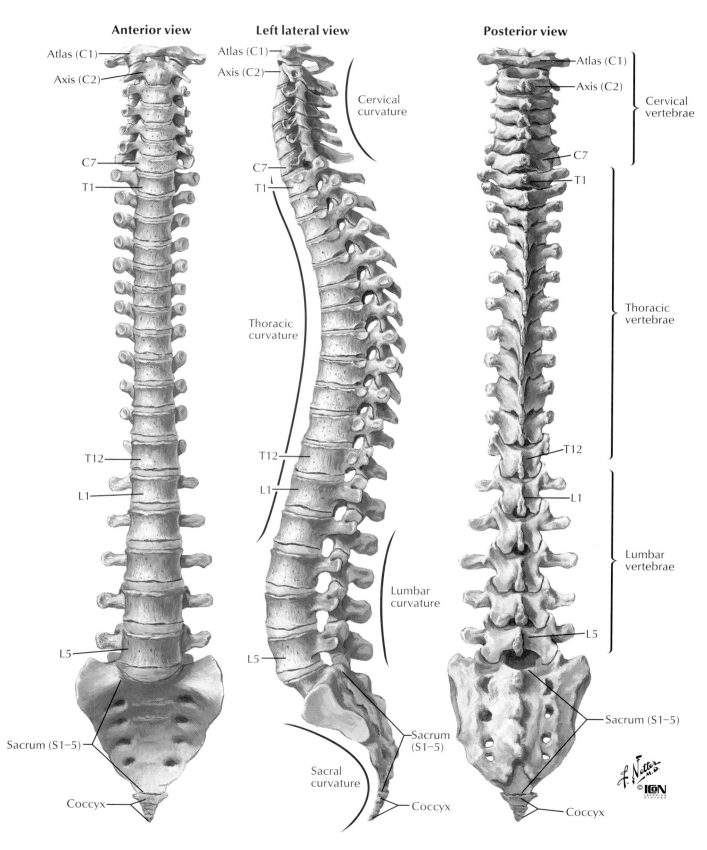

Anterior view

Atlas (C1)
Axis (C2)
C7
T1
T12
L1
L5
Sacrum (S1–5)
Coccyx

Left lateral view

Atlas (C1)
Axis (C2)
Cervical curvature
C7
T1
Thoracic curvature
T12
L1
Lumbar curvature
L5
Sacrum (S1–5)
Sacral curvature
Coccyx

Posterior view

Atlas (C1)
Axis (C2)
Cervical vertebrae
C7
T1
Thoracic vertebrae
T12
L1
Lumbar vertebrae
L5
Sacrum (S1–5)
Coccyx

PLATE 146

BACK AND SPINAL CORD

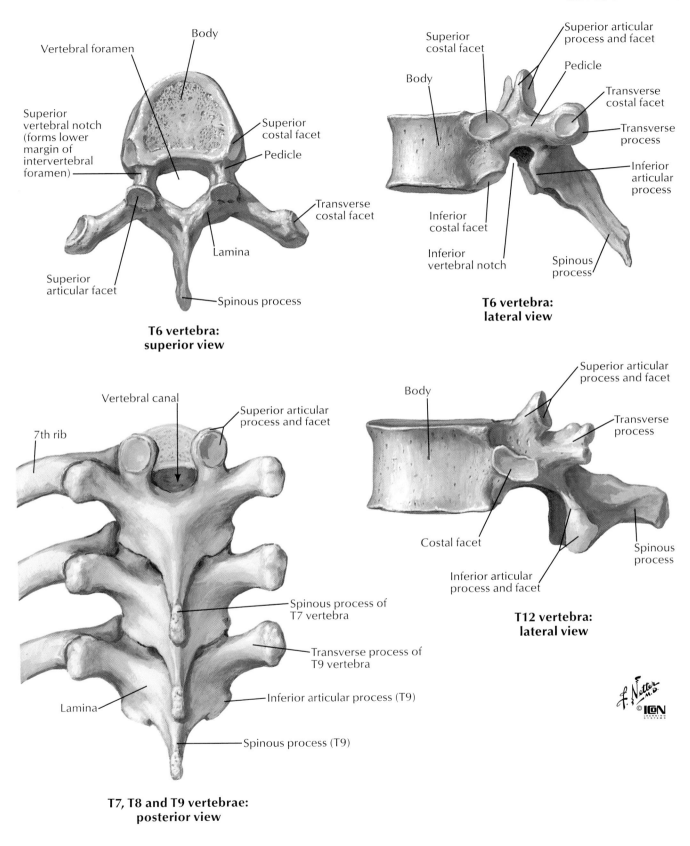

**T6 vertebra:
superior view**

Vertebral foramen

Body

Superior
vertebral notch
(forms lower
margin of
intervertebral
foramen)

Superior
costal facet

Pedicle

Transverse
costal facet

Lamina

Superior
articular facet

Spinous process

**T6 vertebra:
lateral view**

Superior
costal facet

Body

Superior articular
process and facet

Pedicle

Transverse
costal facet

Transverse
process

Inferior
articular
process

Inferior
costal facet

Inferior
vertebral notch

Spinous
process

**T7, T8 and T9 vertebrae:
posterior view**

Vertebral canal

Superior articular
process and facet

7th rib

Spinous process of
T7 vertebra

Transverse process of
T9 vertebra

Inferior articular process (T9)

Lamina

Spinous process (T9)

**T12 vertebra:
lateral view**

Body

Superior articular
process and facet

Transverse
process

Costal facet

Inferior articular
process and facet

Spinous
process

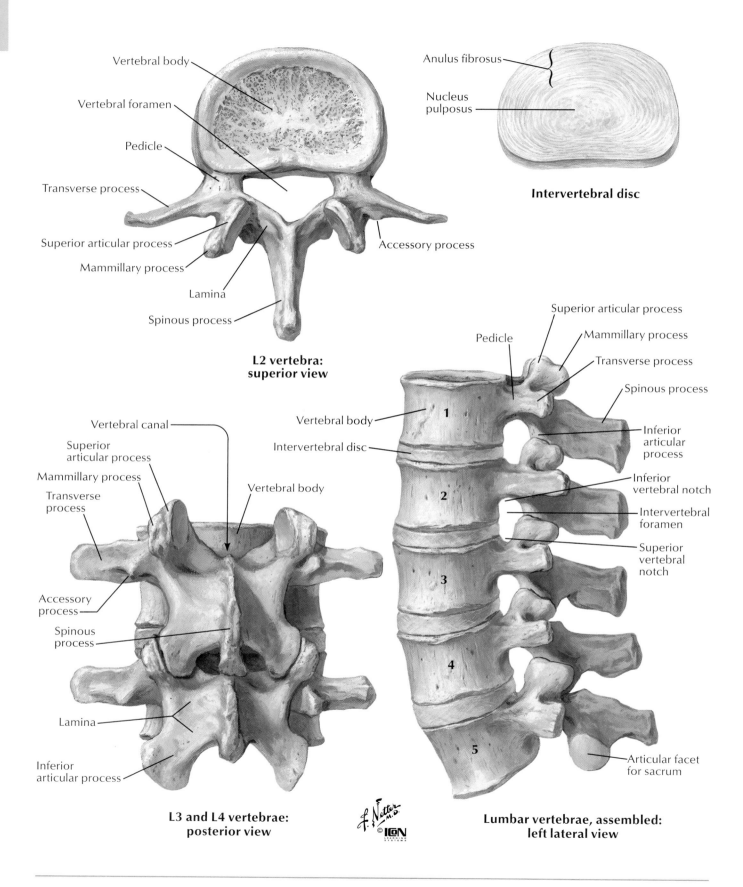

Vertebral body

Vertebral foramen

Pedicle

Transverse process

Superior articular process

Mammillary process

Lamina

Spinous process

**L2 vertebra:
superior view**

Anulus fibrosus

Nucleus pulposus

Intervertebral disc

Vertebral canal

Superior articular process

Mammillary process

Transverse process

Vertebral body

Accessory process

Spinous process

Lamina

Inferior articular process

**L3 and L4 vertebrae:
posterior view**

Superior articular process

Mammillary process

Pedicle

Transverse process

Spinous process

Vertebral body

Intervertebral disc

Inferior articular process

Inferior vertebral notch

Intervertebral foramen

Superior vertebral notch

Articular facet for sacrum

**Lumbar vertebrae, assembled:
left lateral view**

PLATE 148

BACK AND SPINAL CORD

Anteroposterior radiograph

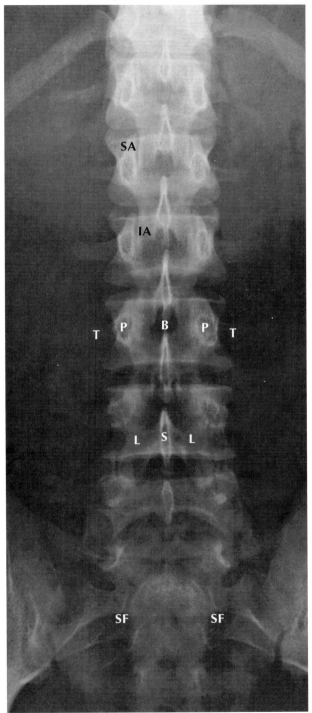

Lateral radiograph

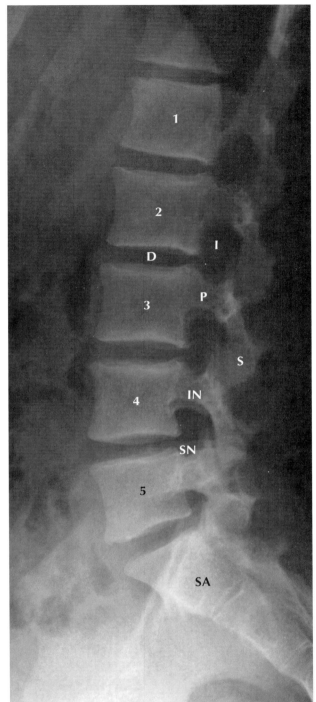

B	Body of L3 vertebra
IA	Inferior articular process of L1 vertebra
L	Lamina of L4 vertebra
P	Pedicle of L3 vertebra
S	Spinous process of L4 vertebra
SA	Superior articular process of L1 vertebra
SF	Sacral foramen
T	Transverse process of L3 vertebra

D	Intervertebral disc space
I	Intervertebral foramen
IN	Inferior vertebral notch of L4 vertebra
P	Pedicle of L3 vertebra
S	Spinous process of L3 vertebra
SA	Sacrum
SN	Superior vertebral notch of L5 vertebra
Note:	The lumbar vertebral bodies are numbered

Sacrum and Coccyx

SEE ALSO PLATES 146, 152, 240, 340—342

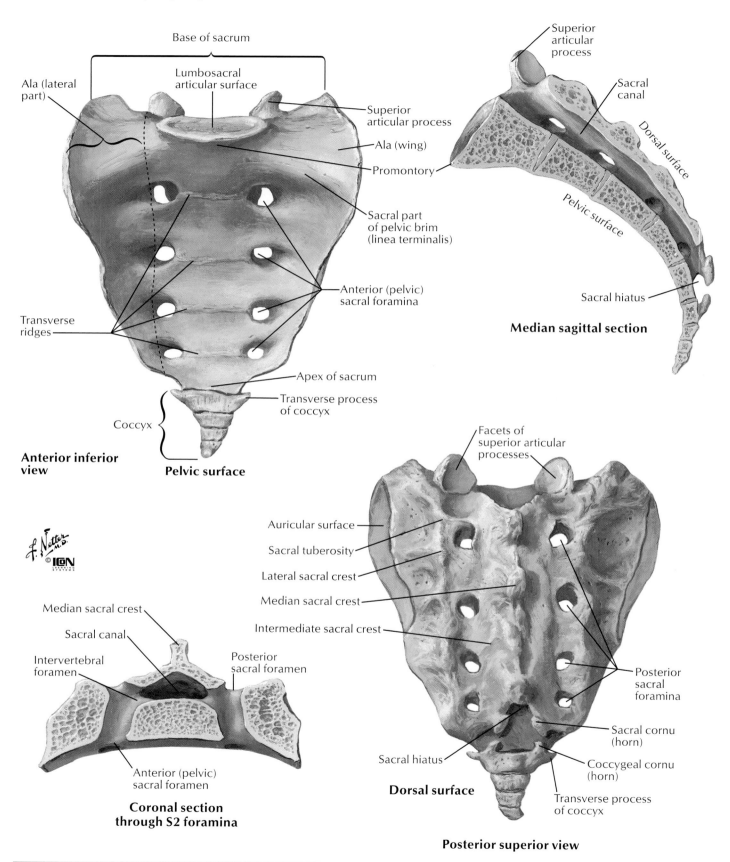

Base of sacrum

Ala (lateral part)

Lumbosacral articular surface

Superior articular process

Ala (wing)

Promontory

Sacral part of pelvic brim (linea terminalis)

Anterior (pelvic) sacral foramina

Transverse ridges

Apex of sacrum

Transverse process of coccyx

Coccyx

Anterior inferior view

Pelvic surface

Superior articular process

Sacral canal

Dorsal surface

Pelvic surface

Sacral hiatus

Median sagittal section

Median sacral crest

Sacral canal

Intervertebral foramen

Posterior sacral foramen

Anterior (pelvic) sacral foramen

Coronal section through S2 foramina

Facets of superior articular processes

Auricular surface

Sacral tuberosity

Lateral sacral crest

Median sacral crest

Intermediate sacral crest

Posterior sacral foramina

Sacral cornu (horn)

Sacral hiatus

Coccygeal cornu (horn)

Transverse process of coccyx

Dorsal surface

Posterior superior view

PLATE 150

BACK AND SPINAL CORD

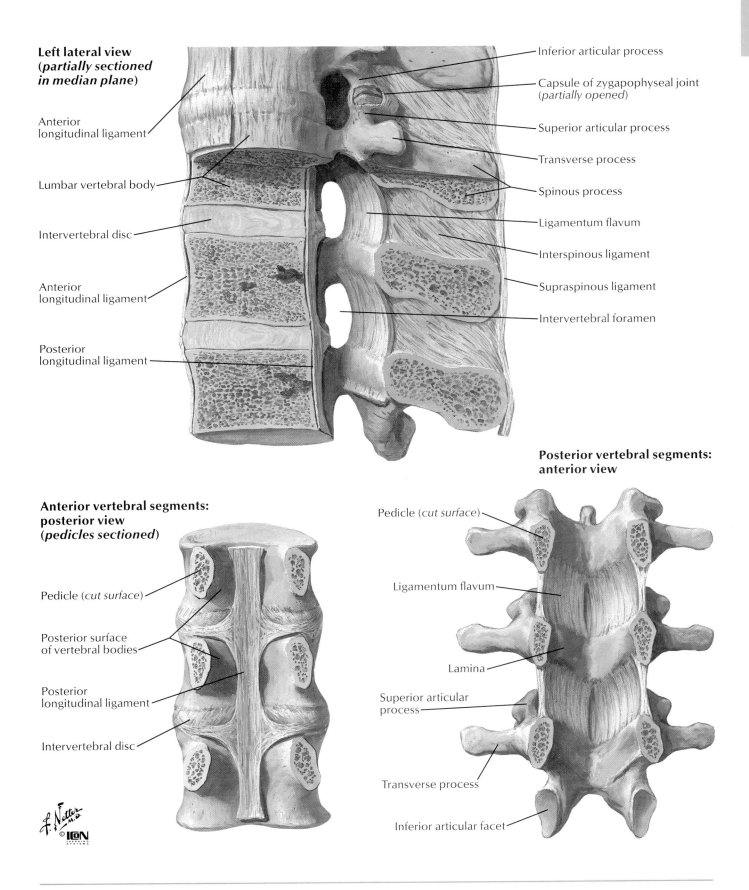

Left lateral view (*partially sectioned in median plane*)

Anterior longitudinal ligament

Lumbar vertebral body

Intervertebral disc

Anterior longitudinal ligament

Posterior longitudinal ligament

Inferior articular process

Capsule of zygapophyseal joint (*partially opened*)

Superior articular process

Transverse process

Spinous process

Ligamentum flavum

Interspinous ligament

Supraspinous ligament

Intervertebral foramen

Posterior vertebral segments: anterior view

Pedicle (*cut surface*)

Ligamentum flavum

Lamina

Superior articular process

Transverse process

Inferior articular facet

Anterior vertebral segments: posterior view (*pedicles sectioned*)

Pedicle (*cut surface*)

Posterior surface of vertebral bodies

Posterior longitudinal ligament

Intervertebral disc

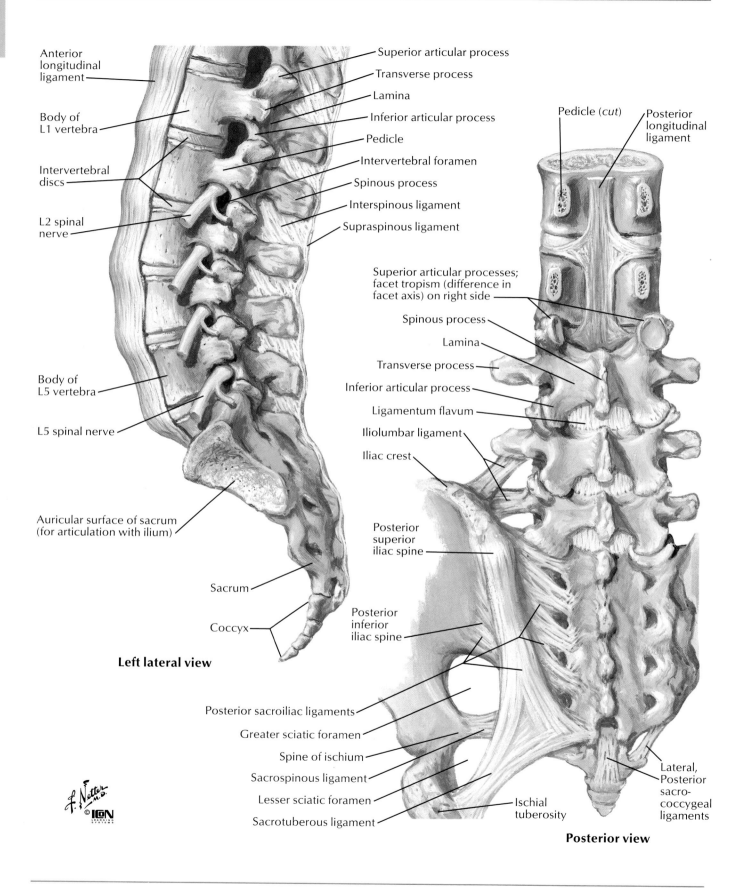

Anterior longitudinal ligament

Body of L1 vertebra

Intervertebral discs

L2 spinal nerve

Body of L5 vertebra

L5 spinal nerve

Auricular surface of sacrum (for articulation with ilium)

Sacrum

Coccyx

Left lateral view

Superior articular process

Transverse process

Lamina

Inferior articular process

Pedicle

Intervertebral foramen

Spinous process

Interspinous ligament

Supraspinous ligament

Pedicle (cut)

Posterior longitudinal ligament

Superior articular processes; facet tropism (difference in facet axis) on right side

Spinous process

Lamina

Transverse process

Inferior articular process

Ligamentum flavum

Iliolumbar ligament

Iliac crest

Posterior superior iliac spine

Posterior inferior iliac spine

Posterior sacroiliac ligaments

Greater sciatic foramen

Spine of ischium

Sacrospinous ligament

Lesser sciatic foramen

Sacrotuberous ligament

Ischial tuberosity

Lateral, Posterior sacro-coccygeal ligaments

Posterior view

PLATE 152

BACK AND SPINAL CORD

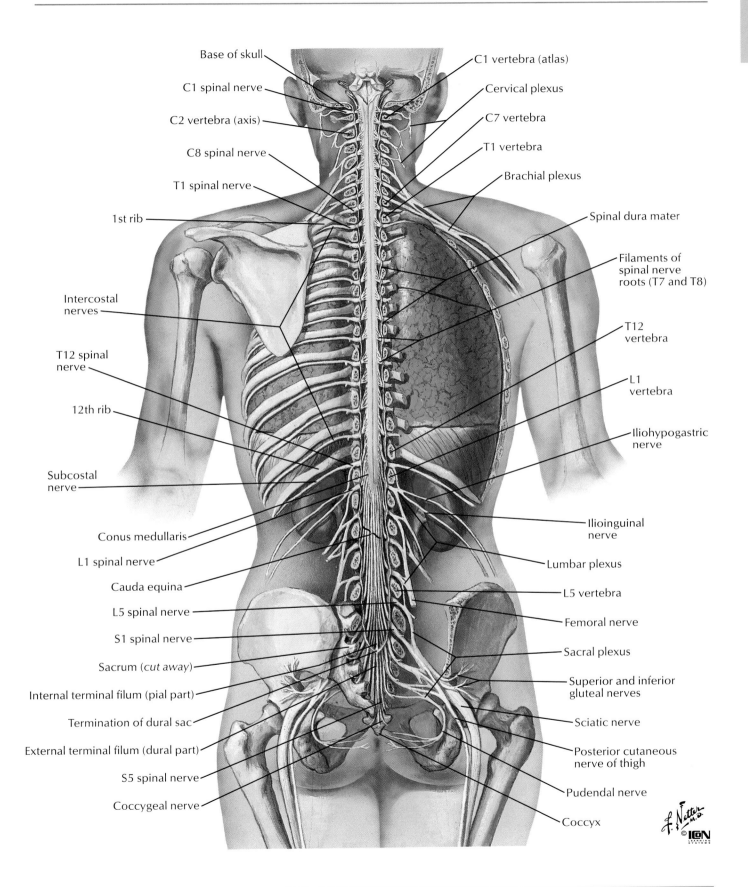

Base of skull

C1 spinal nerve

C2 vertebra (axis)

C8 spinal nerve

T1 spinal nerve

1st rib

Intercostal nerves

T12 spinal nerve

12th rib

Subcostal nerve

Conus medullaris

L1 spinal nerve

Cauda equina

L5 spinal nerve

S1 spinal nerve

Sacrum (*cut away*)

Internal terminal filum (pial part)

Termination of dural sac

External terminal filum (dural part)

S5 spinal nerve

Coccygeal nerve

C1 vertebra (atlas)

Cervical plexus

C7 vertebra

T1 vertebra

Brachial plexus

Spinal dura mater

Filaments of spinal nerve roots (T7 and T8)

T12 vertebra

L1 vertebra

Iliohypogastric nerve

Ilioinguinal nerve

Lumbar plexus

L5 vertebra

Femoral nerve

Sacral plexus

Superior and inferior gluteal nerves

Sciatic nerve

Posterior cutaneous nerve of thigh

Pudendal nerve

Coccyx

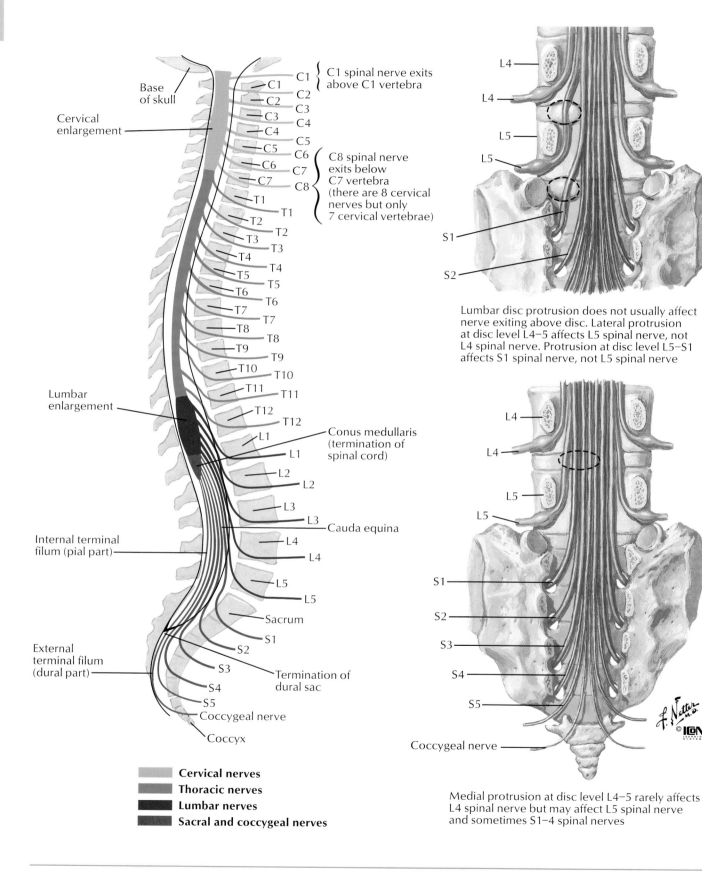

Base of skull

Cervical enlargement

C1 { C1 spinal nerve exits above C1 vertebra

C1
C2
C3
C4
C5
C6
C7
C8

C8 spinal nerve exits below C7 vertebra (there are 8 cervical nerves but only 7 cervical vertebrae)

T1
T2
T3
T4
T5
T6
T7
T8
T9
T10
T11
T12

Lumbar enlargement

Conus medullaris (termination of spinal cord)

L1
L2
L3

Cauda equina

L4
L5

Internal terminal filum (pial part)

Sacrum
S1
S2
S3

Termination of dural sac

External terminal filum (dural part)

S4
S5
Coccygeal nerve
Coccyx

Cervical nerves
Thoracic nerves
Lumbar nerves
Sacral and coccygeal nerves

L4
L4
L5
L5
S1
S2

Lumbar disc protrusion does not usually affect nerve exiting above disc. Lateral protrusion at disc level L4–5 affects L5 spinal nerve, not L4 spinal nerve. Protrusion at disc level L5–S1 affects S1 spinal nerve, not L5 spinal nerve

L4
L4
L5
L5
S1
S2
S3
S4
S5
Coccygeal nerve

Medial protrusion at disc level L4–5 rarely affects L4 spinal nerve but may affect L5 spinal nerve and sometimes S1–4 spinal nerves

PLATE 154

BACK AND SPINAL CORD

Function	Muscles	Segments
Inspiration	Diaphragm	C3, 4, 5
Shoulder abduction	Deltoid	C5
Elbow flexion	Biceps brachii Brachialis	C5, 6
Wrist extension	Extensor carpi radialis longus and brevis	C6, 7
Elbow extension	Triceps brachii	C7, 8
Finger flexion	Flexor digitorum superficialis and profundus	C8
Finger abduction and adduction	Interossei	C8, T1
Thigh adduction	Adductor longus and brevis	L2, 3
Knee extension	Quadriceps	L3, 4
Ankle dorsiflexion	Tibialis anterior	L4, 5
Great toe extension	Extensor hallucis longus	L5, S1
Ankle plantar flexion	Gastrocnemius Soleus	S1, 2
Anal contraction	Sphincter ani externus	S2, 3, 4

Lumbar Disc Herniation: Clinical Manifestations

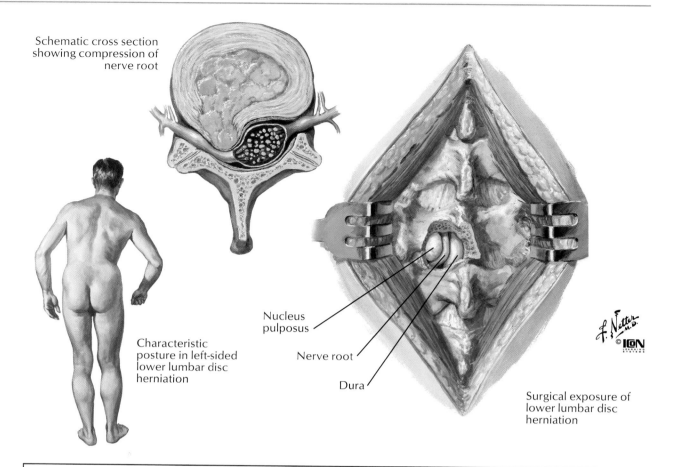

Schematic cross section showing compression of nerve root

Characteristic posture in left-sided lower lumbar disc herniation

Nucleus pulposus

Nerve root

Dura

Surgical exposure of lower lumbar disc herniation

Clinical features of herniated lumbar nucleus pulposus					
Level of herniation	Pain	Numbness	Weakness	Atrophy	Reflexes
L4–5 disc; 5th lumbar nerve root	Over sacro-iliac joint, hip, lateral thigh and leg	Lateral leg, first 3 toes	Dorsiflexion of great toe and foot; difficulty walking on heels; foot drop may occur	Minor	Changes uncommon in knee and ankle jerks, but internal hamstring reflex diminished or absent
L5–S1 disc; 1st sacral nerve root	Over sacro-iliac joint, hip, postero-lateral thigh and leg to heel	Back of calf, lateral heel, foot to toe	Plantar flexion of foot and great toe may be affected; difficulty walking on toes	Gastrocnemius and soleus	Ankle jerk diminished or absent

PLATE 156

BACK AND SPINAL CORD

SEE ALSO PLATES 465, 525; FOR MAPS OF CUTANEOUS NERVES SEE PLATES 20, 455, 457–459, 461, 464, 520–524

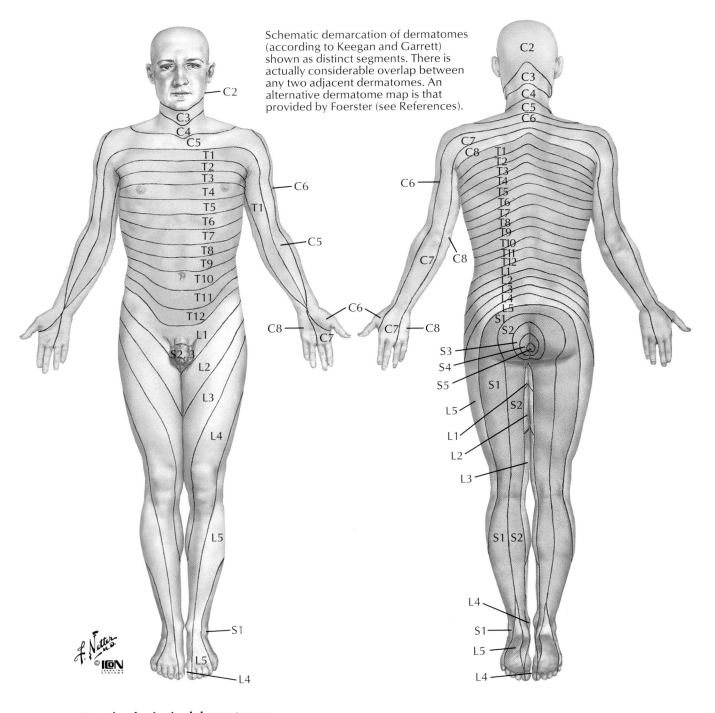

Schematic demarcation of dermatomes (according to Keegan and Garrett) shown as distinct segments. There is actually considerable overlap between any two adjacent dermatomes. An alternative dermatome map is that provided by Foerster (see References).

Levels of principal dermatomes

C5	Clavicles
C5, 6, 7	Lateral parts of upper limbs
C8, T1	Medial sides of upper limbs
C6	Thumb
C6, 7, 8	Hand
C8	Ring and little fingers
T4	Level of nipples
T10	Level of umbilicus
T12	Inguinal or groin regions
L1, 2, 3, 4	Anterior and inner surfaces of lower limbs
L4, 5, S1	Foot
L4	Medial side of great toe
S1, 2, L5	Posterior and outer surfaces of lower limbs
S1	Lateral margin of foot and little toe
S2, 3, 4	Perineum

Spinal Cord Cross Sections: Fiber Tracts

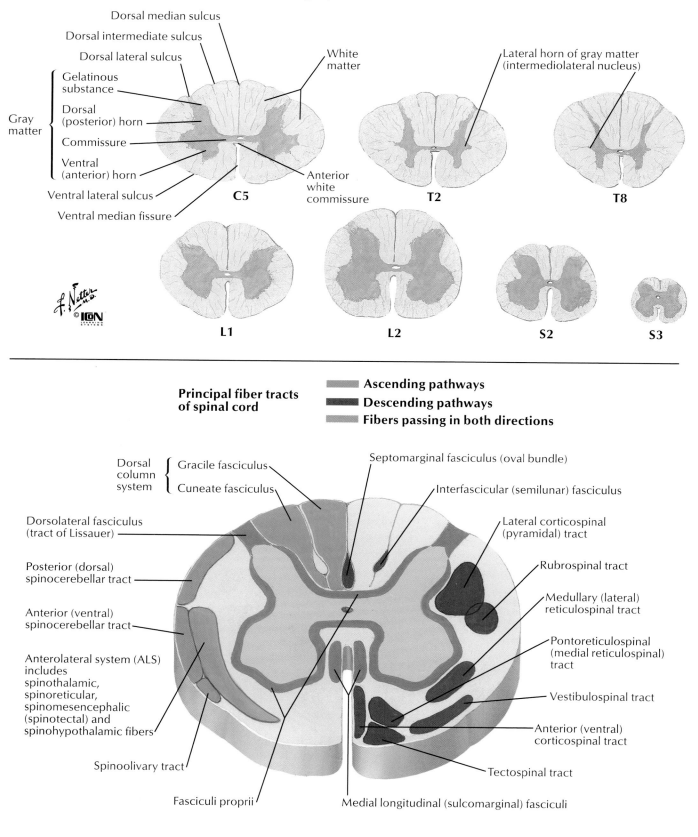

Sections through spinal cord at various levels

Dorsal median sulcus

Dorsal intermediate sulcus

Dorsal lateral sulcus

White matter

Lateral horn of gray matter (intermediolateral nucleus)

Gray matter
- Gelatinous substance
- Dorsal (posterior) horn
- Commissure
- Ventral (anterior) horn

Ventral lateral sulcus

Ventral median fissure

Anterior white commissure

C5　　**T2**　　**T8**

L1　　**L2**　　**S2**　　**S3**

Principal fiber tracts of spinal cord

　　Ascending pathways
　　Descending pathways
　　Fibers passing in both directions

Dorsal column system
- Gracile fasciculus
- Cuneate fasciculus

Septomarginal fasciculus (oval bundle)

Interfascicular (semilunar) fasciculus

Dorsolateral fasciculus (tract of Lissauer)

Posterior (dorsal) spinocerebellar tract

Anterior (ventral) spinocerebellar tract

Anterolateral system (ALS) includes spinothalamic, spinoreticular, spinomesencephalic (spinotectal) and spinohypothalamic fibers

Spinoolivary tract

Fasciculi proprii

Medial longitudinal (sulcomarginal) fasciculi

Lateral corticospinal (pyramidal) tract

Rubrospinal tract

Medullary (lateral) reticulospinal tract

Pontoreticulospinal (medial reticulospinal) tract

Vestibulospinal tract

Anterior (ventral) corticospinal tract

Tectospinal tract

PLATE 158

BACK AND SPINAL CORD

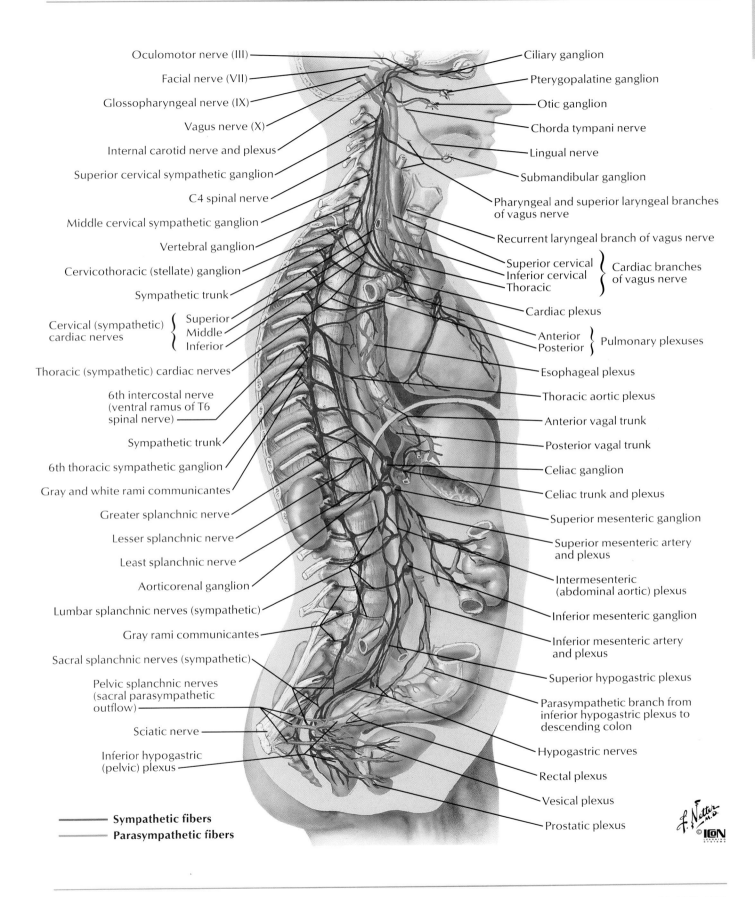

Oculomotor nerve (III)

Facial nerve (VII)

Glossopharyngeal nerve (IX)

Vagus nerve (X)

Internal carotid nerve and plexus

Superior cervical sympathetic ganglion

C4 spinal nerve

Middle cervical sympathetic ganglion

Vertebral ganglion

Cervicothoracic (stellate) ganglion

Sympathetic trunk

Cervical (sympathetic) cardiac nerves { Superior Middle Inferior

Thoracic (sympathetic) cardiac nerves

6th intercostal nerve (ventral ramus of T6 spinal nerve)

Sympathetic trunk

6th thoracic sympathetic ganglion

Gray and white rami communicantes

Greater splanchnic nerve

Lesser splanchnic nerve

Least splanchnic nerve

Aorticorenal ganglion

Lumbar splanchnic nerves (sympathetic)

Gray rami communicantes

Sacral splanchnic nerves (sympathetic)

Pelvic splanchnic nerves (sacral parasympathetic outflow)

Sciatic nerve

Inferior hypogastric (pelvic) plexus

Ciliary ganglion

Pterygopalatine ganglion

Otic ganglion

Chorda tympani nerve

Lingual nerve

Submandibular ganglion

Pharyngeal and superior laryngeal branches of vagus nerve

Recurrent laryngeal branch of vagus nerve

Superior cervical } Inferior cervical } Cardiac branches Thoracic } of vagus nerve

Cardiac plexus

Anterior } Posterior } Pulmonary plexuses

Esophageal plexus

Thoracic aortic plexus

Anterior vagal trunk

Posterior vagal trunk

Celiac ganglion

Celiac trunk and plexus

Superior mesenteric ganglion

Superior mesenteric artery and plexus

Intermesenteric (abdominal aortic) plexus

Inferior mesenteric ganglion

Inferior mesenteric artery and plexus

Superior hypogastric plexus

Parasympathetic branch from inferior hypogastric plexus to descending colon

Hypogastric nerves

Rectal plexus

Vesical plexus

Prostatic plexus

——— **Sympathetic fibers**
——— **Parasympathetic fibers**

Autonomic Nervous System: Schema

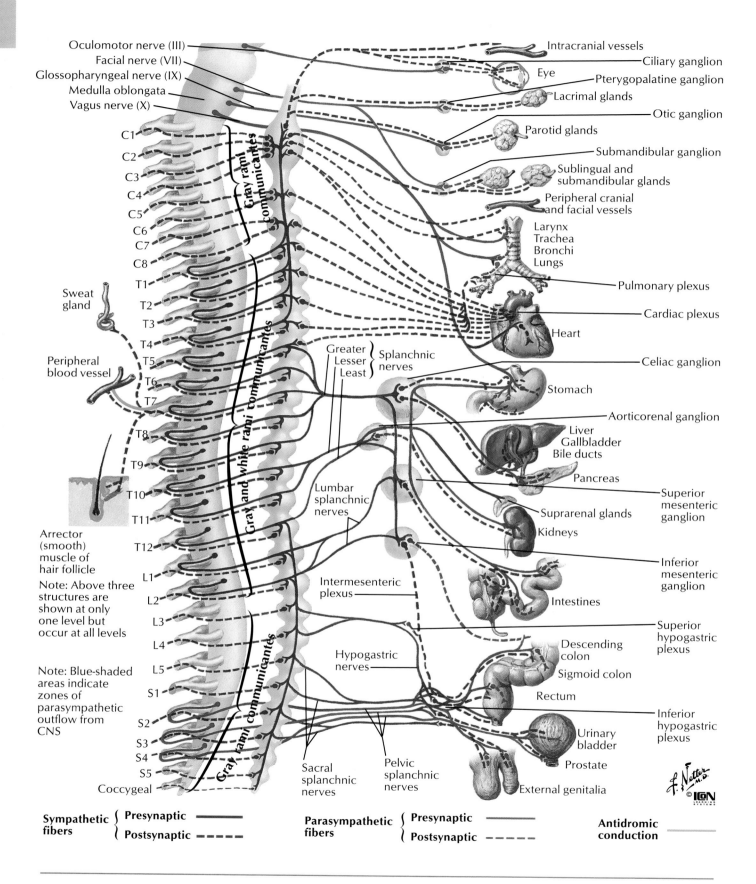

Oculomotor nerve (III)
Facial nerve (VII)
Glossopharyngeal nerve (IX)
Medulla oblongata
Vagus nerve (X)

C1
C2
C3
C4
C5
C6
C7
C8
T1
T2
T3
T4
T5
T6
T7
T8
T9
T10
T11
T12
L1
L2
L3
L4
L5
S1
S2
S3
S4
S5
Coccygeal

Gray rami communicantes

Gray and white rami communicantes

Gray rami communicantes

Sweat gland

Peripheral blood vessel

Arrector (smooth) muscle of hair follicle

Note: Above three structures are shown at only one level but occur at all levels

Note: Blue-shaded areas indicate zones of parasympathetic outflow from CNS

Greater
Lesser
Least
Splanchnic nerves

Lumbar splanchnic nerves

Intermesenteric plexus

Hypogastric nerves

Sacral splanchnic nerves

Pelvic splanchnic nerves

Intracranial vessels
Ciliary ganglion
Eye
Pterygopalatine ganglion
Lacrimal glands
Otic ganglion
Parotid glands
Submandibular ganglion
Sublingual and submandibular glands
Peripheral cranial and facial vessels
Larynx
Trachea
Bronchi
Lungs
Pulmonary plexus
Cardiac plexus
Heart
Celiac ganglion
Stomach
Aorticorenal ganglion
Liver
Gallbladder
Bile ducts
Pancreas
Superior mesenteric ganglion
Suprarenal glands
Kidneys
Inferior mesenteric ganglion
Intestines
Superior hypogastric plexus
Descending colon
Sigmoid colon
Rectum
Inferior hypogastric plexus
Urinary bladder
Prostate
External genitalia

Sympathetic fibers { Presynaptic ——— / Postsynaptic - - - -
Parasympathetic fibers { Presynaptic ——— / Postsynaptic - - - -
Antidromic conduction

f. Netter M.D.
© ICON LEARNING SYSTEMS

PLATE 160

BACK AND SPINAL CORD

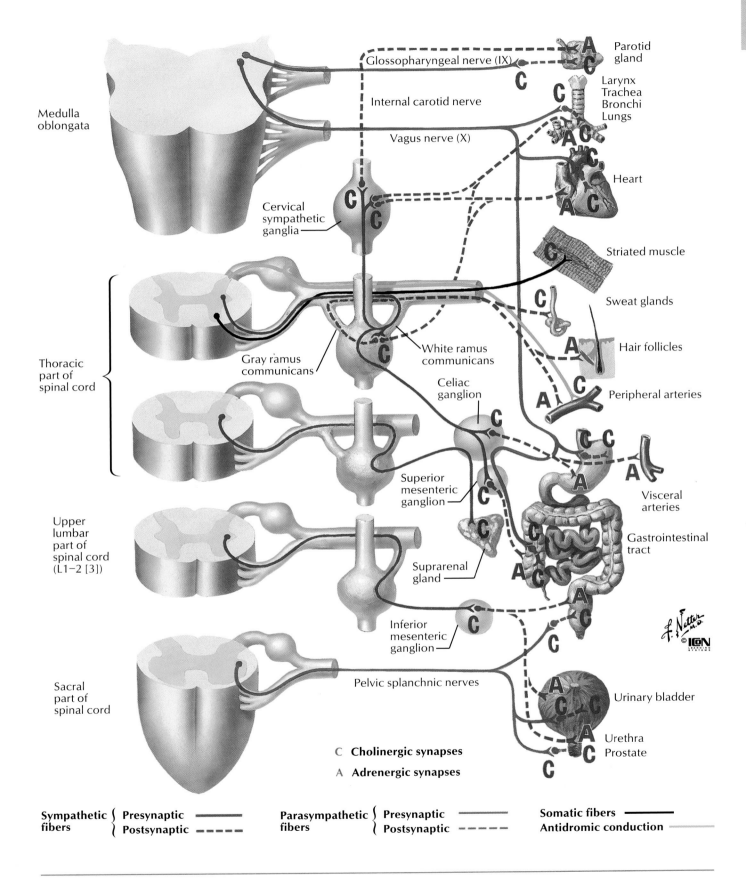

Medulla oblongata

Glossopharyngeal nerve (IX)

Internal carotid nerve

Vagus nerve (X)

Parotid gland

Larynx
Trachea
Bronchi
Lungs

Heart

Cervical sympathetic ganglia

Striated muscle

Sweat glands

Thoracic part of spinal cord

Gray ramus communicans

White ramus communicans

Hair follicles

Celiac ganglion

Peripheral arteries

Superior mesenteric ganglion

Visceral arteries

Upper lumbar part of spinal cord (L1–2 [3])

Gastrointestinal tract

Suprarenal gland

Inferior mesenteric ganglion

Sacral part of spinal cord

Pelvic splanchnic nerves

Urinary bladder

Urethra
Prostate

C **Cholinergic synapses**

A **Adrenergic synapses**

Sympathetic fibers { Presynaptic ——— / Postsynaptic - - - -

Parasympathetic fibers { Presynaptic ——— / Postsynaptic - - - -

Somatic fibers ———
Antidromic conduction ———

Spinal Membranes and Nerve Roots

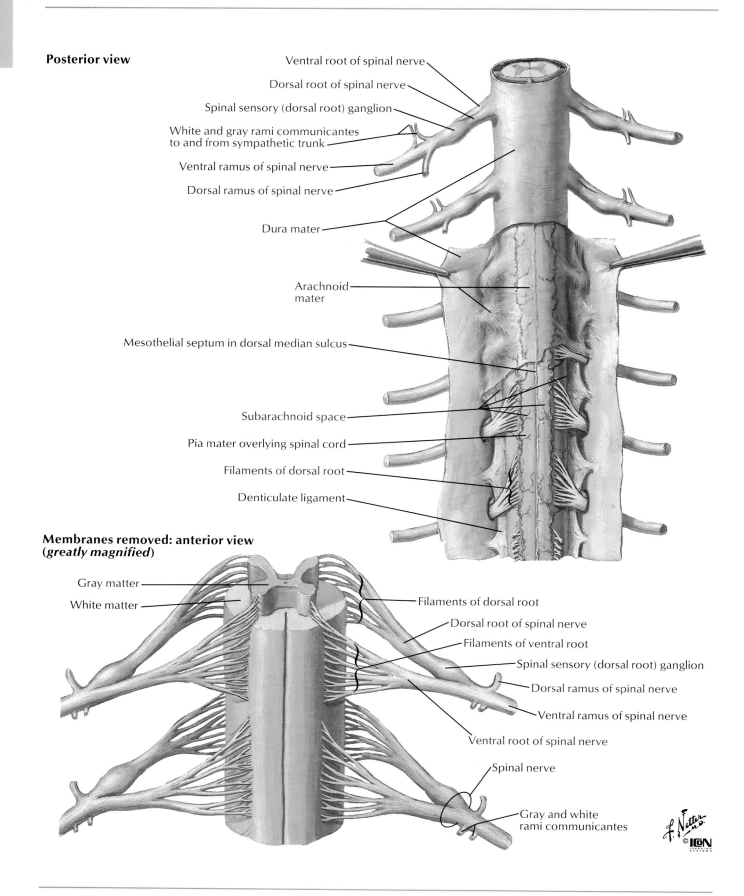

Posterior view

Ventral root of spinal nerve

Dorsal root of spinal nerve

Spinal sensory (dorsal root) ganglion

White and gray rami communicantes to and from sympathetic trunk

Ventral ramus of spinal nerve

Dorsal ramus of spinal nerve

Dura mater

Arachnoid mater

Mesothelial septum in dorsal median sulcus

Subarachnoid space

Pia mater overlying spinal cord

Filaments of dorsal root

Denticulate ligament

Membranes removed: anterior view
(*greatly magnified*)

Gray matter

White matter

Filaments of dorsal root

Dorsal root of spinal nerve

Filaments of ventral root

Spinal sensory (dorsal root) ganglion

Dorsal ramus of spinal nerve

Ventral ramus of spinal nerve

Ventral root of spinal nerve

Spinal nerve

Gray and white rami communicantes

PLATE 162

BACK AND SPINAL CORD

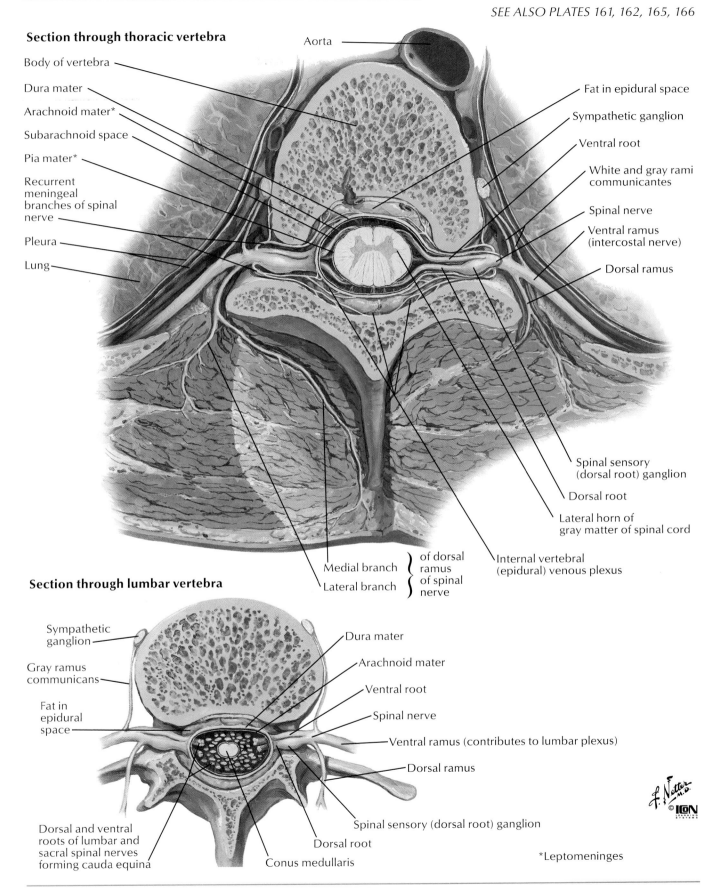

Section through thoracic vertebra

Aorta

Body of vertebra

Dura mater

Arachnoid mater*

Subarachnoid space

Pia mater*

Recurrent meningeal branches of spinal nerve

Pleura

Lung

Fat in epidural space

Sympathetic ganglion

Ventral root

White and gray rami communicantes

Spinal nerve

Ventral ramus (intercostal nerve)

Dorsal ramus

Spinal sensory (dorsal root) ganglion

Dorsal root

Lateral horn of gray matter of spinal cord

Internal vertebral (epidural) venous plexus

Medial branch
Lateral branch
} of dorsal ramus of spinal nerve

Section through lumbar vertebra

Sympathetic ganglion

Gray ramus communicans

Fat in epidural space

Dura mater

Arachnoid mater

Ventral root

Spinal nerve

Ventral ramus (contributes to lumbar plexus)

Dorsal ramus

Spinal sensory (dorsal root) ganglion

Dorsal and ventral roots of lumbar and sacral spinal nerves forming cauda equina

Dorsal root

Conus medullaris

*Leptomeninges

Arteries of Spinal Cord: Schema

SEE ALSO PLATE 131

Anterior view

Posterior view

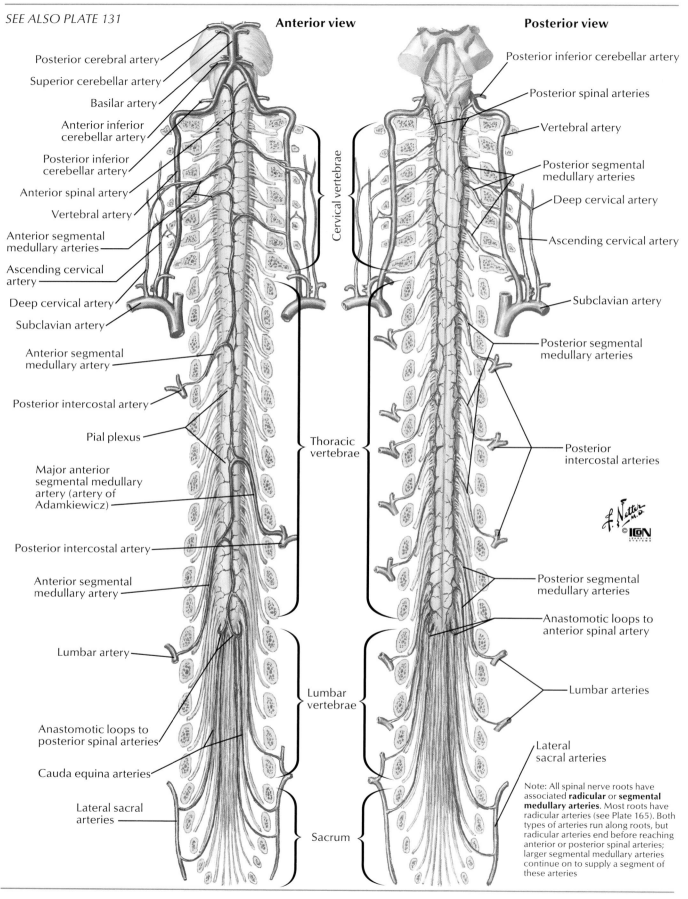

Posterior cerebral artery

Superior cerebellar artery

Basilar artery

Anterior inferior cerebellar artery

Posterior inferior cerebellar artery

Anterior spinal artery

Vertebral artery

Anterior segmental medullary arteries

Ascending cervical artery

Deep cervical artery

Subclavian artery

Anterior segmental medullary artery

Posterior intercostal artery

Pial plexus

Major anterior segmental medullary artery (artery of Adamkiewicz)

Posterior intercostal artery

Anterior segmental medullary artery

Lumbar artery

Anastomotic loops to posterior spinal arteries

Cauda equina arteries

Lateral sacral arteries

Cervical vertebrae

Thoracic vertebrae

Lumbar vertebrae

Sacrum

Posterior inferior cerebellar artery

Posterior spinal arteries

Vertebral artery

Posterior segmental medullary arteries

Deep cervical artery

Ascending cervical artery

Subclavian artery

Posterior segmental medullary arteries

Posterior intercostal arteries

Posterior segmental medullary arteries

Anastomotic loops to anterior spinal artery

Lumbar arteries

Lateral sacral arteries

Note: All spinal nerve roots have associated **radicular** or **segmental medullary arteries**. Most roots have radicular arteries (see Plate 165). Both types of arteries run along roots, but radicular arteries end before reaching anterior or posterior spinal arteries; larger segmental medullary arteries continue on to supply a segment of these arteries

PLATE 164

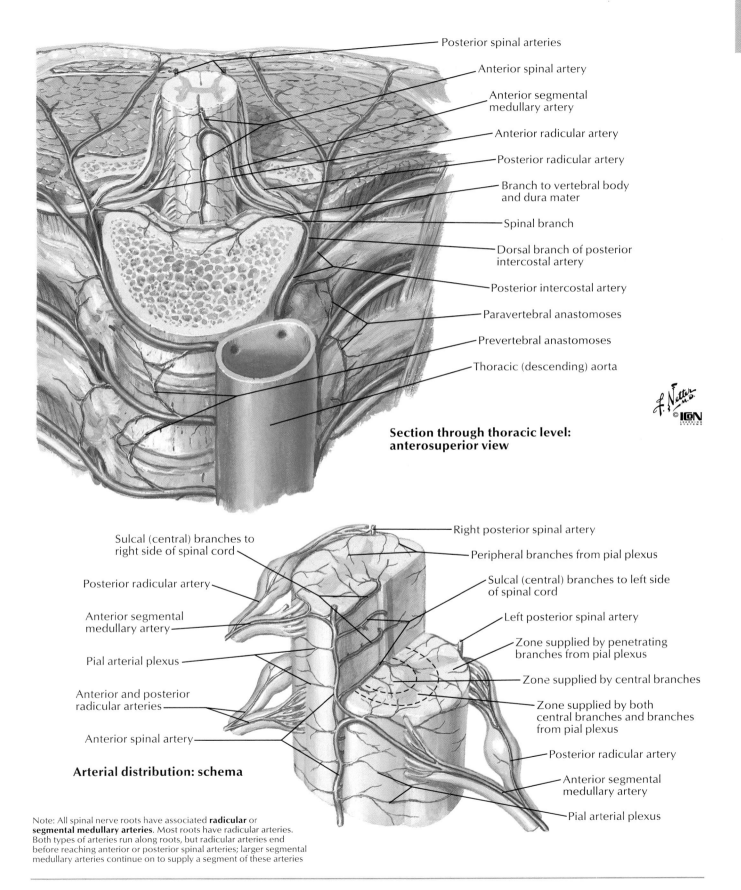

Posterior spinal arteries

Anterior spinal artery

Anterior segmental medullary artery

Anterior radicular artery

Posterior radicular artery

Branch to vertebral body and dura mater

Spinal branch

Dorsal branch of posterior intercostal artery

Posterior intercostal artery

Paravertebral anastomoses

Prevertebral anastomoses

Thoracic (descending) aorta

Section through thoracic level: anterosuperior view

Sulcal (central) branches to right side of spinal cord

Posterior radicular artery

Anterior segmental medullary artery

Pial arterial plexus

Anterior and posterior radicular arteries

Anterior spinal artery

Arterial distribution: schema

Right posterior spinal artery

Peripheral branches from pial plexus

Sulcal (central) branches to left side of spinal cord

Left posterior spinal artery

Zone supplied by penetrating branches from pial plexus

Zone supplied by central branches

Zone supplied by both central branches and branches from pial plexus

Posterior radicular artery

Anterior segmental medullary artery

Pial arterial plexus

Note: All spinal nerve roots have associated **radicular** or **segmental medullary arteries**. Most roots have radicular arteries. Both types of arteries run along roots, but radicular arteries end before reaching anterior or posterior spinal arteries; larger segmental medullary arteries continue on to supply a segment of these arteries

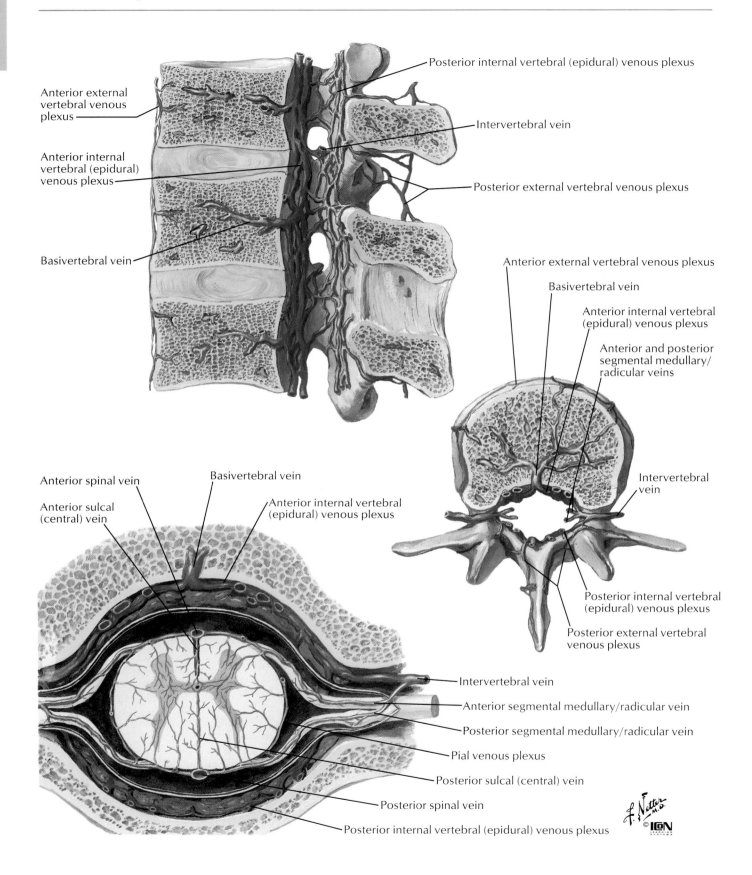

Anterior external vertebral venous plexus

Anterior internal vertebral (epidural) venous plexus

Basivertebral vein

Posterior internal vertebral (epidural) venous plexus

Intervertebral vein

Posterior external vertebral venous plexus

Anterior external vertebral venous plexus

Basivertebral vein

Anterior internal vertebral (epidural) venous plexus

Anterior and posterior segmental medullary/radicular veins

Intervertebral vein

Posterior internal vertebral (epidural) venous plexus

Posterior external vertebral venous plexus

Anterior spinal vein

Anterior sulcal (central) vein

Basivertebral vein

Anterior internal vertebral (epidural) venous plexus

Intervertebral vein

Anterior segmental medullary/radicular vein

Posterior segmental medullary/radicular vein

Pial venous plexus

Posterior sulcal (central) vein

Posterior spinal vein

Posterior internal vertebral (epidural) venous plexus

PLATE 166

BACK AND SPINAL CORD

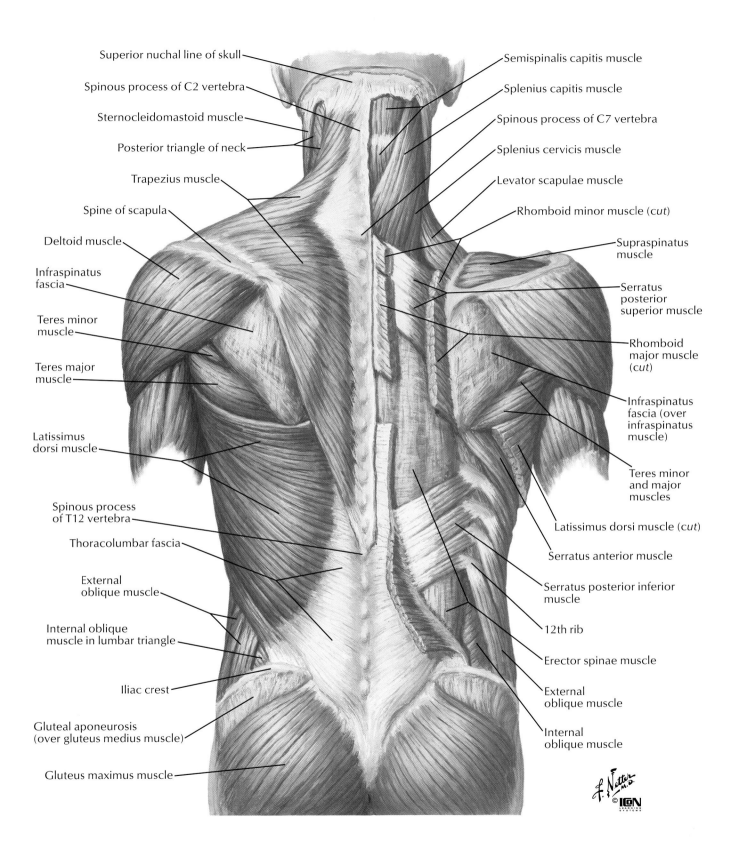

Superior nuchal line of skull

Spinous process of C2 vertebra

Sternocleidomastoid muscle

Posterior triangle of neck

Trapezius muscle

Spine of scapula

Deltoid muscle

Infraspinatus fascia

Teres minor muscle

Teres major muscle

Latissimus dorsi muscle

Spinous process of T12 vertebra

Thoracolumbar fascia

External oblique muscle

Internal oblique muscle in lumbar triangle

Iliac crest

Gluteal aponeurosis (over gluteus medius muscle)

Gluteus maximus muscle

Semispinalis capitis muscle

Splenius capitis muscle

Spinous process of C7 vertebra

Splenius cervicis muscle

Levator scapulae muscle

Rhomboid minor muscle (cut)

Supraspinatus muscle

Serratus posterior superior muscle

Rhomboid major muscle (cut)

Infraspinatus fascia (over infraspinatus muscle)

Teres minor and major muscles

Latissimus dorsi muscle (cut)

Serratus anterior muscle

Serratus posterior inferior muscle

12th rib

Erector spinae muscle

External oblique muscle

Internal oblique muscle

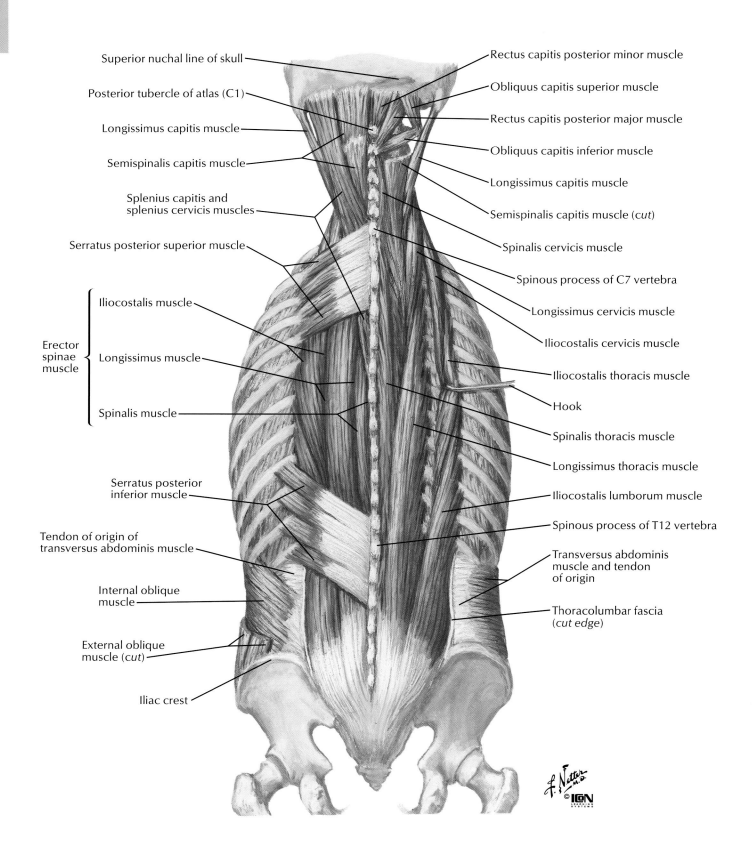

Superior nuchal line of skull

Posterior tubercle of atlas (C1)

Longissimus capitis muscle

Semispinalis capitis muscle

Splenius capitis and splenius cervicis muscles

Serratus posterior superior muscle

Erector spinae muscle
- Iliocostalis muscle
- Longissimus muscle
- Spinalis muscle

Serratus posterior inferior muscle

Tendon of origin of transversus abdominis muscle

Internal oblique muscle

External oblique muscle (cut)

Iliac crest

Rectus capitis posterior minor muscle

Obliquus capitis superior muscle

Rectus capitis posterior major muscle

Obliquus capitis inferior muscle

Longissimus capitis muscle

Semispinalis capitis muscle (cut)

Spinalis cervicis muscle

Spinous process of C7 vertebra

Longissimus cervicis muscle

Iliocostalis cervicis muscle

Iliocostalis thoracis muscle

Hook

Spinalis thoracis muscle

Longissimus thoracis muscle

Iliocostalis lumborum muscle

Spinous process of T12 vertebra

Transversus abdominis muscle and tendon of origin

Thoracolumbar fascia (cut edge)

PLATE 168

BACK AND SPINAL CORD

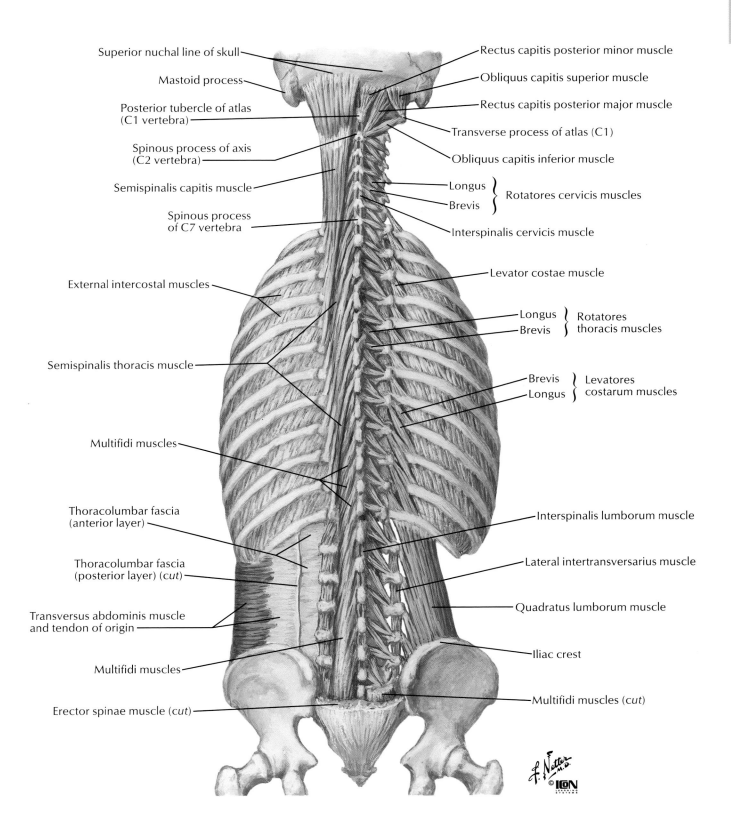

Superior nuchal line of skull

Mastoid process

Posterior tubercle of atlas (C1 vertebra)

Spinous process of axis (C2 vertebra)

Semispinalis capitis muscle

Spinous process of C7 vertebra

External intercostal muscles

Semispinalis thoracis muscle

Multifidi muscles

Thoracolumbar fascia (anterior layer)

Thoracolumbar fascia (posterior layer) (*cut*)

Transversus abdominis muscle and tendon of origin

Multifidi muscles

Erector spinae muscle (*cut*)

Rectus capitis posterior minor muscle

Obliquus capitis superior muscle

Rectus capitis posterior major muscle

Transverse process of atlas (C1)

Obliquus capitis inferior muscle

Longus

Brevis
} Rotatores cervicis muscles

Interspinalis cervicis muscle

Levator costae muscle

Longus

Brevis
} Rotatores thoracis muscles

Brevis

Longus
} Levatores costarum muscles

Interspinalis lumborum muscle

Lateral intertransversarius muscle

Quadratus lumborum muscle

Iliac crest

Multifidi muscles (*cut*)

SEE ALSO PLATES 173, 187, 246, 250

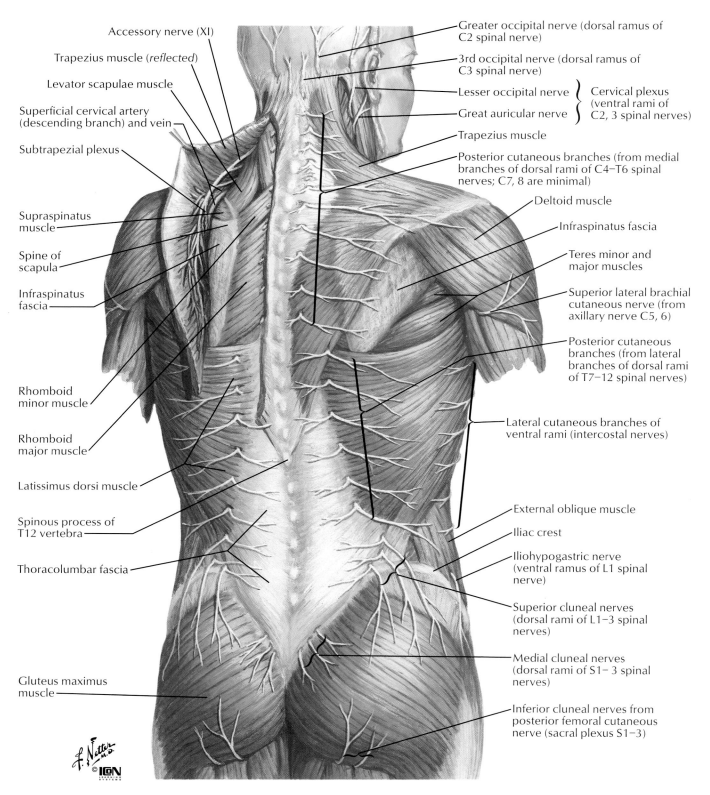

Accessory nerve (XI)

Trapezius muscle (reflected)

Levator scapulae muscle

Superficial cervical artery (descending branch) and vein

Subtrapezial plexus

Supraspinatus muscle

Spine of scapula

Infraspinatus fascia

Rhomboid minor muscle

Rhomboid major muscle

Latissimus dorsi muscle

Spinous process of T12 vertebra

Thoracolumbar fascia

Gluteus maximus muscle

Greater occipital nerve (dorsal ramus of C2 spinal nerve)

3rd occipital nerve (dorsal ramus of C3 spinal nerve)

Lesser occipital nerve

Great auricular nerve

Cervical plexus (ventral rami of C2, 3 spinal nerves)

Trapezius muscle

Posterior cutaneous branches (from medial branches of dorsal rami of C4–T6 spinal nerves; C7, 8 are minimal)

Deltoid muscle

Infraspinatus fascia

Teres minor and major muscles

Superior lateral brachial cutaneous nerve (from axillary nerve C5, 6)

Posterior cutaneous branches (from lateral branches of dorsal rami of T7–12 spinal nerves)

Lateral cutaneous branches of ventral rami (intercostal nerves)

External oblique muscle

Iliac crest

Iliohypogastric nerve (ventral ramus of L1 spinal nerve)

Superior cluneal nerves (dorsal rami of L1–3 spinal nerves)

Medial cluneal nerves (dorsal rami of S1–3 spinal nerves)

Inferior cluneal nerves from posterior femoral cutaneous nerve (sacral plexus S1–3)

PLATE 170

BACK AND SPINAL CORD

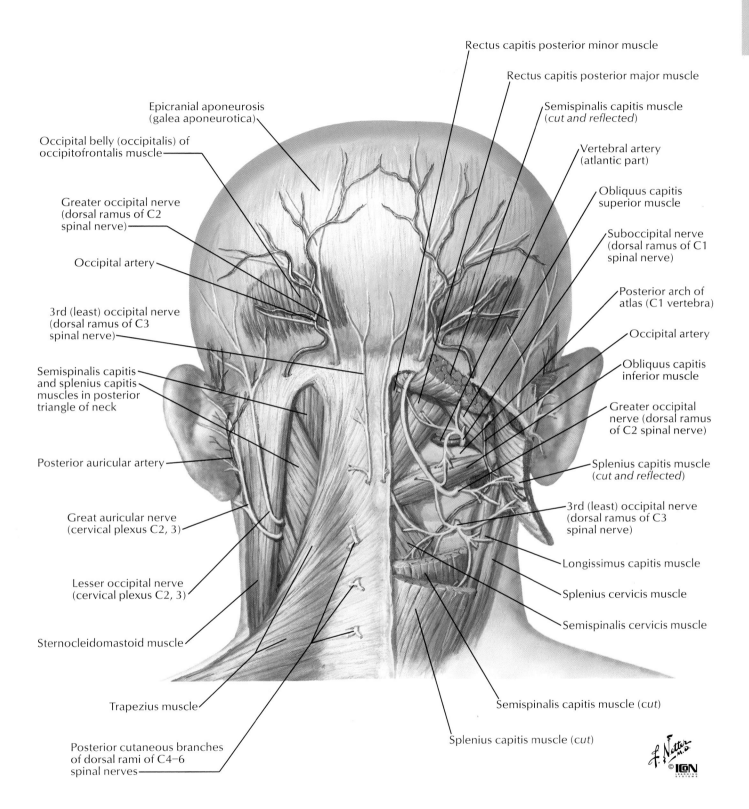

Rectus capitis posterior minor muscle

Rectus capitis posterior major muscle

Semispinalis capitis muscle
(*cut and reflected*)

Epicranial aponeurosis
(galea aponeurotica)

Vertebral artery
(atlantic part)

Occipital belly (occipitalis) of
occipitofrontalis muscle

Obliquus capitis
superior muscle

Greater occipital nerve
(dorsal ramus of C2
spinal nerve)

Suboccipital nerve
(dorsal ramus of C1
spinal nerve)

Occipital artery

Posterior arch of
atlas (C1 vertebra)

3rd (least) occipital nerve
(dorsal ramus of C3
spinal nerve)

Occipital artery

Obliquus capitis
inferior muscle

Semispinalis capitis
and splenius capitis
muscles in posterior
triangle of neck

Greater occipital
nerve (dorsal ramus
of C2 spinal nerve)

Posterior auricular artery

Splenius capitis muscle
(*cut and reflected*)

Great auricular nerve
(cervical plexus C2, 3)

3rd (least) occipital nerve
(dorsal ramus of C3
spinal nerve)

Longissimus capitis muscle

Lesser occipital nerve
(cervical plexus C2, 3)

Splenius cervicis muscle

Semispinalis cervicis muscle

Sternocleidomastoid muscle

Trapezius muscle

Semispinalis capitis muscle (*cut*)

Splenius capitis muscle (*cut*)

Posterior cutaneous branches
of dorsal rami of C4–6
spinal nerves

MUSCLES AND NERVES

PLATE 171

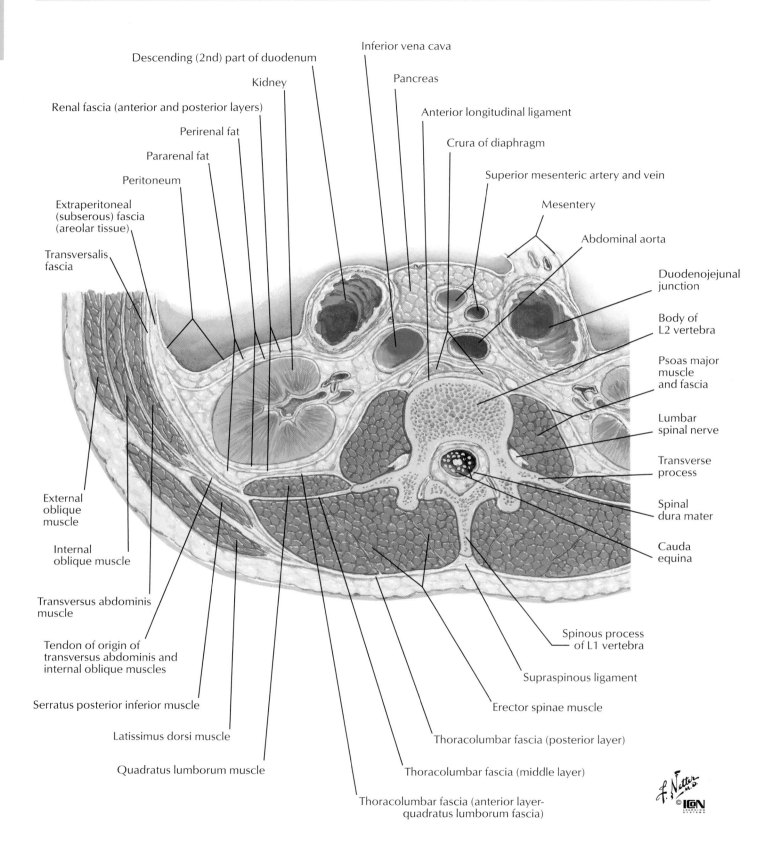

Descending (2nd) part of duodenum

Kidney

Renal fascia (anterior and posterior layers)

Perirenal fat

Pararenal fat

Peritoneum

Extraperitoneal (subserous) fascia (areolar tissue)

Transversalis fascia

Inferior vena cava

Pancreas

Anterior longitudinal ligament

Crura of diaphragm

Superior mesenteric artery and vein

Mesentery

Abdominal aorta

Duodenojejunal junction

Body of L2 vertebra

Psoas major muscle and fascia

Lumbar spinal nerve

Transverse process

Spinal dura mater

Cauda equina

External oblique muscle

Internal oblique muscle

Transversus abdominis muscle

Tendon of origin of transversus abdominis and internal oblique muscles

Serratus posterior inferior muscle

Latissimus dorsi muscle

Quadratus lumborum muscle

Spinous process of L1 vertebra

Supraspinous ligament

Erector spinae muscle

Thoracolumbar fascia (posterior layer)

Thoracolumbar fascia (middle layer)

Thoracolumbar fascia (anterior layer-quadratus lumborum fascia)

PLATE 172

BACK AND SPINAL CORD

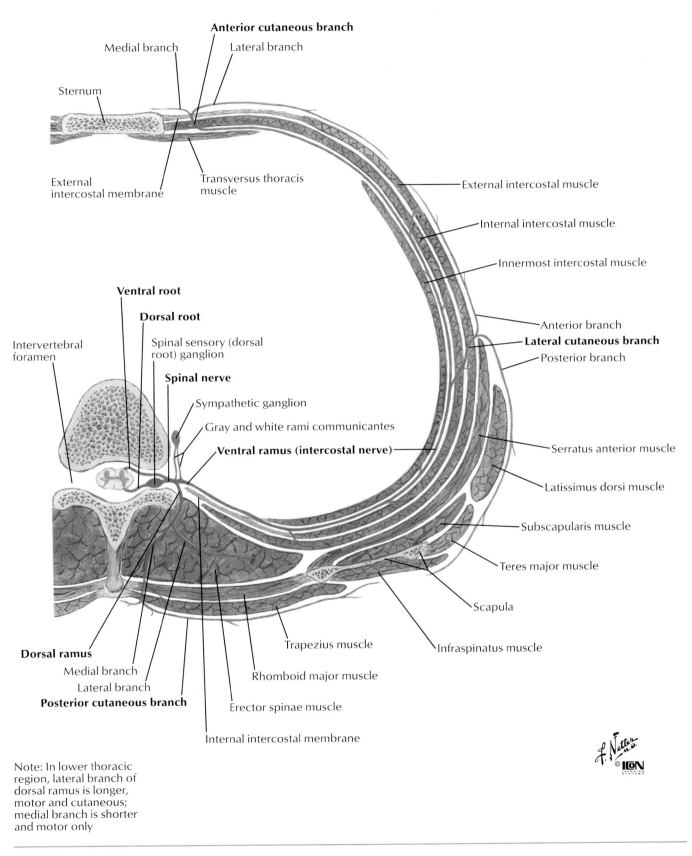

Anterior cutaneous branch

Medial branch

Lateral branch

Sternum

External intercostal muscle

External
intercostal membrane

Transversus thoracis
muscle

Internal intercostal muscle

Innermost intercostal muscle

Ventral root

Dorsal root

Spinal sensory (dorsal
root) ganglion

Anterior branch

Lateral cutaneous branch

Posterior branch

Intervertebral
foramen

Spinal nerve

Sympathetic ganglion

Gray and white rami communicantes

Ventral ramus (intercostal nerve)

Serratus anterior muscle

Latissimus dorsi muscle

Subscapularis muscle

Teres major muscle

Scapula

Infraspinatus muscle

Dorsal ramus

Medial branch

Lateral branch

Posterior cutaneous branch

Trapezius muscle

Rhomboid major muscle

Erector spinae muscle

Internal intercostal membrane

Note: In lower thoracic
region, lateral branch of
dorsal ramus is longer,
motor and cutaneous;
medial branch is shorter
and motor only

Section III
THORAX

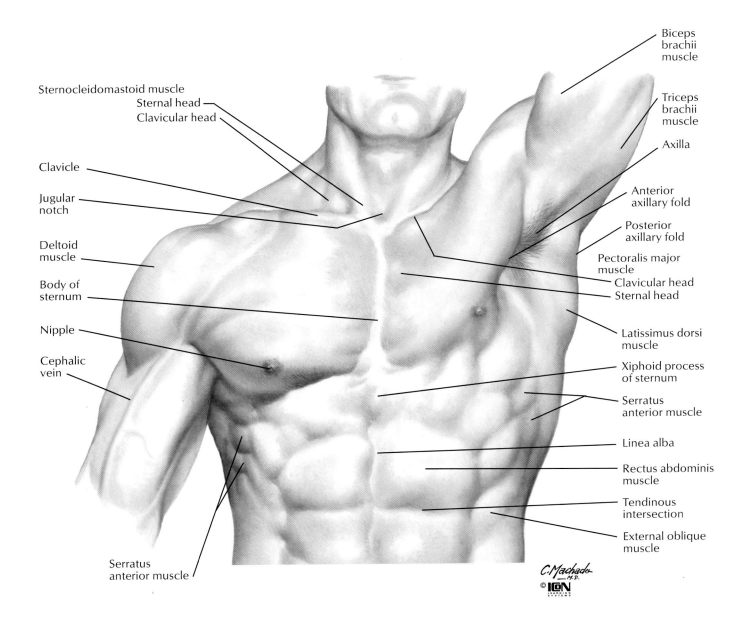

Biceps
brachii
muscle

Sternocleidomastoid muscle
Sternal head
Clavicular head

Triceps
brachii
muscle

Axilla

Clavicle

Anterior
axillary fold

Jugular
notch

Posterior
axillary fold

Deltoid
muscle

Pectoralis major
muscle

Body of
sternum

Clavicular head
Sternal head

Nipple

Latissimus dorsi
muscle

Cephalic
vein

Xiphoid process
of sternum

Serratus
anterior muscle

Linea alba

Rectus abdominis
muscle

Tendinous
intersection

External oblique
muscle

Serratus
anterior muscle

C. Machado
M.D.
© ICON
LEARNING
SYSTEMS

Mammary Gland

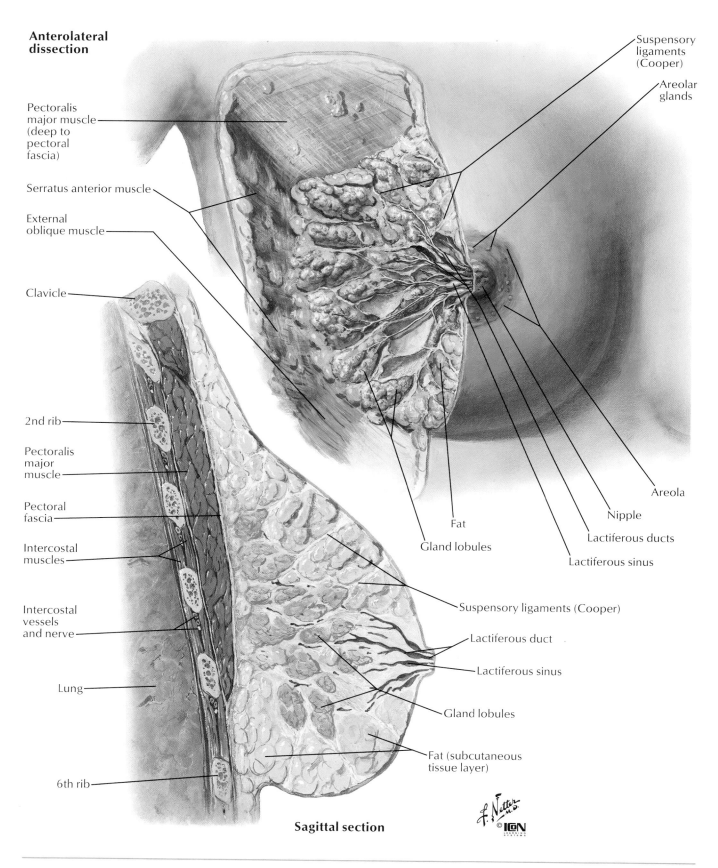

Anterolateral dissection

Pectoralis major muscle (deep to pectoral fascia)

Serratus anterior muscle

External oblique muscle

Clavicle

2nd rib

Pectoralis major muscle

Pectoral fascia

Intercostal muscles

Intercostal vessels and nerve

Lung

6th rib

Suspensory ligaments (Cooper)

Areolar glands

Areola

Nipple

Lactiferous ducts

Lactiferous sinus

Fat

Gland lobules

Suspensory ligaments (Cooper)

Lactiferous duct

Lactiferous sinus

Gland lobules

Fat (subcutaneous tissue layer)

Sagittal section

PLATE 175

THORAX

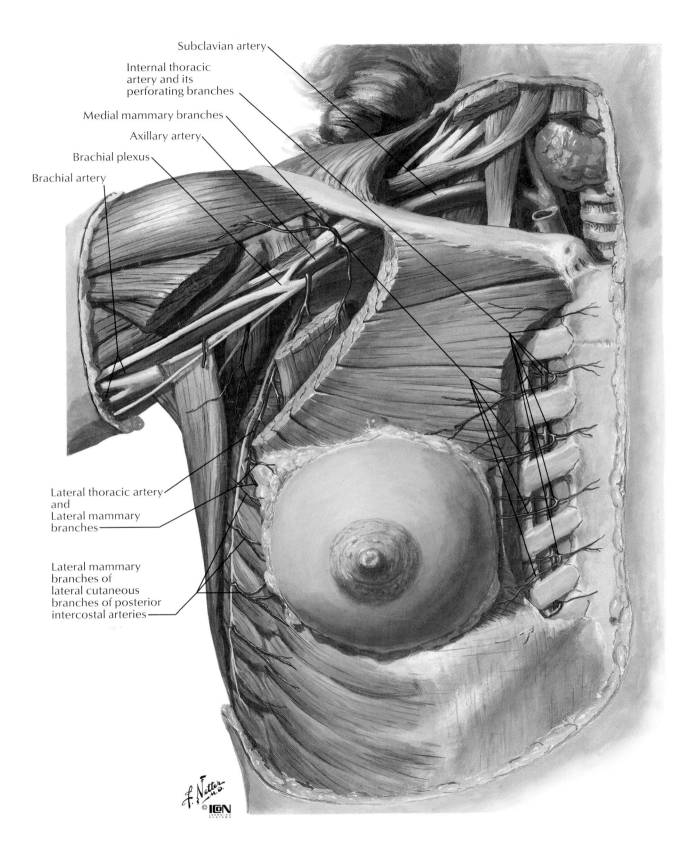

Subclavian artery

Internal thoracic artery and its perforating branches

Medial mammary branches

Axillary artery

Brachial plexus

Brachial artery

Lateral thoracic artery and Lateral mammary branches

Lateral mammary branches of lateral cutaneous branches of posterior intercostal arteries

Lymph Vessels and Nodes of Mammary Gland

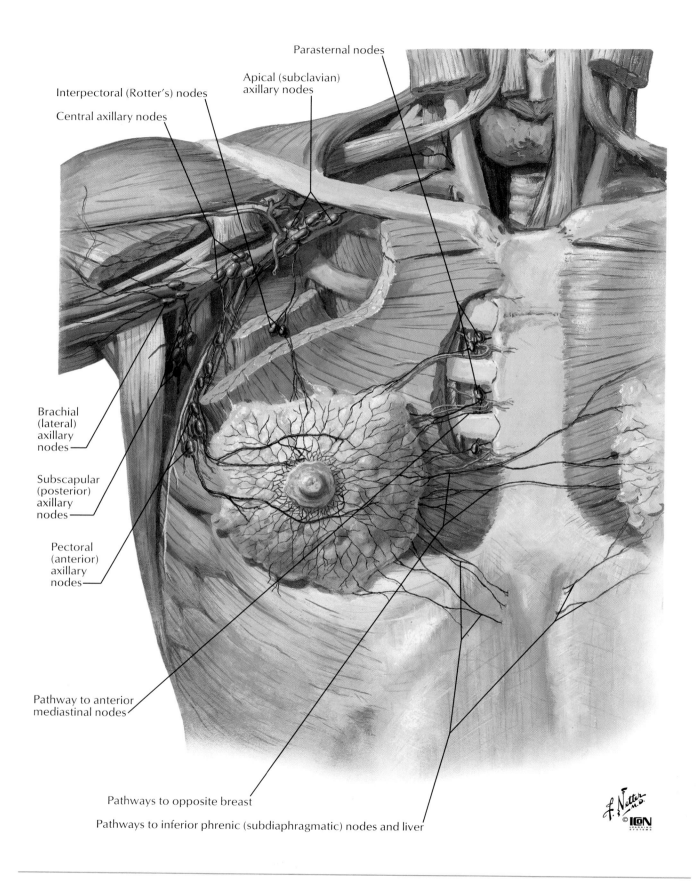

Parasternal nodes

Apical (subclavian) axillary nodes

Interpectoral (Rotter's) nodes

Central axillary nodes

Brachial (lateral) axillary nodes

Subscapular (posterior) axillary nodes

Pectoral (anterior) axillary nodes

Pathway to anterior mediastinal nodes

Pathways to opposite breast

Pathways to inferior phrenic (subdiaphragmatic) nodes and liver

PLATE 177

THORAX

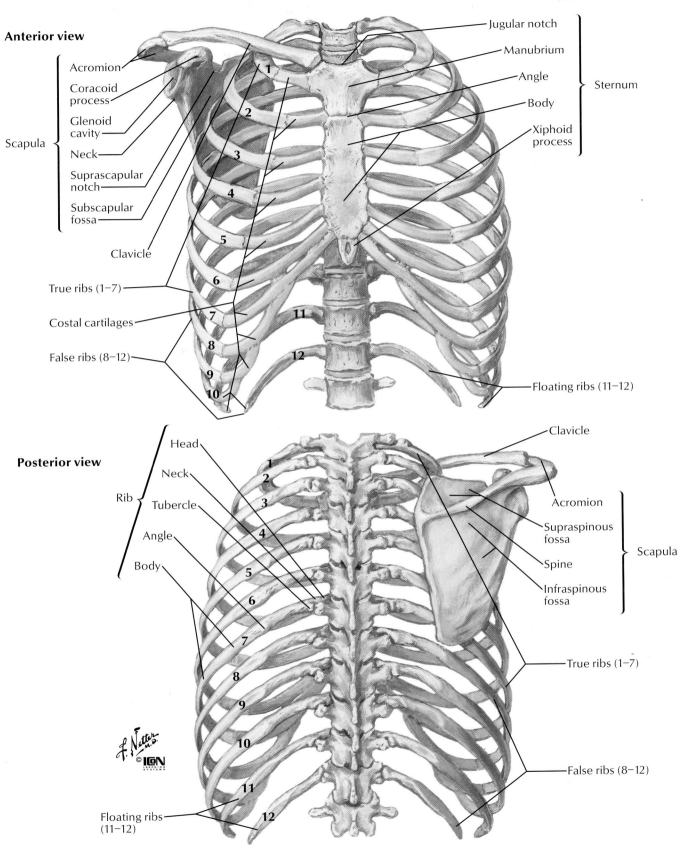

Anterior view

Acromion
Coracoid process
Glenoid cavity
Neck
Suprascapular notch
Subscapular fossa

Scapula

Clavicle

True ribs (1–7)

Costal cartilages

False ribs (8–12)

Jugular notch
Manubrium
Angle
Body
Xiphoid process

Sternum

Floating ribs (11–12)

Posterior view

Head
Neck
Tubercle
Angle
Body

Rib

Clavicle

Acromion
Supraspinous fossa
Spine
Infraspinous fossa

Scapula

True ribs (1–7)

False ribs (8–12)

Floating ribs (11–12)

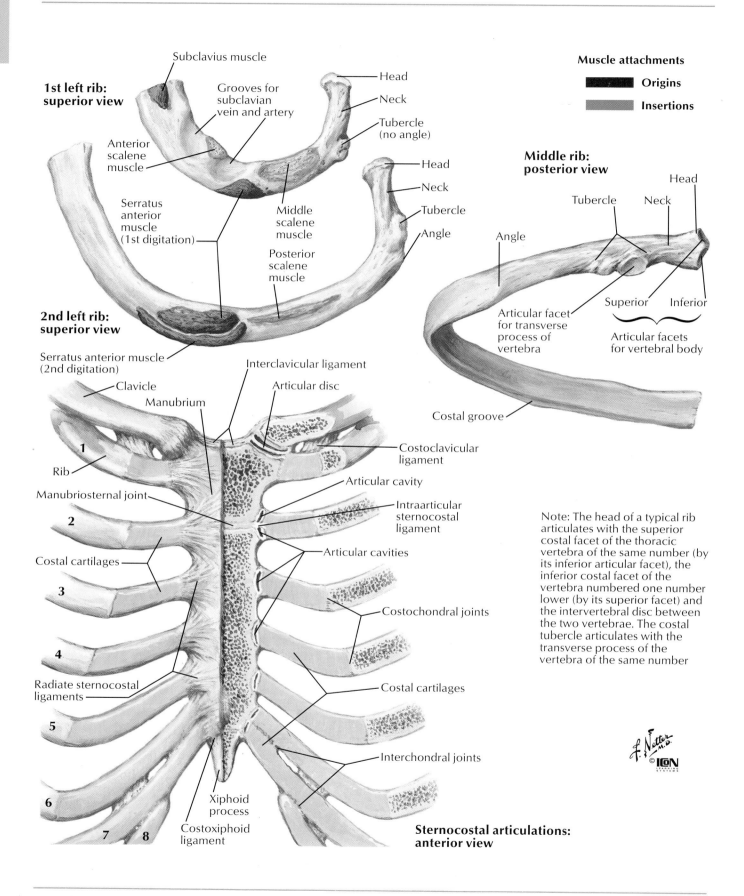

1st left rib: superior view

Subclavius muscle

Grooves for subclavian vein and artery

Anterior scalene muscle

Head

Neck

Tubercle (no angle)

Serratus anterior muscle (1st digitation)

Head

Neck

Tubercle

Angle

Middle scalene muscle

Posterior scalene muscle

2nd left rib: superior view

Serratus anterior muscle (2nd digitation)

Muscle attachments

Origins

Insertions

Middle rib: posterior view

Tubercle

Neck

Head

Angle

Head

Tubercle

Neck

Superior

Inferior

Articular facet for transverse process of vertebra

Articular facets for vertebral body

Costal groove

Clavicle

Manubrium

Interclavicular ligament

Articular disc

1

Rib

Manubriosternal joint

2

Costal cartilages

3

4

Radiate sternocostal ligaments

5

6

7   8

Xiphoid process

Costoxiphoid ligament

Costoclavicular ligament

Articular cavity

Intraarticular sternocostal ligament

Articular cavities

Costochondral joints

Costal cartilages

Interchondral joints

Sternocostal articulations: anterior view

Note: The head of a typical rib articulates with the superior costal facet of the thoracic vertebra of the same number (by its inferior articular facet), the inferior costal facet of the vertebra numbered one number lower (by its superior facet) and the intervertebral disc between the two vertebrae. The costal tubercle articulates with the transverse process of the vertebra of the same number

PLATE 179

THORAX

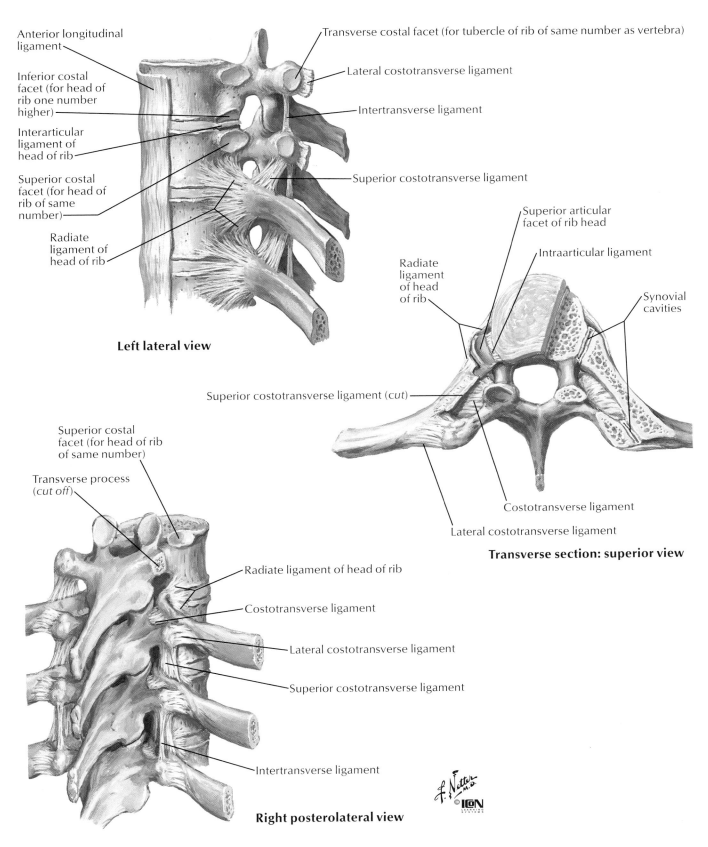

Anterior longitudinal ligament

Inferior costal facet (for head of rib one number higher)

Interarticular ligament of head of rib

Superior costal facet (for head of rib of same number)

Radiate ligament of head of rib

Transverse costal facet (for tubercle of rib of same number as vertebra)

Lateral costotransverse ligament

Intertransverse ligament

Superior costotransverse ligament

Left lateral view

Radiate ligament of head of rib

Superior articular facet of rib head

Intraarticular ligament

Synovial cavities

Superior costotransverse ligament (*cut*)

Costotransverse ligament

Lateral costotransverse ligament

Transverse section: superior view

Superior costal facet (for head of rib of same number)

Transverse process (*cut off*)

Radiate ligament of head of rib

Costotransverse ligament

Lateral costotransverse ligament

Superior costotransverse ligament

Intertransverse ligament

Right posterolateral view

SEE ALSO PLATES 29, 412, 413

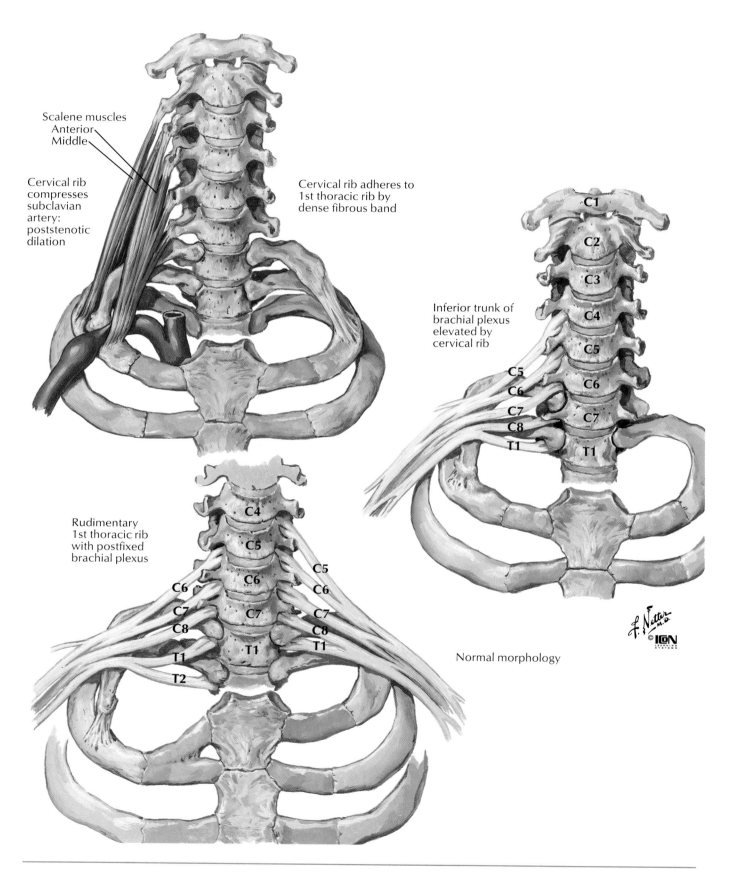

Scalene muscles
Anterior
Middle

Cervical rib compresses subclavian artery: poststenotic dilation

Cervical rib adheres to 1st thoracic rib by dense fibrous band

Inferior trunk of brachial plexus elevated by cervical rib

C1
C2
C3
C4
C5
C6
C7
T1

C5
C6
C7
C8
T1

Rudimentary 1st thoracic rib with postfixed brachial plexus

C4
C5
C6
C7
T1
T2

C6
C7
C8
T1

C5
C6
C7
C8
T1

Normal morphology

PLATE 181

THORAX

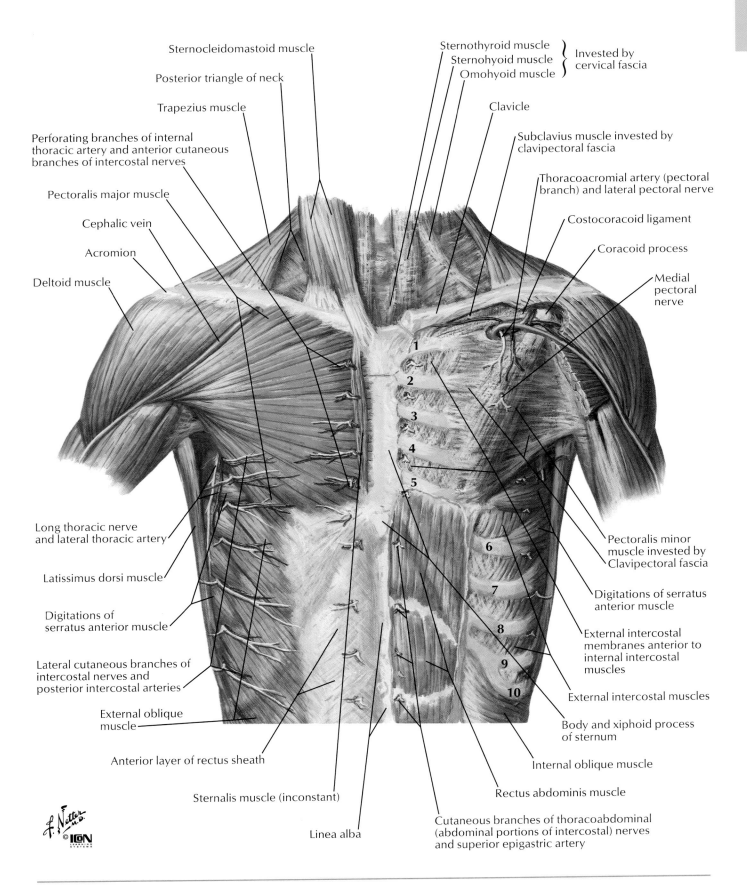

Sternocleidomastoid muscle

Posterior triangle of neck

Trapezius muscle

Perforating branches of internal thoracic artery and anterior cutaneous branches of intercostal nerves

Pectoralis major muscle

Cephalic vein

Acromion

Deltoid muscle

Long thoracic nerve and lateral thoracic artery

Latissimus dorsi muscle

Digitations of serratus anterior muscle

Lateral cutaneous branches of intercostal nerves and posterior intercostal arteries

External oblique muscle

Anterior layer of rectus sheath

Sternalis muscle (inconstant)

Linea alba

Sternothyroid muscle
Sternohyoid muscle } Invested by cervical fascia
Omohyoid muscle

Clavicle

Subclavius muscle invested by clavipectoral fascia

Thoracoacromial artery (pectoral branch) and lateral pectoral nerve

Costocoracoid ligament

Coracoid process

Medial pectoral nerve

Pectoralis minor muscle invested by Clavipectoral fascia

Digitations of serratus anterior muscle

External intercostal membranes anterior to internal intercostal muscles

External intercostal muscles

Body and xiphoid process of sternum

Internal oblique muscle

Rectus abdominis muscle

Cutaneous branches of thoracoabdominal (abdominal portions of intercostal) nerves and superior epigastric artery

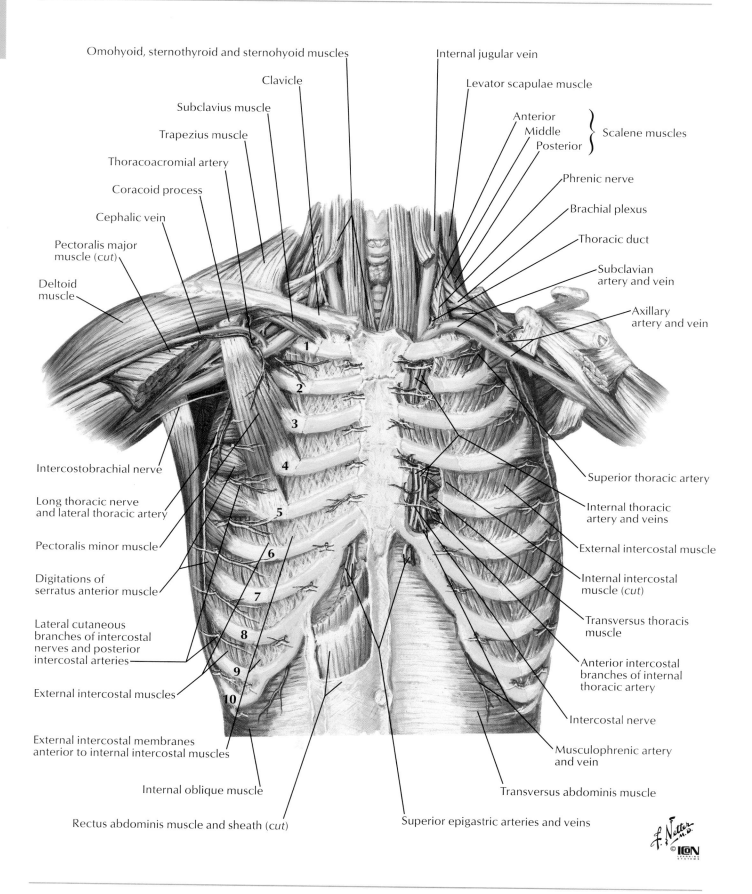

Omohyoid, sternothyroid and sternohyoid muscles

Clavicle

Subclavius muscle

Trapezius muscle

Thoracoacromial artery

Coracoid process

Cephalic vein

Pectoralis major muscle (cut)

Deltoid muscle

Intercostobrachial nerve

Long thoracic nerve and lateral thoracic artery

Pectoralis minor muscle

Digitations of serratus anterior muscle

Lateral cutaneous branches of intercostal nerves and posterior intercostal arteries

External intercostal muscles

External intercostal membranes anterior to internal intercostal muscles

Internal oblique muscle

Rectus abdominis muscle and sheath (cut)

Internal jugular vein

Levator scapulae muscle

Anterior
Middle   } Scalene muscles
Posterior

Phrenic nerve

Brachial plexus

Thoracic duct

Subclavian artery and vein

Axillary artery and vein

Superior thoracic artery

Internal thoracic artery and veins

External intercostal muscle

Internal intercostal muscle (cut)

Transversus thoracis muscle

Anterior intercostal branches of internal thoracic artery

Intercostal nerve

Musculophrenic artery and vein

Transversus abdominis muscle

Superior epigastric arteries and veins

1
2
3
4
5
6
7
8
9
10

PLATE 183

THORAX

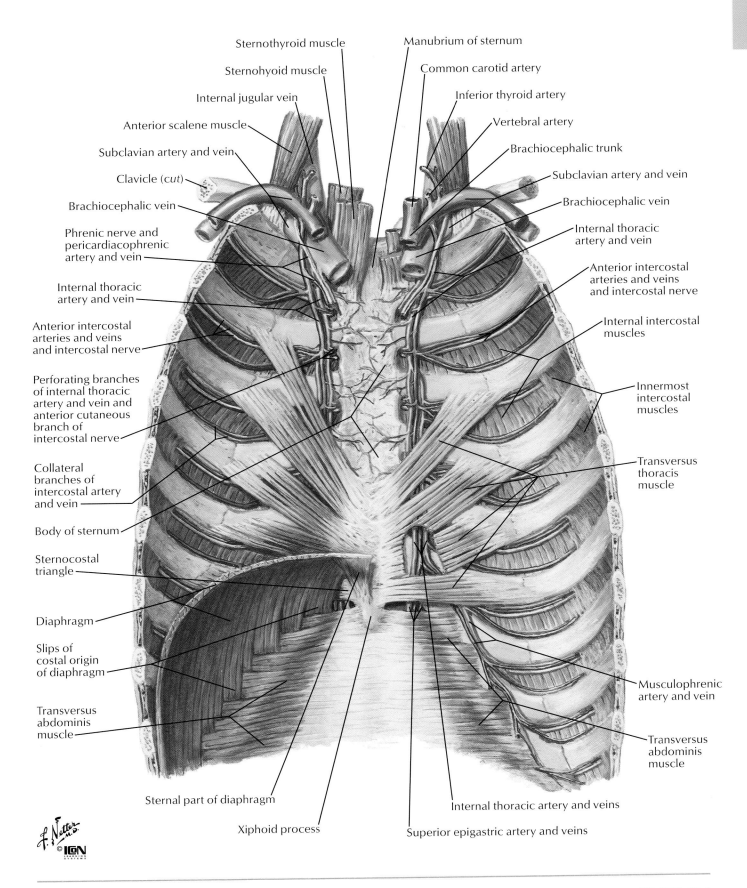

Sternothyroid muscle

Sternohyoid muscle

Internal jugular vein

Anterior scalene muscle

Subclavian artery and vein

Clavicle (cut)

Brachiocephalic vein

Phrenic nerve and pericardiacophrenic artery and vein

Internal thoracic artery and vein

Anterior intercostal arteries and veins and intercostal nerve

Perforating branches of internal thoracic artery and vein and anterior cutaneous branch of intercostal nerve

Collateral branches of intercostal artery and vein

Body of sternum

Sternocostal triangle

Diaphragm

Slips of costal origin of diaphragm

Transversus abdominis muscle

Manubrium of sternum

Common carotid artery

Inferior thyroid artery

Vertebral artery

Brachiocephalic trunk

Subclavian artery and vein

Brachiocephalic vein

Internal thoracic artery and vein

Anterior intercostal arteries and veins and intercostal nerve

Internal intercostal muscles

Innermost intercostal muscles

Transversus thoracis muscle

Musculophrenic artery and vein

Transversus abdominis muscle

Sternal part of diaphragm

Xiphoid process

Internal thoracic artery and veins

Superior epigastric artery and veins

Posterior and Lateral Thoracic Walls

SEE ALSO PLATES 167–169

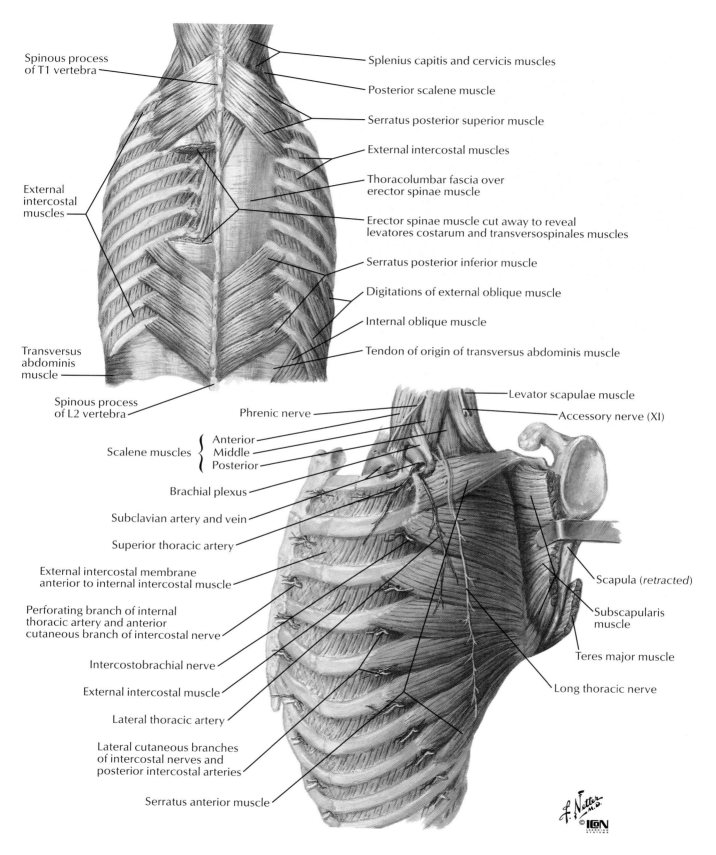

Spinous process of T1 vertebra

Splenius capitis and cervicis muscles

Posterior scalene muscle

Serratus posterior superior muscle

External intercostal muscles

Thoracolumbar fascia over erector spinae muscle

External intercostal muscles

Erector spinae muscle cut away to reveal levatores costarum and transversospinales muscles

Serratus posterior inferior muscle

Digitations of external oblique muscle

Internal oblique muscle

Tendon of origin of transversus abdominis muscle

Transversus abdominis muscle

Spinous process of L2 vertebra

Levator scapulae muscle

Phrenic nerve

Accessory nerve (XI)

Scalene muscles { Anterior Middle Posterior

Brachial plexus

Subclavian artery and vein

Superior thoracic artery

Scapula (retracted)

External intercostal membrane anterior to internal intercostal muscle

Subscapularis muscle

Perforating branch of internal thoracic artery and anterior cutaneous branch of intercostal nerve

Teres major muscle

Intercostobrachial nerve

Long thoracic nerve

External intercostal muscle

Lateral thoracic artery

Lateral cutaneous branches of intercostal nerves and posterior intercostal arteries

Serratus anterior muscle

PLATE 185

THORAX

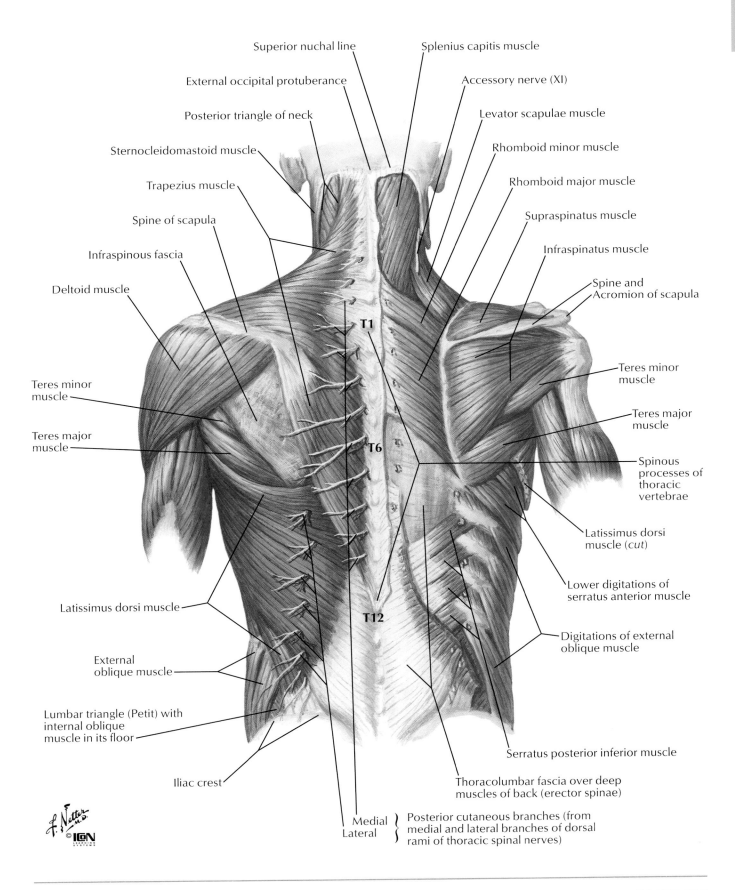

Superior nuchal line

Splenius capitis muscle

External occipital protuberance

Accessory nerve (XI)

Posterior triangle of neck

Levator scapulae muscle

Sternocleidomastoid muscle

Rhomboid minor muscle

Trapezius muscle

Rhomboid major muscle

Spine of scapula

Supraspinatus muscle

Infraspinous fascia

Infraspinatus muscle

Deltoid muscle

Spine and
Acromion of scapula

T1

Teres minor
muscle

Teres minor
muscle

Teres major
muscle

Teres major
muscle

T6

Spinous
processes of
thoracic
vertebrae

Latissimus dorsi
muscle (*cut*)

Latissimus dorsi muscle

T12

Lower digitations of
serratus anterior muscle

External
oblique muscle

Digitations of external
oblique muscle

Lumbar triangle (Petit) with
internal oblique
muscle in its floor

Serratus posterior inferior muscle

Iliac crest

Thoracolumbar fascia over deep
muscles of back (erector spinae)

Medial
Lateral

Posterior cutaneous branches (from
medial and lateral branches of dorsal
rami of thoracic spinal nerves)

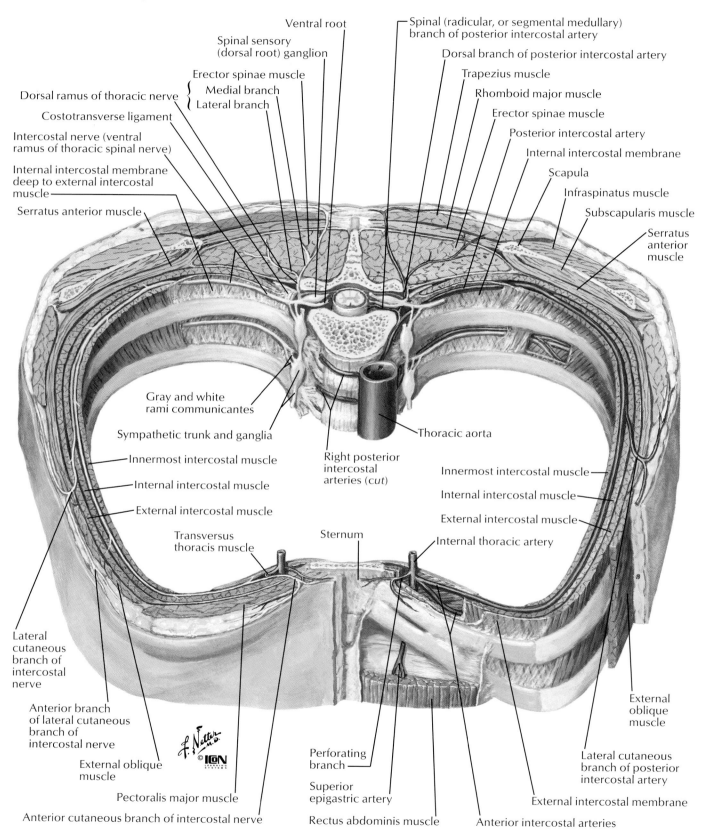

Ventral root

Spinal sensory
(dorsal root) ganglion

Spinal (radicular, or segmental medullary)
branch of posterior intercostal artery

Dorsal branch of posterior intercostal artery

Erector spinae muscle

Dorsal ramus of thoracic nerve { Medial branch
Lateral branch

Trapezius muscle

Rhomboid major muscle

Costotransverse ligament

Erector spinae muscle

Intercostal nerve (ventral
ramus of thoracic spinal nerve)

Posterior intercostal artery

Internal intercostal membrane

Internal intercostal membrane
deep to external intercostal
muscle

Scapula

Infraspinatus muscle

Serratus anterior muscle

Subscapularis muscle

Serratus
anterior
muscle

Gray and white
rami communicantes

Sympathetic trunk and ganglia

Innermost intercostal muscle

Internal intercostal muscle

External intercostal muscle

Thoracic aorta

Right posterior
intercostal
arteries (cut)

Innermost intercostal muscle

Internal intercostal muscle

External intercostal muscle

Transversus
thoracis muscle

Sternum

Internal thoracic artery

Lateral
cutaneous
branch of
intercostal
nerve

Anterior branch
of lateral cutaneous
branch of
intercostal nerve

External oblique
muscle

Pectoralis major muscle

Perforating
branch

Superior
epigastric artery

Anterior cutaneous branch of intercostal nerve

Rectus abdominis muscle

External
oblique
muscle

Lateral cutaneous
branch of posterior
intercostal artery

External intercostal membrane

Anterior intercostal arteries

F. Netter, M.D.
©ICON

PLATE 187

THORAX

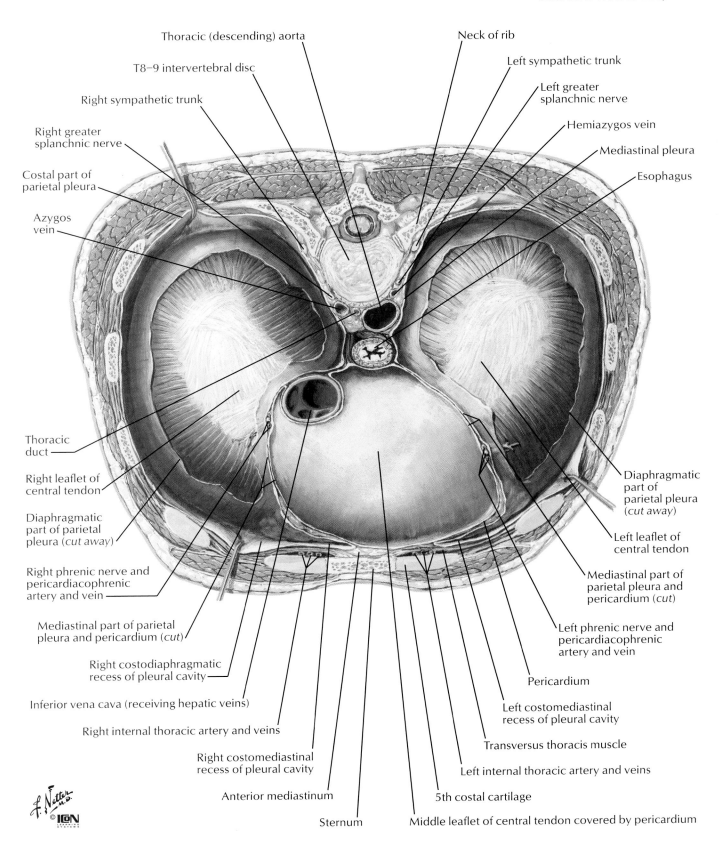

Thoracic (descending) aorta

T8–9 intervertebral disc

Right sympathetic trunk

Right greater
splanchnic nerve

Costal part of
parietal pleura

Azygos
vein

Thoracic
duct

Right leaflet of
central tendon

Diaphragmatic
part of parietal
pleura (*cut away*)

Right phrenic nerve and
pericardiacophrenic
artery and vein

Mediastinal part of parietal
pleura and pericardium (*cut*)

Right costodiaphragmatic
recess of pleural cavity

Inferior vena cava (receiving hepatic veins)

Right internal thoracic artery and veins

Right costomediastinal
recess of pleural cavity

Anterior mediastinum

Sternum

Neck of rib

Left sympathetic trunk

Left greater
splanchnic nerve

Hemiazygos vein

Mediastinal pleura

Esophagus

Diaphragmatic
part of
parietal pleura
(*cut away*)

Left leaflet of
central tendon

Mediastinal part of
parietal pleura and
pericardium (*cut*)

Left phrenic nerve and
pericardiacophrenic
artery and vein

Pericardium

Left costomediastinal
recess of pleural cavity

Transversus thoracis muscle

Left internal thoracic artery and veins

5th costal cartilage

Middle leaflet of central tendon covered by pericardium

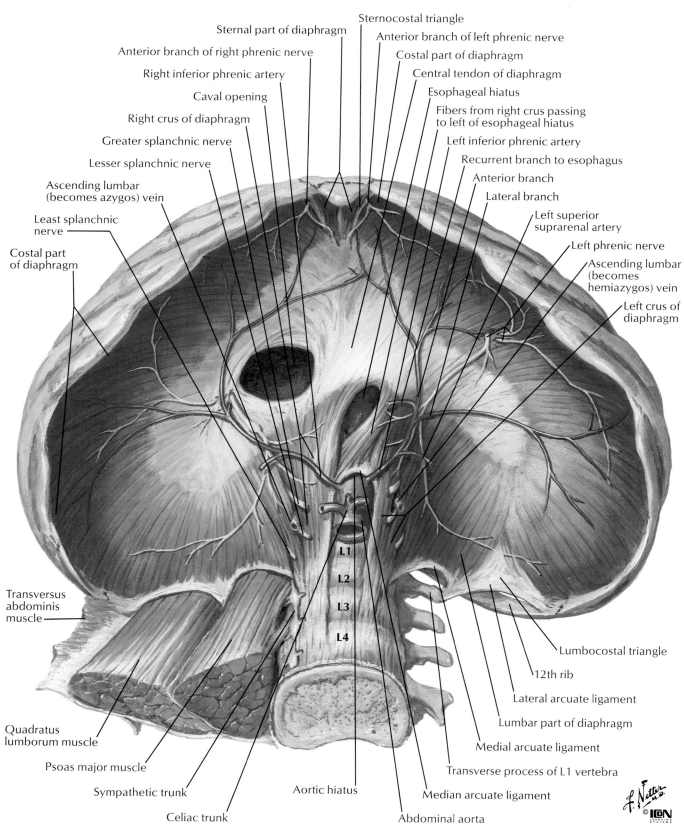

Sternocostal triangle

Sternal part of diaphragm

Anterior branch of left phrenic nerve

Anterior branch of right phrenic nerve

Costal part of diaphragm

Right inferior phrenic artery

Central tendon of diaphragm

Caval opening

Esophageal hiatus

Right crus of diaphragm

Fibers from right crus passing to left of esophageal hiatus

Greater splanchnic nerve

Left inferior phrenic artery

Lesser splanchnic nerve

Recurrent branch to esophagus

Ascending lumbar (becomes azygos) vein

Anterior branch

Lateral branch

Least splanchnic nerve

Left superior suprarenal artery

Costal part of diaphragm

Left phrenic nerve

Ascending lumbar (becomes hemiazygos) vein

Left crus of diaphragm

L1

L2

L3

L4

Transversus abdominis muscle

Lumbocostal triangle

12th rib

Lateral arcuate ligament

Quadratus lumborum muscle

Lumbar part of diaphragm

Psoas major muscle

Medial arcuate ligament

Sympathetic trunk

Transverse process of L1 vertebra

Celiac trunk

Aortic hiatus

Median arcuate ligament

Abdominal aorta

PLATE 189

THORAX

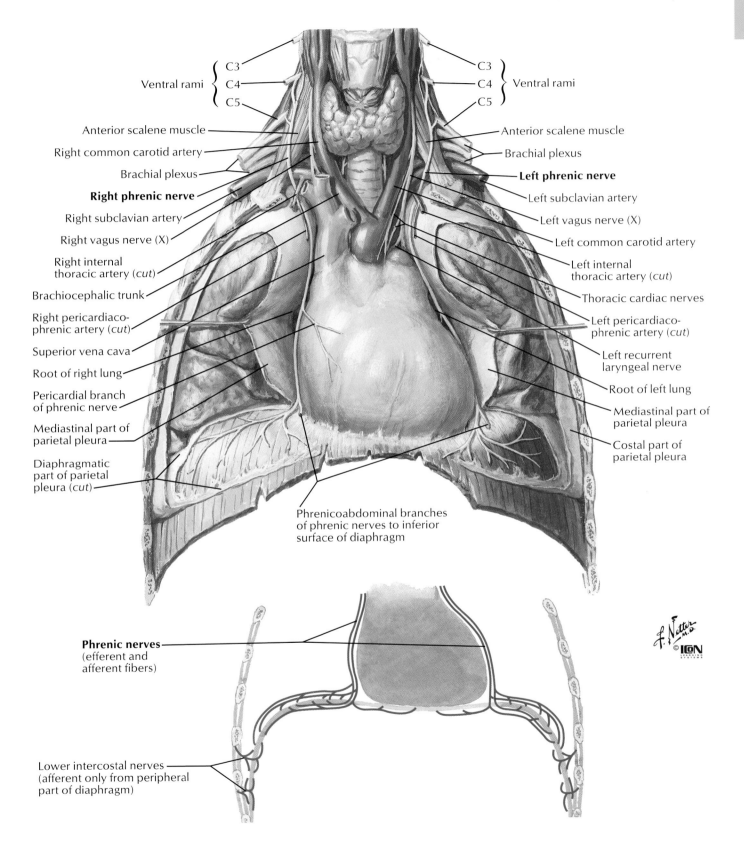

C3

Ventral rami { C4
C5

C3

C4 } Ventral rami
C5

Anterior scalene muscle

Right common carotid artery

Brachial plexus

Right phrenic nerve

Right subclavian artery

Right vagus nerve (X)

Right internal thoracic artery (*cut*)

Brachiocephalic trunk

Right pericardiaco-phrenic artery (*cut*)

Superior vena cava

Root of right lung

Pericardial branch of phrenic nerve

Mediastinal part of parietal pleura

Diaphragmatic part of parietal pleura (*cut*)

Anterior scalene muscle

Brachial plexus

Left phrenic nerve

Left subclavian artery

Left vagus nerve (X)

Left common carotid artery

Left internal thoracic artery (*cut*)

Thoracic cardiac nerves

Left pericardiaco-phrenic artery (*cut*)

Left recurrent laryngeal nerve

Root of left lung

Mediastinal part of parietal pleura

Costal part of parietal pleura

Phrenicoabdominal branches of phrenic nerves to inferior surface of diaphragm

Phrenic nerves (efferent and afferent fibers)

Lower intercostal nerves (afferent only from peripheral part of diaphragm)

Muscles of Respiration

FOR ADDITIONAL MUSCLES OF INSPIRATION SEE PLATES 169, 185

Muscles of inspiration

Muscles of expiration

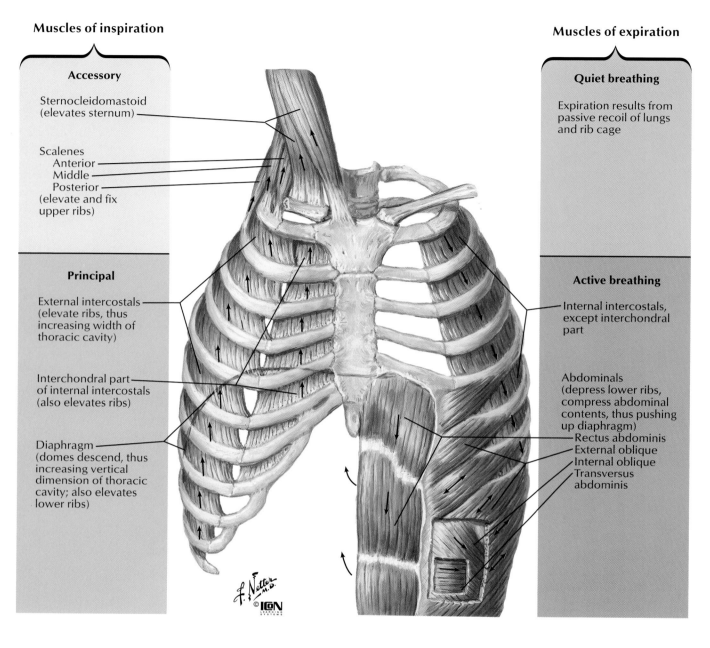

Accessory

Sternocleidomastoid
(elevates sternum)

Scalenes
    Anterior
    Middle
    Posterior
(elevate and fix
upper ribs)

Principal

External intercostals
(elevate ribs, thus
increasing width of
thoracic cavity)

Interchondral part
of internal intercostals
(also elevates ribs)

Diaphragm
(domes descend, thus
increasing vertical
dimension of thoracic
cavity; also elevates
lower ribs)

Quiet breathing

Expiration results from
passive recoil of lungs
and rib cage

Active breathing

Internal intercostals,
except interchondral
part

Abdominals
(depress lower ribs,
compress abdominal
contents, thus pushing
up diaphragm)
    Rectus abdominis
    External oblique
    Internal oblique
    Transversus
    abdominis

PLATE 191

THORAX

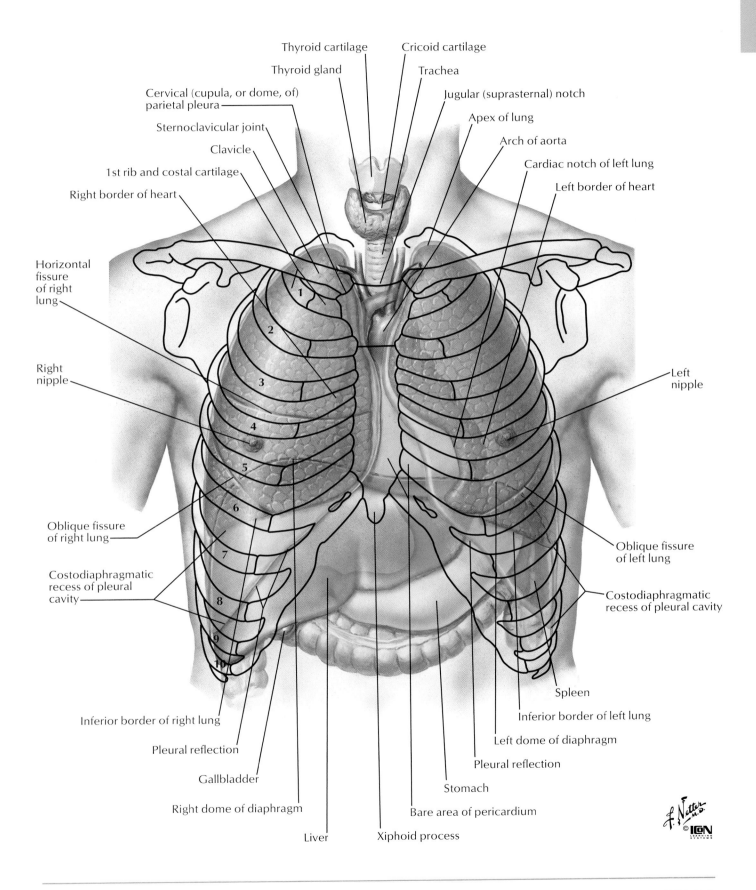

Thyroid cartilage

Thyroid gland

Cricoid cartilage

Trachea

Cervical (cupula, or dome, of) parietal pleura

Jugular (suprasternal) notch

Sternoclavicular joint

Apex of lung

Clavicle

Arch of aorta

1st rib and costal cartilage

Cardiac notch of left lung

Right border of heart

Left border of heart

Horizontal fissure of right lung

Right nipple

Left nipple

Oblique fissure of right lung

Oblique fissure of left lung

Costodiaphragmatic recess of pleural cavity

Costodiaphragmatic recess of pleural cavity

Inferior border of right lung

Spleen

Inferior border of left lung

Pleural reflection

Left dome of diaphragm

Gallbladder

Pleural reflection

Right dome of diaphragm

Stomach

Liver

Bare area of pericardium

Xiphoid process

Topography of Lungs: Posterior View

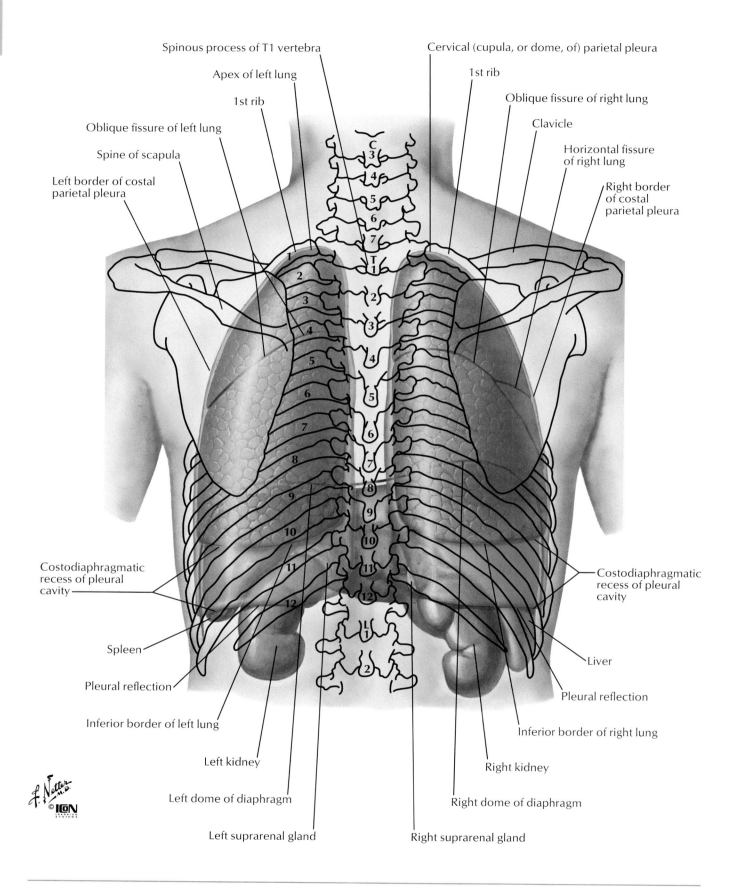

Spinous process of T1 vertebra

Apex of left lung

1st rib

Oblique fissure of left lung

Spine of scapula

Left border of costal parietal pleura

Cervical (cupula, or dome, of) parietal pleura

1st rib

Oblique fissure of right lung

Clavicle

Horizontal fissure of right lung

Right border of costal parietal pleura

Costodiaphragmatic recess of pleural cavity

Spleen

Pleural reflection

Inferior border of left lung

Left kidney

Left dome of diaphragm

Left suprarenal gland

Costodiaphragmatic recess of pleural cavity

Liver

Pleural reflection

Inferior border of right lung

Right kidney

Right dome of diaphragm

Right suprarenal gland

PLATE 193

THORAX

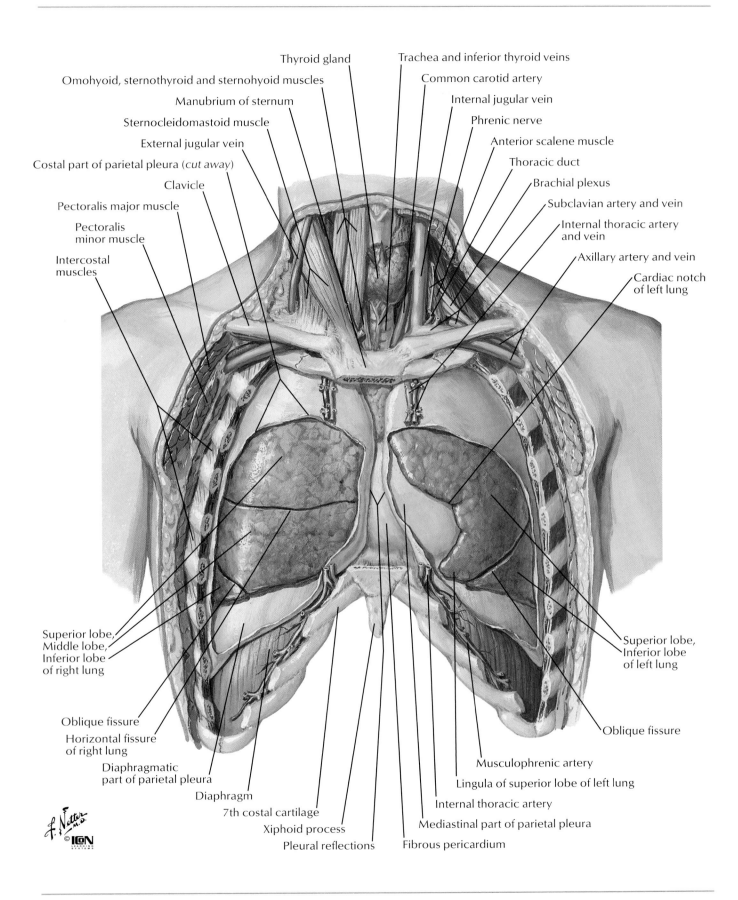

Thyroid gland

Trachea and inferior thyroid veins

Omohyoid, sternothyroid and sternohyoid muscles

Common carotid artery

Manubrium of sternum

Internal jugular vein

Sternocleidomastoid muscle

Phrenic nerve

External jugular vein

Anterior scalene muscle

Costal part of parietal pleura (*cut away*)

Thoracic duct

Clavicle

Brachial plexus

Pectoralis major muscle

Subclavian artery and vein

Pectoralis minor muscle

Internal thoracic artery and vein

Intercostal muscles

Axillary artery and vein

Cardiac notch of left lung

Superior lobe, Middle lobe, Inferior lobe of right lung

Superior lobe, Inferior lobe of left lung

Oblique fissure

Oblique fissure

Horizontal fissure of right lung

Diaphragmatic part of parietal pleura

Musculophrenic artery

Lingula of superior lobe of left lung

Diaphragm

Internal thoracic artery

7th costal cartilage

Mediastinal part of parietal pleura

Xiphoid process

Pleural reflections

Fibrous pericardium

Lungs: Medial Views

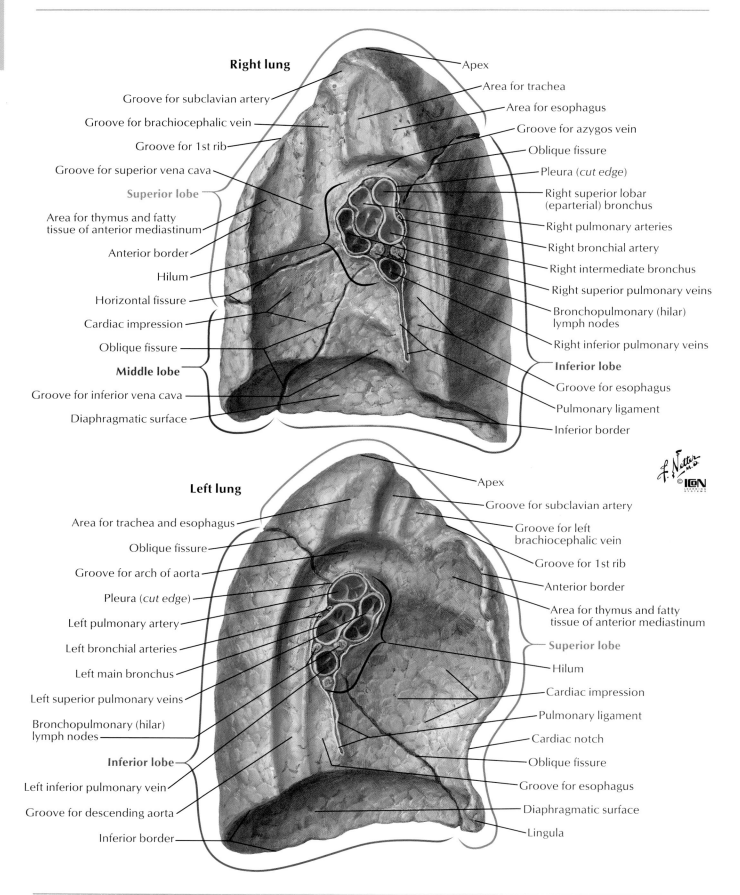

Right lung

Groove for subclavian artery
Groove for brachiocephalic vein
Groove for 1st rib
Groove for superior vena cava
Superior lobe
Area for thymus and fatty tissue of anterior mediastinum
Anterior border
Hilum
Horizontal fissure
Cardiac impression
Oblique fissure
Middle lobe
Groove for inferior vena cava
Diaphragmatic surface

Apex
Area for trachea
Area for esophagus
Groove for azygos vein
Oblique fissure
Pleura (*cut edge*)
Right superior lobar (eparterial) bronchus
Right pulmonary arteries
Right bronchial artery
Right intermediate bronchus
Right superior pulmonary veins
Bronchopulmonary (hilar) lymph nodes
Right inferior pulmonary veins
Inferior lobe
Groove for esophagus
Pulmonary ligament
Inferior border

Left lung

Area for trachea and esophagus
Oblique fissure
Groove for arch of aorta
Pleura (*cut edge*)
Left pulmonary artery
Left bronchial arteries
Left main bronchus
Left superior pulmonary veins
Bronchopulmonary (hilar) lymph nodes
Inferior lobe
Left inferior pulmonary vein
Groove for descending aorta
Inferior border

Apex
Groove for subclavian artery
Groove for left brachiocephalic vein
Groove for 1st rib
Anterior border
Area for thymus and fatty tissue of anterior mediastinum
Superior lobe
Hilum
Cardiac impression
Pulmonary ligament
Cardiac notch
Oblique fissure
Groove for esophagus
Diaphragmatic surface
Lingula

PLATE 195

THORAX

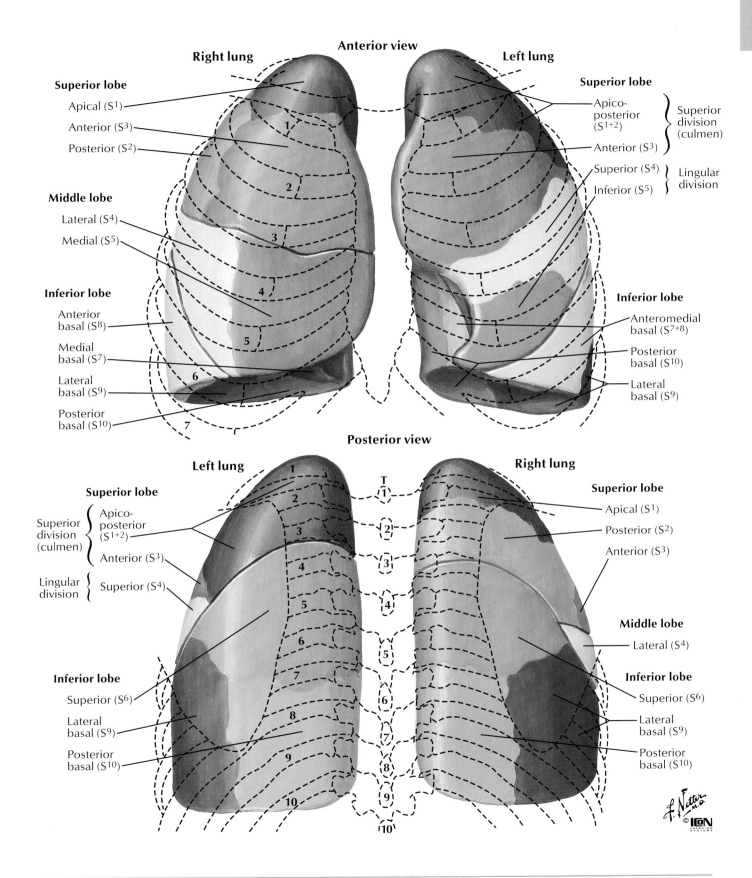

Anterior view

Right lung

Superior lobe
- Apical (S^1)
- Anterior (S^3)
- Posterior (S^2)

Middle lobe
- Lateral (S^4)
- Medial (S^5)

Inferior lobe
- Anterior basal (S^8)
- Medial basal (S^7)
- Lateral basal (S^9)
- Posterior basal (S^{10})

Left lung

Superior lobe
- Apico-posterior (S^{1+2}) } Superior division (culmen)
- Anterior (S^3) }
- Superior (S^4) } Lingular
- Inferior (S^5) } division

Inferior lobe
- Anteromedial basal (S^{7+8})
- Posterior basal (S^{10})
- Lateral basal (S^9)

Posterior view

Left lung

Superior lobe
- Superior division (culmen) { Apico-posterior (S^{1+2})
- { Anterior (S^3)
- Lingular division { Superior (S^4)

Inferior lobe
- Superior (S^6)
- Lateral basal (S^9)
- Posterior basal (S^{10})

Right lung

Superior lobe
- Apical (S^1)
- Posterior (S^2)
- Anterior (S^3)

Middle lobe
- Lateral (S^4)

Inferior lobe
- Superior (S^6)
- Lateral basal (S^9)
- Posterior basal (S^{10})

Bronchopulmonary Segments (continued)

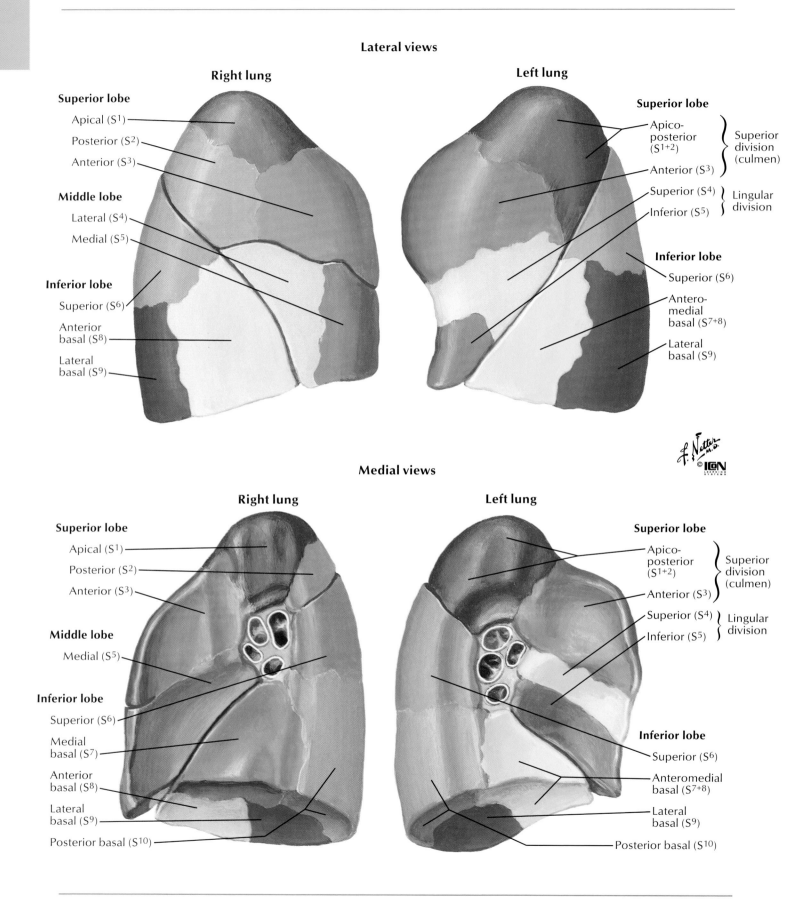

Lateral views

Right lung

Superior lobe
- Apical (S^1)
- Posterior (S^2)
- Anterior (S^3)

Middle lobe
- Lateral (S^4)
- Medial (S^5)

Inferior lobe
- Superior (S^6)
- Anterior basal (S^8)
- Lateral basal (S^9)

Left lung

Superior lobe
- Apico-posterior (S^{1+2}) } Superior division (culmen)
- Anterior (S^3)
- Superior (S^4) } Lingular division
- Inferior (S^5)

Inferior lobe
- Superior (S^6)
- Antero-medial basal (S^{7+8})
- Lateral basal (S^9)

Medial views

Right lung

Superior lobe
- Apical (S^1)
- Posterior (S^2)
- Anterior (S^3)

Middle lobe
- Medial (S^5)

Inferior lobe
- Superior (S^6)
- Medial basal (S^7)
- Anterior basal (S^8)
- Lateral basal (S^9)
- Posterior basal (S^{10})

Left lung

Superior lobe
- Apico-posterior (S^{1+2}) } Superior division (culmen)
- Anterior (S^3)
- Superior (S^4) } Lingular division
- Inferior (S^5)

Inferior lobe
- Superior (S^6)
- Anteromedial basal (S^{7+8})
- Lateral basal (S^9)
- Posterior basal (S^{10})

PLATE 197

THORAX

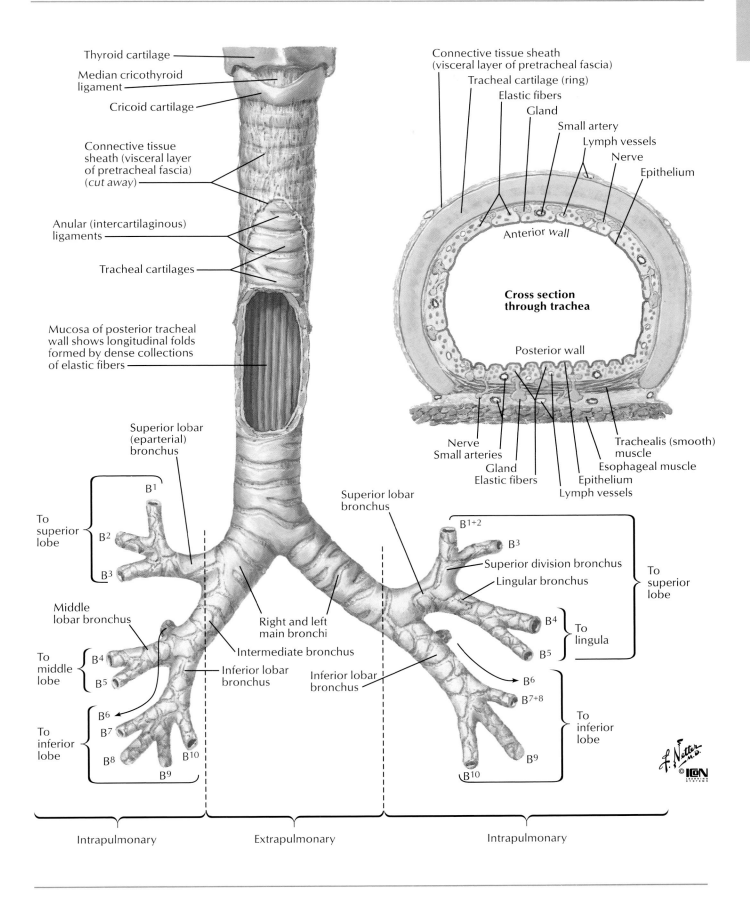

Thyroid cartilage

Median cricothyroid ligament

Cricoid cartilage

Connective tissue sheath (visceral layer of pretracheal fascia) (*cut away*)

Anular (intercartilaginous) ligaments

Tracheal cartilages

Mucosa of posterior tracheal wall shows longitudinal folds formed by dense collections of elastic fibers

Superior lobar (eparterial) bronchus

To superior lobe

B¹

B²

B³

Middle lobar bronchus

To middle lobe

B⁴

B⁵

To inferior lobe

B⁶

B⁷

B⁸   B¹⁰

B⁹

Right and left main bronchi

Intermediate bronchus

Inferior lobar bronchus

Connective tissue sheath (visceral layer of pretracheal fascia)

Tracheal cartilage (ring)

Elastic fibers

Gland

Small artery

Lymph vessels

Nerve

Epithelium

Anterior *wall*

Cross section through trachea

Posterior wall

Nerve
Small arteries

Gland
Elastic fibers

Trachealis (smooth) muscle

Esophageal muscle

Epithelium

Lymph vessels

Superior lobar bronchus

B¹⁺²

B³

Superior division bronchus

Lingular bronchus

To superior lobe

B⁴

To lingula

B⁵

Inferior lobar bronchus

B⁶

B⁷⁺⁸

To inferior lobe

B⁹

B¹⁰

Intrapulmonary

Extrapulmonary

Intrapulmonary

Nomenclature of Bronchi: Schema

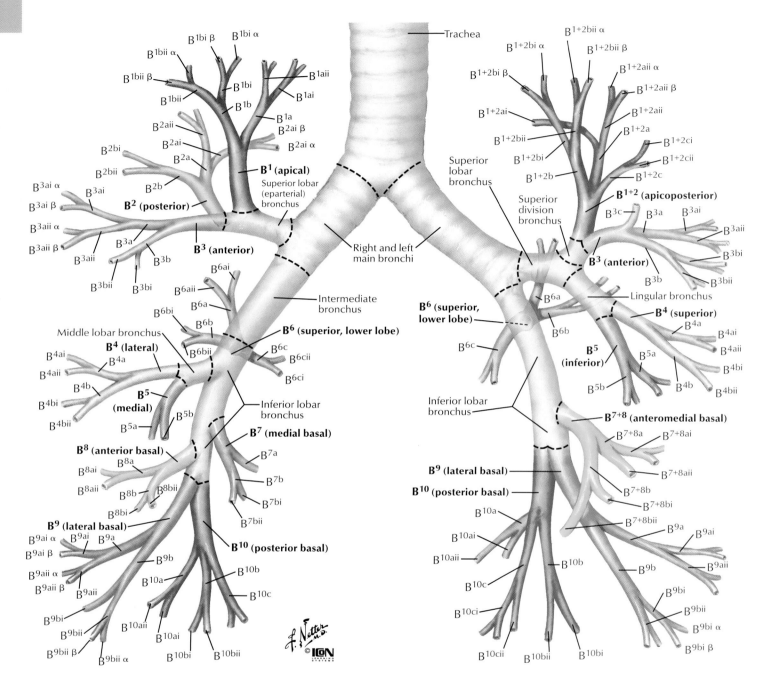

Trachea

B^{1bi} β   B^{1bi} α
B^{1bii} α   B^{1aii}
B^{1bii} β   B^{1bi} B^{1ai}
B^{1bii} B^{1b} B^{1a}
B^{2aii} B^{2ai} β
B^{2ai} B^{2ai} α
B^{2bi} B^{2a}
B^{2bii} B^{2b} **B^{1} (apical)**
B^{3ai} α   B^{3ai} Superior lobar
B^{3ai} β   (eparterial)
B^{3aii} α   bronchus
B^{3aii} β   B^{3a} **B^{2} (posterior)**
B^{3aii} B^{3b} **B^{3} (anterior)**
B^{3bii} B^{3bi}

B^{1+2bi} α   B^{1+2bii} α
B^{1+2bi} β   B^{1+2bii} β
B^{1+2ai} B^{1+2aii} α
B^{1+2bii} B^{1+2aii} β
B^{1+2bi} B^{1+2aii}
B^{1+2b} B^{1+2a} B^{1+2ci}
Superior   B^{1+2ci}
lobar   B^{1+2cii}
bronchus   B^{1+2c}
Superior   **B^{1+2} (apicoposterior)**
division
bronchus   B^{3c} B^{3a} B^{3ai}
    B^{3aii}
B^{3} (anterior)   B^{3bi}
B^{3b} B^{3bii}

Right and left
main bronchi

B^{6ai}
B^{6aii} B^{6a}
B^{6bi} Intermediate bronchus
B^{6b} **B^{6} (superior, lower lobe)**
Middle lobar bronchus   B^{6bii} B^{6c}
B^{4} (lateral)   B^{6cii}
B^{4ai} B^{4a} B^{6ci}
B^{4aii} Inferior lobar
B^{4b} bronchus
B^{4bi} **B^{5}**
    (medial)
B^{4bii} B^{5b}
B^{5a}
B^{8} (anterior basal)   **B^{7} (medial basal)**
B^{8ai} B^{8a} B^{7a}
B^{8aii} B^{7b}
B^{8b} B^{8bii} B^{7bi}
B^{8bi} B^{7bii}
B^{9} (lateral basal)   **B^{10} (posterior basal)**
B^{9ai} α   B^{9ai} B^{9a}
B^{9ai} β   B^{9b} B^{10b}
B^{9aii} α   B^{9aii} B^{10a}
B^{9aii} β   B^{10c}
B^{9bi} B^{10aii}
B^{9bii} B^{10ai}
B^{9bii} β   B^{9bii} α   B^{10bi} B^{10bii}

B^{6} (superior, lower lobe)   Lingular bronchus
B^{6a} **B^{4} (superior)**
B^{6b} B^{4a}
B^{6c} **B^{5}**   B^{4ai}
    (inferior)   B^{5a} B^{4aii}
B^{5b} B^{4b} B^{4bi}
Inferior lobar   B^{4bii}
bronchus   **B^{7+8} (anteromedial basal)**
B^{7+8a} B^{7+8ai}
B^{9} (lateral basal)   B^{7+8aii}
B^{10} (posterior basal)   B^{7+8b}
B^{10a} B^{7+8bi}
B^{10ai} B^{7+8bii} B^{9a}
B^{10aii} B^{9ai}
B^{10b} B^{9b} B^{9aii}
B^{10c} B^{9bi}
B^{10ci} B^{9bii}
B^{10cii} B^{10bii} B^{10bi} B^{9bi} α
B^{9bi} β

Nomenclature in common usage for bronchopulmonary segments (Plates 196 and 197) is that of Jackson and Huber, and segmental bronchi are named accordingly. Ikeda proposed nomenclature (as demonstrated here) for bronchial subdivisions as far as 6th generation. For simplification on this illustration, only some bronchial subdivisions are labeled as far as 5th or 6th generation. Segmental bronchi (B) are numbered from 1 to 10 in each lung, corresponding to pulmonary segments. In left lung,

B^{1} and B^{2} are combined as are B^{7} and B^{8}. Subsegmental, or 4th order, bronchi are indicated by addition of lower-case letters a, b or c when an additional branch is present. Fifth order bronchi are designated by Roman numerals i (anterior) or ii (posterior) and 6th order bronchi by Greek letters α or β. Several texts use alternate numbers (as proposed by Boyden) for segmental bronchi.

Variations of standard bronchial pattern shown here are common, especially in peripheral airways.

PLATE 199   **THORAX**

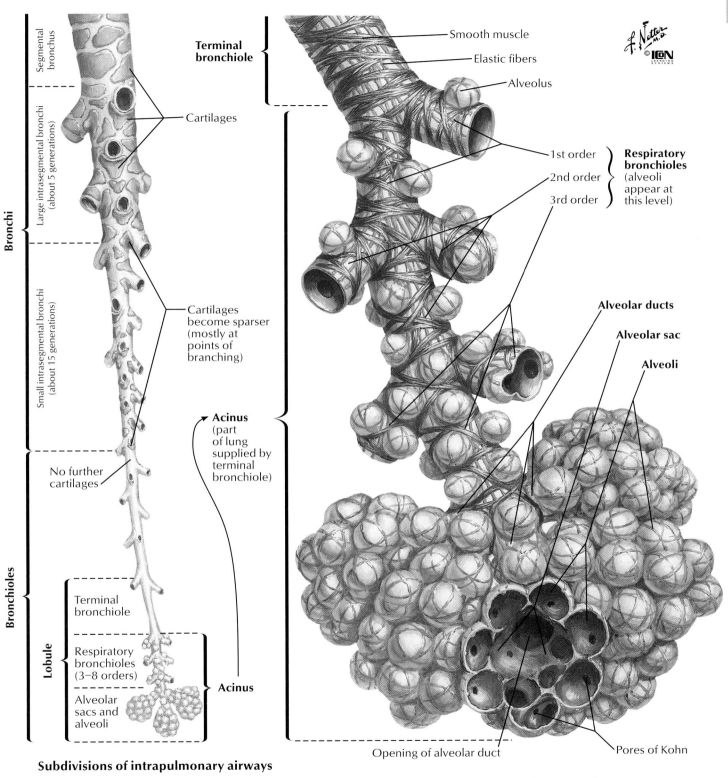

Terminal bronchiole

Cartilages

Cartilages become sparser (mostly at points of branching)

No further cartilages

Acinus (part of lung supplied by terminal bronchiole)

Segmental bronchus

Large intrasegmental bronchi (about 5 generations)

Small intrasegmental bronchi (about 15 generations)

Bronchi

Bronchioles

Lobule

Terminal bronchiole

Respiratory bronchioles (3–8 orders)

Alveolar sacs and alveoli

Acinus

Subdivisions of intrapulmonary airways

Smooth muscle

Elastic fibers

Alveolus

1st order

2nd order

3rd order

Respiratory bronchioles (alveoli appear at this level)

Alveolar ducts

Alveolar sac

Alveoli

Opening of alveolar duct

Pores of Kohn

Structure of intrapulmonary airways

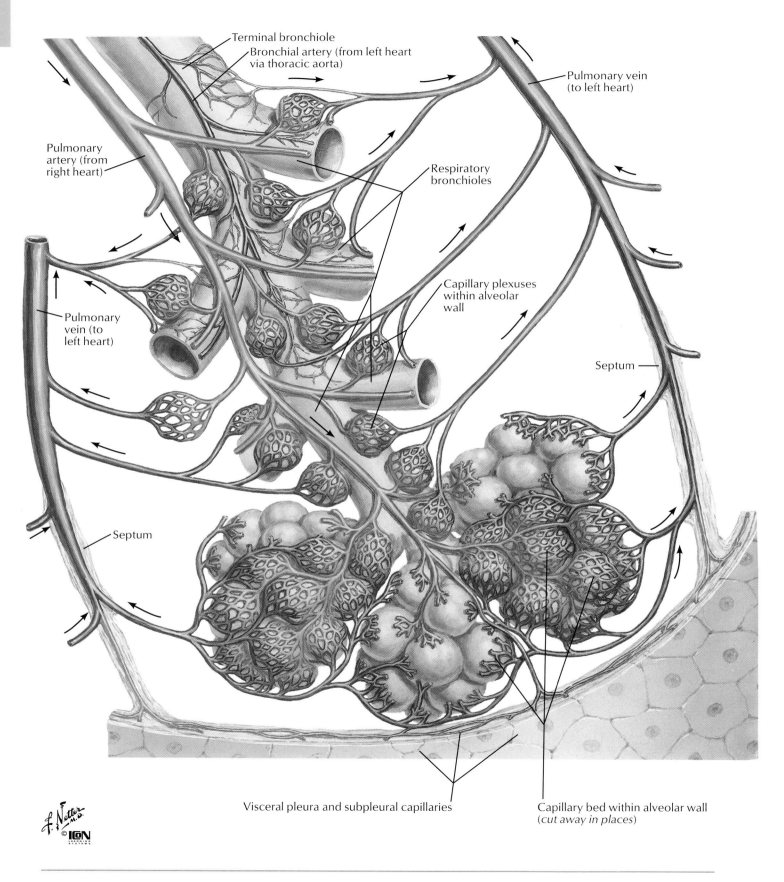

Terminal bronchiole

Bronchial artery (from left heart via thoracic aorta)

Pulmonary vein (to left heart)

Pulmonary artery (from right heart)

Respiratory bronchioles

Capillary plexuses within alveolar wall

Pulmonary vein (to left heart)

Septum

Septum

Visceral pleura and subpleural capillaries

Capillary bed within alveolar wall (*cut away in places*)

PLATE 201

THORAX

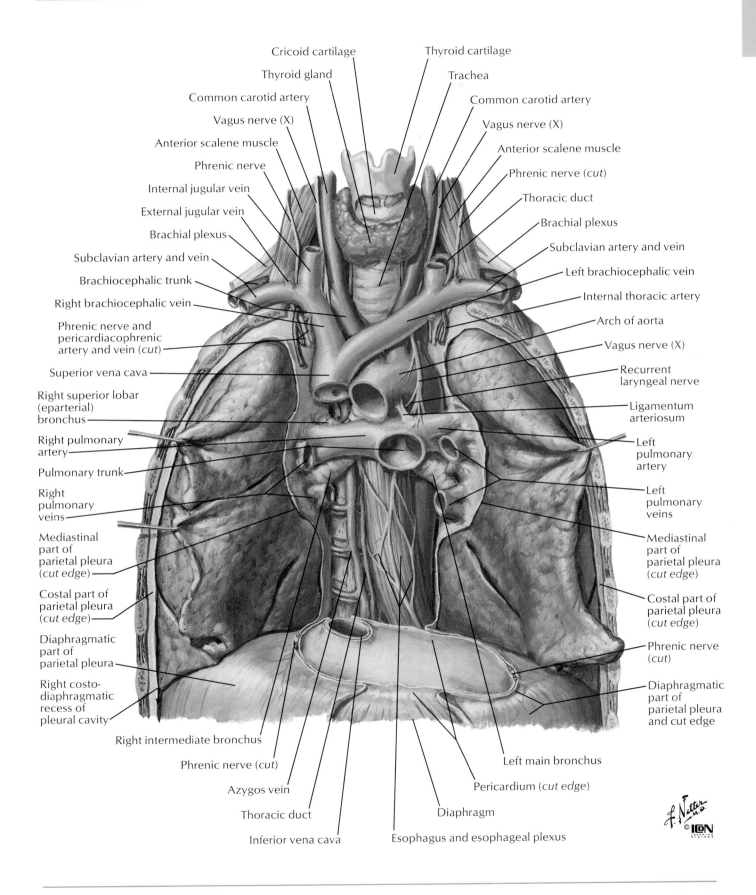

Cricoid cartilage

Thyroid cartilage

Thyroid gland

Trachea

Common carotid artery

Common carotid artery

Vagus nerve (X)

Vagus nerve (X)

Anterior scalene muscle

Anterior scalene muscle

Phrenic nerve

Phrenic nerve (*cut*)

Internal jugular vein

Thoracic duct

External jugular vein

Brachial plexus

Brachial plexus

Subclavian artery and vein

Subclavian artery and vein

Left brachiocephalic vein

Brachiocephalic trunk

Internal thoracic artery

Right brachiocephalic vein

Arch of aorta

Phrenic nerve and
pericardiacophrenic
artery and vein (*cut*)

Vagus nerve (X)

Superior vena cava

Recurrent
laryngeal nerve

Right superior lobar
(eparterial)
bronchus

Ligamentum
arteriosum

Right pulmonary
artery

Left
pulmonary
artery

Pulmonary trunk

Right
pulmonary
veins

Left
pulmonary
veins

Mediastinal
part of
parietal pleura
(*cut edge*)

Mediastinal
part of
parietal pleura
(*cut edge*)

Costal part of
parietal pleura
(*cut edge*)

Costal part of
parietal pleura
(*cut edge*)

Diaphragmatic
part of
parietal pleura

Phrenic nerve
(*cut*)

Right costo-
diaphragmatic
recess of
pleural cavity

Diaphragmatic
part of
parietal pleura
and cut edge

Right intermediate bronchus

Phrenic nerve (*cut*)

Left main bronchus

Azygos vein

Pericardium (*cut edge*)

Thoracic duct

Diaphragm

Inferior vena cava

Esophagus and esophageal plexus

Bronchial Arteries and Veins

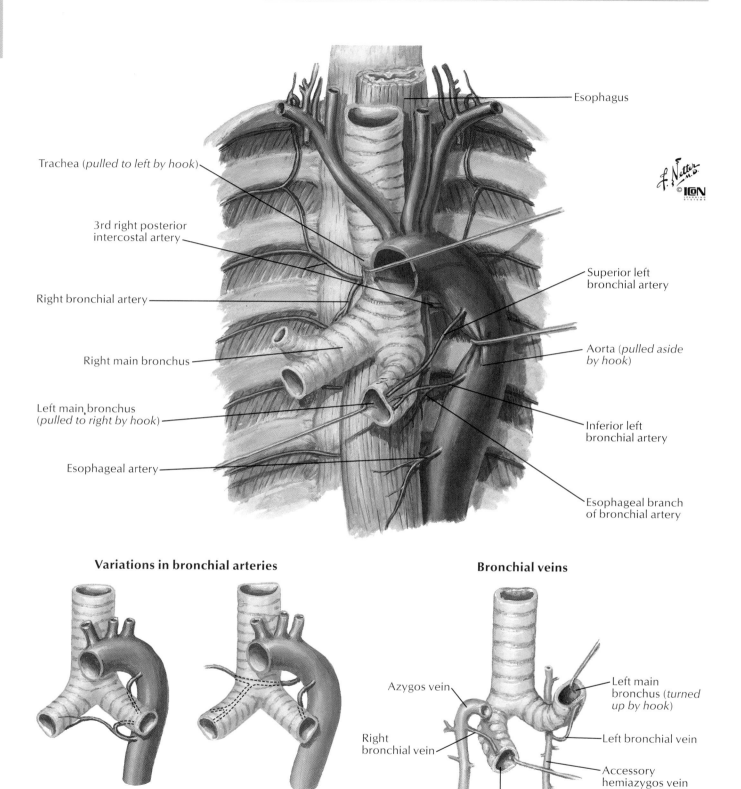

Esophagus

Trachea (*pulled to left by hook*)

3rd right posterior intercostal artery

Right bronchial artery

Right main bronchus

Left main bronchus (*pulled to right by hook*)

Esophageal artery

Superior left bronchial artery

Aorta (*pulled aside by hook*)

Inferior left bronchial artery

Esophageal branch of bronchial artery

Variations in bronchial arteries

Right and left bronchial arteries originating from aorta by single stem

Only single bronchial artery to each bronchus (normally, two to left bronchus)

Bronchial veins

Azygos vein

Right bronchial vein

Left main bronchus (*turned up by hook*)

Left bronchial vein

Accessory hemiazygos vein

Right main bronchus (*pulled to left and rotated by hook*)

PLATE 203

THORAX

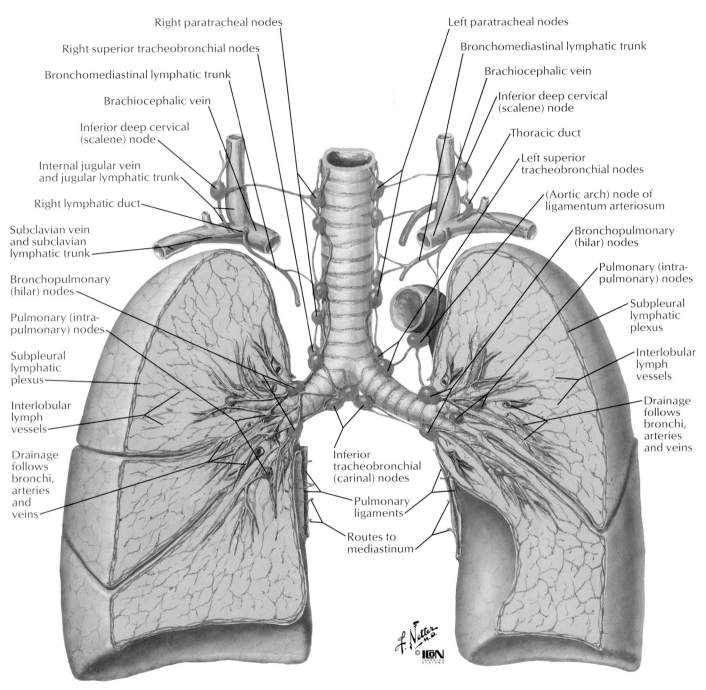

Right paratracheal nodes

Right superior tracheobronchial nodes

Bronchomediastinal lymphatic trunk

Brachiocephalic vein

Inferior deep cervical (scalene) node

Internal jugular vein and jugular lymphatic trunk

Right lymphatic duct

Subclavian vein and subclavian lymphatic trunk

Bronchopulmonary (hilar) nodes

Pulmonary (intra-pulmonary) nodes

Subpleural lymphatic plexus

Interlobular lymph vessels

Drainage follows bronchi, arteries and veins

Left paratracheal nodes

Bronchomediastinal lymphatic trunk

Brachiocephalic vein

Inferior deep cervical (scalene) node

Thoracic duct

Left superior tracheobronchial nodes

(Aortic arch) node of ligamentum arteriosum

Bronchopulmonary (hilar) nodes

Pulmonary (intra-pulmonary) nodes

Subpleural lymphatic plexus

Interlobular lymph vessels

Drainage follows bronchi, arteries and veins

Inferior tracheobronchial (carinal) nodes

Pulmonary ligaments

Routes to mediastinum

Drainage routes

Right lung: All lobes drain to pulmonary and broncho-pulmonary (hilar) nodes, then to inferior tracheobronchial (carinal) nodes, right superior tracheobronchial nodes and to right paratracheal nodes on way to brachiocephalic vein via bronchomediastinal lymphatic trunk and/or inferior deep cervical (scalene) node.

Left lung: Superior lobe drains to pulmonary and broncho-pulmonary (hilar) nodes, inferior tracheobronchial (carinal) nodes, left superior tracheobronchial nodes, left paratracheal nodes and/or (aortic arch) node of ligamentum arteriosum, then to brachiocephalic vein via left bronchomediastinal trunk and thoracic duct. Left inferior lobe drains also to pulmonary and bronchopulmonary (hilar) nodes and to inferior tracheo-bronchial (carinal) nodes, but then mostly to right superior tracheobronchial nodes, where it follows same route as lymph from right lung.

SEE ALSO PLATES 124, 125, 159, 308

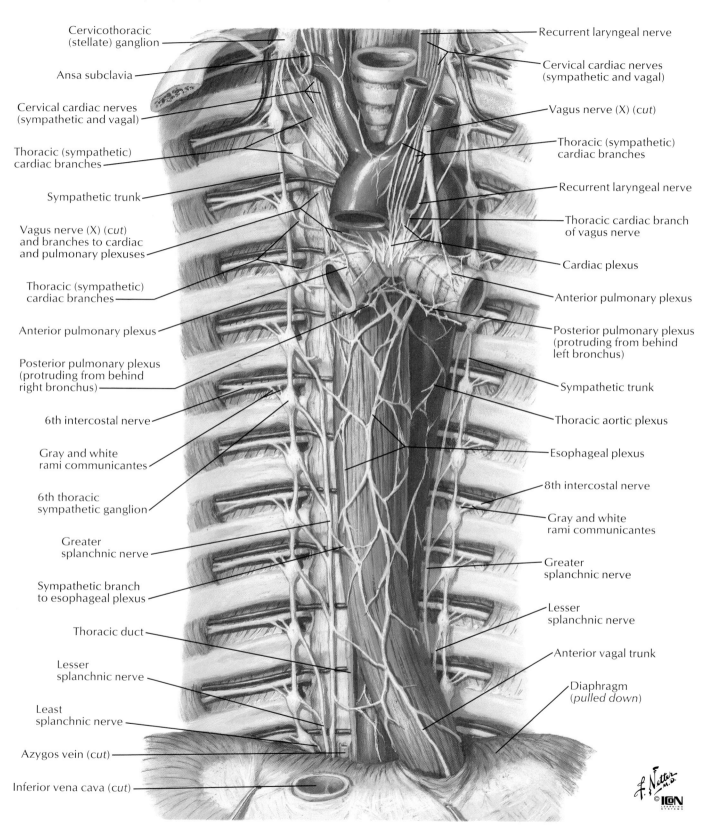

Cervicothoracic (stellate) ganglion

Ansa subclavia

Cervical cardiac nerves (sympathetic and vagal)

Thoracic (sympathetic) cardiac branches

Sympathetic trunk

Vagus nerve (X) (*cut*) and branches to cardiac and pulmonary plexuses

Thoracic (sympathetic) cardiac branches

Anterior pulmonary plexus

Posterior pulmonary plexus (protruding from behind right bronchus)

6th intercostal nerve

Gray and white rami communicantes

6th thoracic sympathetic ganglion

Greater splanchnic nerve

Sympathetic branch to esophageal plexus

Thoracic duct

Lesser splanchnic nerve

Least splanchnic nerve

Azygos vein (*cut*)

Inferior vena cava (*cut*)

Recurrent laryngeal nerve

Cervical cardiac nerves (sympathetic and vagal)

Vagus nerve (X) (*cut*)

Thoracic (sympathetic) cardiac branches

Recurrent laryngeal nerve

Thoracic cardiac branch of vagus nerve

Cardiac plexus

Anterior pulmonary plexus

Posterior pulmonary plexus (protruding from behind left bronchus)

Sympathetic trunk

Thoracic aortic plexus

Esophageal plexus

8th intercostal nerve

Gray and white rami communicantes

Greater splanchnic nerve

Lesser splanchnic nerve

Anterior vagal trunk

Diaphragm (*pulled down*)

PLATE 205

THORAX

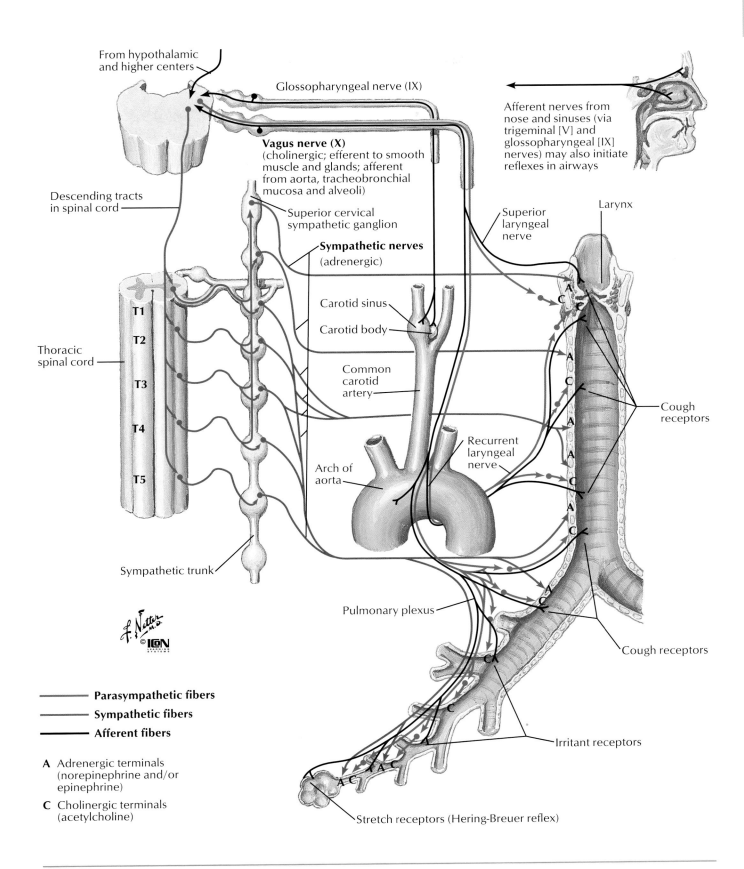

From hypothalamic and higher centers

Glossopharyngeal nerve (IX)

Afferent nerves from nose and sinuses (via trigeminal [V] and glossopharyngeal [IX] nerves) may also initiate reflexes in airways

Vagus nerve (X) (cholinergic; efferent to smooth muscle and glands; afferent from aorta, tracheobronchial mucosa and alveoli)

Descending tracts in spinal cord

Superior cervical sympathetic ganglion

Sympathetic nerves (adrenergic)

Superior laryngeal nerve

Larynx

T1

T2

Carotid sinus

Carotid body

Thoracic spinal cord

T3

Common carotid artery

Cough receptors

T4

Recurrent laryngeal nerve

T5

Arch of aorta

Cough receptors

Sympathetic trunk

Pulmonary plexus

Cough receptors

Irritant receptors

——— **Parasympathetic fibers**

——— **Sympathetic fibers**

——— **Afferent fibers**

A Adrenergic terminals (norepinephrine and/or epinephrine)

C Cholinergic terminals (acetylcholine)

Stretch receptors (Hering-Breuer reflex)

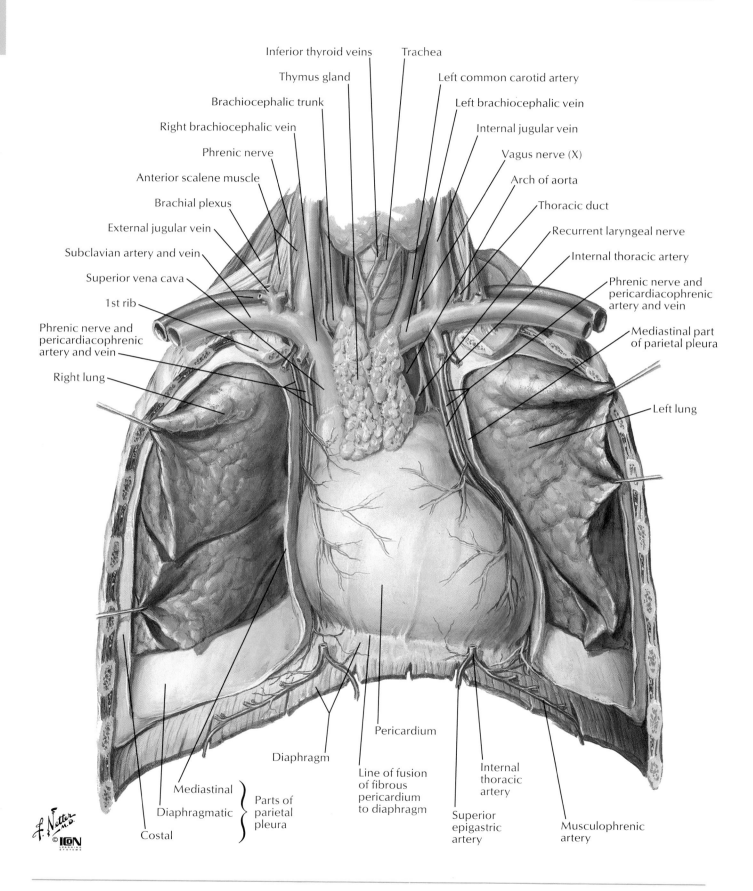

Inferior thyroid veins

Thymus gland

Brachiocephalic trunk

Right brachiocephalic vein

Phrenic nerve

Anterior scalene muscle

Brachial plexus

External jugular vein

Subclavian artery and vein

Superior vena cava

1st rib

Phrenic nerve and pericardiacophrenic artery and vein

Right lung

Trachea

Left common carotid artery

Left brachiocephalic vein

Internal jugular vein

Vagus nerve (X)

Arch of aorta

Thoracic duct

Recurrent laryngeal nerve

Internal thoracic artery

Phrenic nerve and pericardiacophrenic artery and vein

Mediastinal part of parietal pleura

Left lung

Mediastinal ⎫
Diaphragmatic ⎬ Parts of parietal pleura
Costal ⎭

Diaphragm

Line of fusion of fibrous pericardium to diaphragm

Pericardium

Superior epigastric artery

Internal thoracic artery

Musculophrenic artery

F. Netter M.D.
© ICON LEARNING SYSTEMS

PLATE 207

THORAX

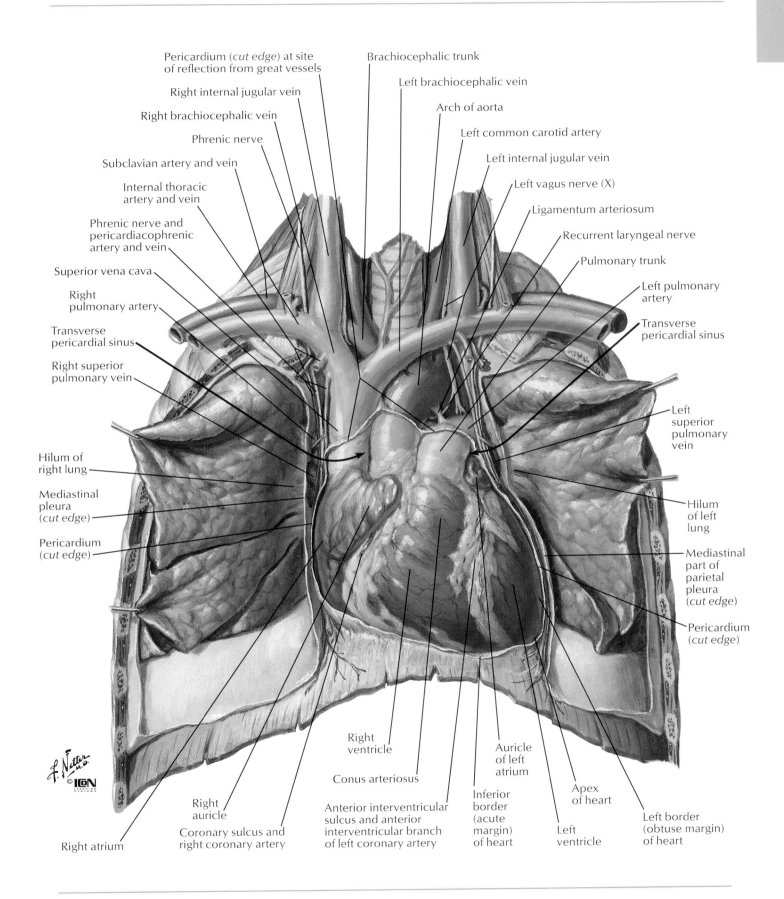

Pericardium (*cut edge*) at site of reflection from great vessels

Right internal jugular vein

Right brachiocephalic vein

Phrenic nerve

Subclavian artery and vein

Internal thoracic artery and vein

Phrenic nerve and pericardiacophrenic artery and vein

Superior vena cava

Right pulmonary artery

Transverse pericardial sinus

Right superior pulmonary vein

Hilum of right lung

Mediastinal pleura (*cut edge*)

Pericardium (*cut edge*)

Brachiocephalic trunk

Left brachiocephalic vein

Arch of aorta

Left common carotid artery

Left internal jugular vein

Left vagus nerve (X)

Ligamentum arteriosum

Recurrent laryngeal nerve

Pulmonary trunk

Left pulmonary artery

Transverse pericardial sinus

Left superior pulmonary vein

Hilum of left lung

Mediastinal part of parietal pleura (*cut edge*)

Pericardium (*cut edge*)

Right ventricle

Conus arteriosus

Right auricle

Coronary sulcus and right coronary artery

Anterior interventricular sulcus and anterior interventricular branch of left coronary artery

Right atrium

Auricle of left atrium

Inferior border (acute margin) of heart

Left ventricle

Apex of heart

Left border (obtuse margin) of heart

Radiograph of Chest

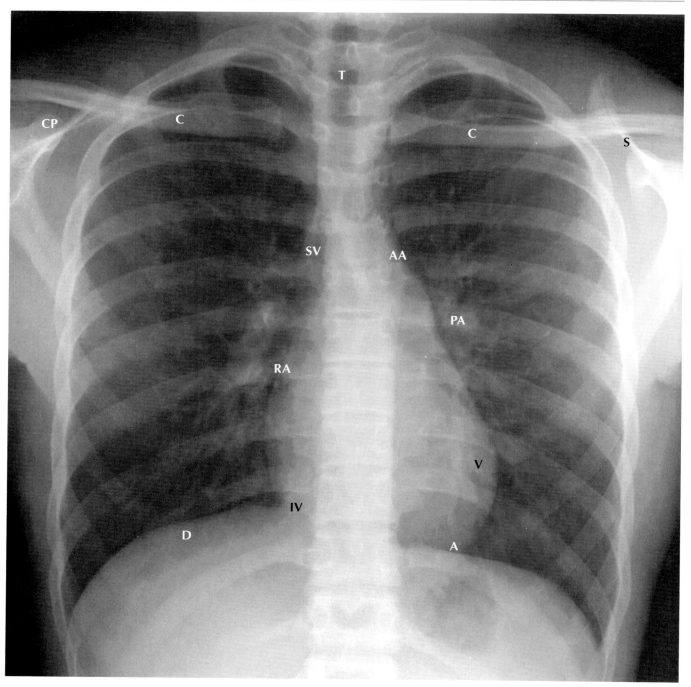

A	Apex of heart
AA	Aortic arch
C	Clavicle
CP	Coracoid process of scapula
D	Dome of diaphragm (right)
IV	Inferior vena cava
PA	Pulmonary artery (left)
RA	Right atrium
S	Spine of scapula
SV	Superior vena cava
T	Trachea (air)
V	Left ventricle

PLATE 209

THORAX

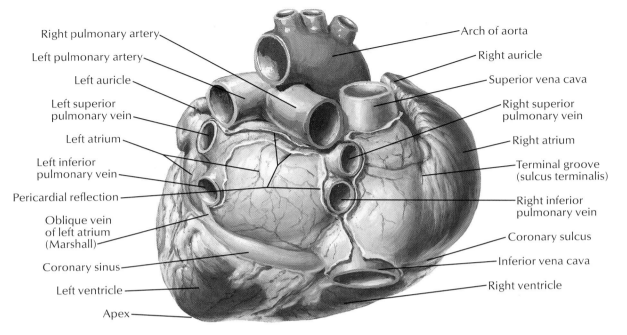

Right pulmonary artery

Left pulmonary artery

Left auricle

Left superior pulmonary vein

Left atrium

Left inferior pulmonary vein

Pericardial reflection

Oblique vein of left atrium (Marshall)

Coronary sinus

Left ventricle

Apex

Arch of aorta

Right auricle

Superior vena cava

Right superior pulmonary vein

Right atrium

Terminal groove (sulcus terminalis)

Right inferior pulmonary vein

Coronary sulcus

Inferior vena cava

Right ventricle

Base of heart: posterior view

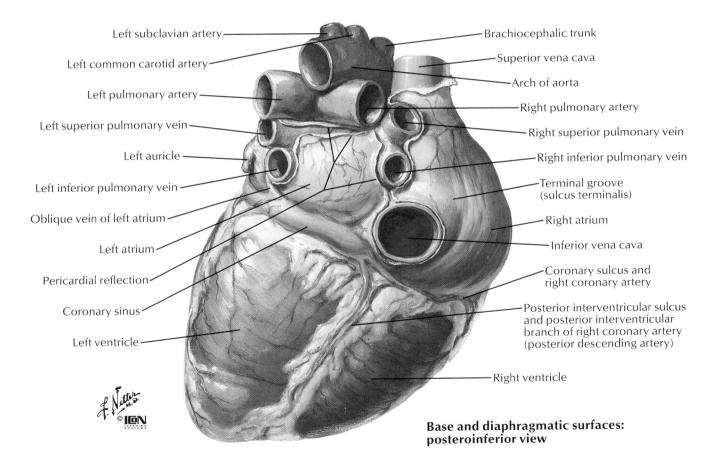

Left subclavian artery

Left common carotid artery

Left pulmonary artery

Left superior pulmonary vein

Left auricle

Left inferior pulmonary vein

Oblique vein of left atrium

Left atrium

Pericardial reflection

Coronary sinus

Left ventricle

Brachiocephalic trunk

Superior vena cava

Arch of aorta

Right pulmonary artery

Right superior pulmonary vein

Right inferior pulmonary vein

Terminal groove (sulcus terminalis)

Right atrium

Inferior vena cava

Coronary sulcus and right coronary artery

Posterior interventricular sulcus and posterior interventricular branch of right coronary artery (posterior descending artery)

Right ventricle

Base and diaphragmatic surfaces: posteroinferior view

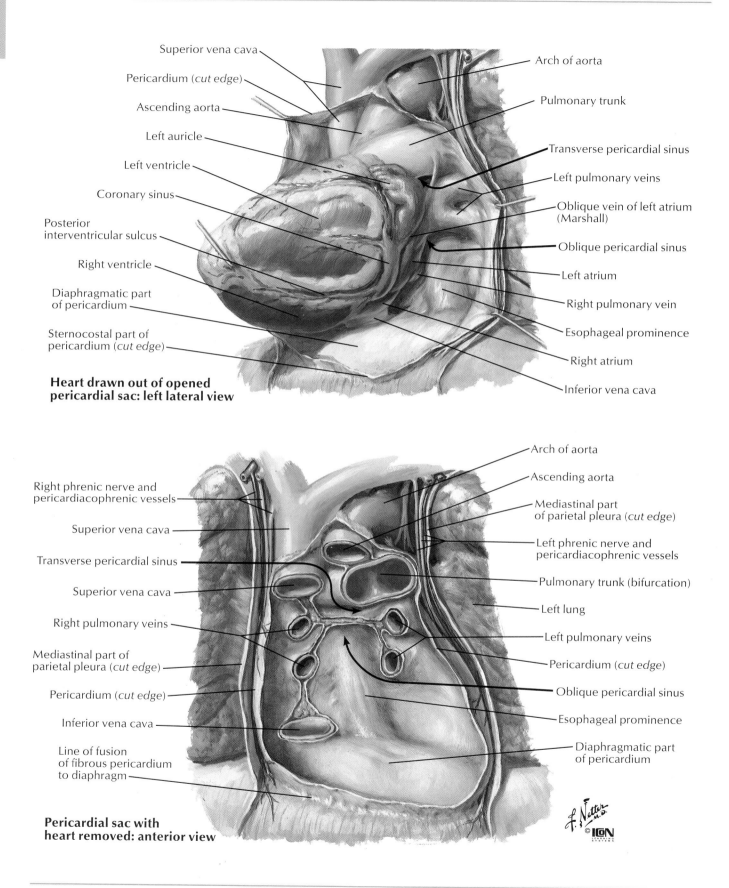

Superior vena cava

Pericardium (*cut edge*)

Ascending aorta

Left auricle

Left ventricle

Coronary sinus

Posterior interventricular sulcus

Right ventricle

Diaphragmatic part of pericardium

Sternocostal part of pericardium (*cut edge*)

Arch of aorta

Pulmonary trunk

Transverse pericardial sinus

Left pulmonary veins

Oblique vein of left atrium (Marshall)

Oblique pericardial sinus

Left atrium

Right pulmonary vein

Esophageal prominence

Right atrium

Inferior vena cava

Heart drawn out of opened pericardial sac: left lateral view

Right phrenic nerve and pericardiacophrenic vessels

Superior vena cava

Transverse pericardial sinus

Superior vena cava

Right pulmonary veins

Mediastinal part of parietal pleura (*cut edge*)

Pericardium (*cut edge*)

Inferior vena cava

Line of fusion of fibrous pericardium to diaphragm

Arch of aorta

Ascending aorta

Mediastinal part of parietal pleura (*cut edge*)

Left phrenic nerve and pericardiacophrenic vessels

Pulmonary trunk (bifurcation)

Left lung

Left pulmonary veins

Pericardium (*cut edge*)

Oblique pericardial sinus

Esophageal prominence

Diaphragmatic part of pericardium

Pericardial sac with heart removed: anterior view

PLATE 211

THORAX

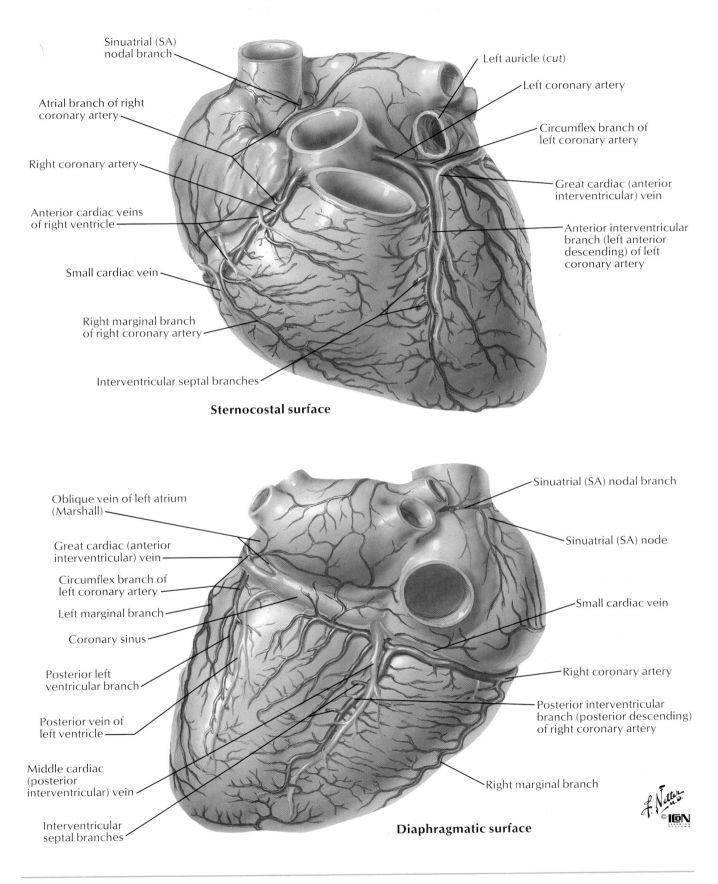

Sinuatrial (SA) nodal branch

Atrial branch of right coronary artery

Right coronary artery

Anterior cardiac veins of right ventricle

Small cardiac vein

Right marginal branch of right coronary artery

Interventricular septal branches

Left auricle (*cut*)

Left coronary artery

Circumflex branch of left coronary artery

Great cardiac (anterior interventricular) vein

Anterior interventricular branch (left anterior descending) of left coronary artery

Sternocostal surface

Oblique vein of left atrium (Marshall)

Great cardiac (anterior interventricular) vein

Circumflex branch of left coronary artery

Left marginal branch

Coronary sinus

Posterior left ventricular branch

Posterior vein of left ventricle

Middle cardiac (posterior interventricular) vein

Interventricular septal branches

Sinuatrial (SA) nodal branch

Sinuatrial (SA) node

Small cardiac vein

Right coronary artery

Posterior interventricular branch (posterior descending) of right coronary artery

Right marginal branch

Diaphragmatic surface

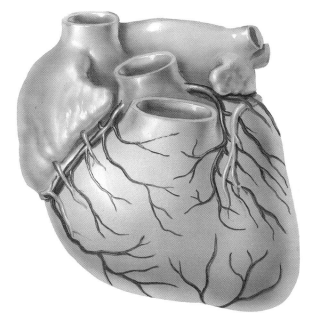

Anterior interventricular (left anterior descending) branch of left coronary artery very short. Apical part of anterior (sternocostal) surface supplied by branches from posterior interventricular (posterior descending) branch of right coronary artery curving around apex

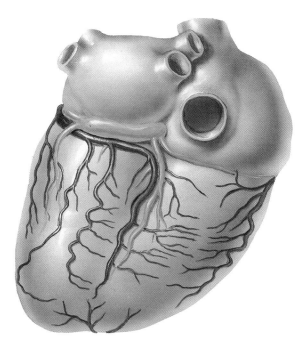

Posterior interventricular (posterior descending) branch derived from circumflex branch of left coronary artery instead of from right coronary artery

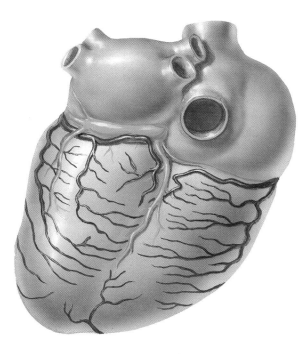

Posterior interventricular (posterior descending) branch absent. Area supplied chiefly by small branches from circumflex branch of left coronary artery and from right coronary artery

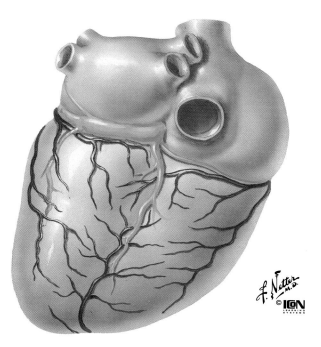

Posterior interventricular (posterior descending) branch absent. Area supplied chiefly by elongated anterior interventricular (left anterior descending) branch curving around apex

PLATE 213

THORAX

Right coronary artery: left anterior oblique view

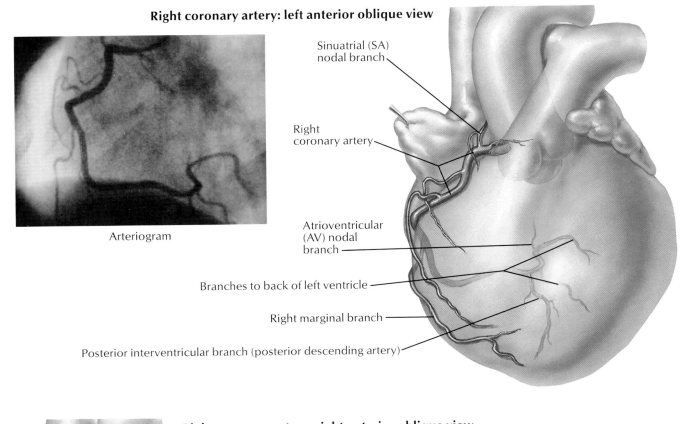

Arteriogram

Sinuatrial (SA) nodal branch

Right coronary artery

Atrioventricular (AV) nodal branch

Branches to back of left ventricle

Right marginal branch

Posterior interventricular branch (posterior descending artery)

Right coronary artery: right anterior oblique view

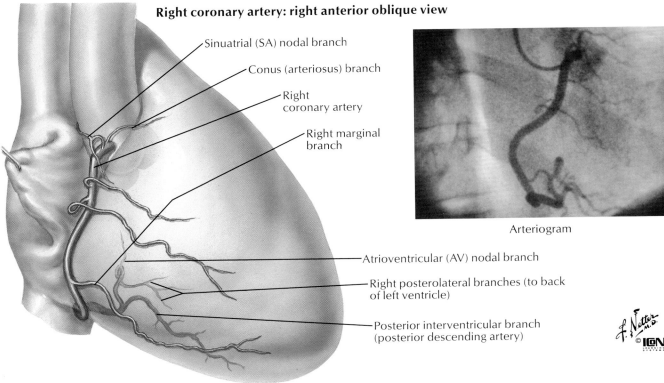

Sinuatrial (SA) nodal branch

Conus (arteriosus) branch

Right coronary artery

Right marginal branch

Arteriogram

Atrioventricular (AV) nodal branch

Right posterolateral branches (to back of left ventricle)

Posterior interventricular branch (posterior descending artery)

Coronary Arteries: Arteriographic Views (continued)

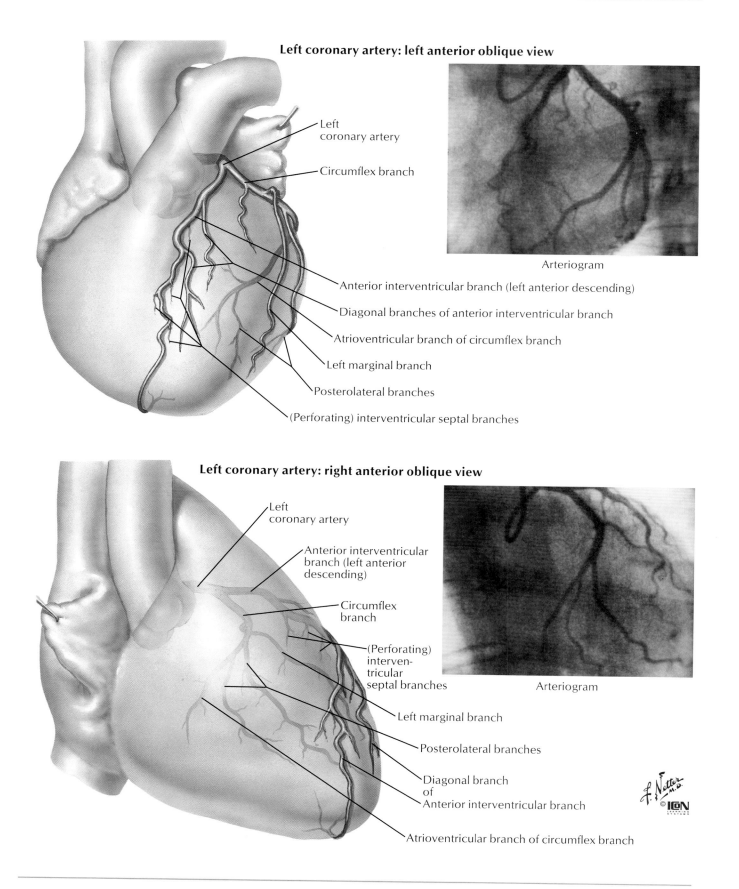

Left coronary artery: left anterior oblique view

Left coronary artery

Circumflex branch

Anterior interventricular branch (left anterior descending)

Diagonal branches of anterior interventricular branch

Atrioventricular branch of circumflex branch

Left marginal branch

Posterolateral branches

(Perforating) interventricular septal branches

Arteriogram

Left coronary artery: right anterior oblique view

Left coronary artery

Anterior interventricular branch (left anterior descending)

Circumflex branch

(Perforating) interventricular septal branches

Left marginal branch

Posterolateral branches

Diagonal branch of Anterior interventricular branch

Atrioventricular branch of circumflex branch

Arteriogram

PLATE 215

THORAX

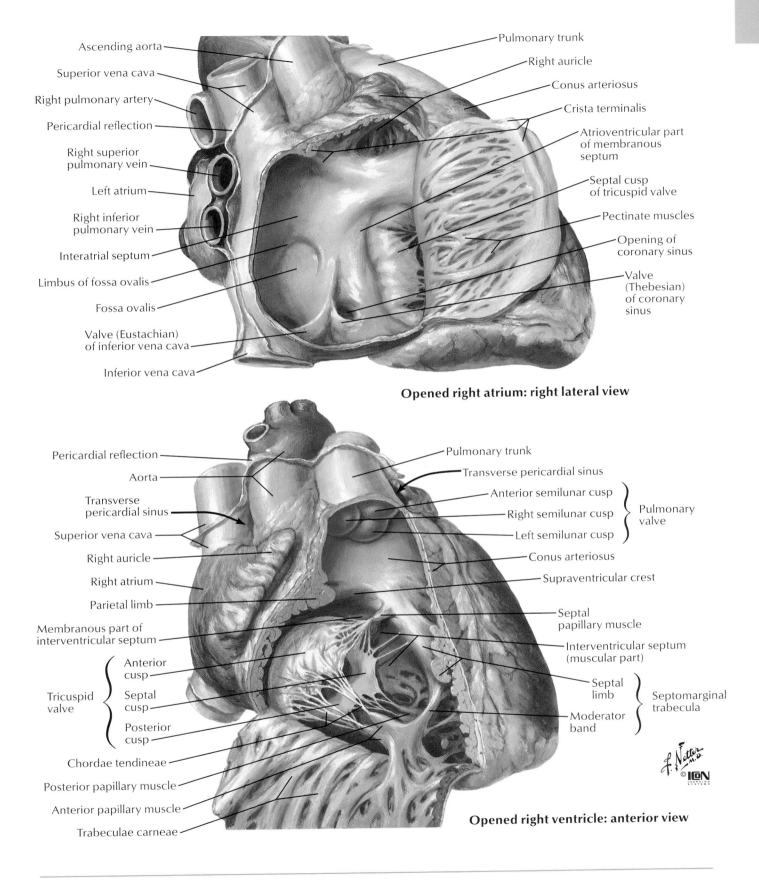

Ascending aorta

Superior vena cava

Right pulmonary artery

Pericardial reflection

Right superior pulmonary vein

Left atrium

Right inferior pulmonary vein

Interatrial septum

Limbus of fossa ovalis

Fossa ovalis

Valve (Eustachian) of inferior vena cava

Inferior vena cava

Pulmonary trunk

Right auricle

Conus arteriosus

Crista terminalis

Atrioventricular part of membranous septum

Septal cusp of tricuspid valve

Pectinate muscles

Opening of coronary sinus

Valve (Thebesian) of coronary sinus

Opened right atrium: right lateral view

Pericardial reflection

Aorta

Transverse pericardial sinus

Superior vena cava

Right auricle

Right atrium

Parietal limb

Membranous part of interventricular septum

Tricuspid valve { Anterior cusp

Septal cusp

Posterior cusp }

Chordae tendineae

Posterior papillary muscle

Anterior papillary muscle

Trabeculae carneae

Pulmonary trunk

Transverse pericardial sinus

Anterior semilunar cusp

Right semilunar cusp

Left semilunar cusp

} Pulmonary valve

Conus arteriosus

Supraventricular crest

Septal papillary muscle

Interventricular septum (muscular part)

Septal limb

Moderator band

} Septomarginal trabecula

Opened right ventricle: anterior view

HEART

PLATE 216

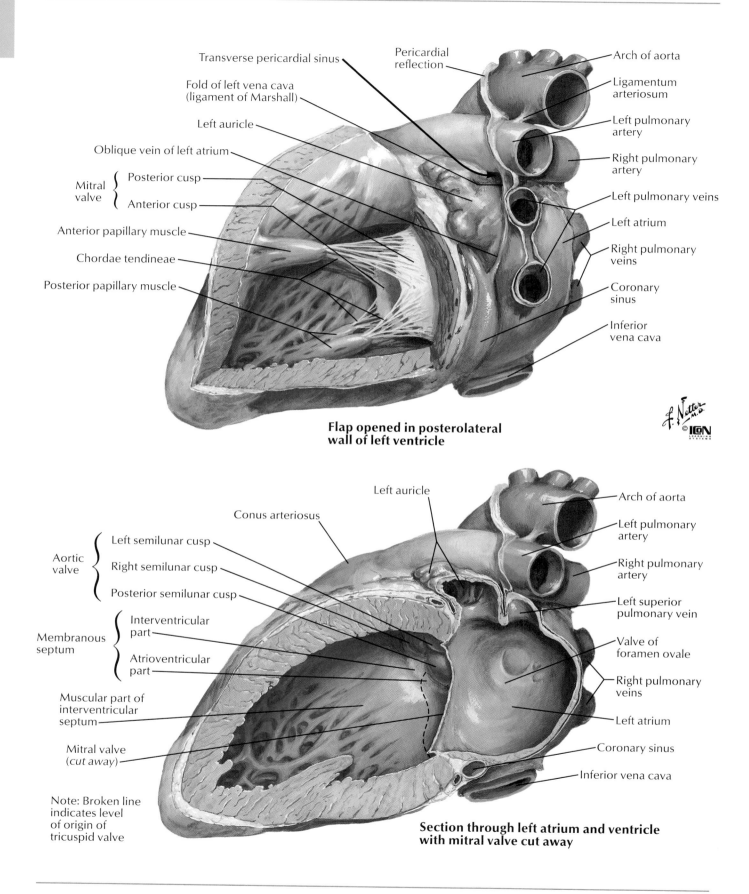

Transverse pericardial sinus

Pericardial reflection

Arch of aorta

Ligamentum arteriosum

Fold of left vena cava (ligament of Marshall)

Left pulmonary artery

Left auricle

Right pulmonary artery

Oblique vein of left atrium

Mitral valve { Posterior cusp

Anterior cusp

Left pulmonary veins

Left atrium

Anterior papillary muscle

Right pulmonary veins

Chordae tendineae

Posterior papillary muscle

Coronary sinus

Inferior vena cava

Flap opened in posterolateral wall of left ventricle

Left auricle

Conus arteriosus

Arch of aorta

Left pulmonary artery

Aortic valve { Left semilunar cusp

Right semilunar cusp

Posterior semilunar cusp

Right pulmonary artery

Membranous septum { Interventricular part

Atrioventricular part

Left superior pulmonary vein

Valve of foramen ovale

Right pulmonary veins

Muscular part of interventricular septum

Left atrium

Mitral valve (*cut away*)

Coronary sinus

Inferior vena cava

Note: Broken line indicates level of origin of tricuspid valve

Section through left atrium and ventricle with mitral valve cut away

PLATE 217

THORAX

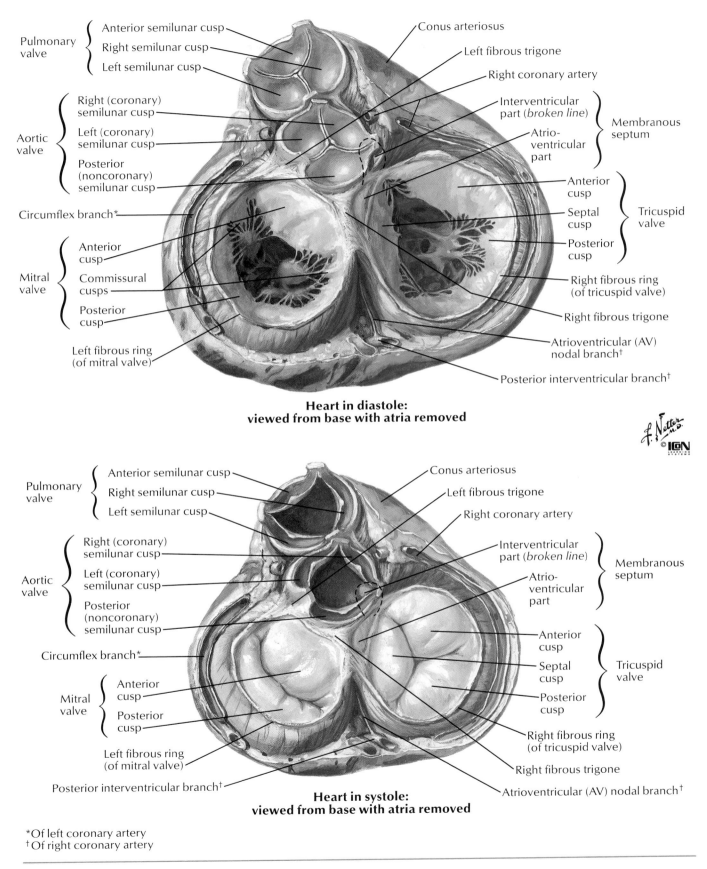

Pulmonary valve
- Anterior semilunar cusp
- Right semilunar cusp
- Left semilunar cusp

Aortic valve
- Right (coronary) semilunar cusp
- Left (coronary) semilunar cusp
- Posterior (noncoronary) semilunar cusp

Circumflex branch*

Mitral valve
- Anterior cusp
- Commissural cusps
- Posterior cusp

Left fibrous ring (of mitral valve)

Conus arteriosus
Left fibrous trigone
Right coronary artery

Membranous septum
- Interventricular part (*broken line*)
- Atrio-ventricular part

Tricuspid valve
- Anterior cusp
- Septal cusp
- Posterior cusp

Right fibrous ring (of tricuspid valve)
Right fibrous trigone
Atrioventricular (AV) nodal branch†
Posterior interventricular branch†

Heart in diastole: viewed from base with atria removed

Pulmonary valve
- Anterior semilunar cusp
- Right semilunar cusp
- Left semilunar cusp

Aortic valve
- Right (coronary) semilunar cusp
- Left (coronary) semilunar cusp
- Posterior (noncoronary) semilunar cusp

Circumflex branch*

Mitral valve
- Anterior cusp
- Posterior cusp

Left fibrous ring (of mitral valve)

Posterior interventricular branch†

Conus arteriosus
Left fibrous trigone
Right coronary artery

Membranous septum
- Interventricular part (*broken line*)
- Atrio-ventricular part

Tricuspid valve
- Anterior cusp
- Septal cusp
- Posterior cusp

Right fibrous ring (of tricuspid valve)
Right fibrous trigone
Atrioventricular (AV) nodal branch†

Heart in systole: viewed from base with atria removed

*Of left coronary artery
†Of right coronary artery

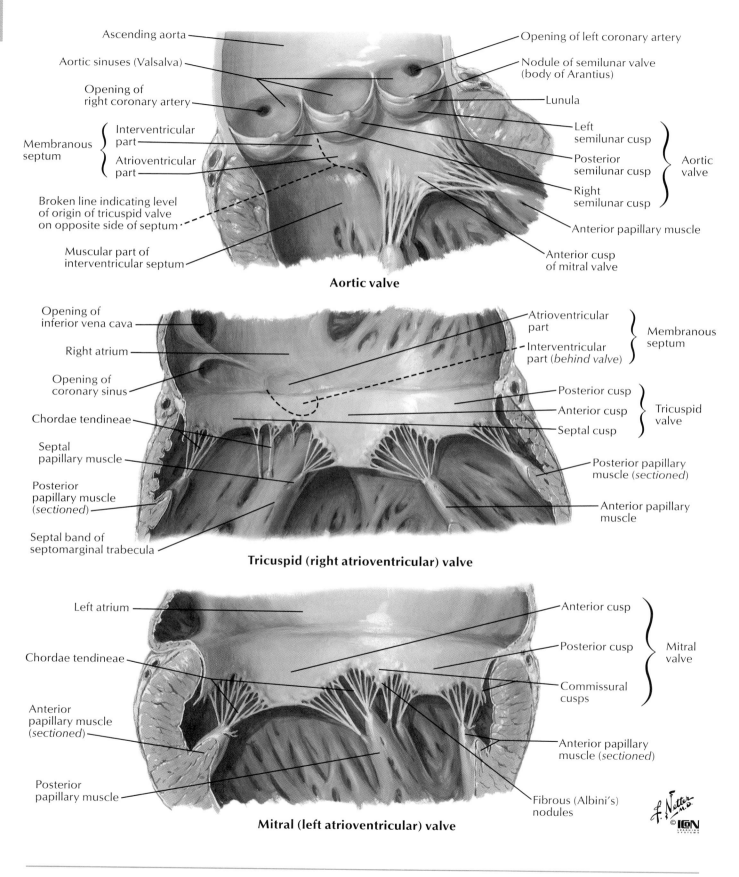

Ascending aorta

Aortic sinuses (Valsalva)

Opening of right coronary artery

Membranous septum
- Interventricular part
- Atrioventricular part

Broken line indicating level of origin of tricuspid valve on opposite side of septum

Muscular part of interventricular septum

Opening of left coronary artery

Nodule of semilunar valve (body of Arantius)

Lunula

Left semilunar cusp

Posterior semilunar cusp — Aortic valve

Right semilunar cusp

Anterior papillary muscle

Anterior cusp of mitral valve

Aortic valve

Opening of inferior vena cava

Right atrium

Opening of coronary sinus

Chordae tendineae

Septal papillary muscle

Posterior papillary muscle (sectioned)

Septal band of septomarginal trabecula

Atrioventricular part

Interventricular part (behind valve) — Membranous septum

Posterior cusp

Anterior cusp — Tricuspid valve

Septal cusp

Posterior papillary muscle (sectioned)

Anterior papillary muscle

Tricuspid (right atrioventricular) valve

Left atrium

Chordae tendineae

Anterior papillary muscle (sectioned)

Posterior papillary muscle

Anterior cusp

Posterior cusp — Mitral valve

Commissural cusps

Anterior papillary muscle (sectioned)

Fibrous (Albini's) nodules

Mitral (left atrioventricular) valve

PLATE 219

THORAX

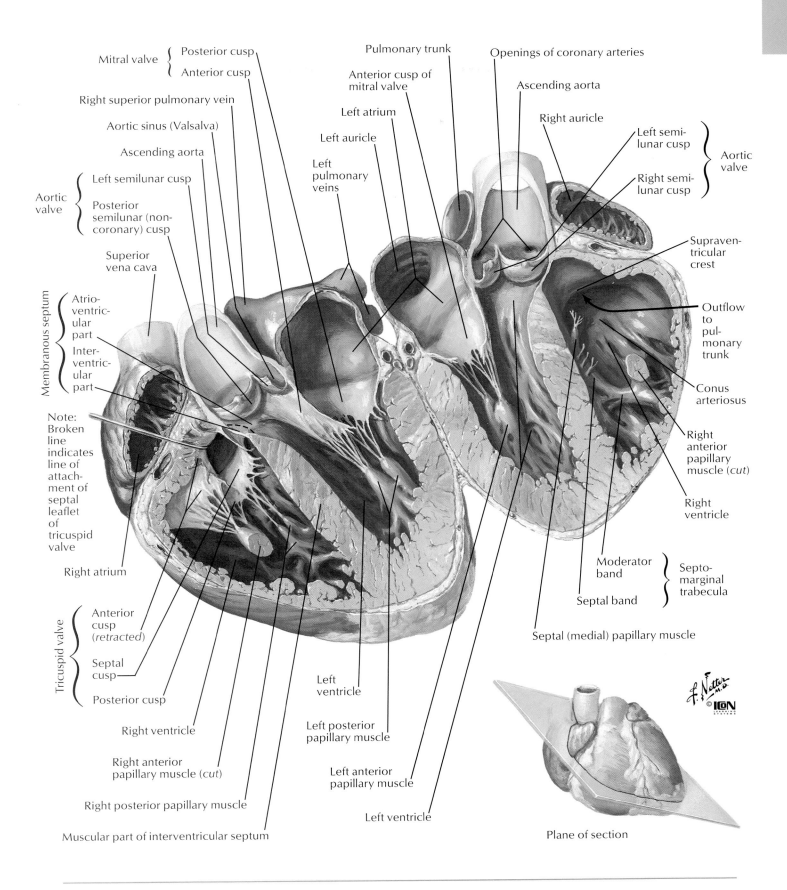

Mitral valve { Posterior cusp
Anterior cusp

Right superior pulmonary vein

Aortic sinus (Valsalva)

Ascending aorta

Aortic valve { Left semilunar cusp
Posterior semilunar (non-coronary) cusp

Superior vena cava

Membranous septum {
Atrio-ventricular part
Inter-ventricular part

Note: Broken line indicates line of attachment of septal leaflet of tricuspid valve

Right atrium

Tricuspid valve {
Anterior cusp (retracted)
Septal cusp
Posterior cusp

Right ventricle

Right anterior papillary muscle (cut)

Right posterior papillary muscle

Muscular part of interventricular septum

Pulmonary trunk

Anterior cusp of mitral valve

Left atrium

Left auricle

Left pulmonary veins

Openings of coronary arteries

Ascending aorta

Right auricle

Left semilunar cusp

Right semilunar cusp

Aortic valve

Supraventricular crest

Outflow to pulmonary trunk

Conus arteriosus

Right anterior papillary muscle (cut)

Right ventricle

Moderator band

Septal band

Septomarginal trabecula

Septal (medial) papillary muscle

Left ventricle

Left posterior papillary muscle

Left anterior papillary muscle

Left ventricle

Plane of section

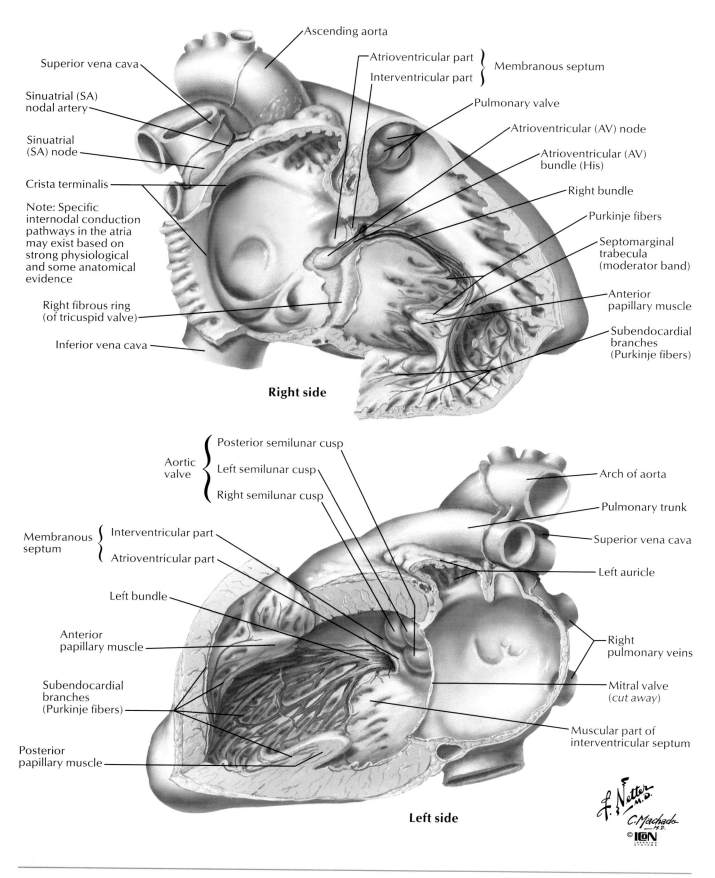

Ascending aorta

Superior vena cava

Atrioventricular part ⎱
Interventricular part ⎰ Membranous septum

Sinuatrial (SA) nodal artery

Pulmonary valve

Sinuatrial (SA) node

Atrioventricular (AV) node

Crista terminalis

Atrioventricular (AV) bundle (His)

Note: Specific internodal conduction pathways in the atria may exist based on strong physiological and some anatomical evidence

Right bundle

Purkinje fibers

Septomarginal trabecula (moderator band)

Anterior papillary muscle

Right fibrous ring (of tricuspid valve)

Subendocardial branches (Purkinje fibers)

Inferior vena cava

Right side

Aortic valve ⎰ Posterior semilunar cusp
Left semilunar cusp
Right semilunar cusp

Arch of aorta

Pulmonary trunk

Superior vena cava

Membranous septum ⎱ Interventricular part
Atrioventricular part

Left auricle

Left bundle

Anterior papillary muscle

Right pulmonary veins

Subendocardial branches (Purkinje fibers)

Mitral valve (*cut away*)

Posterior papillary muscle

Muscular part of interventricular septum

Left side

PLATE 221

THORAX

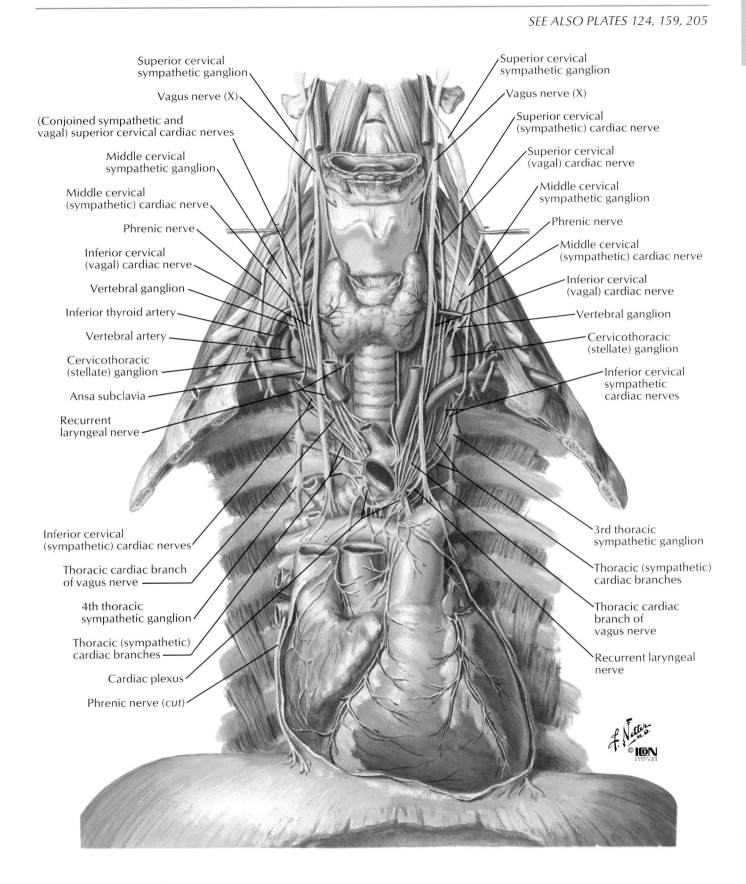

Superior cervical
sympathetic ganglion

Vagus nerve (X)

(Conjoined sympathetic and
vagal) superior cervical cardiac nerves

Middle cervical
sympathetic ganglion

Middle cervical
(sympathetic) cardiac nerve

Phrenic nerve

Inferior cervical
(vagal) cardiac nerve

Vertebral ganglion

Inferior thyroid artery

Vertebral artery

Cervicothoracic
(stellate) ganglion

Ansa subclavia

Recurrent
laryngeal nerve

Inferior cervical
(sympathetic) cardiac nerves

Thoracic cardiac branch
of vagus nerve

4th thoracic
sympathetic ganglion

Thoracic (sympathetic)
cardiac branches

Cardiac plexus

Phrenic nerve (*cut*)

Superior cervical
sympathetic ganglion

Vagus nerve (X)

Superior cervical
(sympathetic) cardiac nerve

Superior cervical
(vagal) cardiac nerve

Middle cervical
sympathetic ganglion

Phrenic nerve

Middle cervical
(sympathetic) cardiac nerve

Inferior cervical
(vagal) cardiac nerve

Vertebral ganglion

Cervicothoracic
(stellate) ganglion

Inferior cervical
sympathetic
cardiac nerves

3rd thoracic
sympathetic ganglion

Thoracic (sympathetic)
cardiac branches

Thoracic cardiac
branch of
vagus nerve

Recurrent laryngeal
nerve

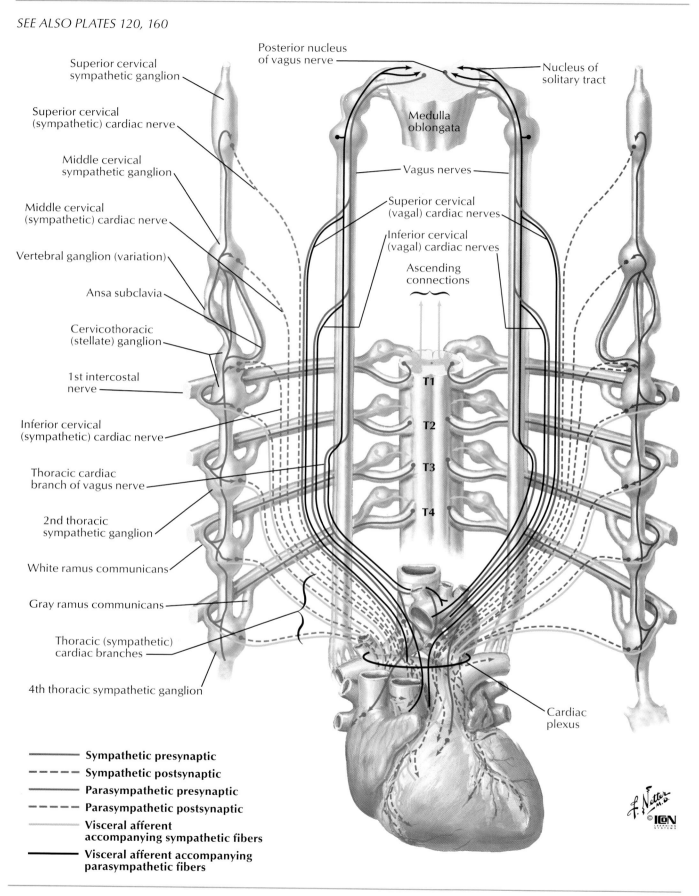

Superior cervical sympathetic ganglion

Superior cervical (sympathetic) cardiac nerve

Middle cervical sympathetic ganglion

Middle cervical (sympathetic) cardiac nerve

Vertebral ganglion (variation)

Ansa subclavia

Cervicothoracic (stellate) ganglion

1st intercostal nerve

Inferior cervical (sympathetic) cardiac nerve

Thoracic cardiac branch of vagus nerve

2nd thoracic sympathetic ganglion

White ramus communicans

Gray ramus communicans

Thoracic (sympathetic) cardiac branches

4th thoracic sympathetic ganglion

Posterior nucleus of vagus nerve

Nucleus of solitary tract

Medulla oblongata

Vagus nerves

Superior cervical (vagal) cardiac nerves

Inferior cervical (vagal) cardiac nerves

Ascending connections

T1

T2

T3

T4

Cardiac plexus

— Sympathetic presynaptic

---- Sympathetic postsynaptic

— Parasympathetic presynaptic

---- Parasympathetic postsynaptic

— Visceral afferent accompanying sympathetic fibers

— Visceral afferent accompanying parasympathetic fibers

PLATE 223

THORAX

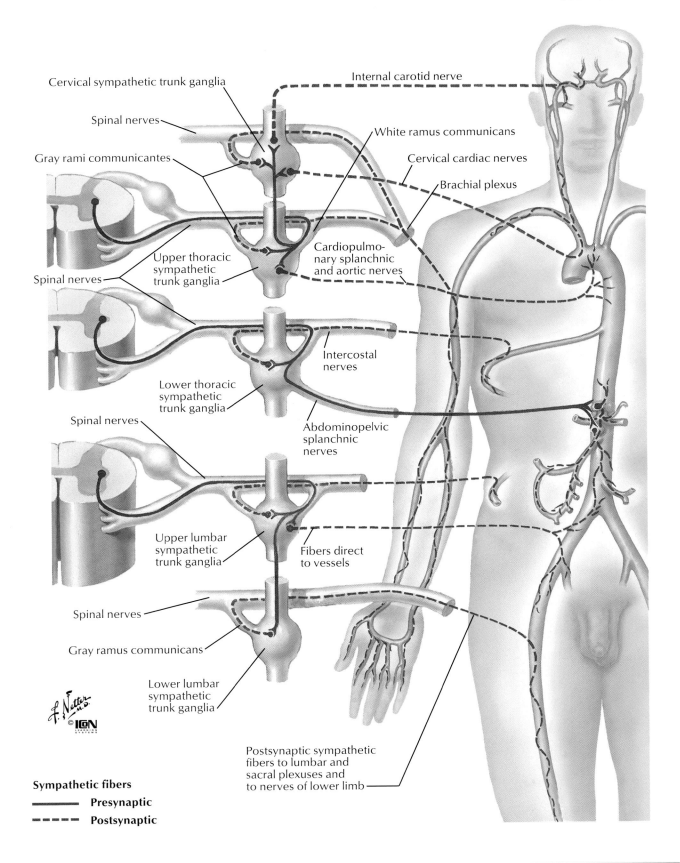

Cervical sympathetic trunk ganglia

Internal carotid nerve

Spinal nerves

White ramus communicans

Gray rami communicantes

Cervical cardiac nerves

Brachial plexus

Upper thoracic sympathetic trunk ganglia

Cardiopulmonary splanchnic and aortic nerves

Spinal nerves

Intercostal nerves

Lower thoracic sympathetic trunk ganglia

Abdominopelvic splanchnic nerves

Spinal nerves

Upper lumbar sympathetic trunk ganglia

Fibers direct to vessels

Spinal nerves

Gray ramus communicans

Lower lumbar sympathetic trunk ganglia

Postsynaptic sympathetic fibers to lumbar and sacral plexuses and to nerves of lower limb

Sympathetic fibers

———— **Presynaptic**

– – – – **Postsynaptic**

Prenatal and Postnatal Circulation

FOR OCCLUDED PART OF UMBILICAL VESSELS SEE PLATE 245

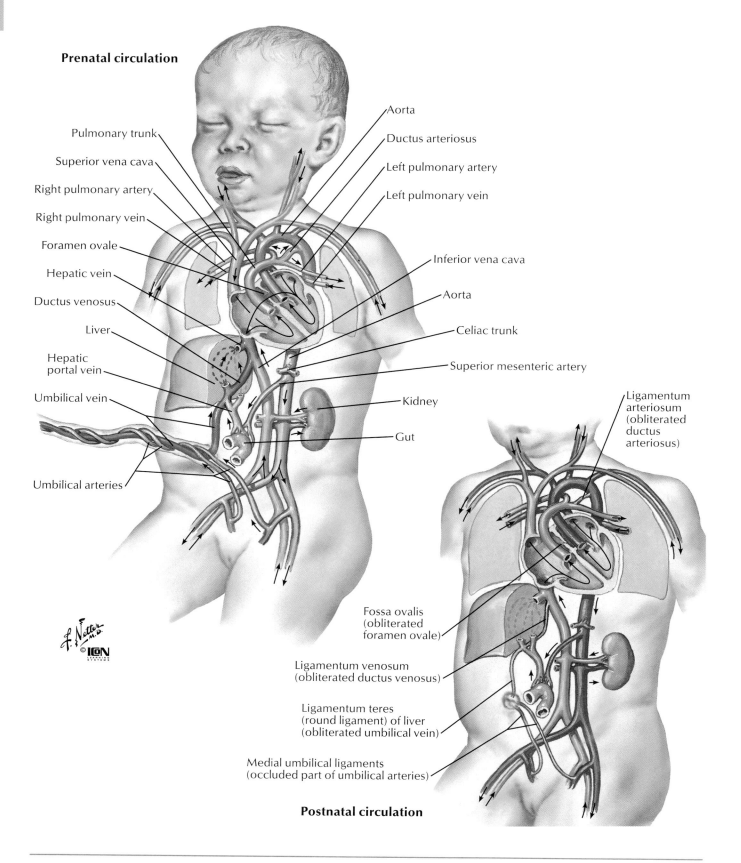

Prenatal circulation

Pulmonary trunk

Superior vena cava

Right pulmonary artery

Right pulmonary vein

Foramen ovale

Hepatic vein

Ductus venosus

Liver

Hepatic portal vein

Umbilical vein

Umbilical arteries

Aorta

Ductus arteriosus

Left pulmonary artery

Left pulmonary vein

Inferior vena cava

Aorta

Celiac trunk

Superior mesenteric artery

Kidney

Gut

Ligamentum arteriosum (obliterated ductus arteriosus)

Fossa ovalis (obliterated foramen ovale)

Ligamentum venosum (obliterated ductus venosus)

Ligamentum teres (round ligament) of liver (obliterated umbilical vein)

Medial umbilical ligaments (occluded part of umbilical arteries)

Postnatal circulation

PLATE 225

THORAX

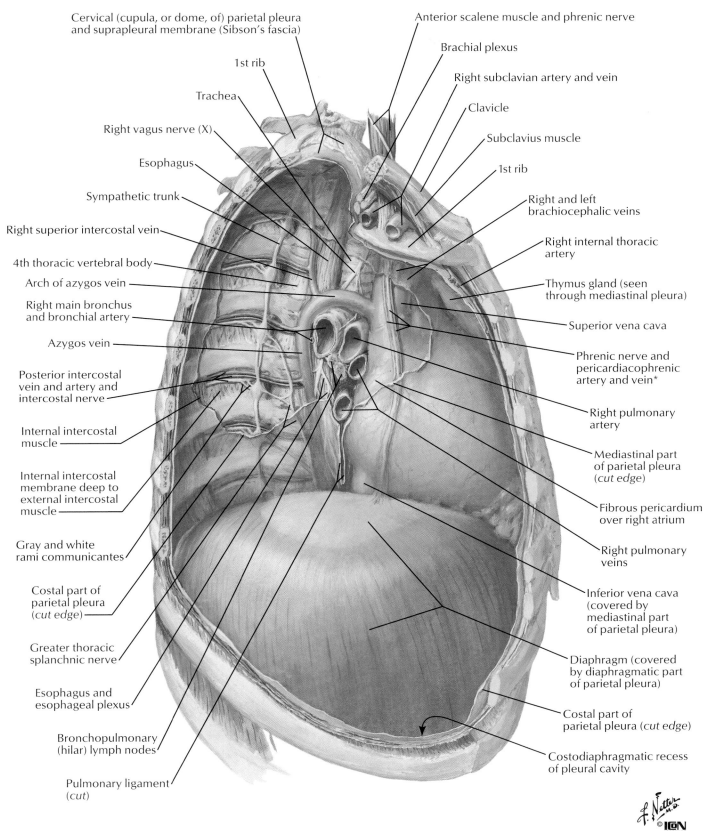

Cervical (cupula, or dome, of) parietal pleura and suprapleural membrane (Sibson's fascia)

Anterior scalene muscle and phrenic nerve

1st rib

Brachial plexus

Trachea

Right subclavian artery and vein

Right vagus nerve (X)

Clavicle

Esophagus

Subclavius muscle

Sympathetic trunk

1st rib

Right superior intercostal vein

Right and left brachiocephalic veins

4th thoracic vertebral body

Right internal thoracic artery

Arch of azygos vein

Thymus gland (seen through mediastinal pleura)

Right main bronchus and bronchial artery

Superior vena cava

Azygos vein

Phrenic nerve and pericardiacophrenic artery and vein*

Posterior intercostal vein and artery and intercostal nerve

Right pulmonary artery

Internal intercostal muscle

Mediastinal part of parietal pleura (*cut edge*)

Internal intercostal membrane deep to external intercostal muscle

Fibrous pericardium over right atrium

Gray and white rami communicantes

Right pulmonary veins

Costal part of parietal pleura (*cut edge*)

Inferior vena cava (covered by mediastinal part of parietal pleura)

Greater thoracic splanchnic nerve

Diaphragm (covered by diaphragmatic part of parietal pleura)

Esophagus and esophageal plexus

Costal part of parietal pleura (*cut edge*)

Bronchopulmonary (hilar) lymph nodes

Costodiaphragmatic recess of pleural cavity

Pulmonary ligament (*cut*)

*Nerve and vessels commonly run independently

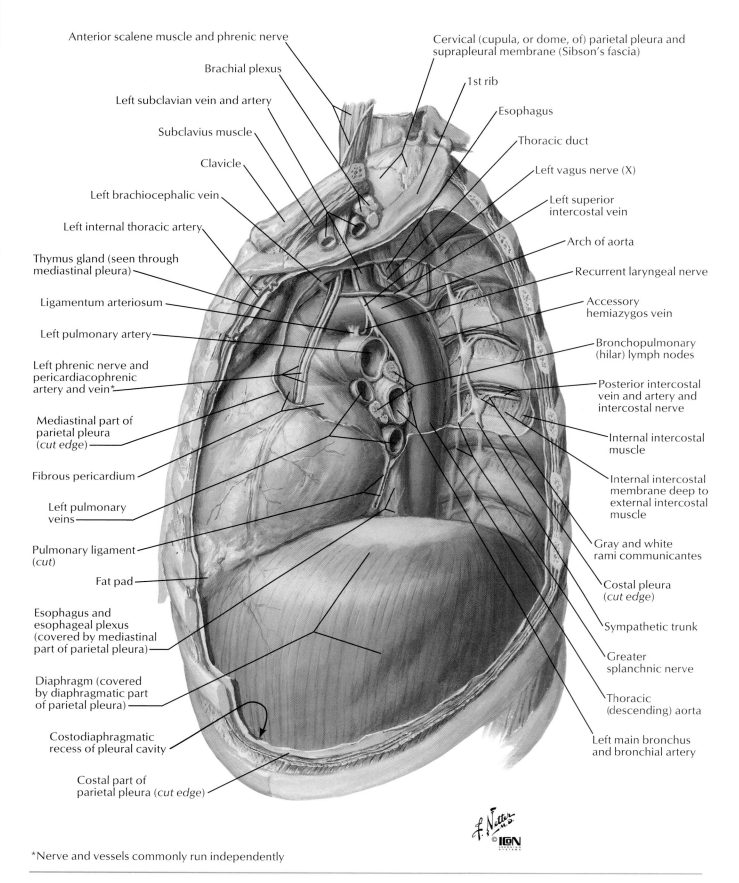

Anterior scalene muscle and phrenic nerve

Brachial plexus

Left subclavian vein and artery

Subclavius muscle

Clavicle

Left brachiocephalic vein

Left internal thoracic artery

Thymus gland (seen through mediastinal pleura)

Ligamentum arteriosum

Left pulmonary artery

Left phrenic nerve and pericardiacophrenic artery and vein*

Mediastinal part of parietal pleura (*cut edge*)

Fibrous pericardium

Left pulmonary veins

Pulmonary ligament (*cut*)

Fat pad

Esophagus and esophageal plexus (covered by mediastinal part of parietal pleura)

Diaphragm (covered by diaphragmatic part of parietal pleura)

Costodiaphragmatic recess of pleural cavity

Costal part of parietal pleura (*cut edge*)

Cervical (cupula, or dome, of) parietal pleura and suprapleural membrane (Sibson's fascia)

1st rib

Esophagus

Thoracic duct

Left vagus nerve (X)

Left superior intercostal vein

Arch of aorta

Recurrent laryngeal nerve

Accessory hemiazygos vein

Bronchopulmonary (hilar) lymph nodes

Posterior intercostal vein and artery and intercostal nerve

Internal intercostal muscle

Internal intercostal membrane deep to external intercostal muscle

Gray and white rami communicantes

Costal pleura (*cut edge*)

Sympathetic trunk

Greater splanchnic nerve

Thoracic (descending) aorta

Left main bronchus and bronchial artery

*Nerve and vessels commonly run independently

PLATE 227

THORAX

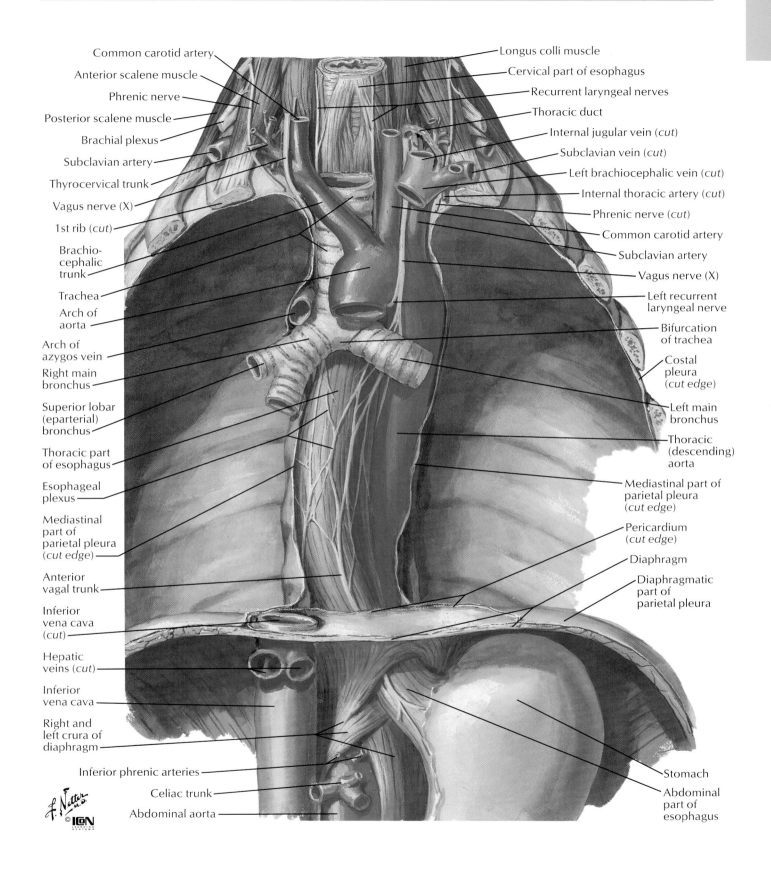

Common carotid artery

Anterior scalene muscle

Phrenic nerve

Posterior scalene muscle

Brachial plexus

Subclavian artery

Thyrocervical trunk

Vagus nerve (X)

1st rib (*cut*)

Brachio-cephalic trunk

Trachea

Arch of aorta

Arch of azygos vein

Right main bronchus

Superior lobar (eparterial) bronchus

Thoracic part of esophagus

Esophageal plexus

Mediastinal part of parietal pleura (*cut edge*)

Anterior vagal trunk

Inferior vena cava (*cut*)

Hepatic veins (*cut*)

Inferior vena cava

Right and left crura of diaphragm

Inferior phrenic arteries

Celiac trunk

Abdominal aorta

Longus colli muscle

Cervical part of esophagus

Recurrent laryngeal nerves

Thoracic duct

Internal jugular vein (*cut*)

Subclavian vein (*cut*)

Left brachiocephalic vein (*cut*)

Internal thoracic artery (*cut*)

Phrenic nerve (*cut*)

Common carotid artery

Subclavian artery

Vagus nerve (X)

Left recurrent laryngeal nerve

Bifurcation of trachea

Costal pleura (*cut edge*)

Left main bronchus

Thoracic (descending) aorta

Mediastinal part of parietal pleura (*cut edge*)

Pericardium (*cut edge*)

Diaphragm

Diaphragmatic part of parietal pleura

Stomach

Abdominal part of esophagus

Topography and Constrictions of Esophagus

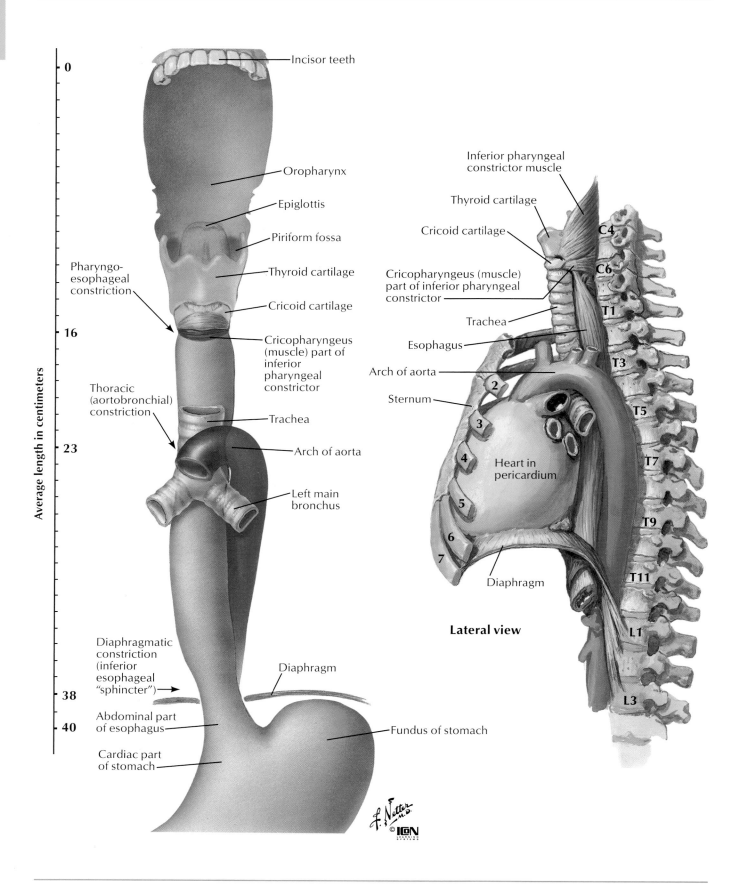

Incisor teeth

Oropharynx

Epiglottis

Piriform fossa

Thyroid cartilage

Cricoid cartilage

Cricopharyngeus (muscle) part of inferior pharyngeal constrictor

Trachea

Arch of aorta

Left main bronchus

Pharyngo-esophageal constriction

Thoracic (aortobronchial) constriction

Diaphragmatic constriction (inferior esophageal "sphincter")

Abdominal part of esophagus

Cardiac part of stomach

Diaphragm

Fundus of stomach

Average length in centimeters

0

16

23

38

40

Inferior pharyngeal constrictor muscle

Thyroid cartilage

Cricoid cartilage

Cricopharyngeus (muscle) part of inferior pharyngeal constrictor

Trachea

Esophagus

Arch of aorta

Sternum

Heart in pericardium

Diaphragm

C4

C6

T1

T3

T5

T7

T9

T11

L1

L3

2

3

4

5

6

7

Lateral view

PLATE 229

THORAX

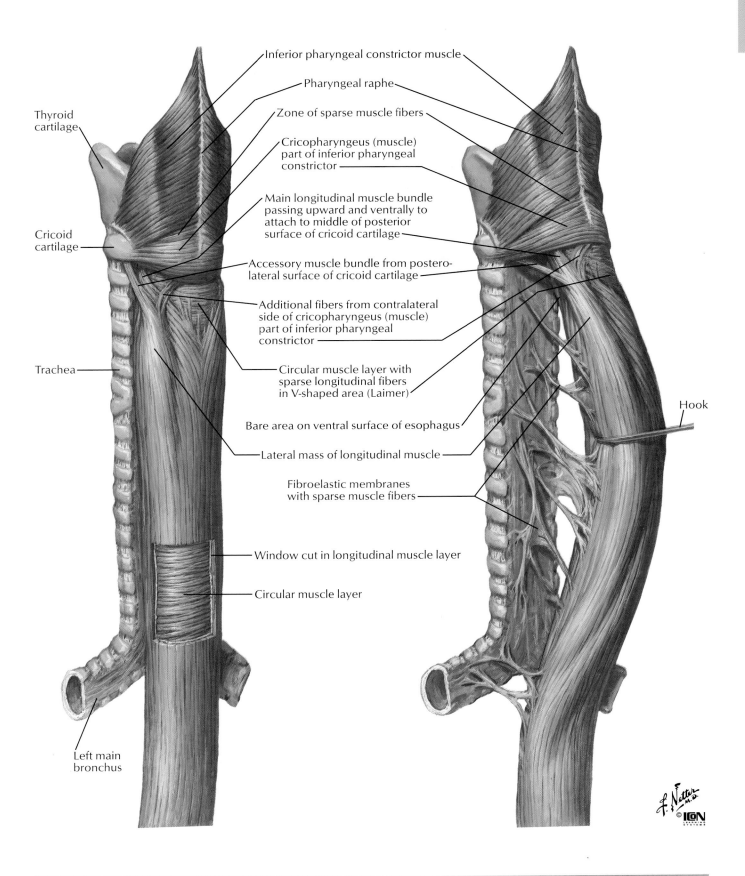

Inferior pharyngeal constrictor muscle

Pharyngeal raphe

Zone of sparse muscle fibers

Thyroid cartilage

Cricopharyngeus (muscle) part of inferior pharyngeal constrictor

Main longitudinal muscle bundle passing upward and ventrally to attach to middle of posterior surface of cricoid cartilage

Cricoid cartilage

Accessory muscle bundle from postero-lateral surface of cricoid cartilage

Additional fibers from contralateral side of cricopharyngeus (muscle) part of inferior pharyngeal constrictor

Trachea

Circular muscle layer with sparse longitudinal fibers in V-shaped area (Laimer)

Bare area on ventral surface of esophagus

Lateral mass of longitudinal muscle

Hook

Fibroelastic membranes with sparse muscle fibers

Window cut in longitudinal muscle layer

Circular muscle layer

Left main bronchus

Pharyngoesophageal Junction

SEE ALSO PLATE 63

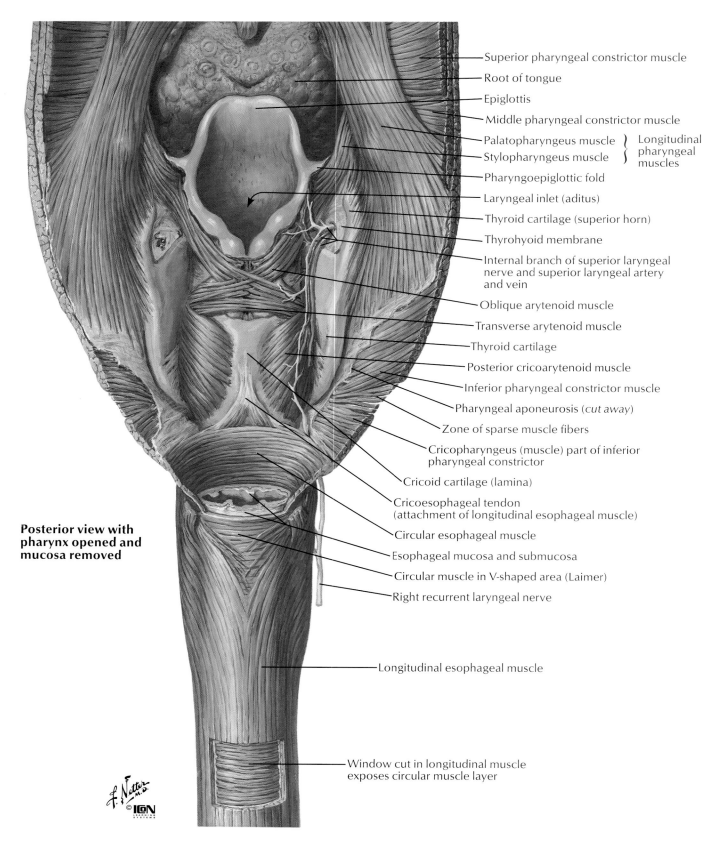

Superior pharyngeal constrictor muscle

Root of tongue

Epiglottis

Middle pharyngeal constrictor muscle

Palatopharyngeus muscle } Longitudinal

Stylopharyngeus muscle } pharyngeal muscles

Pharyngoepiglottic fold

Laryngeal inlet (aditus)

Thyroid cartilage (superior horn)

Thyrohyoid membrane

Internal branch of superior laryngeal nerve and superior laryngeal artery and vein

Oblique arytenoid muscle

Transverse arytenoid muscle

Thyroid cartilage

Posterior cricoarytenoid muscle

Inferior pharyngeal constrictor muscle

Pharyngeal aponeurosis (*cut away*)

Zone of sparse muscle fibers

Cricopharyngeus (muscle) part of inferior pharyngeal constrictor

Cricoid cartilage (lamina)

Cricoesophageal tendon (attachment of longitudinal esophageal muscle)

Circular esophageal muscle

Esophageal mucosa and submucosa

Circular muscle in V-shaped area (Laimer)

Right recurrent laryngeal nerve

Longitudinal esophageal muscle

Window cut in longitudinal muscle exposes circular muscle layer

Posterior view with pharynx opened and mucosa removed

PLATE 231

THORAX

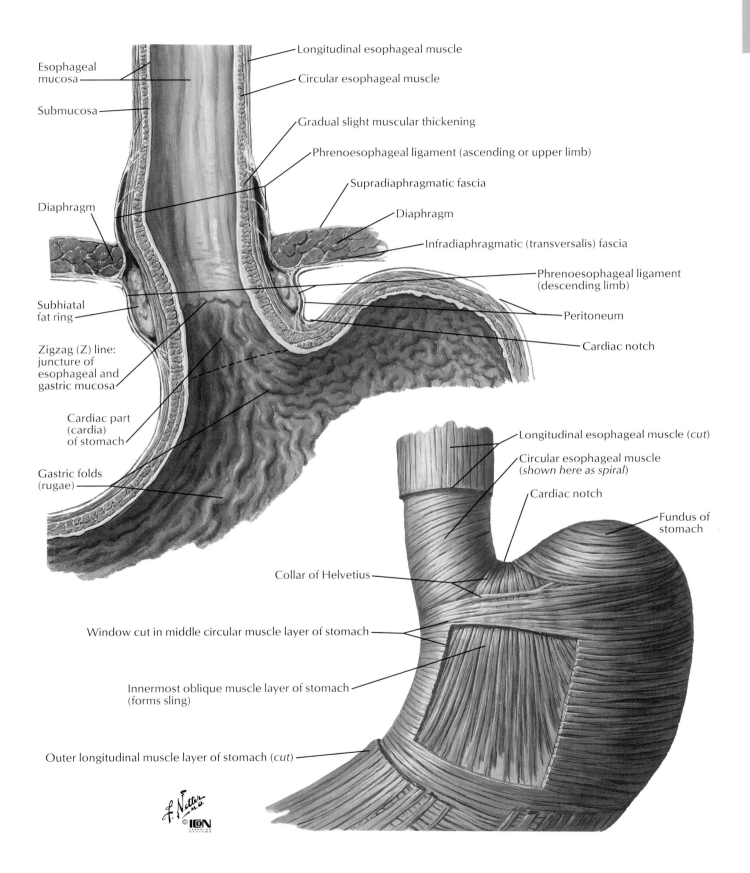

Esophageal mucosa

Submucosa

Diaphragm

Subhiatal fat ring

Zigzag (Z) line: juncture of esophageal and gastric mucosa

Cardiac part (cardia) of stomach

Gastric folds (rugae)

Longitudinal esophageal muscle

Circular esophageal muscle

Gradual slight muscular thickening

Phrenoesophageal ligament (ascending or upper limb)

Supradiaphragmatic fascia

Diaphragm

Infradiaphragmatic (transversalis) fascia

Phrenoesophageal ligament (descending limb)

Peritoneum

Cardiac notch

Longitudinal esophageal muscle (*cut*)

Circular esophageal muscle (*shown here as spiral*)

Cardiac notch

Fundus of stomach

Collar of Helvetius

Window cut in middle circular muscle layer of stomach

Innermost oblique muscle layer of stomach (forms sling)

Outer longitudinal muscle layer of stomach (*cut*)

SEE ALSO PLATES 290, 291

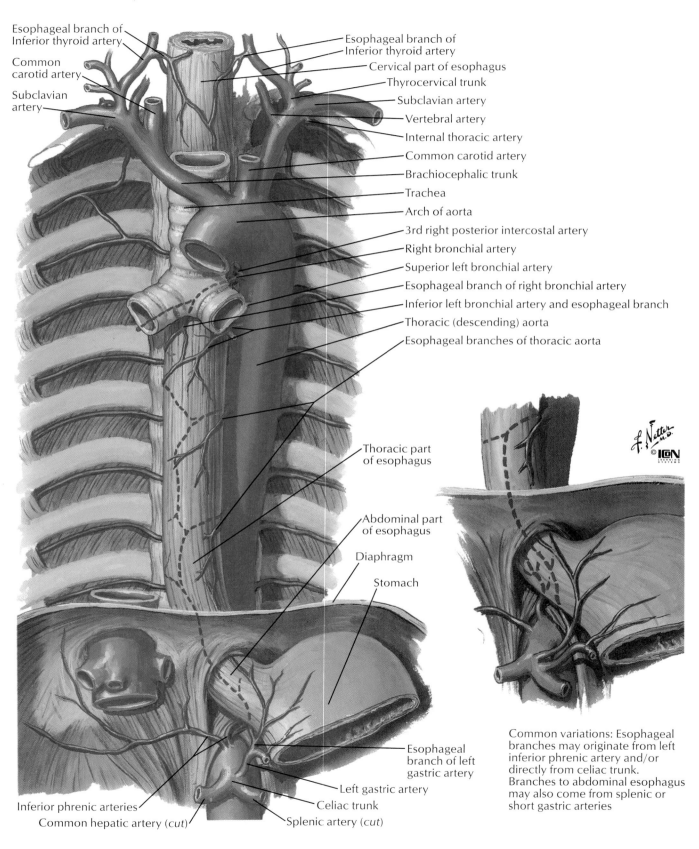

Esophageal branch of
Inferior thyroid artery

Common
carotid artery

Subclavian
artery

Esophageal branch of
Inferior thyroid artery

Cervical part of esophagus

Thyrocervical trunk

Subclavian artery

Vertebral artery

Internal thoracic artery

Common carotid artery

Brachiocephalic trunk

Trachea

Arch of aorta

3rd right posterior intercostal artery

Right bronchial artery

Superior left bronchial artery

Esophageal branch of right bronchial artery

Inferior left bronchial artery and esophageal branch

Thoracic (descending) aorta

Esophageal branches of thoracic aorta

Thoracic part
of esophagus

Abdominal part
of esophagus

Diaphragm

Stomach

Esophageal
branch of left
gastric artery

Left gastric artery

Celiac trunk

Splenic artery (*cut*)

Inferior phrenic arteries

Common hepatic artery (*cut*)

Common variations: Esophageal
branches may originate from left
inferior phrenic artery and/or
directly from celiac trunk.
Branches to abdominal esophagus
may also come from splenic or
short gastric arteries

PLATE 233

THORAX

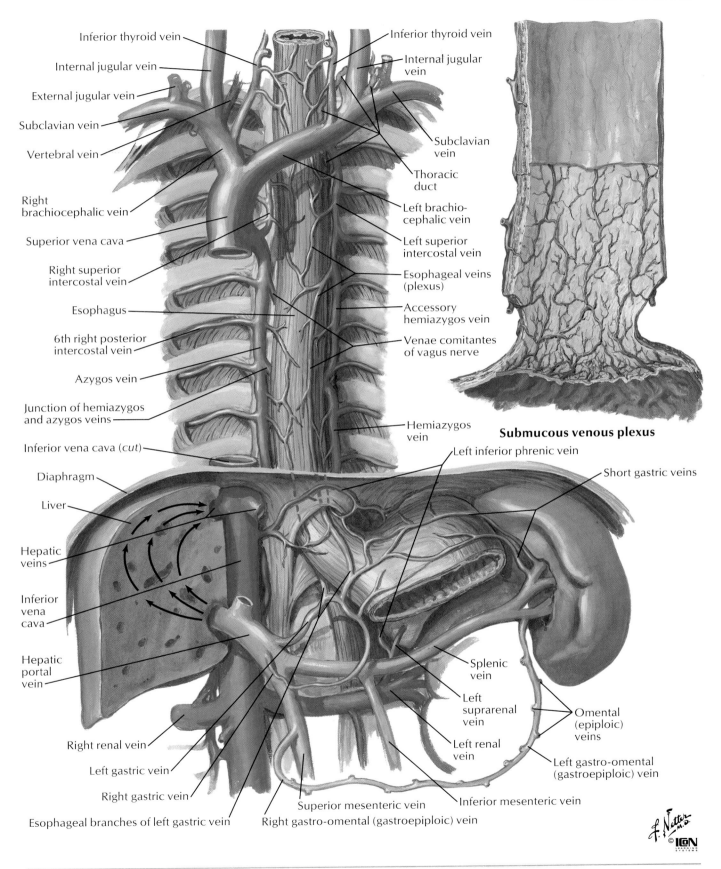

Inferior thyroid vein

Internal jugular vein

External jugular vein

Subclavian vein

Vertebral vein

Right brachiocephalic vein

Superior vena cava

Right superior intercostal vein

Esophagus

6th right posterior intercostal vein

Azygos vein

Junction of hemiazygos and azygos veins

Inferior vena cava (*cut*)

Diaphragm

Liver

Hepatic veins

Inferior vena cava

Hepatic portal vein

Right renal vein

Left gastric vein

Right gastric vein

Esophageal branches of left gastric vein

Inferior thyroid vein

Internal jugular vein

Subclavian vein

Thoracic duct

Left brachiocephalic vein

Left superior intercostal vein

Esophageal veins (plexus)

Accessory hemiazygos vein

Venae comitantes of vagus nerve

Hemiazygos vein

Submucous venous plexus

Left inferior phrenic vein

Short gastric veins

Splenic vein

Left suprarenal vein

Left renal vein

Omental (epiploic) veins

Left gastro-omental (gastroepiploic) vein

Inferior mesenteric vein

Superior mesenteric vein

Right gastro-omental (gastroepiploic) vein

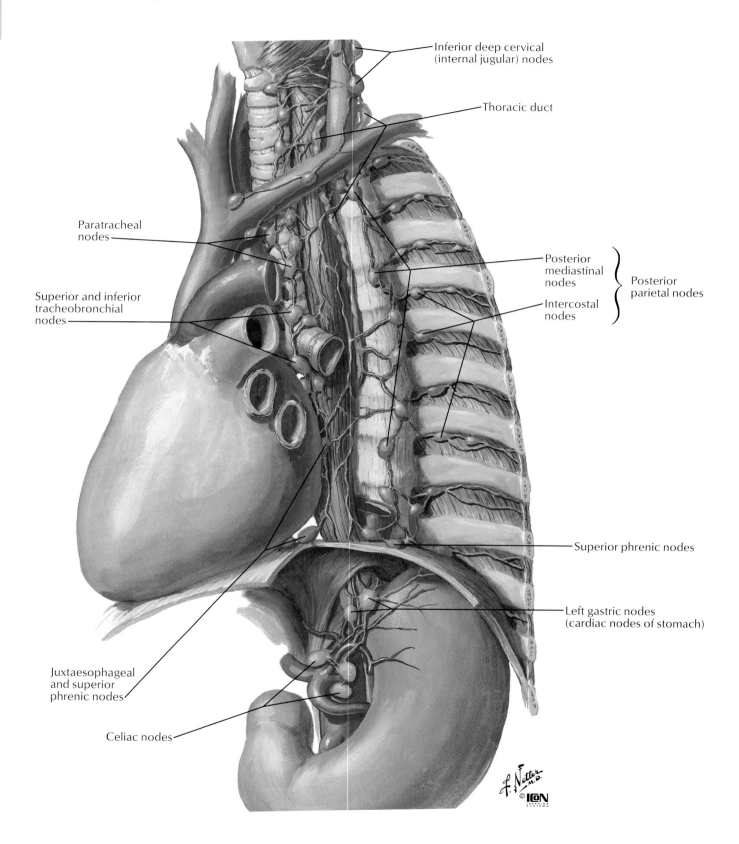

Inferior deep cervical
(internal jugular) nodes

Thoracic duct

Paratracheal
nodes

Posterior
mediastinal
nodes

Posterior
parietal nodes

Superior and inferior
tracheobronchial
nodes

Intercostal
nodes

Superior phrenic nodes

Left gastric nodes
(cardiac nodes of stomach)

Juxtaesophageal
and superior
phrenic nodes

Celiac nodes

PLATE 235

THORAX

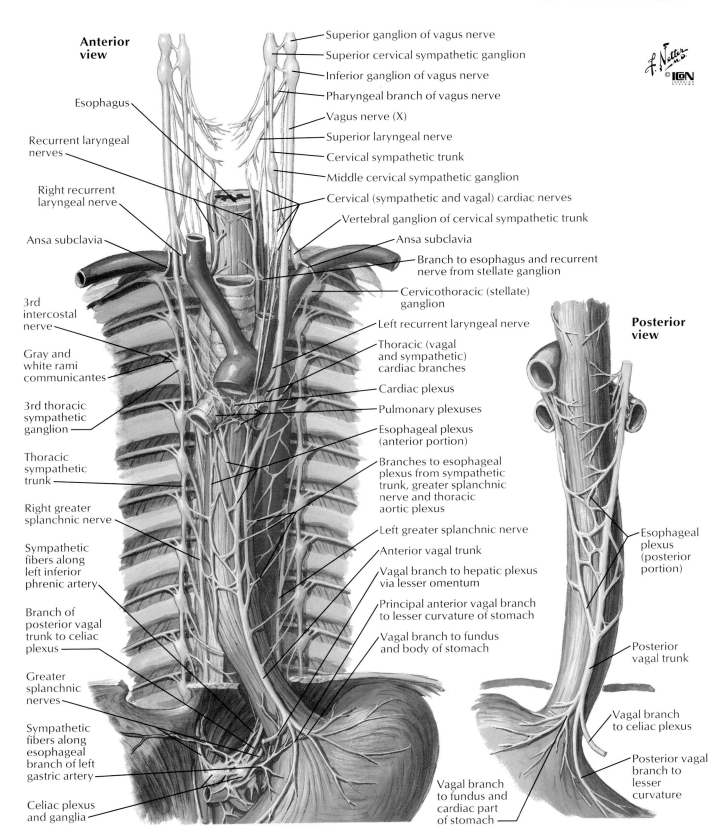

Anterior view

Esophagus

Recurrent laryngeal nerves

Right recurrent laryngeal nerve

Ansa subclavia

3rd intercostal nerve

Gray and white rami communicantes

3rd thoracic sympathetic ganglion

Thoracic sympathetic trunk

Right greater splanchnic nerve

Sympathetic fibers along left inferior phrenic artery

Branch of posterior vagal trunk to celiac plexus

Greater splanchnic nerves

Sympathetic fibers along esophageal branch of left gastric artery

Celiac plexus and ganglia

Superior ganglion of vagus nerve

Superior cervical sympathetic ganglion

Inferior ganglion of vagus nerve

Pharyngeal branch of vagus nerve

Vagus nerve (X)

Superior laryngeal nerve

Cervical sympathetic trunk

Middle cervical sympathetic ganglion

Cervical (sympathetic and vagal) cardiac nerves

Vertebral ganglion of cervical sympathetic trunk

Ansa subclavia

Branch to esophagus and recurrent nerve from stellate ganglion

Cervicothoracic (stellate) ganglion

Left recurrent laryngeal nerve

Thoracic (vagal and sympathetic) cardiac branches

Cardiac plexus

Pulmonary plexuses

Esophageal plexus (anterior portion)

Branches to esophageal plexus from sympathetic trunk, greater splanchnic nerve and thoracic aortic plexus

Left greater splanchnic nerve

Anterior vagal trunk

Vagal branch to hepatic plexus via lesser omentum

Principal anterior vagal branch to lesser curvature of stomach

Vagal branch to fundus and body of stomach

Vagal branch to fundus and cardiac part of stomach

Posterior view

Esophageal plexus (posterior portion)

Posterior vagal trunk

Vagal branch to celiac plexus

Posterior vagal branch to lesser curvature

SEE ALSO PLATE 533

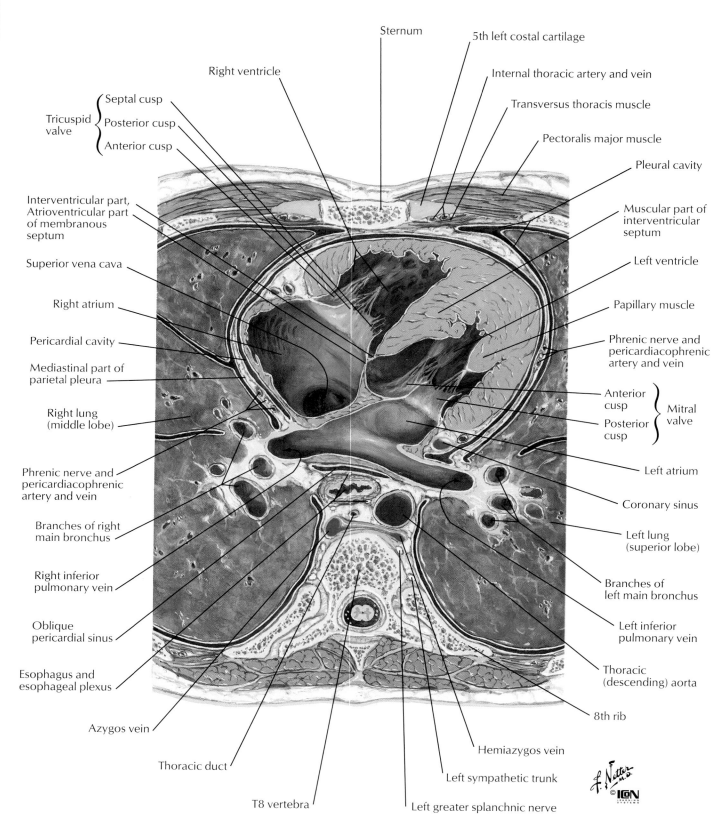

Sternum

5th left costal cartilage

Right ventricle

Internal thoracic artery and vein

Transversus thoracis muscle

Septal cusp

Tricuspid valve — Posterior cusp

Anterior cusp

Pectoralis major muscle

Pleural cavity

Interventricular part, Atrioventricular part of membranous septum

Muscular part of interventricular septum

Superior vena cava

Left ventricle

Right atrium

Papillary muscle

Pericardial cavity

Phrenic nerve and pericardiacophrenic artery and vein

Mediastinal part of parietal pleura

Anterior cusp — Mitral valve

Posterior cusp

Right lung (middle lobe)

Phrenic nerve and pericardiacophrenic artery and vein

Left atrium

Coronary sinus

Branches of right main bronchus

Left lung (superior lobe)

Right inferior pulmonary vein

Branches of left main bronchus

Oblique pericardial sinus

Left inferior pulmonary vein

Esophagus and esophageal plexus

Thoracic (descending) aorta

8th rib

Azygos vein

Hemiazygos vein

Thoracic duct

Left sympathetic trunk

T8 vertebra

Left greater splanchnic nerve

PLATE 237

THORAX

Series of chest axial CT images from superior (A) to inferior (C)

A

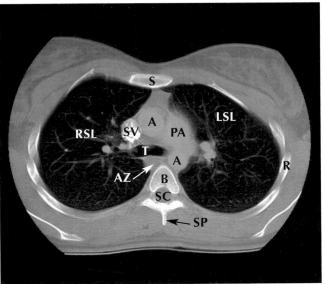

A	Aorta
AZ	Azygos vein
B	Body of vertebra
IV	Inferior vena cava
L	Liver
LB	Left bronchus
LSL	Left superior lobe of lung
LV	Left ventricle
PA	Pulmonary artery
R	Rib
RB	Right bronchus
RSL	Right superior lobe of lung
RV	Right ventricle
S	Sternum
SC	Spinal cord
SP	Spinous process of vertebra
SV	Superior vena cava
T	Trachea (bifurcation)

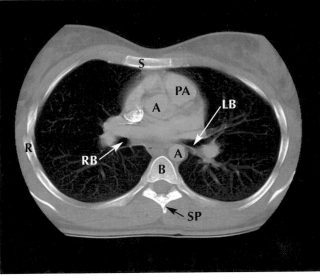

B

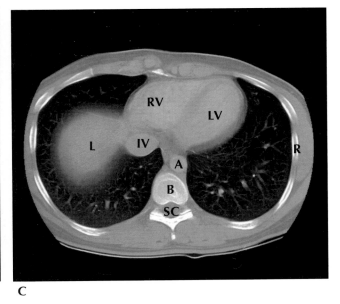

C

Section IV
ABDOMEN

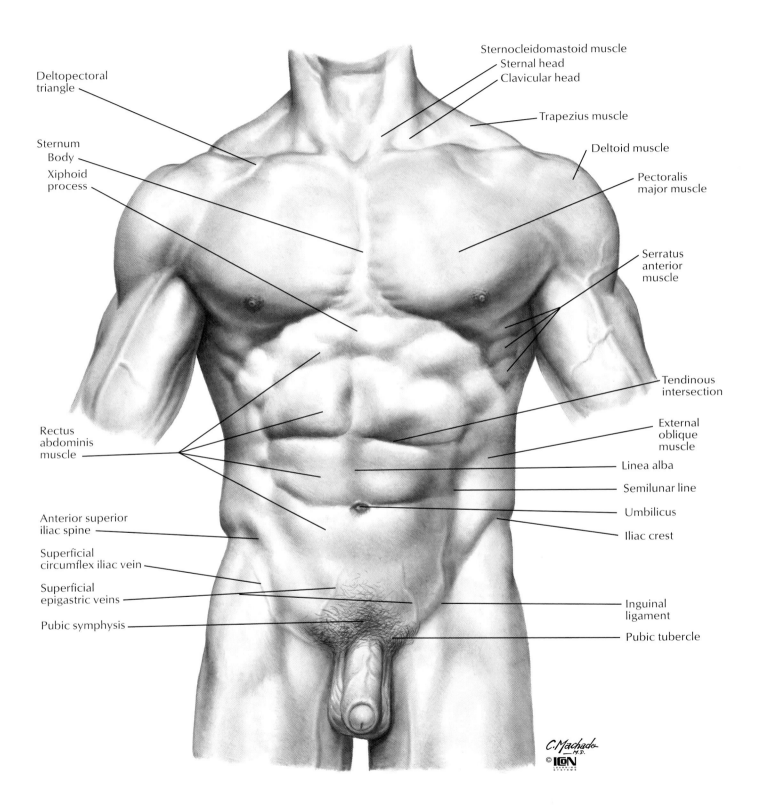

Deltopectoral triangle

Sternum
Body
Xiphoid process

Rectus abdominis muscle

Anterior superior iliac spine

Superficial circumflex iliac vein

Superficial epigastric veins

Pubic symphysis

Sternocleidomastoid muscle
Sternal head
Clavicular head

Trapezius muscle

Deltoid muscle

Pectoralis major muscle

Serratus anterior muscle

Tendinous intersection

External oblique muscle

Linea alba

Semilunar line

Umbilicus

Iliac crest

Inguinal ligament

Pubic tubercle

C.Machado
_M.D.
© ICON

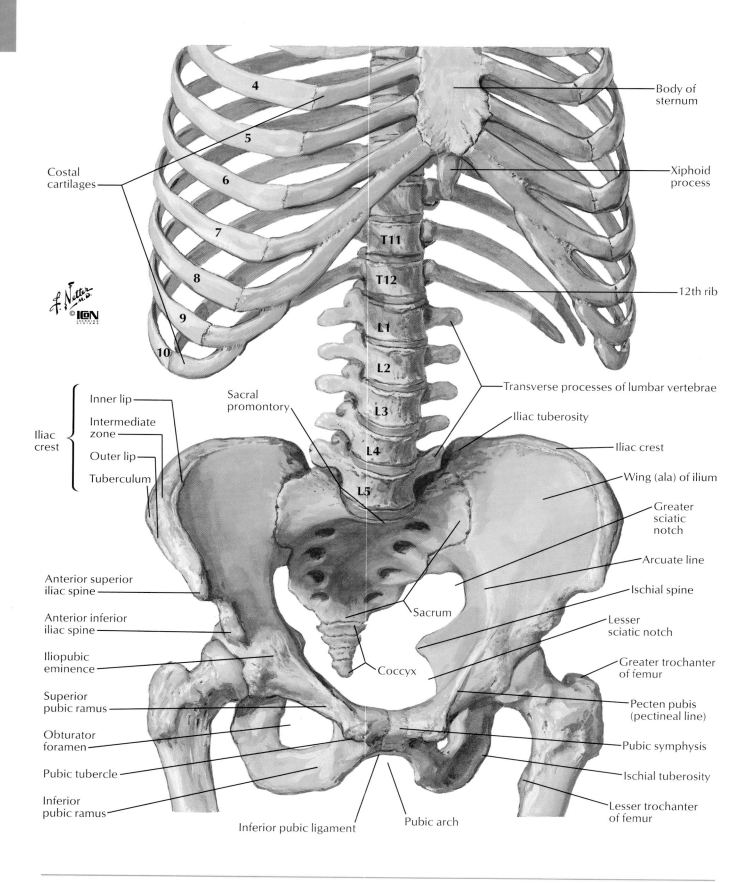

Body of sternum

Xiphoid process

12th rib

Costal cartilages

4

5

6

7

8

9

10

T11

T12

L1

L2

L3

L4

L5

Transverse processes of lumbar vertebrae

Iliac tuberosity

Iliac crest

Wing (ala) of ilium

Greater sciatic notch

Arcuate line

Ischial spine

Lesser sciatic notch

Greater trochanter of femur

Pecten pubis (pectineal line)

Pubic symphysis

Ischial tuberosity

Lesser trochanter of femur

Iliac crest
- Inner lip
- Intermediate zone
- Outer lip
- Tuberculum

Sacral promontory

Anterior superior iliac spine

Anterior inferior iliac spine

Iliopubic eminence

Superior pubic ramus

Obturator foramen

Pubic tubercle

Inferior pubic ramus

Sacrum

Coccyx

Inferior pubic ligament

Pubic arch

PLATE 240

ABDOMEN

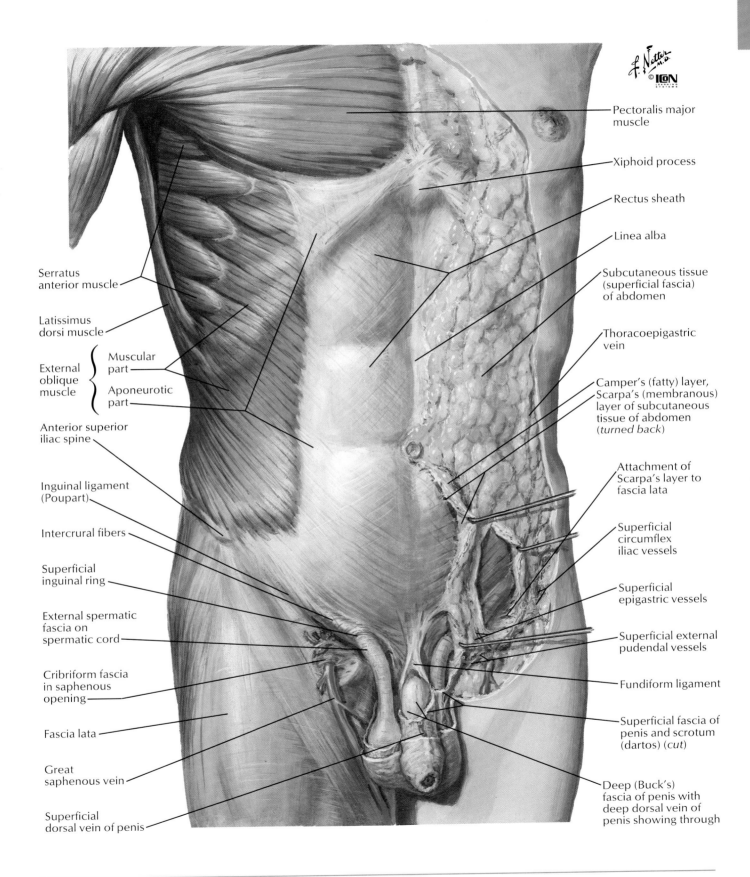

Pectoralis major muscle

Xiphoid process

Rectus sheath

Linea alba

Subcutaneous tissue (superficial fascia) of abdomen

Thoracoepigastric vein

Camper's (fatty) layer, Scarpa's (membranous) layer of subcutaneous tissue of abdomen (*turned back*)

Attachment of Scarpa's layer to fascia lata

Superficial circumflex iliac vessels

Superficial epigastric vessels

Superficial external pudendal vessels

Fundiform ligament

Superficial fascia of penis and scrotum (dartos) (*cut*)

Deep (Buck's) fascia of penis with deep dorsal vein of penis showing through

Serratus anterior muscle

Latissimus dorsi muscle

External oblique muscle
- Muscular part
- Aponeurotic part

Anterior superior iliac spine

Inguinal ligament (Poupart)

Intercrural fibers

Superficial inguinal ring

External spermatic fascia on spermatic cord

Cribriform fascia in saphenous opening

Fascia lata

Great saphenous vein

Superficial dorsal vein of penis

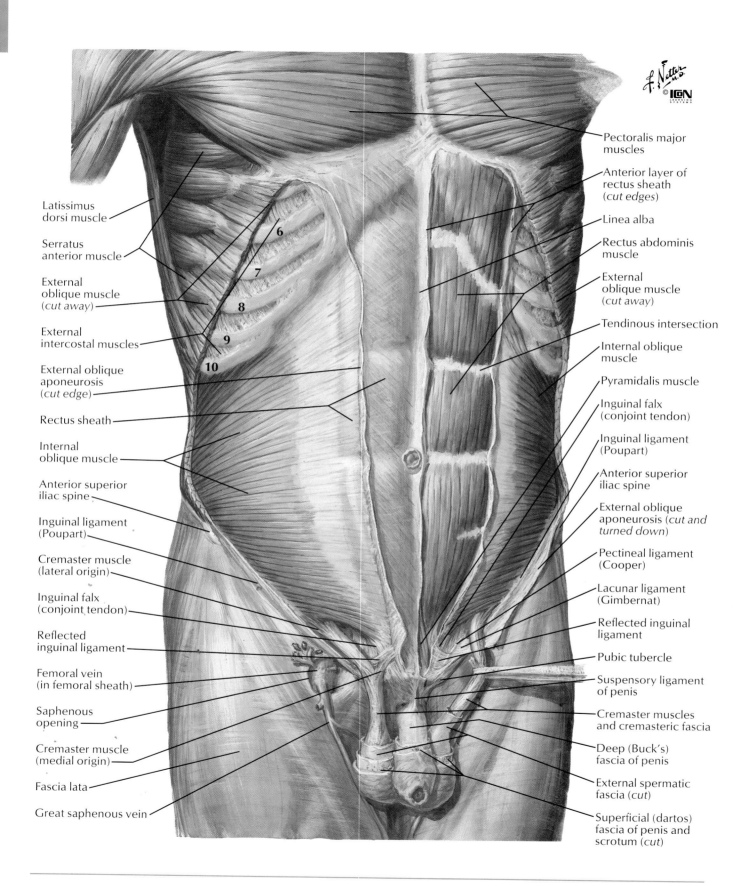

Latissimus
dorsi muscle

Serratus
anterior muscle

External
oblique muscle
(cut away)

External
intercostal muscles

External oblique
aponeurosis
(cut edge)

Rectus sheath

Internal
oblique muscle

Anterior superior
iliac spine

Inguinal ligament
(Poupart)

Cremaster muscle
(lateral origin)

Inguinal falx
(conjoint tendon)

Reflected
inguinal ligament

Femoral vein
(in femoral sheath)

Saphenous
opening

Cremaster muscle
(medial origin)

Fascia lata

Great saphenous vein

Pectoralis major
muscles

Anterior layer of
rectus sheath
(cut edges)

Linea alba

Rectus abdominis
muscle

External
oblique muscle
(cut away)

Tendinous intersection

Internal oblique
muscle

Pyramidalis muscle

Inguinal falx
(conjoint tendon)

Inguinal ligament
(Poupart)

Anterior superior
iliac spine

External oblique
aponeurosis (cut and
turned down)

Pectineal ligament
(Cooper)

Lacunar ligament
(Gimbernat)

Reflected inguinal
ligament

Pubic tubercle

Suspensory ligament
of penis

Cremaster muscles
and cremasteric fascia

Deep (Buck's)
fascia of penis

External spermatic
fascia (cut)

Superficial (dartos)
fascia of penis and
scrotum (cut)

6

7

8

9

10

PLATE 242

ABDOMEN

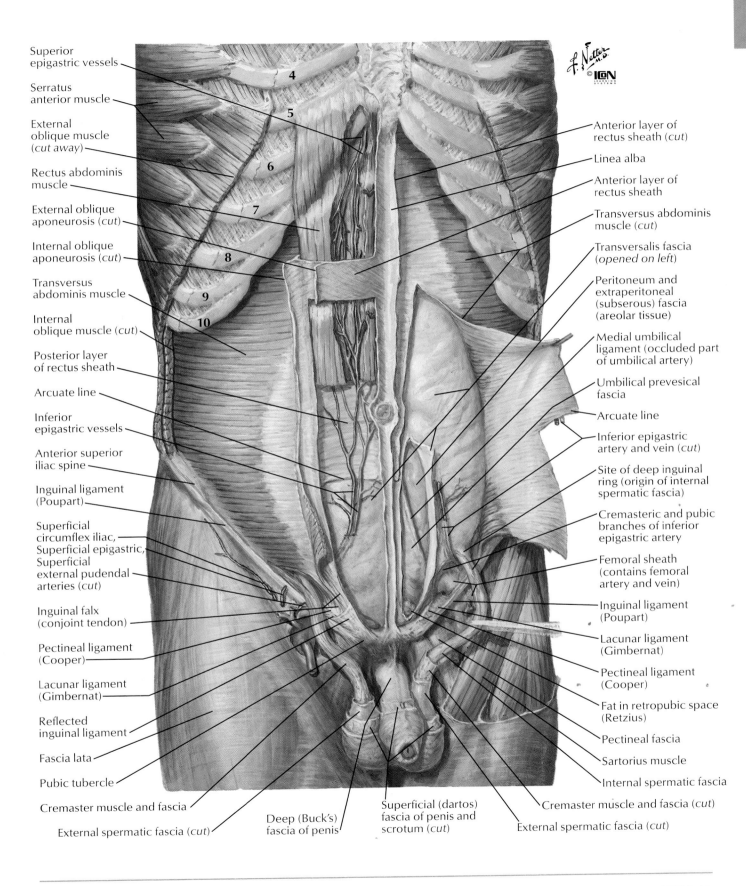

Superior epigastric vessels

Serratus anterior muscle

External oblique muscle (*cut away*)

Rectus abdominis muscle

External oblique aponeurosis (*cut*)

Internal oblique aponeurosis (*cut*)

Transversus abdominis muscle

Internal oblique muscle (*cut*)

Posterior layer of rectus sheath

Arcuate line

Inferior epigastric vessels

Anterior superior iliac spine

Inguinal ligament (Poupart)

Superficial circumflex iliac, Superficial epigastric, Superficial external pudendal arteries (*cut*)

Inguinal falx (conjoint tendon)

Pectineal ligament (Cooper)

Lacunar ligament (Gimbernat)

Reflected inguinal ligament

Fascia lata

Pubic tubercle

Cremaster muscle and fascia

External spermatic fascia (*cut*)

Deep (Buck's) fascia of penis

Superficial (dartos) fascia of penis and scrotum (*cut*)

Anterior layer of rectus sheath (*cut*)

Linea alba

Anterior layer of rectus sheath

Transversus abdominis muscle (*cut*)

Transversalis fascia (*opened on left*)

Peritoneum and extraperitoneal (subserous) fascia (areolar tissue)

Medial umbilical ligament (occluded part of umbilical artery)

Umbilical prevesical fascia

Arcuate line

Inferior epigastric artery and vein (*cut*)

Site of deep inguinal ring (origin of internal spermatic fascia)

Cremasteric and pubic branches of inferior epigastric artery

Femoral sheath (contains femoral artery and vein)

Inguinal ligament (Poupart)

Lacunar ligament (Gimbernat)

Pectineal ligament (Cooper)

Fat in retropubic space (Retzius)

Pectineal fascia

Sartorius muscle

Internal spermatic fascia

Cremaster muscle and fascia (*cut*)

External spermatic fascia (*cut*)

Rectus Sheath: Cross Sections

Section above arcuate line

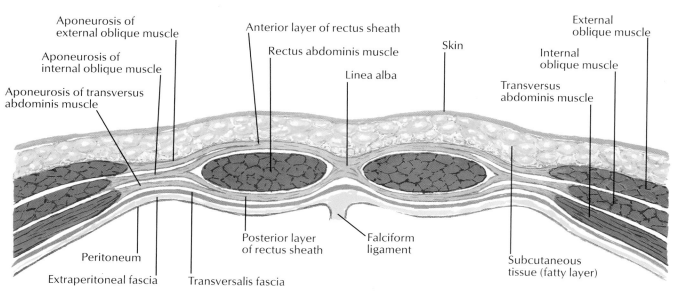

Aponeurosis of external oblique muscle

Aponeurosis of internal oblique muscle

Aponeurosis of transversus abdominis muscle

Anterior layer of rectus sheath

Rectus abdominis muscle

Linea alba

Skin

External oblique muscle

Internal oblique muscle

Transversus abdominis muscle

Peritoneum

Extraperitoneal fascia

Transversalis fascia

Posterior layer of rectus sheath

Falciform ligament

Subcutaneous tissue (fatty layer)

Aponeurosis of internal oblique muscle splits to form anterior and posterior layers of rectus sheath. Aponeurosis of external oblique muscle joins anterior layer of sheath; aponeurosis of transversus abdominis muscle joins posterior layer. Anterior and posterior layers of rectus sheath unite medially to form linea alba

Section below arcuate line

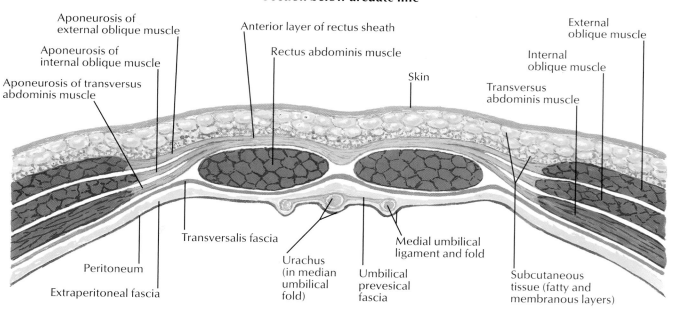

Aponeurosis of external oblique muscle

Aponeurosis of internal oblique muscle

Aponeurosis of transversus abdominis muscle

Anterior layer of rectus sheath

Rectus abdominis muscle

Skin

External oblique muscle

Internal oblique muscle

Transversus abdominis muscle

Transversalis fascia

Urachus (in median umbilical fold)

Umbilical prevesical fascia

Medial umbilical ligament and fold

Peritoneum

Extraperitoneal fascia

Subcutaneous tissue (fatty and membranous layers)

Aponeurosis of internal oblique muscle does not split at this level but passes completely anterior to rectus abdominis muscle and is fused there with both aponeurosis of external oblique muscle and that of transversus abdominis muscle. Thus, posterior wall of rectus sheath is absent below arcuate line and rectus abdominis muscle lies on transversalis fascia

PLATE 244

ABDOMEN

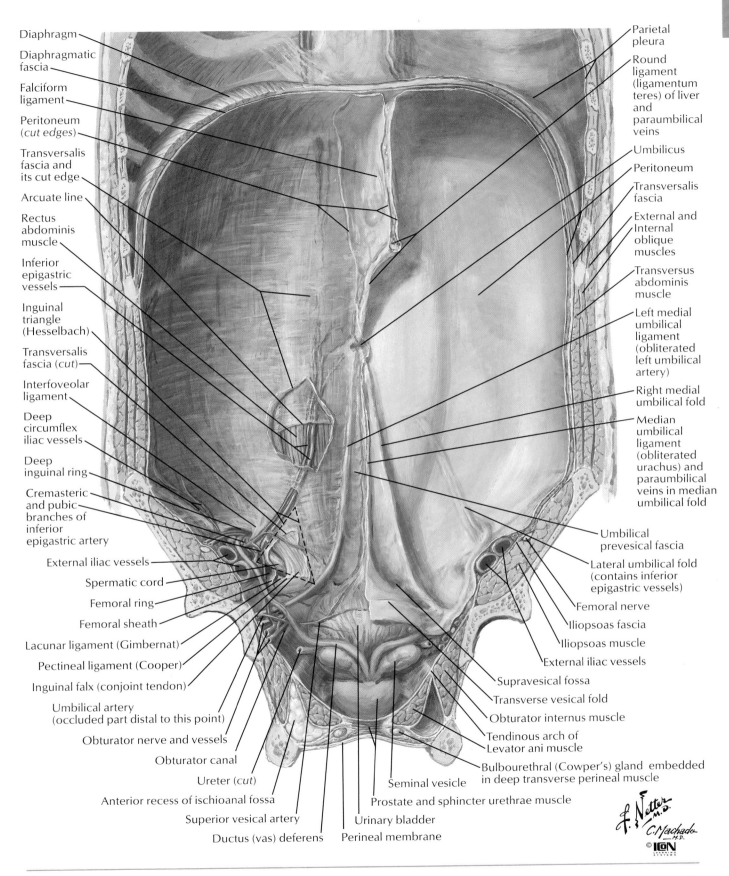

Diaphragm

Diaphragmatic fascia

Falciform ligament

Peritoneum (*cut edges*)

Transversalis fascia and its cut edge

Arcuate line

Rectus abdominis muscle

Inferior epigastric vessels

Inguinal triangle (Hesselbach)

Transversalis fascia (*cut*)

Interfoveolar ligament

Deep circumflex iliac vessels

Deep inguinal ring

Cremasteric and pubic branches of inferior epigastric artery

External iliac vessels

Spermatic cord

Femoral ring

Femoral sheath

Lacunar ligament (Gimbernat)

Pectineal ligament (Cooper)

Inguinal falx (conjoint tendon)

Umbilical artery (occluded part distal to this point)

Obturator nerve and vessels

Obturator canal

Ureter (*cut*)

Anterior recess of ischioanal fossa

Superior vesical artery

Ductus (vas) deferens

Parietal pleura

Round ligament (ligamentum teres) of liver and paraumbilical veins

Umbilicus

Peritoneum

Transversalis fascia

External and Internal oblique muscles

Transversus abdominis muscle

Left medial umbilical ligament (obliterated left umbilical artery)

Right medial umbilical fold

Median umbilical ligament (obliterated urachus) and paraumbilical veins in median umbilical fold

Umbilical prevesical fascia

Lateral umbilical fold (contains inferior epigastric vessels)

Femoral nerve

Iliopsoas fascia

Iliopsoas muscle

External iliac vessels

Supravesical fossa

Transverse vesical fold

Obturator internus muscle

Tendinous arch of Levator ani muscle

Bulbourethral (Cowper's) gland embedded in deep transverse perineal muscle

Seminal vesicle

Prostate and sphincter urethrae muscle

Urinary bladder

Perineal membrane

SEE ALSO PLATES 167, 170, 172, 173, 250

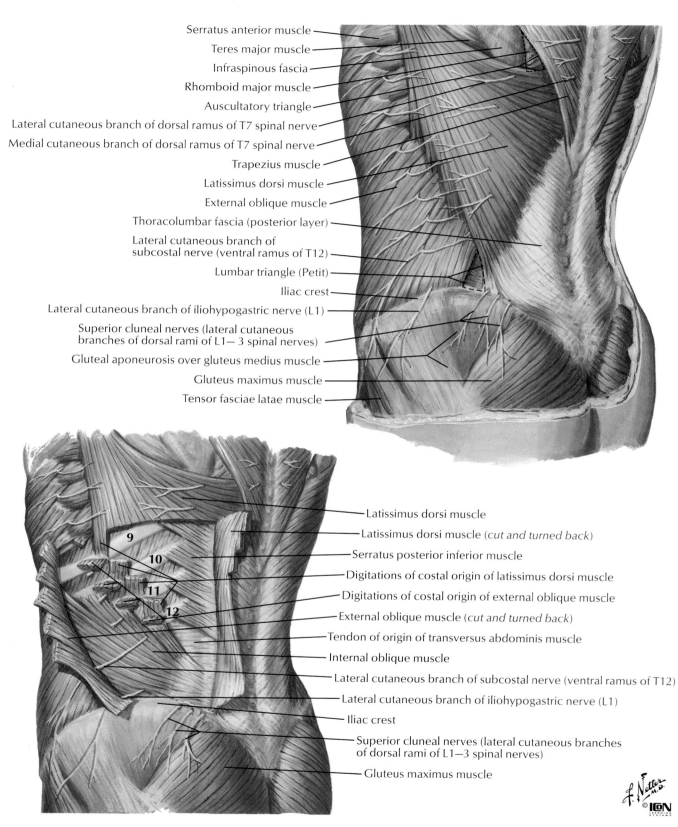

Serratus anterior muscle

Teres major muscle

Infraspinous fascia

Rhomboid major muscle

Auscultatory triangle

Lateral cutaneous branch of dorsal ramus of T7 spinal nerve

Medial cutaneous branch of dorsal ramus of T7 spinal nerve

Trapezius muscle

Latissimus dorsi muscle

External oblique muscle

Thoracolumbar fascia (posterior layer)

Lateral cutaneous branch of subcostal nerve (ventral ramus of T12)

Lumbar triangle (Petit)

Iliac crest

Lateral cutaneous branch of iliohypogastric nerve (L1)

Superior cluneal nerves (lateral cutaneous branches of dorsal rami of L1— 3 spinal nerves)

Gluteal aponeurosis over gluteus medius muscle

Gluteus maximus muscle

Tensor fasciae latae muscle

Latissimus dorsi muscle

Latissimus dorsi muscle (*cut and turned back*)

Serratus posterior inferior muscle

Digitations of costal origin of latissimus dorsi muscle

Digitations of costal origin of external oblique muscle

External oblique muscle (*cut and turned back*)

Tendon of origin of transversus abdominis muscle

Internal oblique muscle

Lateral cutaneous branch of subcostal nerve (ventral ramus of T12)

Lateral cutaneous branch of iliohypogastric nerve (L1)

Iliac crest

Superior cluneal nerves (lateral cutaneous branches of dorsal rami of L1—3 spinal nerves)

Gluteus maximus muscle

PLATE 246

ABDOMEN

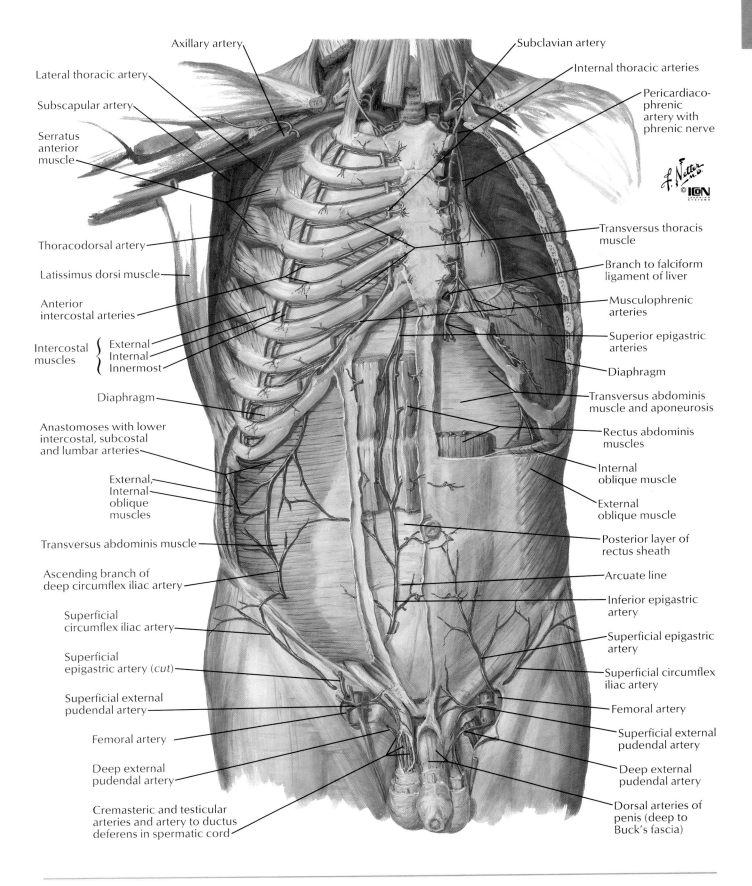

Axillary artery

Subclavian artery

Lateral thoracic artery

Internal thoracic arteries

Subscapular artery

Pericardiaco-phrenic artery with phrenic nerve

Serratus anterior muscle

Thoracodorsal artery

Latissimus dorsi muscle

Anterior intercostal arteries

Intercostal muscles { External Internal Innermost

Transversus thoracis muscle

Branch to falciform ligament of liver

Musculophrenic arteries

Superior epigastric arteries

Diaphragm

Transversus abdominis muscle and aponeurosis

Diaphragm

Anastomoses with lower intercostal, subcostal and lumbar arteries

Rectus abdominis muscles

External, Internal oblique muscles

Internal oblique muscle

Transversus abdominis muscle

External oblique muscle

Ascending branch of deep circumflex iliac artery

Posterior layer of rectus sheath

Arcuate line

Inferior epigastric artery

Superficial circumflex iliac artery

Superficial epigastric artery (cut)

Superficial epigastric artery

Superficial circumflex iliac artery

Superficial external pudendal artery

Femoral artery

Femoral artery

Superficial external pudendal artery

Deep external pudendal artery

Deep external pudendal artery

Cremasteric and testicular arteries and artery to ductus deferens in spermatic cord

Dorsal arteries of penis (deep to Buck's fascia)

BODY WALL

PLATE 247

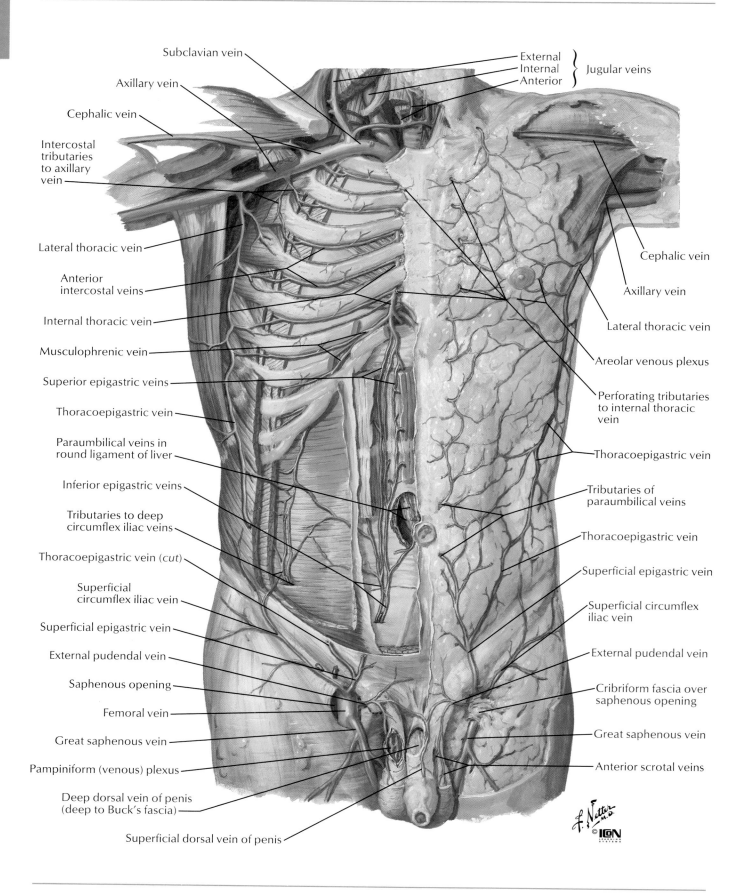

Subclavian vein

External
Internal } Jugular veins
Anterior

Axillary vein

Cephalic vein

Intercostal
tributaries
to axillary
vein

Lateral thoracic vein

Cephalic vein

Anterior
intercostal veins

Axillary vein

Internal thoracic vein

Lateral thoracic vein

Musculophrenic vein

Areolar venous plexus

Superior epigastric veins

Perforating tributaries
to internal thoracic
vein

Thoracoepigastric vein

Paraumbilical veins in
round ligament of liver

Thoracoepigastric vein

Inferior epigastric veins

Tributaries of
paraumbilical veins

Tributaries to deep
circumflex iliac veins

Thoracoepigastric vein

Thoracoepigastric vein (cut)

Superficial epigastric vein

Superficial
circumflex iliac vein

Superficial circumflex
iliac vein

Superficial epigastric vein

External pudendal vein

External pudendal vein

Saphenous opening

Cribriform fascia over
saphenous opening

Femoral vein

Great saphenous vein

Great saphenous vein

Pampiniform (venous) plexus

Anterior scrotal veins

Deep dorsal vein of penis
(deep to Buck's fascia)

Superficial dorsal vein of penis

PLATE 248

ABDOMEN

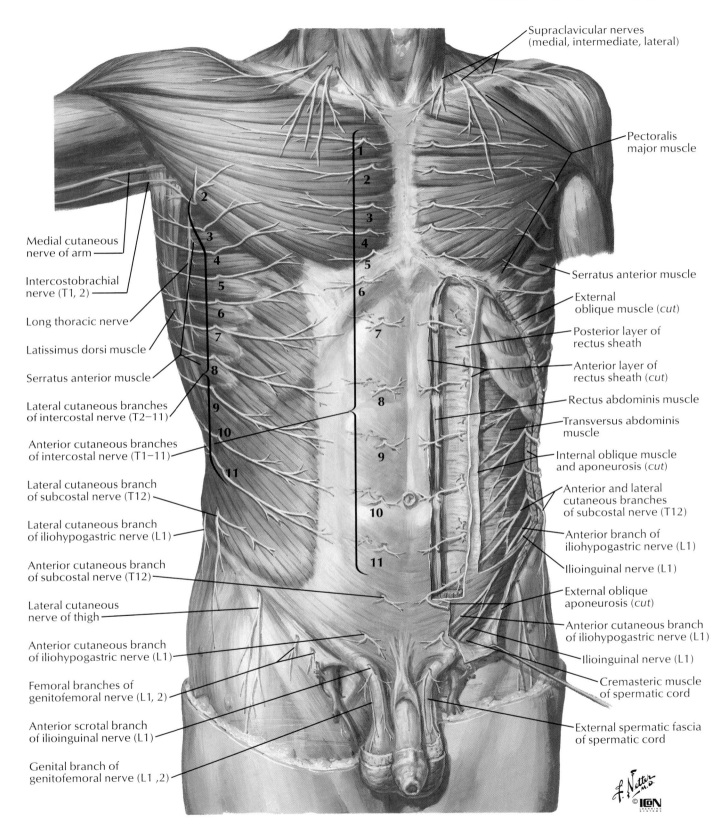

Supraclavicular nerves (medial, intermediate, lateral)

Pectoralis major muscle

Medial cutaneous nerve of arm

Intercostobrachial nerve (T1, 2)

Long thoracic nerve

Latissimus dorsi muscle

Serratus anterior muscle

Lateral cutaneous branches of intercostal nerve (T2–11)

Anterior cutaneous branches of intercostal nerve (T1–11)

Lateral cutaneous branch of subcostal nerve (T12)

Lateral cutaneous branch of iliohypogastric nerve (L1)

Anterior cutaneous branch of subcostal nerve (T12)

Lateral cutaneous nerve of thigh

Anterior cutaneous branch of iliohypogastric nerve (L1)

Femoral branches of genitofemoral nerve (L1, 2)

Anterior scrotal branch of ilioinguinal nerve (L1)

Genital branch of genitofemoral nerve (L1 ,2)

Serratus anterior muscle

External oblique muscle (*cut*)

Posterior layer of rectus sheath

Anterior layer of rectus sheath (*cut*)

Rectus abdominis muscle

Transversus abdominis muscle

Internal oblique muscle and aponeurosis (*cut*)

Anterior and lateral cutaneous branches of subcostal nerve (T12)

Anterior branch of iliohypogastric nerve (L1)

Ilioinguinal nerve (L1)

External oblique aponeurosis (*cut*)

Anterior cutaneous branch of iliohypogastric nerve (L1)

Ilioinguinal nerve (L1)

Cremasteric muscle of spermatic cord

External spermatic fascia of spermatic cord

Thoracoabdominal Nerves

SEE ALSO PLATES 173, 187

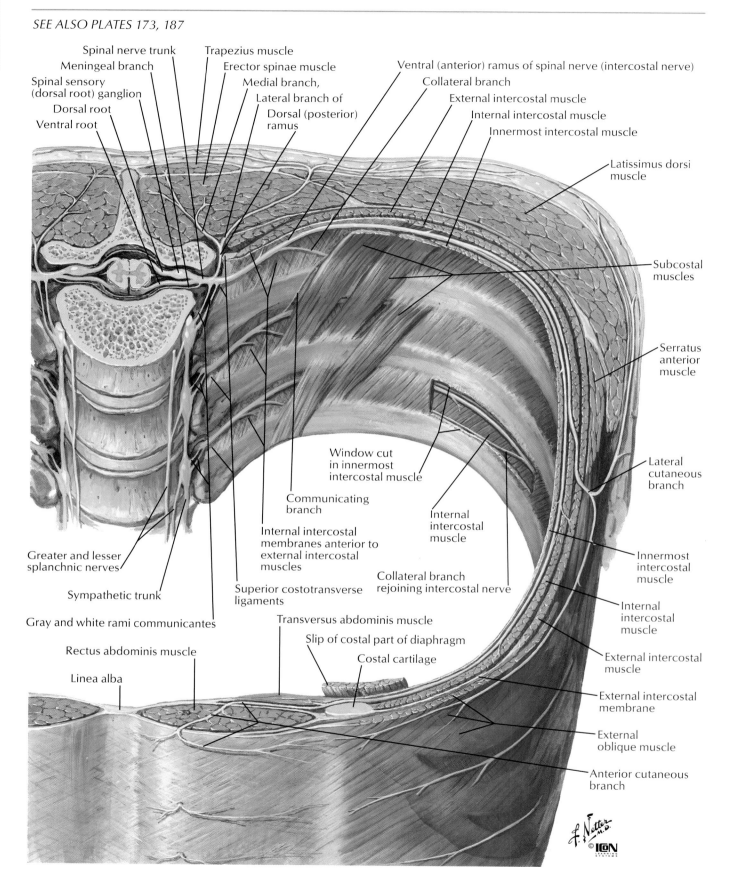

Spinal nerve trunk
Meningeal branch
Spinal sensory (dorsal root) ganglion
Dorsal root
Ventral root
Trapezius muscle
Erector spinae muscle
Medial branch,
Lateral branch of
Dorsal (posterior) ramus
Ventral (anterior) ramus of spinal nerve (intercostal nerve)
Collateral branch
External intercostal muscle
Internal intercostal muscle
Innermost intercostal muscle
Latissimus dorsi muscle
Subcostal muscles
Serratus anterior muscle
Window cut in innermost intercostal muscle
Lateral cutaneous branch
Communicating branch
Internal intercostal muscle
Internal intercostal membranes anterior to external intercostal muscles
Collateral branch rejoining intercostal nerve
Innermost intercostal muscle
Greater and lesser splanchnic nerves
Superior costotransverse ligaments
Internal intercostal muscle
Sympathetic trunk
Transversus abdominis muscle
External intercostal muscle
Gray and white rami communicantes
Slip of costal part of diaphragm
External intercostal membrane
Rectus abdominis muscle
Costal cartilage
Linea alba
External oblique muscle
Anterior cutaneous branch

f. Netter
© ICON LEARNING SYSTEMS

PLATE 250

ABDOMEN

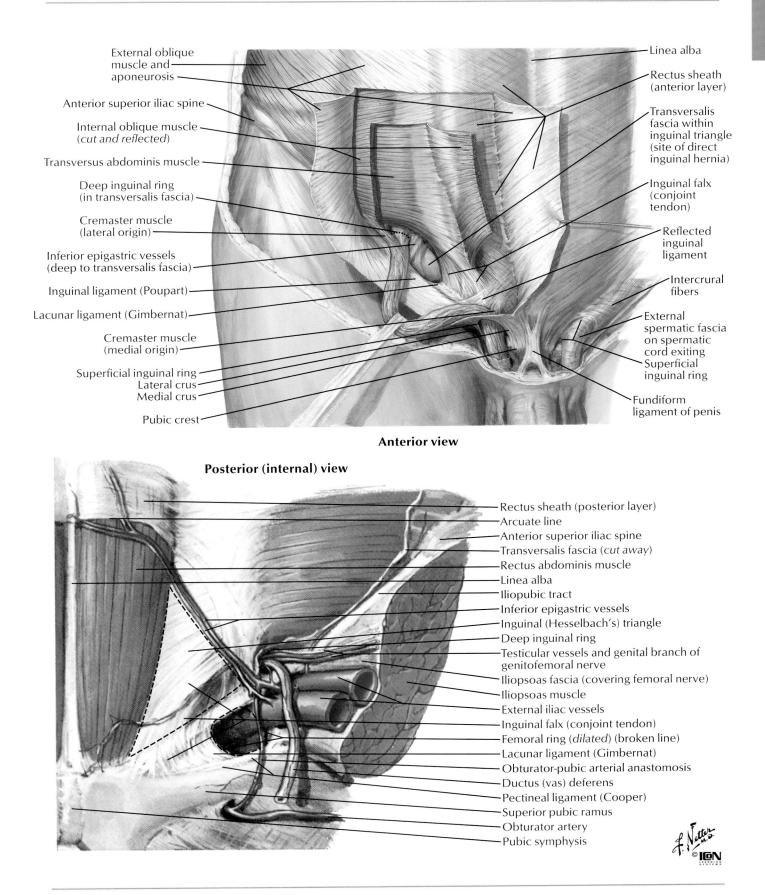

External oblique muscle and aponeurosis

Anterior superior iliac spine

Internal oblique muscle (*cut and reflected*)

Transversus abdominis muscle

Deep inguinal ring (in transversalis fascia)

Cremaster muscle (lateral origin)

Inferior epigastric vessels (deep to transversalis fascia)

Inguinal ligament (Poupart)

Lacunar ligament (Gimbernat)

Cremaster muscle (medial origin)

Superficial inguinal ring
Lateral crus
Medial crus

Pubic crest

Linea alba

Rectus sheath (anterior layer)

Transversalis fascia within inguinal triangle (site of direct inguinal hernia)

Inguinal falx (conjoint tendon)

Reflected inguinal ligament

Intercrural fibers

External spermatic fascia on spermatic cord exiting Superficial inguinal ring

Fundiform ligament of penis

Anterior view

Posterior (internal) view

Rectus sheath (posterior layer)
Arcuate line
Anterior superior iliac spine
Transversalis fascia (*cut away*)
Rectus abdominis muscle
Linea alba
Iliopubic tract
Inferior epigastric vessels
Inguinal (Hesselbach's) triangle
Deep inguinal ring
Testicular vessels and genital branch of genitofemoral nerve
Iliopsoas fascia (covering femoral nerve)
Iliopsoas muscle
External iliac vessels
Inguinal falx (conjoint tendon)
Femoral ring (*dilated*) (broken line)
Lacunar ligament (Gimbernat)
Obturator-pubic arterial anastomosis
Ductus (vas) deferens
Pectineal ligament (Cooper)
Superior pubic ramus
Obturator artery
Pubic symphysis

BODY WALL

PLATE 251

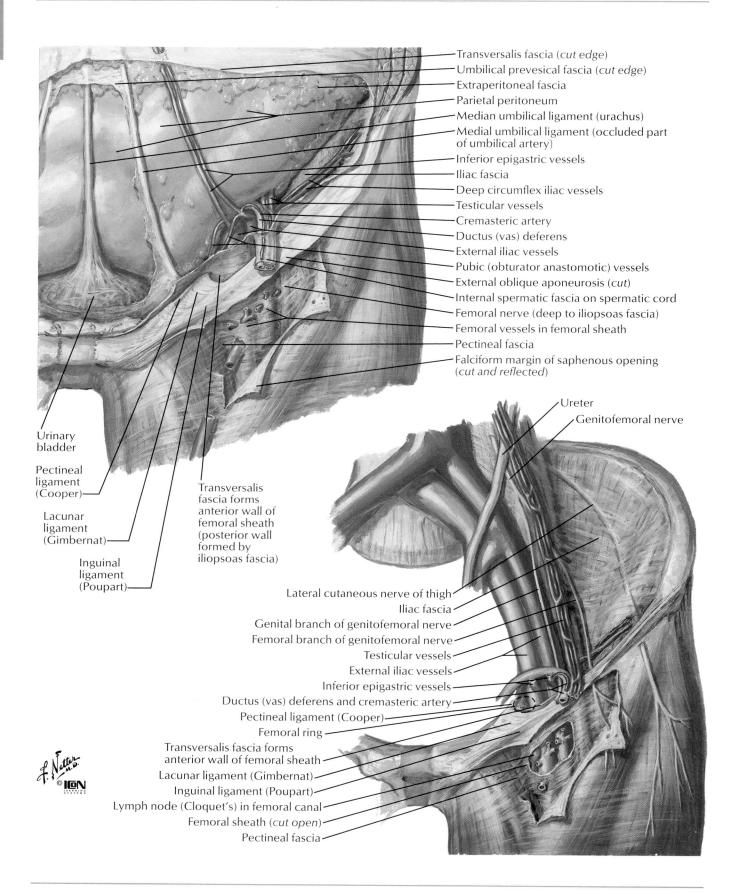

Transversalis fascia (*cut edge*)
Umbilical prevesical fascia (*cut edge*)
Extraperitoneal fascia
Parietal peritoneum
Median umbilical ligament (urachus)
Medial umbilical ligament (occluded part of umbilical artery)
Inferior epigastric vessels
Iliac fascia
Deep circumflex iliac vessels
Testicular vessels
Cremasteric artery
Ductus (vas) deferens
External iliac vessels
Pubic (obturator anastomotic) vessels
External oblique aponeurosis (*cut*)
Internal spermatic fascia on spermatic cord
Femoral nerve (deep to iliopsoas fascia)
Femoral vessels in femoral sheath
Pectineal fascia
Falciform margin of saphenous opening (*cut and reflected*)

Urinary bladder

Pectineal ligament (Cooper)

Lacunar ligament (Gimbernat)

Inguinal ligament (Poupart)

Transversalis fascia forms anterior wall of femoral sheath (posterior wall formed by iliopsoas fascia)

Ureter
Genitofemoral nerve

Lateral cutaneous nerve of thigh
Iliac fascia
Genital branch of genitofemoral nerve
Femoral branch of genitofemoral nerve
Testicular vessels
External iliac vessels
Inferior epigastric vessels
Ductus (vas) deferens and cremasteric artery
Pectineal ligament (Cooper)
Femoral ring
Transversalis fascia forms anterior wall of femoral sheath
Lacunar ligament (Gimbernat)
Inguinal ligament (Poupart)
Lymph node (Cloquet's) in femoral canal
Femoral sheath (*cut open*)
Pectineal fascia

PLATE 252

ABDOMEN

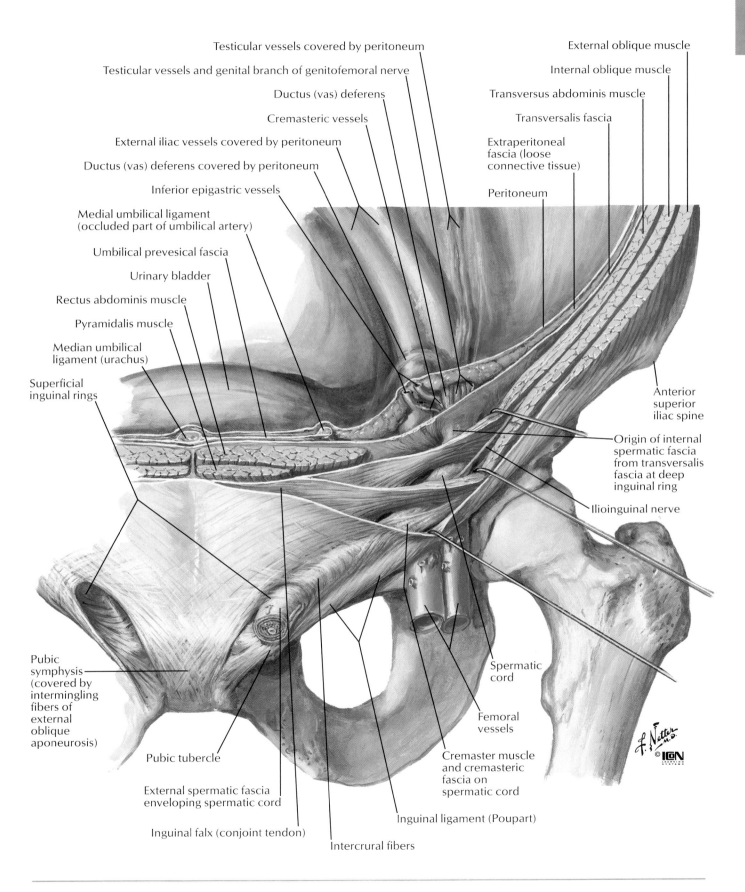

Testicular vessels covered by peritoneum

Testicular vessels and genital branch of genitofemoral nerve

Ductus (vas) deferens

Cremasteric vessels

External iliac vessels covered by peritoneum

Ductus (vas) deferens covered by peritoneum

Inferior epigastric vessels

Medial umbilical ligament (occluded part of umbilical artery)

Umbilical prevesical fascia

Urinary bladder

Rectus abdominis muscle

Pyramidalis muscle

Median umbilical ligament (urachus)

Superficial inguinal rings

Pubic symphysis (covered by intermingling fibers of external oblique aponeurosis)

Pubic tubercle

External spermatic fascia enveloping spermatic cord

Inguinal falx (conjoint tendon)

Intercrural fibers

External oblique muscle

Internal oblique muscle

Transversus abdominis muscle

Transversalis fascia

Extraperitoneal fascia (loose connective tissue)

Peritoneum

Anterior superior iliac spine

Origin of internal spermatic fascia from transversalis fascia at deep inguinal ring

Ilioinguinal nerve

Spermatic cord

Femoral vessels

Cremaster muscle and cremasteric fascia on spermatic cord

Inguinal ligament (Poupart)

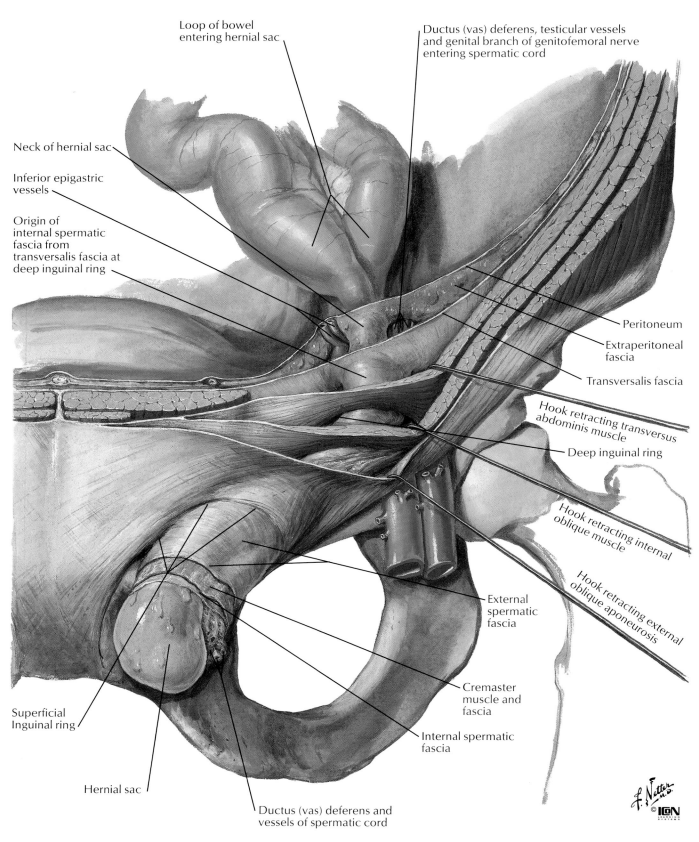

Loop of bowel entering hernial sac

Ductus (vas) deferens, testicular vessels and genital branch of genitofemoral nerve entering spermatic cord

Neck of hernial sac

Inferior epigastric vessels

Origin of internal spermatic fascia from transversalis fascia at deep inguinal ring

Peritoneum

Extraperitoneal fascia

Transversalis fascia

Hook retracting transversus abdominis muscle

Deep inguinal ring

Hook retracting internal oblique muscle

Hook retracting external oblique aponeurosis

External spermatic fascia

Cremaster muscle and fascia

Internal spermatic fascia

Superficial Inguinal ring

Hernial sac

Ductus (vas) deferens and vessels of spermatic cord

PLATE 254

ABDOMEN

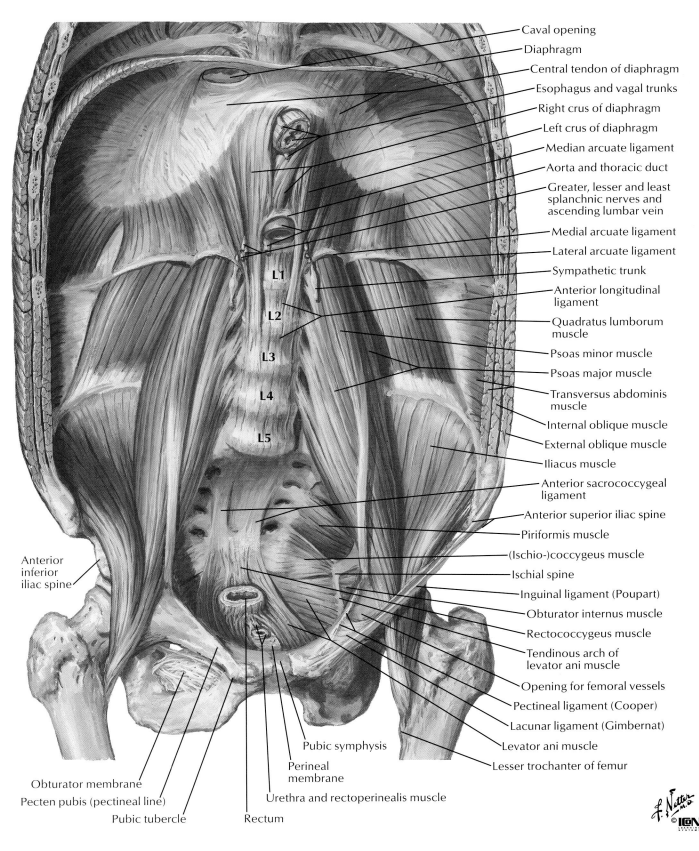

Caval opening
Diaphragm
Central tendon of diaphragm
Esophagus and vagal trunks
Right crus of diaphragm
Left crus of diaphragm
Median arcuate ligament
Aorta and thoracic duct
Greater, lesser and least splanchnic nerves and ascending lumbar vein
Medial arcuate ligament
Lateral arcuate ligament
Sympathetic trunk
Anterior longitudinal ligament
Quadratus lumborum muscle
Psoas minor muscle
Psoas major muscle
Transversus abdominis muscle
Internal oblique muscle
External oblique muscle
Iliacus muscle
Anterior sacrococcygeal ligament
Anterior superior iliac spine
Piriformis muscle
(Ischio-)coccygeus muscle
Ischial spine
Inguinal ligament (Poupart)
Obturator internus muscle
Rectococcygeus muscle
Tendinous arch of levator ani muscle
Opening for femoral vessels
Pectineal ligament (Cooper)
Lacunar ligament (Gimbernat)
Levator ani muscle
Lesser trochanter of femur

L1
L2
L3
L4
L5

Anterior inferior iliac spine

Obturator membrane
Pecten pubis (pectineal line)
Pubic tubercle
Rectum
Perineal membrane
Pubic symphysis
Urethra and rectoperinealis muscle

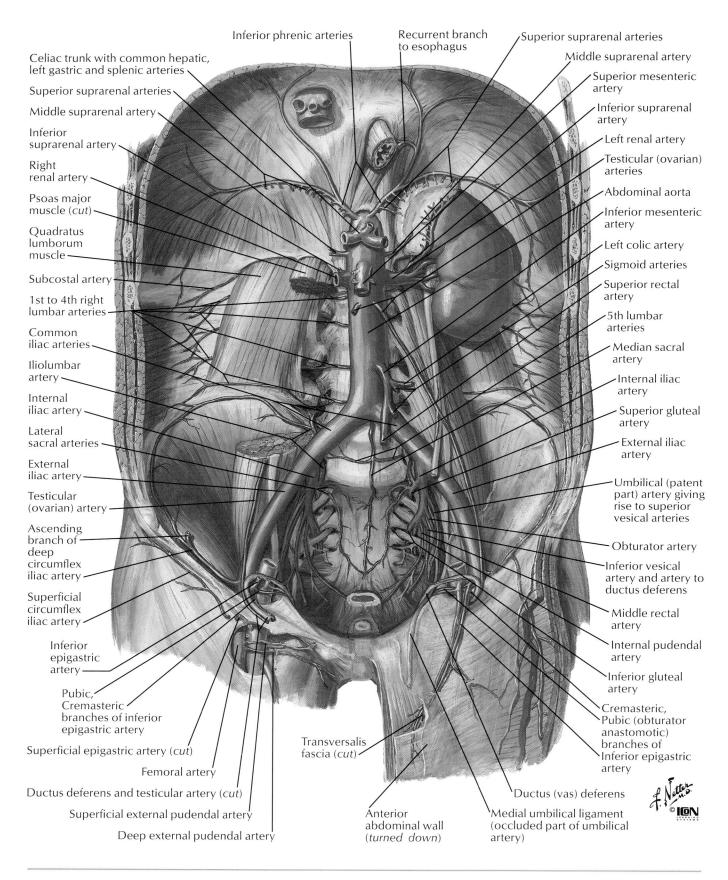

Inferior phrenic arteries

Recurrent branch to esophagus

Superior suprarenal arteries

Celiac trunk with common hepatic, left gastric and splenic arteries

Middle suprarenal artery

Superior suprarenal arteries

Superior mesenteric artery

Middle suprarenal artery

Inferior suprarenal artery

Inferior suprarenal artery

Left renal artery

Right renal artery

Testicular (ovarian) arteries

Psoas major muscle (cut)

Abdominal aorta

Inferior mesenteric artery

Quadratus lumborum muscle

Left colic artery

Sigmoid arteries

Subcostal artery

Superior rectal artery

1st to 4th right lumbar arteries

5th lumbar arteries

Common iliac arteries

Median sacral artery

Iliolumbar artery

Internal iliac artery

Internal iliac artery

Superior gluteal artery

Lateral sacral arteries

External iliac artery

External iliac artery

Testicular (ovarian) artery

Umbilical (patent part) artery giving rise to superior vesical arteries

Ascending branch of deep circumflex iliac artery

Obturator artery

Inferior vesical artery and artery to ductus deferens

Superficial circumflex iliac artery

Middle rectal artery

Internal pudendal artery

Inferior epigastric artery

Inferior gluteal artery

Pubic, Cremasteric branches of inferior epigastric artery

Cremasteric, Pubic (obturator anastomotic) branches of Inferior epigastric artery

Superficial epigastric artery (cut)

Transversalis fascia (cut)

Femoral artery

Ductus (vas) deferens

Ductus deferens and testicular artery (cut)

Superficial external pudendal artery

Anterior abdominal wall (turned down)

Medial umbilical ligament (occluded part of umbilical artery)

Deep external pudendal artery

PLATE 256

ABDOMEN

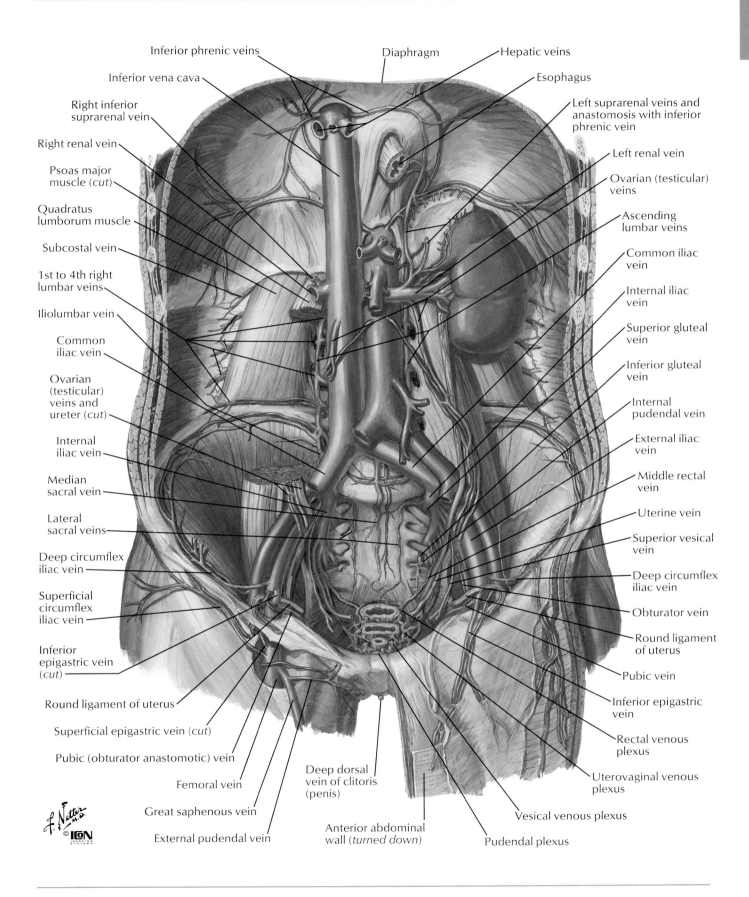

Inferior phrenic veins

Diaphragm

Hepatic veins

Inferior vena cava

Esophagus

Right inferior suprarenal vein

Left suprarenal veins and anastomosis with inferior phrenic vein

Right renal vein

Left renal vein

Psoas major muscle (*cut*)

Ovarian (testicular) veins

Quadratus lumborum muscle

Ascending lumbar veins

Subcostal vein

Common iliac vein

1st to 4th right lumbar veins

Internal iliac vein

Iliolumbar vein

Superior gluteal vein

Common iliac vein

Inferior gluteal vein

Ovarian (testicular) veins and ureter (*cut*)

Internal pudendal vein

Internal iliac vein

External iliac vein

Median sacral vein

Middle rectal vein

Lateral sacral veins

Uterine vein

Deep circumflex iliac vein

Superior vesical vein

Superficial circumflex iliac vein

Deep circumflex iliac vein

Inferior epigastric vein (*cut*)

Obturator vein

Round ligament of uterus

Round ligament of uterus

Pubic vein

Superficial epigastric vein (*cut*)

Inferior epigastric vein

Pubic (obturator anastomotic) vein

Rectal venous plexus

Femoral vein

Uterovaginal venous plexus

Great saphenous vein

Deep dorsal vein of clitoris (penis)

External pudendal vein

Vesical venous plexus

Anterior abdominal wall (*turned down*)

Pudendal plexus

SEE ALSO PLATE 387

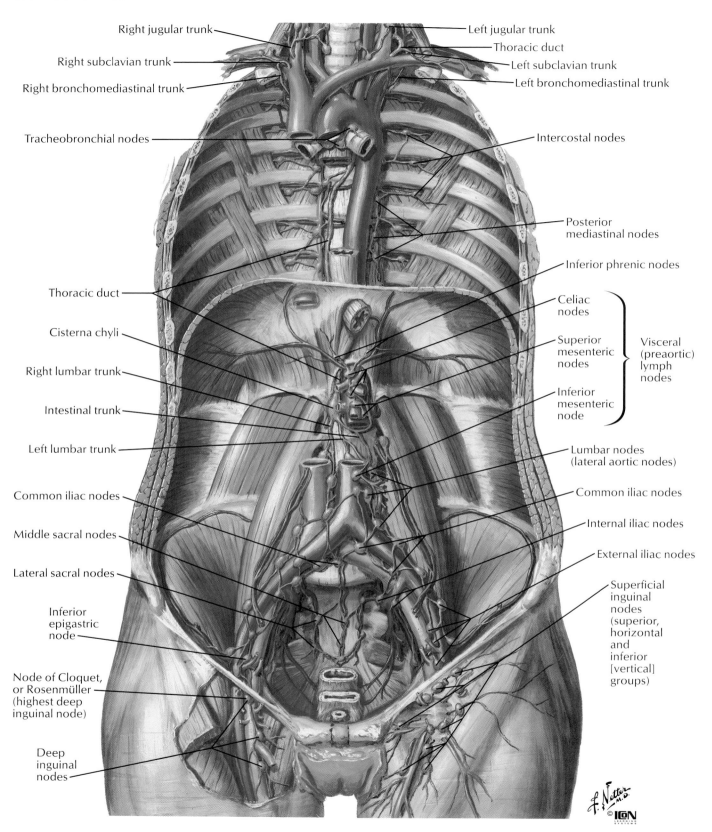

Right jugular trunk

Right subclavian trunk

Right bronchomediastinal trunk

Tracheobronchial nodes

Thoracic duct

Cisterna chyli

Right lumbar trunk

Intestinal trunk

Left lumbar trunk

Common iliac nodes

Middle sacral nodes

Lateral sacral nodes

Inferior epigastric node

Node of Cloquet, or Rosenmüller (highest deep inguinal node)

Deep inguinal nodes

Left jugular trunk

Thoracic duct

Left subclavian trunk

Left bronchomediastinal trunk

Intercostal nodes

Posterior mediastinal nodes

Inferior phrenic nodes

Celiac nodes

Superior mesenteric nodes

Inferior mesenteric node

Visceral (preaortic) lymph nodes

Lumbar nodes (lateral aortic nodes)

Common iliac nodes

Internal iliac nodes

External iliac nodes

Superficial inguinal nodes (superior, horizontal and inferior [vertical] groups)

PLATE 258

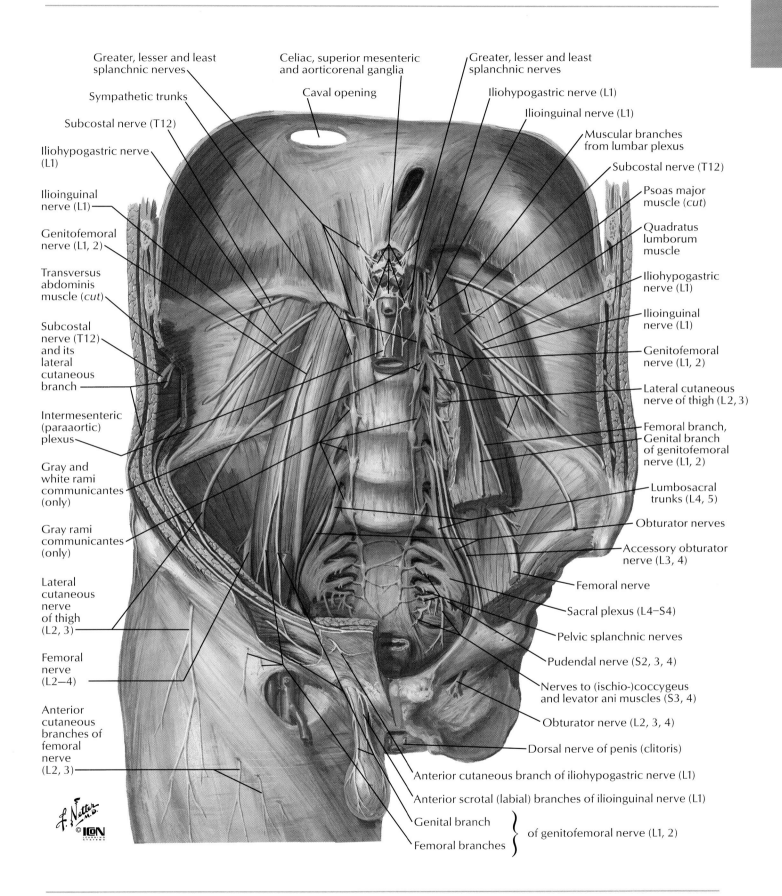

Greater, lesser and least splanchnic nerves

Celiac, superior mesenteric and aorticorenal ganglia

Caval opening

Greater, lesser and least splanchnic nerves

Sympathetic trunks

Iliohypogastric nerve (L1)

Subcostal nerve (T12)

Ilioinguinal nerve (L1)

Iliohypogastric nerve (L1)

Muscular branches from lumbar plexus

Ilioinguinal nerve (L1)

Subcostal nerve (T12)

Genitofemoral nerve (L1, 2)

Psoas major muscle (cut)

Transversus abdominis muscle (cut)

Quadratus lumborum muscle

Subcostal nerve (T12) and its lateral cutaneous branch

Iliohypogastric nerve (L1)

Ilioinguinal nerve (L1)

Genitofemoral nerve (L1, 2)

Intermesenteric (paraaortic) plexus

Lateral cutaneous nerve of thigh (L2, 3)

Gray and white rami communicantes (only)

Femoral branch, Genital branch of genitofemoral nerve (L1, 2)

Gray rami communicantes (only)

Lumbosacral trunks (L4, 5)

Obturator nerves

Lateral cutaneous nerve of thigh (L2, 3)

Accessory obturator nerve (L3, 4)

Femoral nerve

Sacral plexus (L4–S4)

Femoral nerve (L2–4)

Pelvic splanchnic nerves

Pudendal nerve (S2, 3, 4)

Anterior cutaneous branches of femoral nerve (L2, 3)

Nerves to (ischio-)coccygeus and levator ani muscles (S3, 4)

Obturator nerve (L2, 3, 4)

Dorsal nerve of penis (clitoris)

Anterior cutaneous branch of iliohypogastric nerve (L1)

Anterior scrotal (labial) branches of ilioinguinal nerve (L1)

Genital branch

Femoral branches

} of genitofemoral nerve (L1, 2)

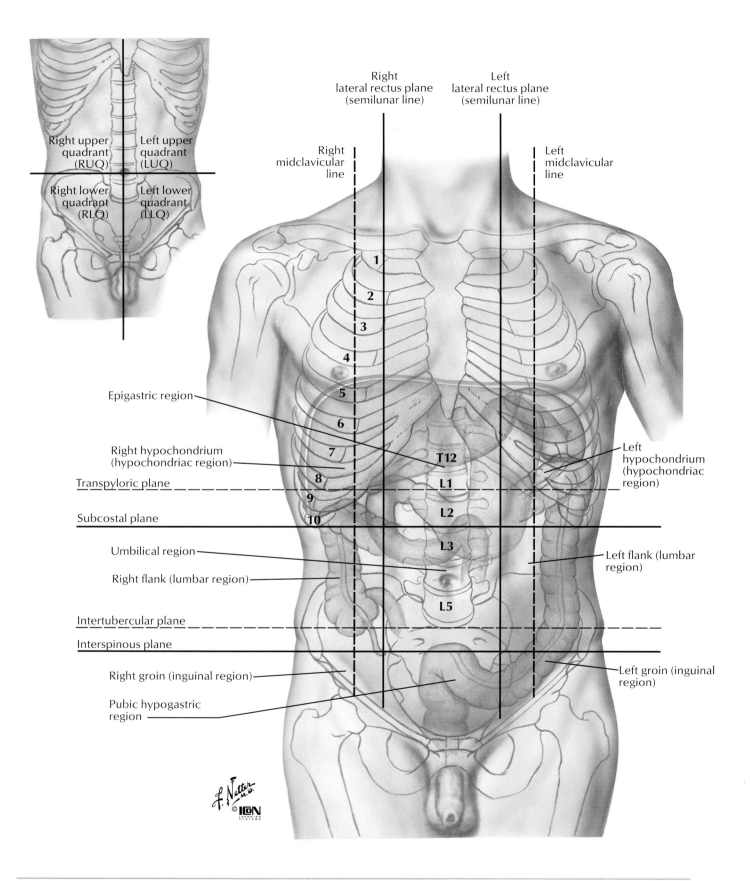

Right upper quadrant (RUQ)

Left upper quadrant (LUQ)

Right lower quadrant (RLQ)

Left lower quadrant (LLQ)

Right lateral rectus plane (semilunar line)

Left lateral rectus plane (semilunar line)

Right midclavicular line

Left midclavicular line

Epigastric region

Left hypochondrium (hypochondriac region)

Right hypochondrium (hypochondriac region)

Transpyloric plane

Subcostal plane

Umbilical region

Left flank (lumbar region)

Right flank (lumbar region)

Intertubercular plane

Interspinous plane

Right groin (inguinal region)

Left groin (inguinal region)

Pubic hypogastric region

T12
L1
L2
L3
L5

PLATE 260

ABDOMEN

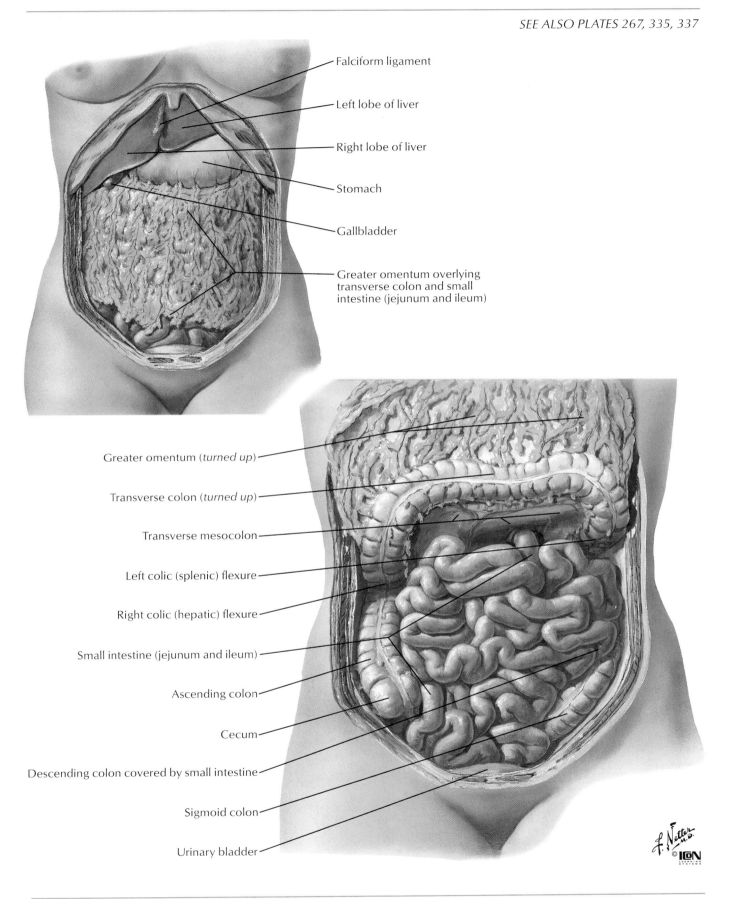

Falciform ligament

Left lobe of liver

Right lobe of liver

Stomach

Gallbladder

Greater omentum overlying transverse colon and small intestine (jejunum and ileum)

Greater omentum (*turned up*)

Transverse colon (*turned up*)

Transverse mesocolon

Left colic (splenic) flexure

Right colic (hepatic) flexure

Small intestine (jejunum and ileum)

Ascending colon

Cecum

Descending colon covered by small intestine

Sigmoid colon

Urinary bladder

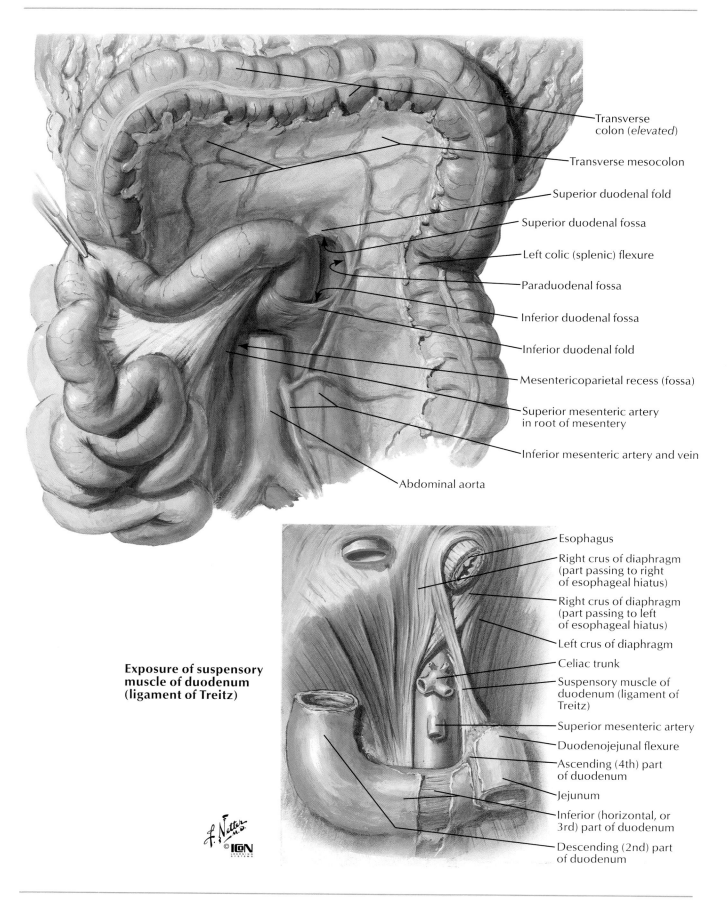

Transverse colon (*elevated*)

Transverse mesocolon

Superior duodenal fold

Superior duodenal fossa

Left colic (splenic) flexure

Paraduodenal fossa

Inferior duodenal fossa

Inferior duodenal fold

Mesentericoparietal recess (fossa)

Superior mesenteric artery in root of mesentery

Inferior mesenteric artery and vein

Abdominal aorta

Exposure of suspensory muscle of duodenum (ligament of Treitz)

Esophagus

Right crus of diaphragm (part passing to right of esophageal hiatus)

Right crus of diaphragm (part passing to left of esophageal hiatus)

Left crus of diaphragm

Celiac trunk

Suspensory muscle of duodenum (ligament of Treitz)

Superior mesenteric artery

Duodenojejunal flexure

Ascending (4th) part of duodenum

Jejunum

Inferior (horizontal, or 3rd) part of duodenum

Descending (2nd) part of duodenum

PLATE 262

ABDOMEN

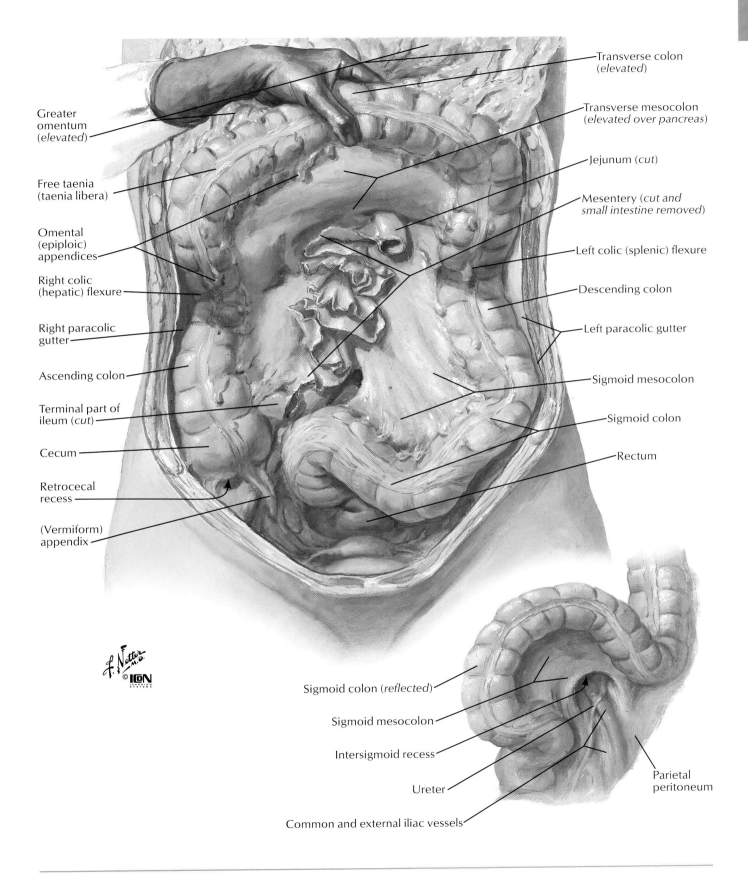

Greater omentum (*elevated*)

Free taenia (taenia libera)

Omental (epiploic) appendices

Right colic (hepatic) flexure

Right paracolic gutter

Ascending colon

Terminal part of ileum (*cut*)

Cecum

Retrocecal recess

(Vermiform) appendix

Transverse colon (*elevated*)

Transverse mesocolon (*elevated over pancreas*)

Jejunum (*cut*)

Mesentery (*cut and small intestine removed*)

Left colic (splenic) flexure

Descending colon

Left paracolic gutter

Sigmoid mesocolon

Sigmoid colon

Rectum

Sigmoid colon (*reflected*)

Sigmoid mesocolon

Intersigmoid recess

Ureter

Common and external iliac vessels

Parietal peritoneum

Omental Bursa: Stomach Reflected

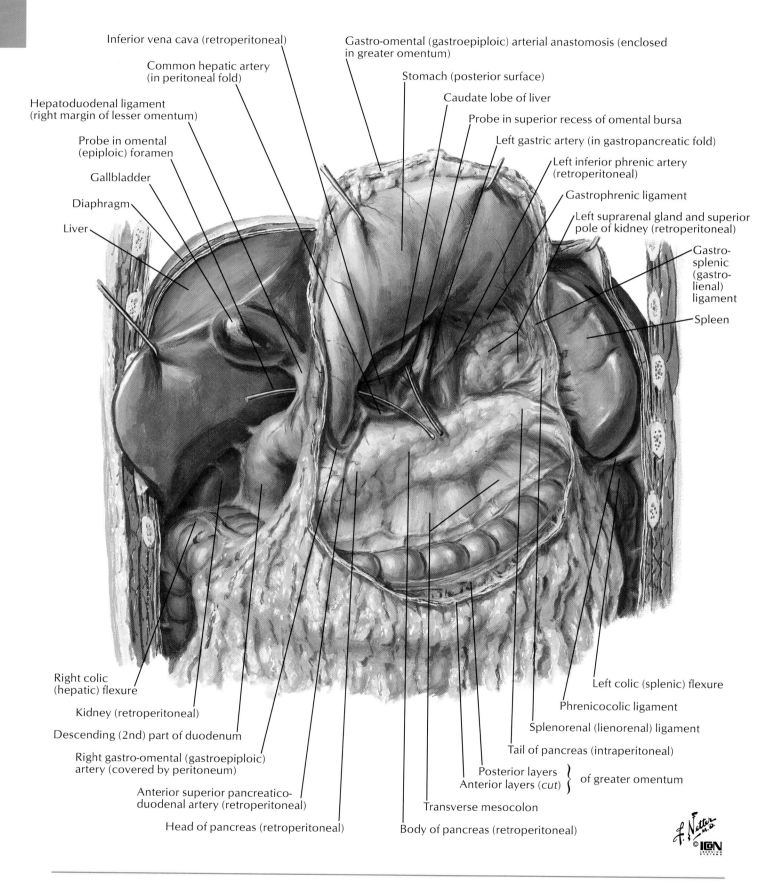

Inferior vena cava (retroperitoneal)

Common hepatic artery (in peritoneal fold)

Hepatoduodenal ligament (right margin of lesser omentum)

Probe in omental (epiploic) foramen

Gallbladder

Diaphragm

Liver

Gastro-omental (gastroepiploic) arterial anastomosis (enclosed in greater omentum)

Stomach (posterior surface)

Caudate lobe of liver

Probe in superior recess of omental bursa

Left gastric artery (in gastropancreatic fold)

Left inferior phrenic artery (retroperitoneal)

Gastrophrenic ligament

Left suprarenal gland and superior pole of kidney (retroperitoneal)

Gastro-splenic (gastro-lienal) ligament

Spleen

Right colic (hepatic) flexure

Kidney (retroperitoneal)

Descending (2nd) part of duodenum

Right gastro-omental (gastroepiploic) artery (covered by peritoneum)

Anterior superior pancreatico-duodenal artery (retroperitoneal)

Head of pancreas (retroperitoneal)

Posterior layers
Anterior layers (cut) } of greater omentum

Transverse mesocolon

Body of pancreas (retroperitoneal)

Tail of pancreas (intraperitoneal)

Splenorenal (lienorenal) ligament

Phrenicocolic ligament

Left colic (splenic) flexure

PLATE 264

ABDOMEN

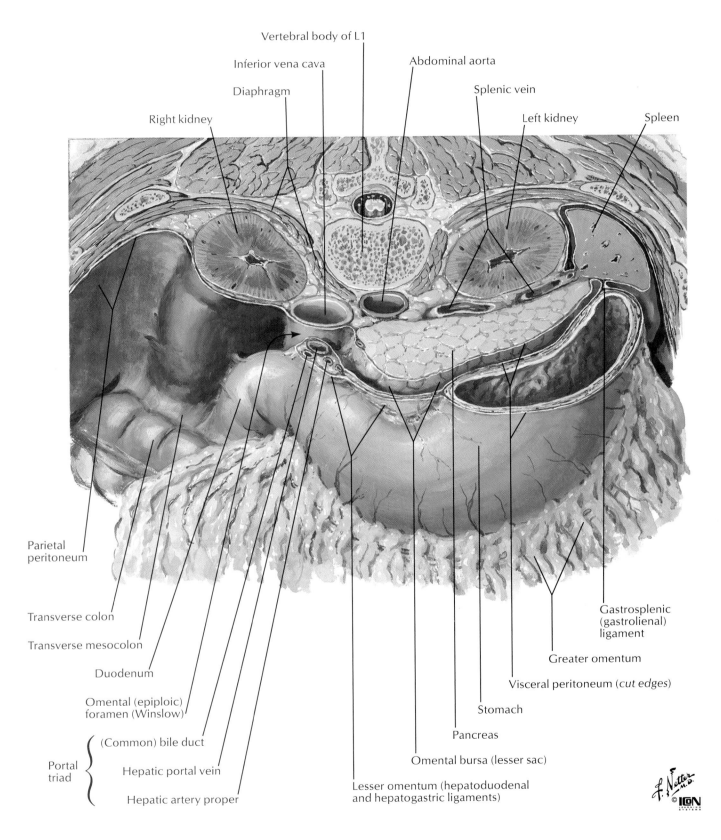

Vertebral body of L1

Inferior vena cava

Diaphragm

Right kidney

Abdominal aorta

Splenic vein

Left kidney

Spleen

Parietal peritoneum

Transverse colon

Transverse mesocolon

Duodenum

Omental (epiploic) foramen (Winslow)

Portal triad { (Common) bile duct

Hepatic portal vein

Hepatic artery proper

Lesser omentum (hepatoduodenal and hepatogastric ligaments)

Omental bursa (lesser sac)

Pancreas

Stomach

Visceral peritoneum (*cut edges*)

Greater omentum

Gastrosplenic (gastrolienal) ligament

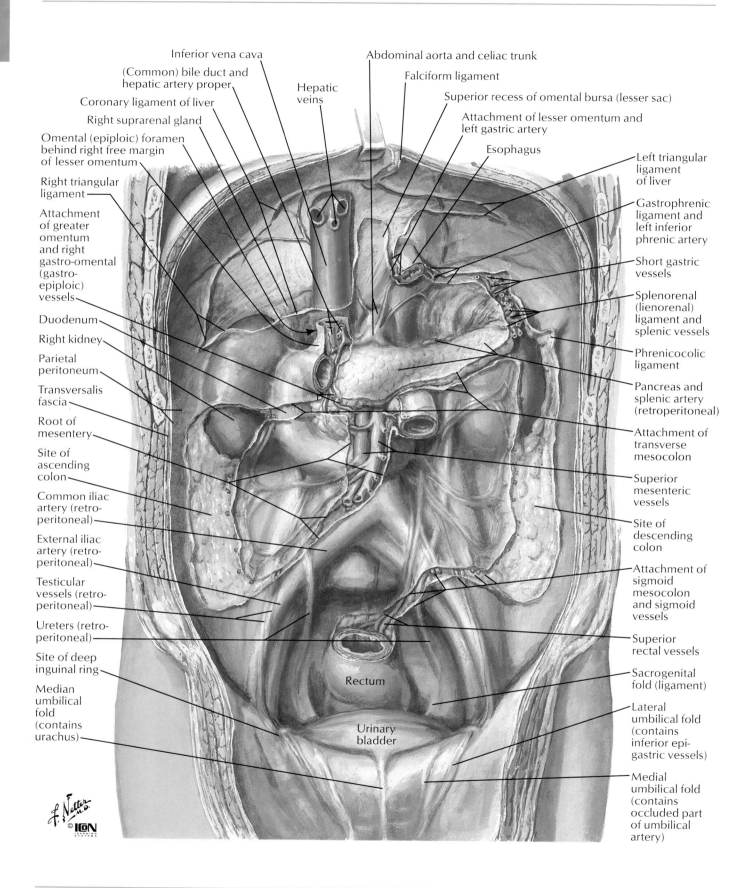

Inferior vena cava

(Common) bile duct and hepatic artery proper

Coronary ligament of liver

Right suprarenal gland

Omental (epiploic) foramen behind right free margin of lesser omentum

Right triangular ligament

Attachment of greater omentum and right gastro-omental (gastro-epiploic) vessels

Duodenum

Right kidney

Parietal peritoneum

Transversalis fascia

Root of mesentery

Site of ascending colon

Common iliac artery (retro-peritoneal)

External iliac artery (retro-peritoneal)

Testicular vessels (retro-peritoneal)

Ureters (retro-peritoneal)

Site of deep inguinal ring

Median umbilical fold (contains urachus)

Hepatic veins

Abdominal aorta and celiac trunk

Falciform ligament

Superior recess of omental bursa (lesser sac)

Attachment of lesser omentum and left gastric artery

Esophagus

Left triangular ligament of liver

Gastrophrenic ligament and left inferior phrenic artery

Short gastric vessels

Splenorenal (lienorenal) ligament and splenic vessels

Phrenicocolic ligament

Pancreas and splenic artery (retroperitoneal)

Attachment of transverse mesocolon

Superior mesenteric vessels

Site of descending colon

Attachment of sigmoid mesocolon and sigmoid vessels

Superior rectal vessels

Sacrogenital fold (ligament)

Lateral umbilical fold (contains inferior epi-gastric vessels)

Medial umbilical fold (contains occluded part of umbilical artery)

Rectum

Urinary bladder

PLATE 266

ABDOMEN

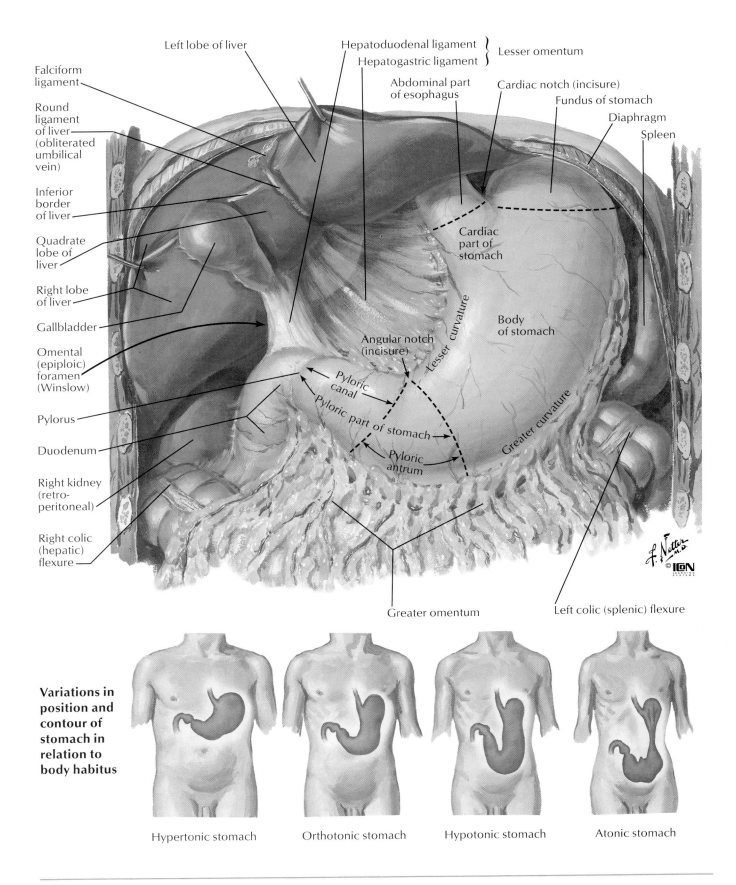

Left lobe of liver

Hepatoduodenal ligament ⎫ Lesser omentum
Hepatogastric ligament ⎭

Falciform ligament

Abdominal part of esophagus

Cardiac notch (incisure)

Fundus of stomach

Round ligament of liver (obliterated umbilical vein)

Diaphragm

Spleen

Inferior border of liver

Cardiac part of stomach

Quadrate lobe of liver

Body of stomach

Right lobe of liver

Lesser curvature

Gallbladder

Angular notch (incisure)

Omental (epiploic) foramen (Winslow)

Pyloric canal

Pyloric part of stomach

Pylorus

Greater curvature

Duodenum

Pyloric antrum

Right kidney (retro-peritoneal)

Right colic (hepatic) flexure

Greater omentum

Left colic (splenic) flexure

Variations in position and contour of stomach in relation to body habitus

Hypertonic stomach

Orthotonic stomach

Hypotonic stomach

Atonic stomach

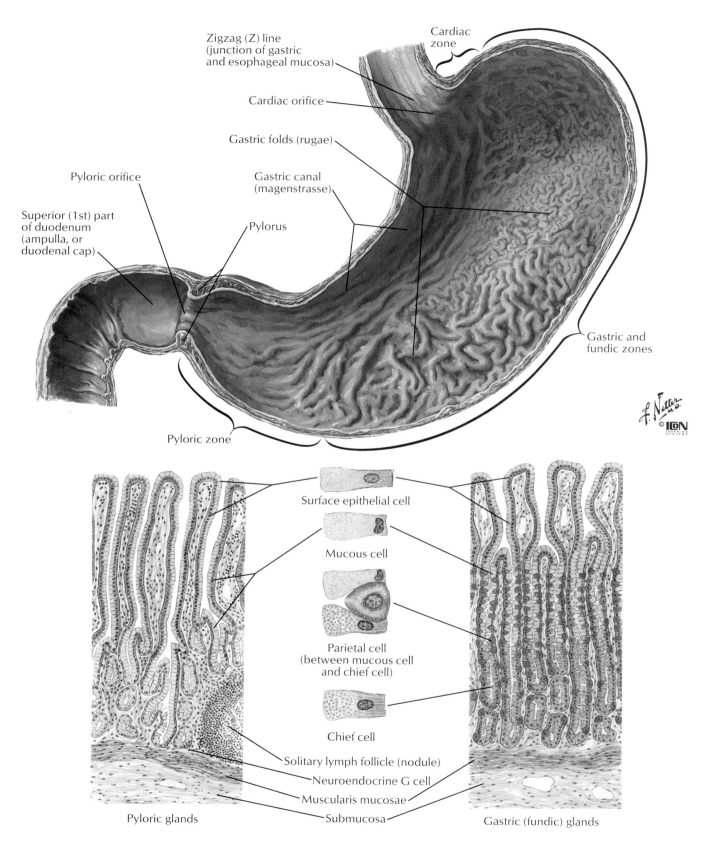

Zigzag (Z) line (junction of gastric and esophageal mucosa)

Cardiac zone

Cardiac orifice

Gastric folds (rugae)

Pyloric orifice

Gastric canal (magenstrasse)

Superior (1st) part of duodenum (ampulla, or duodenal cap)

Pylorus

Gastric and fundic zones

Pyloric zone

Surface epithelial cell

Mucous cell

Parietal cell (between mucous cell and chief cell)

Chief cell

Solitary lymph follicle (nodule)

Neuroendocrine G cell

Muscularis mucosae

Submucosa

Pyloric glands

Gastric (fundic) glands

PLATE 268

ABDOMEN

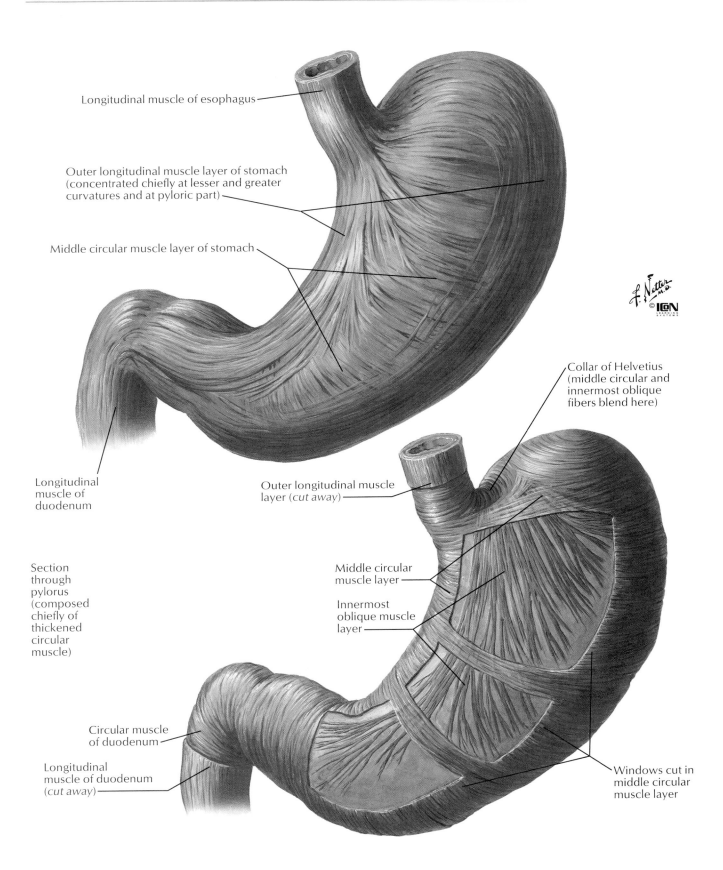

Longitudinal muscle of esophagus

Outer longitudinal muscle layer of stomach (concentrated chiefly at lesser and greater curvatures and at pyloric part)

Middle circular muscle layer of stomach

Longitudinal muscle of duodenum

Section through pylorus (composed chiefly of thickened circular muscle)

Circular muscle of duodenum

Longitudinal muscle of duodenum (*cut away*)

Collar of Helvetius (middle circular and innermost oblique fibers blend here)

Outer longitudinal muscle layer (*cut away*)

Middle circular muscle layer

Innermost oblique muscle layer

Windows cut in middle circular muscle layer

Duodenum In Situ

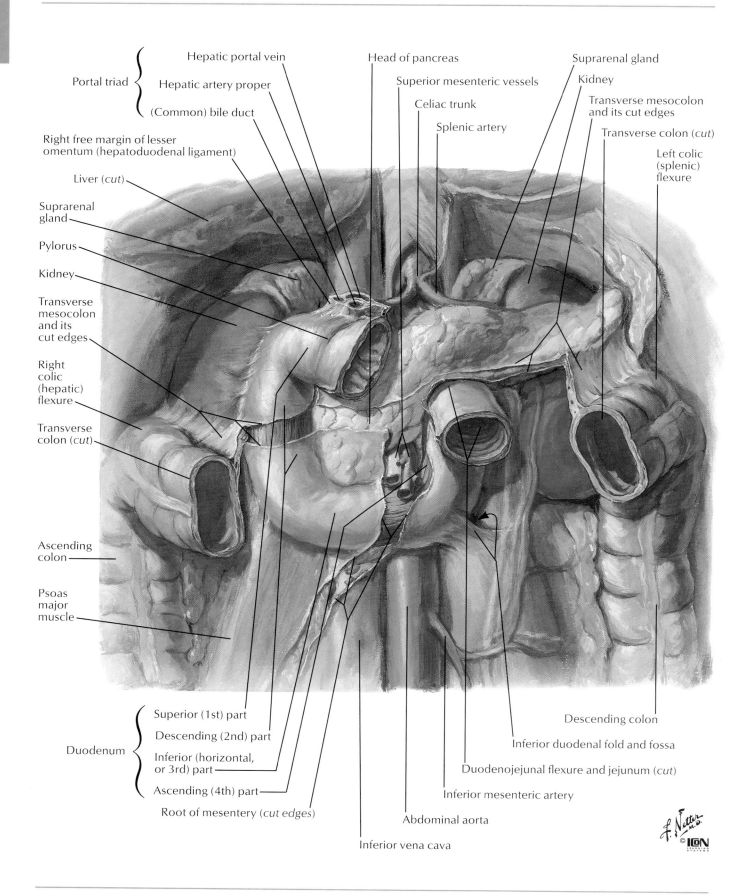

Portal triad {
Hepatic portal vein
Hepatic artery proper
(Common) bile duct

Head of pancreas
Superior mesenteric vessels
Celiac trunk
Splenic artery

Suprarenal gland
Kidney
Transverse mesocolon and its cut edges
Transverse colon (cut)
Left colic (splenic) flexure

Right free margin of lesser omentum (hepatoduodenal ligament)

Liver (cut)

Suprarenal gland

Pylorus

Kidney

Transverse mesocolon and its cut edges

Right colic (hepatic) flexure

Transverse colon (cut)

Ascending colon

Psoas major muscle

Duodenum {
Superior (1st) part
Descending (2nd) part
Inferior (horizontal, or 3rd) part
Ascending (4th) part
Root of mesentery (cut edges)

Descending colon

Inferior duodenal fold and fossa

Duodenojejunal flexure and jejunum (cut)

Inferior mesenteric artery

Abdominal aorta

Inferior vena cava

PLATE 270

ABDOMEN

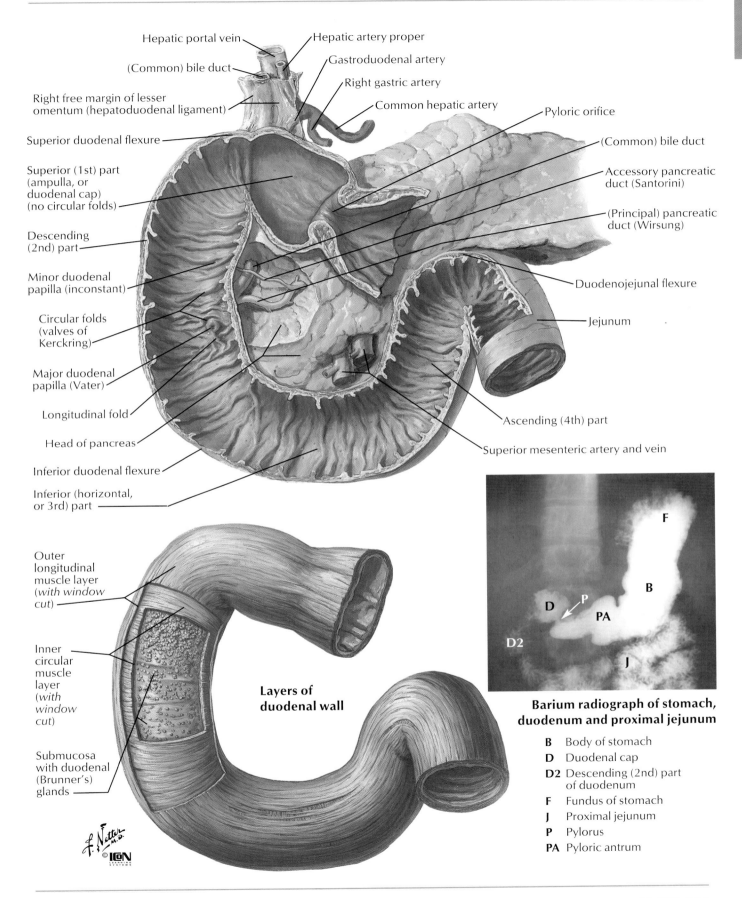

Hepatic portal vein

(Common) bile duct

Right free margin of lesser omentum (hepatoduodenal ligament)

Superior duodenal flexure

Superior (1st) part (ampulla, or duodenal cap) (no circular folds)

Descending (2nd) part

Minor duodenal papilla (inconstant)

Circular folds (valves of Kerckring)

Major duodenal papilla (Vater)

Longitudinal fold

Head of pancreas

Inferior duodenal flexure

Inferior (horizontal, or 3rd) part

Hepatic artery proper

Gastroduodenal artery

Right gastric artery

Common hepatic artery

Pyloric orifice

(Common) bile duct

Accessory pancreatic duct (Santorini)

(Principal) pancreatic duct (Wirsung)

Duodenojejunal flexure

Jejunum

Ascending (4th) part

Superior mesenteric artery and vein

Outer longitudinal muscle layer (*with window cut*)

Inner circular muscle layer (*with window cut*)

Submucosa with duodenal (Brunner's) glands

Layers of duodenal wall

Barium radiograph of stomach, duodenum and proximal jejunum

B   Body of stomach
D   Duodenal cap
D2 Descending (2nd) part of duodenum
F   Fundus of stomach
J   Proximal jejunum
P   Pylorus
PA Pyloric antrum

Mucosa and Musculature of Small Intestine

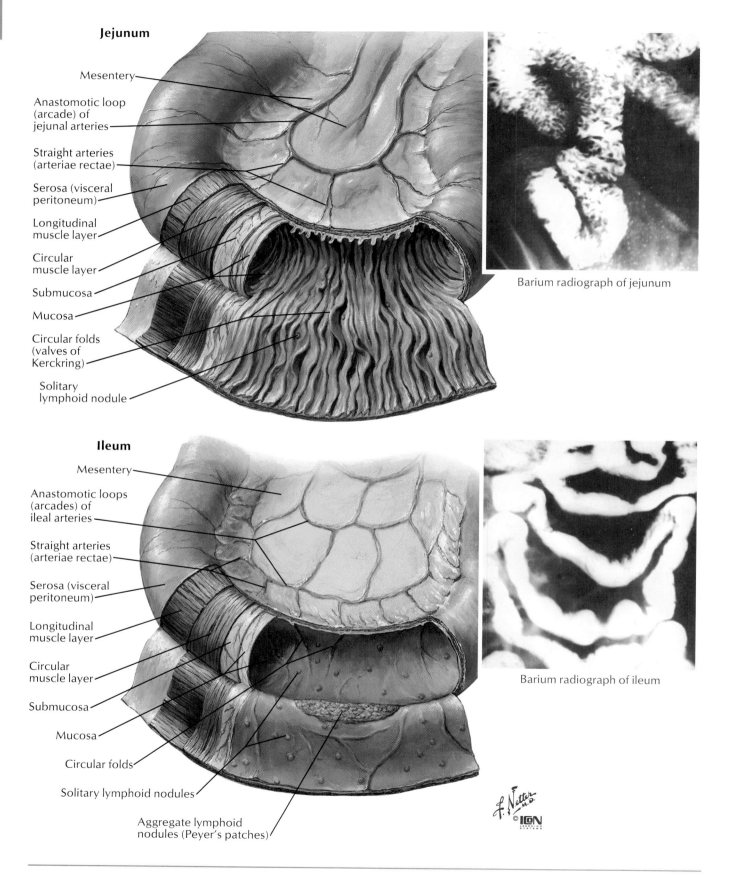

Jejunum

- Mesentery
- Anastomotic loop (arcade) of jejunal arteries
- Straight arteries (arteriae rectae)
- Serosa (visceral peritoneum)
- Longitudinal muscle layer
- Circular muscle layer
- Submucosa
- Mucosa
- Circular folds (valves of Kerckring)
- Solitary lymphoid nodule

Barium radiograph of jejunum

Ileum

- Mesentery
- Anastomotic loops (arcades) of ileal arteries
- Straight arteries (arteriae rectae)
- Serosa (visceral peritoneum)
- Longitudinal muscle layer
- Circular muscle layer
- Submucosa
- Mucosa
- Circular folds
- Solitary lymphoid nodules
- Aggregate lymphoid nodules (Peyer's patches)

Barium radiograph of ileum

PLATE 272

ABDOMEN

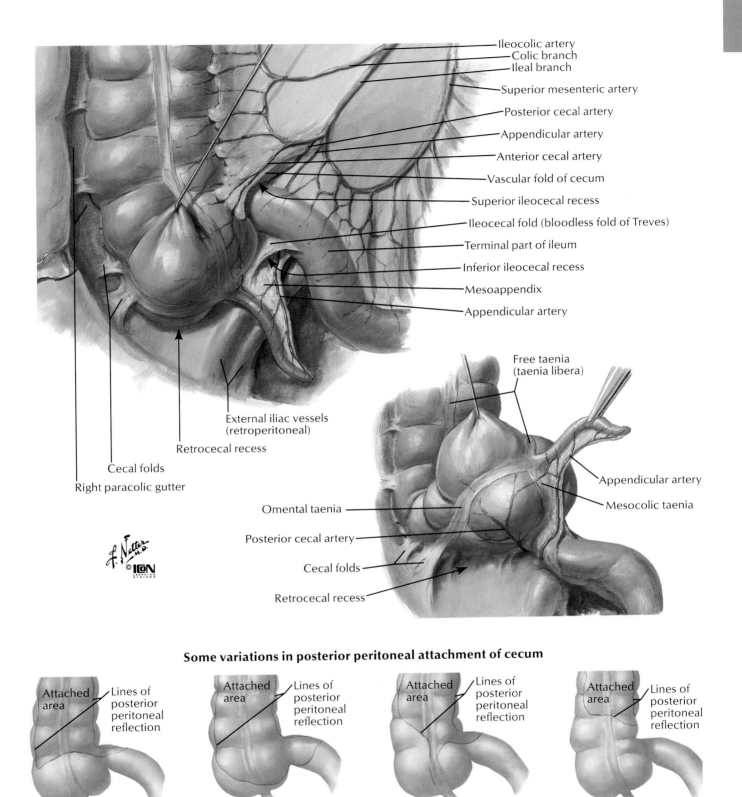

Ileocolic artery
Colic branch
Ileal branch
Superior mesenteric artery
Posterior cecal artery
Appendicular artery
Anterior cecal artery
Vascular fold of cecum
Superior ileocecal recess
Ileocecal fold (bloodless fold of Treves)
Terminal part of ileum
Inferior ileocecal recess
Mesoappendix
Appendicular artery

External iliac vessels (retroperitoneal)

Retrocecal recess

Cecal folds

Right paracolic gutter

Free taenia (taenia libera)

Appendicular artery

Mesocolic taenia

Omental taenia

Posterior cecal artery

Cecal folds

Retrocecal recess

Some variations in posterior peritoneal attachment of cecum

Attached area — Lines of posterior peritoneal reflection

Attached area — Lines of posterior peritoneal reflection

Attached area — Lines of posterior peritoneal reflection

Attached area — Lines of posterior peritoneal reflection

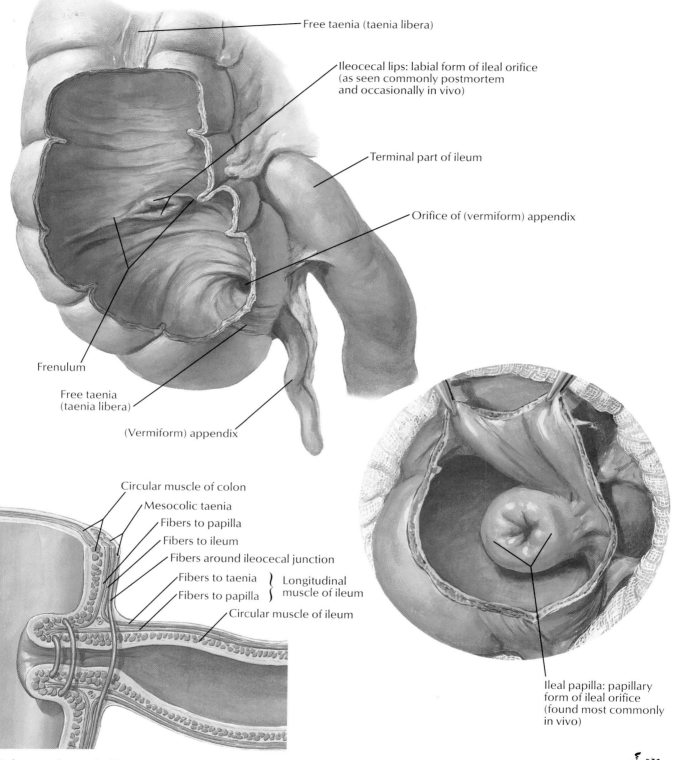

Free taenia (taenia libera)

Ileocecal lips: labial form of ileal orifice
(as seen commonly postmortem
and occasionally in vivo)

Terminal part of ileum

Orifice of (vermiform) appendix

Frenulum

Free taenia
(taenia libera)

(Vermiform) appendix

Circular muscle of colon
Mesocolic taenia
Fibers to papilla
Fibers to ileum
Fibers around ileocecal junction
Fibers to taenia
Fibers to papilla
} Longitudinal
muscle of ileum
Circular muscle of ileum

Ileal papilla: papillary
form of ileal orifice
(found most commonly
in vivo)

Schema of muscle fibers at ileal orifice

PLATE 274

ABDOMEN

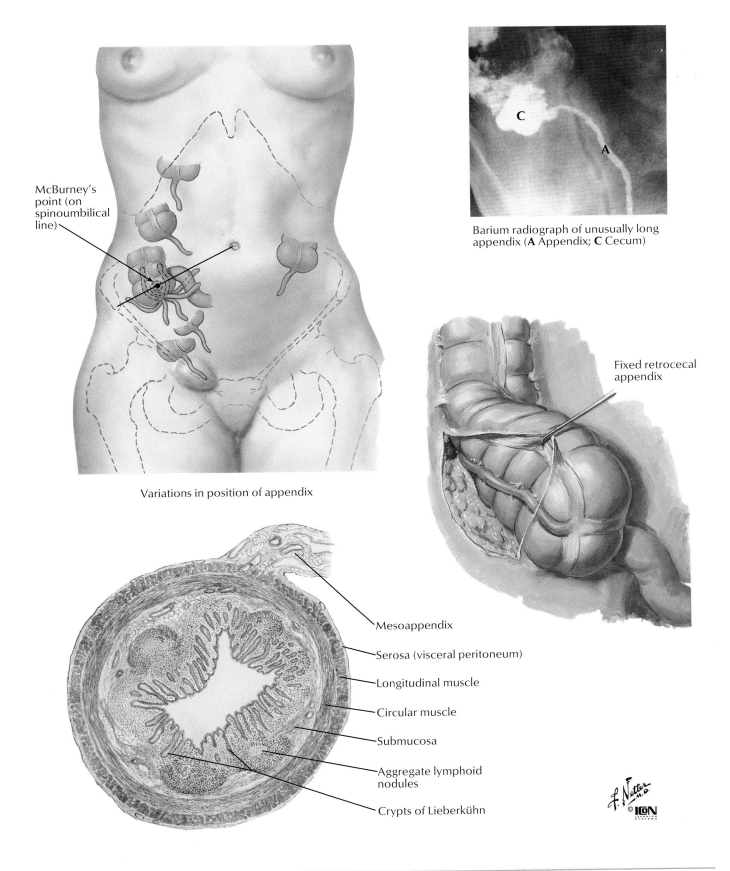

McBurney's point (on spinoumbilical line)

Variations in position of appendix

Barium radiograph of unusually long appendix (**A** Appendix; **C** Cecum)

Fixed retrocecal appendix

Mesoappendix

Serosa (visceral peritoneum)

Longitudinal muscle

Circular muscle

Submucosa

Aggregate lymphoid nodules

Crypts of Lieberkühn

Mucosa and Musculature of Large Intestine

FOR RECTUM AND ANAL CANAL SEE PLATES 372–377

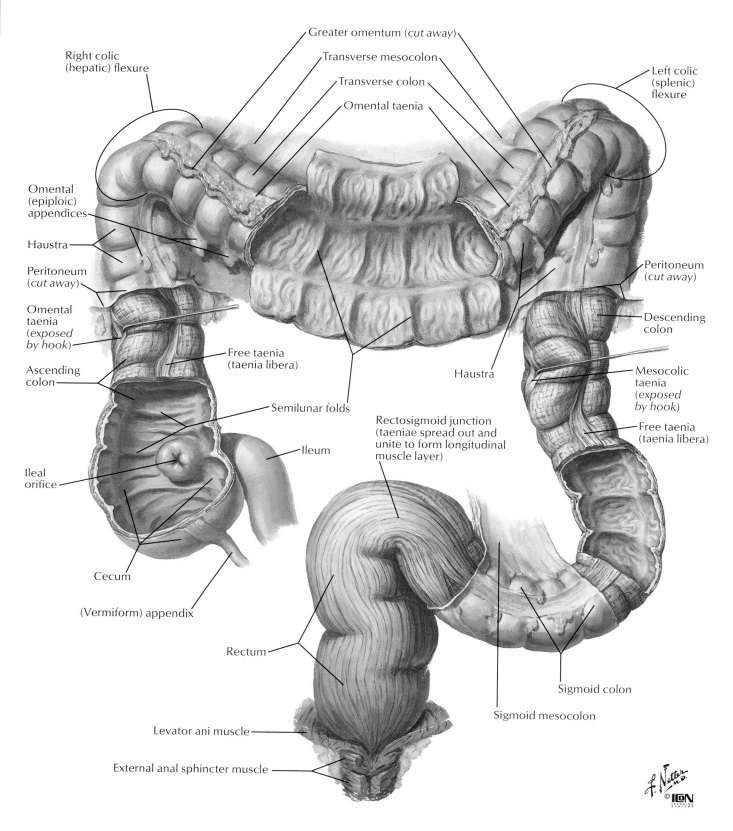

Right colic (hepatic) flexure

Omental (epiploic) appendices

Haustra

Peritoneum (cut away)

Omental taenia (exposed by hook)

Ascending colon

Ileal orifice

Cecum

(Vermiform) appendix

Rectum

Levator ani muscle

External anal sphincter muscle

Greater omentum (cut away)

Transverse mesocolon

Transverse colon

Omental taenia

Free taenia (taenia libera)

Semilunar folds

Ileum

Rectosigmoid junction (taeniae spread out and unite to form longitudinal muscle layer)

Left colic (splenic) flexure

Peritoneum (cut away)

Descending colon

Haustra

Mesocolic taenia (exposed by hook)

Free taenia (taenia libera)

Sigmoid colon

Sigmoid mesocolon

PLATE 276

ABDOMEN

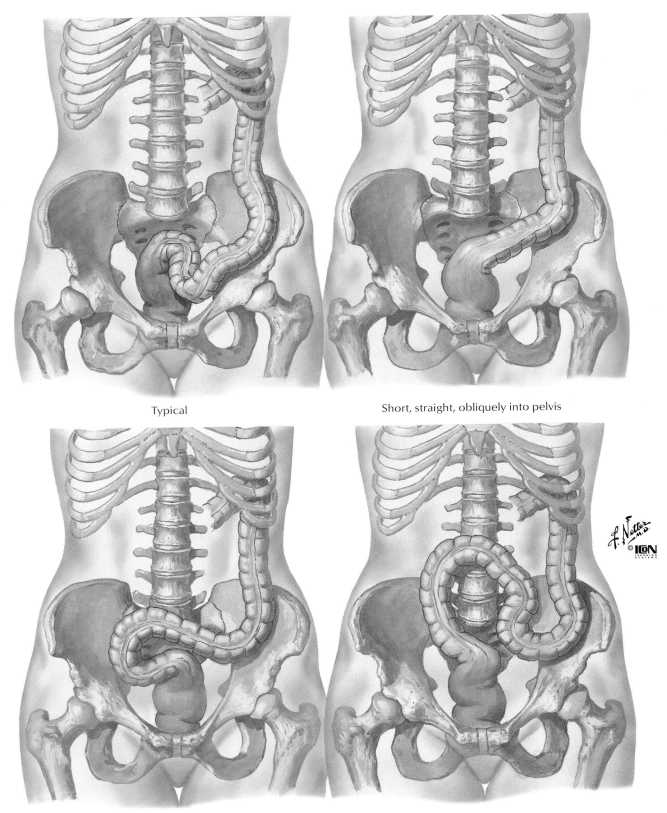

Typical

Short, straight, obliquely into pelvis

Looping to right side

Ascending high into abdomen

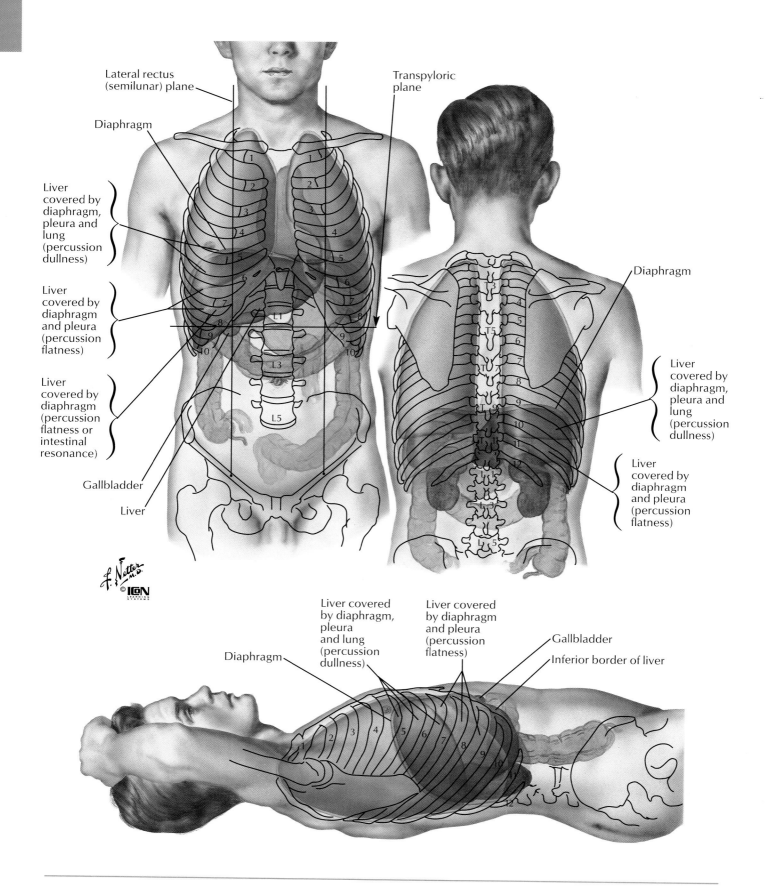

Lateral rectus (semilunar) plane

Transpyloric plane

Diaphragm

Liver covered by diaphragm, pleura and lung (percussion dullness)

Liver covered by diaphragm and pleura (percussion flatness)

Liver covered by diaphragm (percussion flatness or intestinal resonance)

Gallbladder

Liver

Diaphragm

Liver covered by diaphragm, pleura and lung (percussion dullness)

Liver covered by diaphragm and pleura (percussion flatness)

Liver covered by diaphragm, pleura and lung (percussion dullness)

Liver covered by diaphragm and pleura (percussion flatness)

Diaphragm

Gallbladder

Inferior border of liver

PLATE 278

ABDOMEN

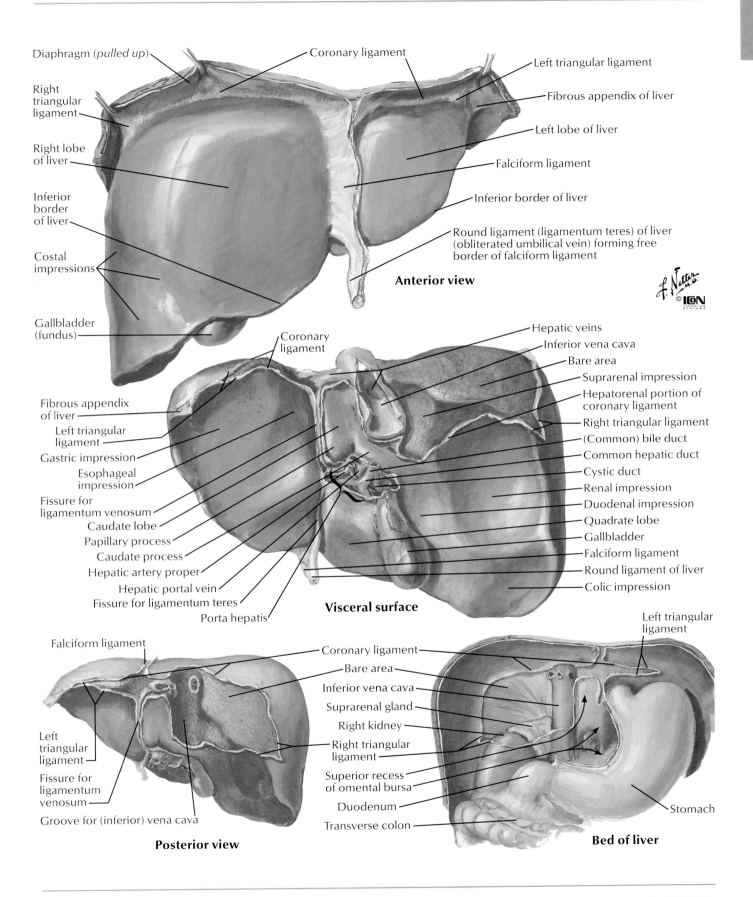

Diaphragm (*pulled up*)
Coronary ligament
Left triangular ligament
Right triangular ligament
Fibrous appendix of liver
Left lobe of liver
Right lobe of liver
Falciform ligament
Inferior border of liver
Inferior border of liver
Costal impressions
Round ligament (ligamentum teres) of liver (obliterated umbilical vein) forming free border of falciform ligament
Gallbladder (fundus)

Anterior view

Coronary ligament
Hepatic veins
Inferior vena cava
Bare area
Suprarenal impression
Hepatorenal portion of coronary ligament
Fibrous appendix of liver
Left triangular ligament
Gastric impression
Right triangular ligament
Esophageal impression
(Common) bile duct
Fissure for ligamentum venosum
Common hepatic duct
Caudate lobe
Cystic duct
Papillary process
Renal impression
Caudate process
Duodenal impression
Hepatic artery proper
Quadrate lobe
Hepatic portal vein
Gallbladder
Fissure for ligamentum teres
Falciform ligament
Porta hepatis
Round ligament of liver
Colic impression

Visceral surface

Falciform ligament
Coronary ligament
Left triangular ligament
Bare area
Inferior vena cava
Suprarenal gland
Right kidney
Left triangular ligament
Fissure for ligamentum venosum
Right triangular ligament
Superior recess of omental bursa
Groove for (inferior) vena cava
Duodenum
Transverse colon
Stomach

Posterior view

Bed of liver

Liver In Situ and Variations in Form

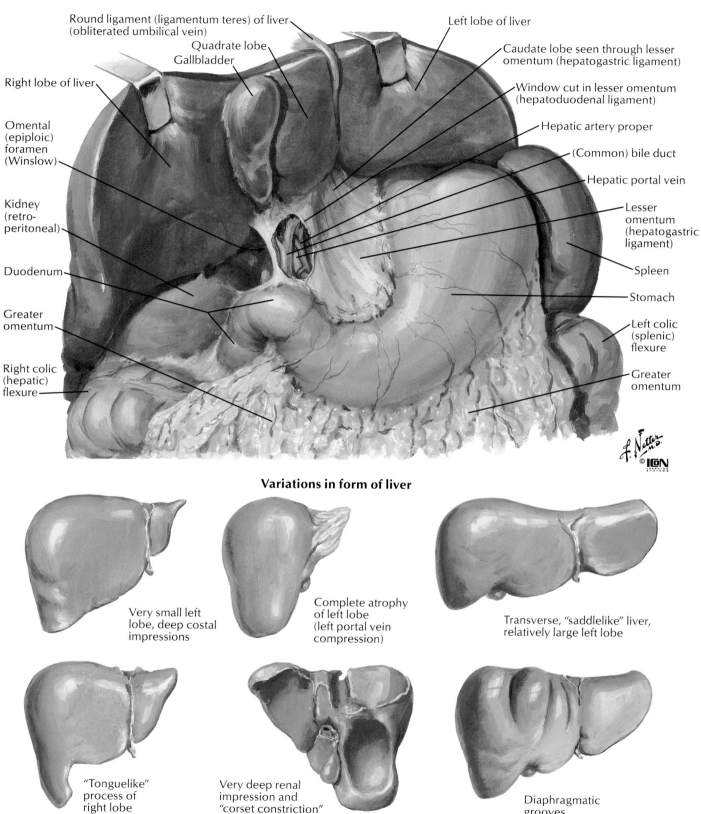

Round ligament (ligamentum teres) of liver (obliterated umbilical vein)

Quadrate lobe

Gallbladder

Left lobe of liver

Caudate lobe seen through lesser omentum (hepatogastric ligament)

Right lobe of liver

Window cut in lesser omentum (hepatoduodenal ligament)

Omental (epiploic) foramen (Winslow)

Hepatic artery proper

(Common) bile duct

Hepatic portal vein

Kidney (retro-peritoneal)

Lesser omentum (hepatogastric ligament)

Duodenum

Spleen

Greater omentum

Stomach

Left colic (splenic) flexure

Right colic (hepatic) flexure

Greater omentum

Variations in form of liver

Very small left lobe, deep costal impressions

Complete atrophy of left lobe (left portal vein compression)

Transverse, "saddlelike" liver, relatively large left lobe

"Tonguelike" process of right lobe

Very deep renal impression and "corset constriction"

Diaphragmatic grooves

PLATE 280

ABDOMEN

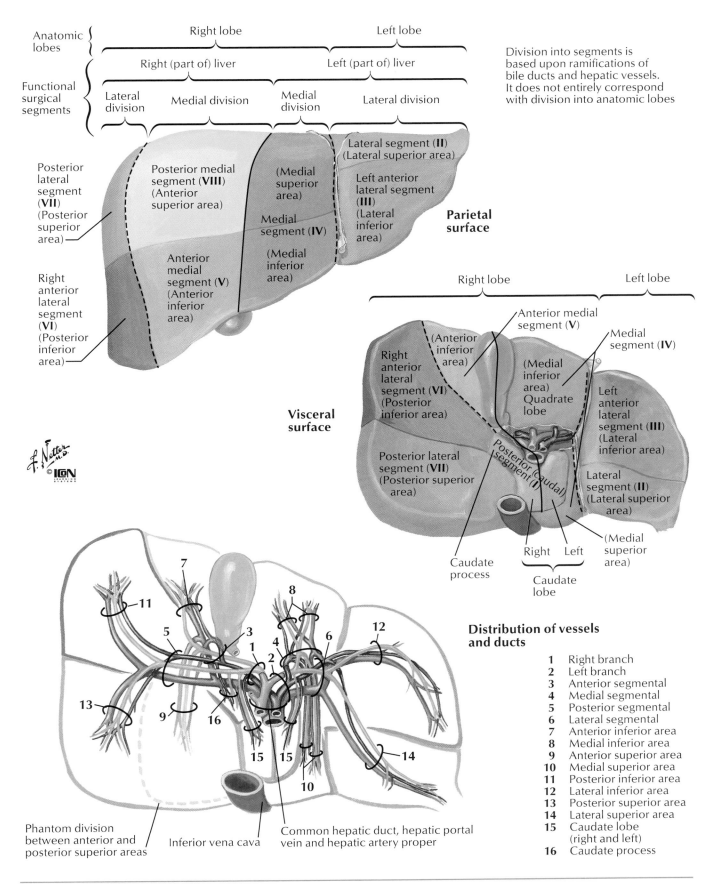

Anatomic lobes

Right lobe

Left lobe

Functional surgical segments

Right (part of) liver

Left (part of) liver

Lateral division

Medial division

Medial division

Lateral division

Division into segments is based upon ramifications of bile ducts and hepatic vessels. It does not entirely correspond with division into anatomic lobes

Posterior lateral segment (**VII**) (Posterior superior area)

Right anterior lateral segment (**VI**) (Posterior inferior area)

Posterior medial segment (**VIII**) (Anterior superior area)

Anterior medial segment (**V**) (Anterior inferior area)

(Medial superior area)

Medial segment (**IV**)

(Medial inferior area)

Lateral segment (**II**) (Lateral superior area)

Left anterior lateral segment (**III**) (Lateral inferior area)

Parietal surface

Visceral surface

Right lobe

Left lobe

Anterior medial segment (**V**)

(Anterior inferior area)

Right anterior lateral segment (**VI**) (Posterior inferior area)

Posterior lateral segment (**VII**) (Posterior superior area)

Posterior Caudal segment (**I**)

(Medial inferior area) Quadrate lobe

Medial segment (**IV**)

Left anterior lateral segment (**III**) (Lateral inferior area)

Lateral segment (**II**) (Lateral superior area)

(Medial superior area)

Right   Left

Caudate lobe

Caudate process

Distribution of vessels and ducts

1	Right branch
2	Left branch
3	Anterior segmental
4	Medial segmental
5	Posterior segmental
6	Lateral segmental
7	Anterior inferior area
8	Medial inferior area
9	Anterior superior area
10	Medial superior area
11	Posterior inferior area
12	Lateral inferior area
13	Posterior superior area
14	Lateral superior area
15	Caudate lobe (right and left)
16	Caudate process

Phantom division between anterior and posterior superior areas

Inferior vena cava

Common hepatic duct, hepatic portal vein and hepatic artery proper

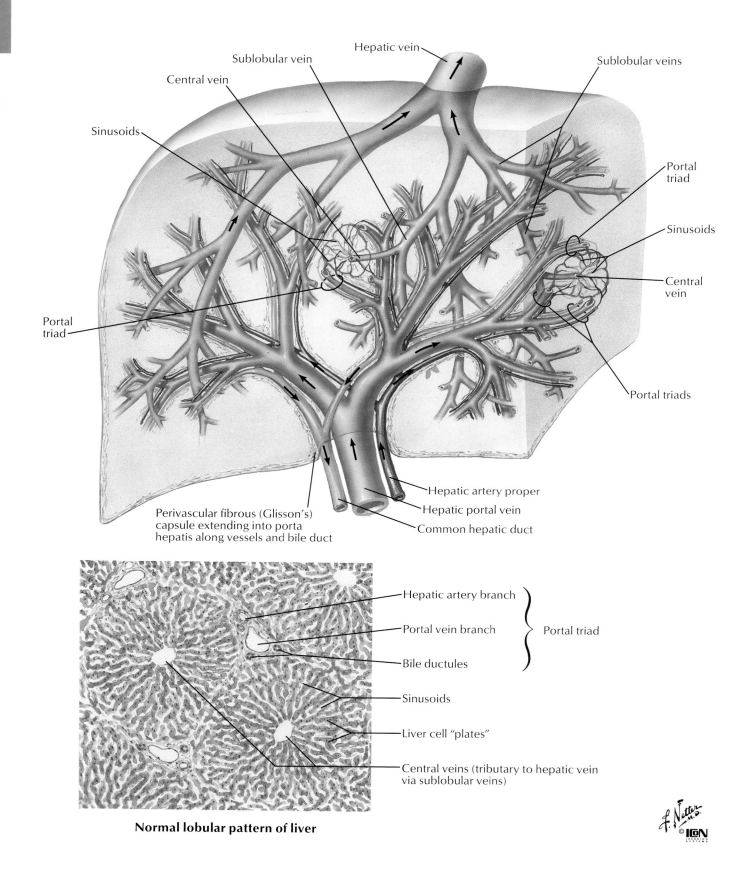

Hepatic vein

Sublobular vein

Central vein

Sinusoids

Sublobular veins

Portal triad

Sinusoids

Central vein

Portal triad

Portal triads

Perivascular fibrous (Glisson's) capsule extending into porta hepatis along vessels and bile duct

Hepatic artery proper

Hepatic portal vein

Common hepatic duct

Hepatic artery branch

Portal vein branch   } Portal triad

Bile ductules

Sinusoids

Liver cell "plates"

Central veins (tributary to hepatic vein via sublobular veins)

Normal lobular pattern of liver

PLATE 282

ABDOMEN

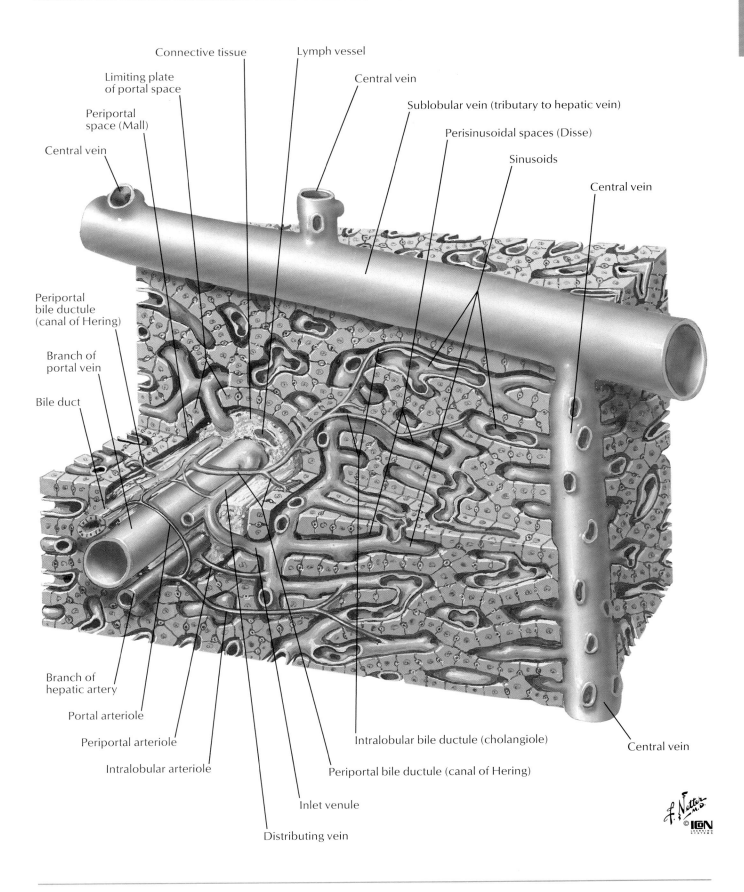

Connective tissue

Lymph vessel

Limiting plate
of portal space

Central vein

Periportal
space (Mall)

Sublobular vein (tributary to hepatic vein)

Central vein

Perisinusoidal spaces (Disse)

Sinusoids

Central vein

Periportal
bile ductule
(canal of Hering)

Branch of
portal vein

Bile duct

Branch of
hepatic artery

Portal arteriole

Peripheral arteriole

Intralobular arteriole

Intralobular bile ductule (cholangiole)

Periportal bile ductule (canal of Hering)

Central vein

Inlet venule

Distributing vein

Intrahepatic Biliary System: Schema

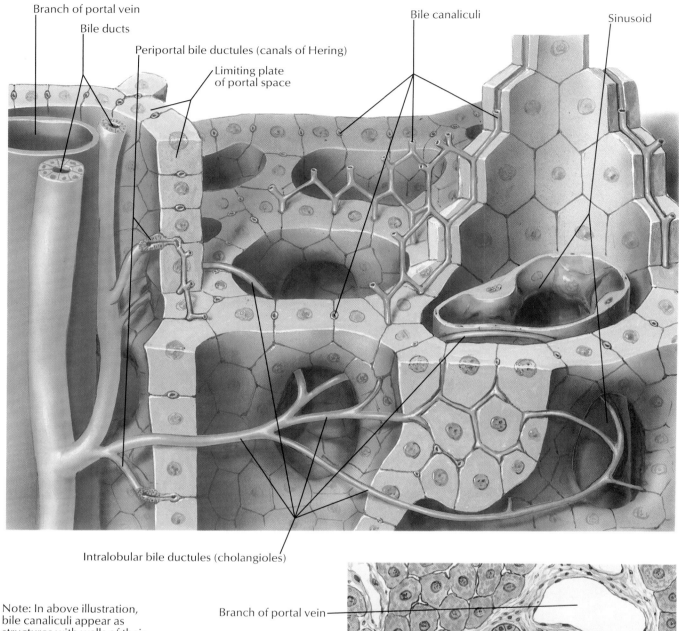

Branch of portal vein

Bile ducts

Periportal bile ductules (canals of Hering)

Limiting plate of portal space

Bile canaliculi

Sinusoid

Intralobular bile ductules (cholangioles)

Note: In above illustration, bile canaliculi appear as structures with walls of their own. However, as shown in histologic section at right, boundaries of canaliculi are actually a specialization of surface membranes of adjoining liver parenchymal cells

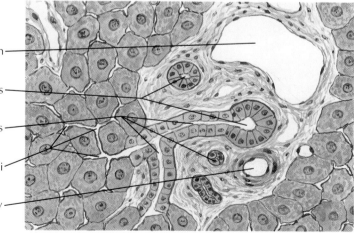

Branch of portal vein

Bile ducts

Bile ductules

Bile canaliculi

Branch of hepatic artery

Low-power section of liver

PLATE 284

ABDOMEN

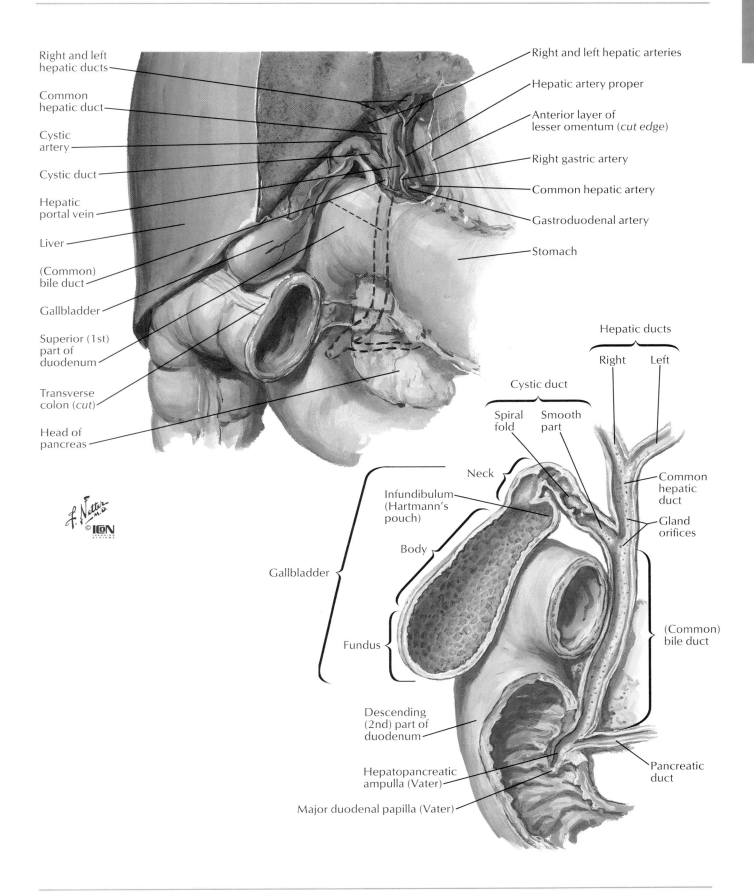

Right and left hepatic ducts

Common hepatic duct

Cystic artery

Cystic duct

Hepatic portal vein

Liver

(Common) bile duct

Gallbladder

Superior (1st) part of duodenum

Transverse colon (cut)

Head of pancreas

Right and left hepatic arteries

Hepatic artery proper

Anterior layer of lesser omentum (cut edge)

Right gastric artery

Common hepatic artery

Gastroduodenal artery

Stomach

Hepatic ducts

Right   Left

Cystic duct

Spiral fold   Smooth part

Neck

Common hepatic duct

Infundibulum (Hartmann's pouch)

Gland orifices

Body

Gallbladder

Fundus

(Common) bile duct

Descending (2nd) part of duodenum

Hepatopancreatic ampulla (Vater)

Major duodenal papilla (Vater)

Pancreatic duct

Variations in Cystic and Hepatic Ducts

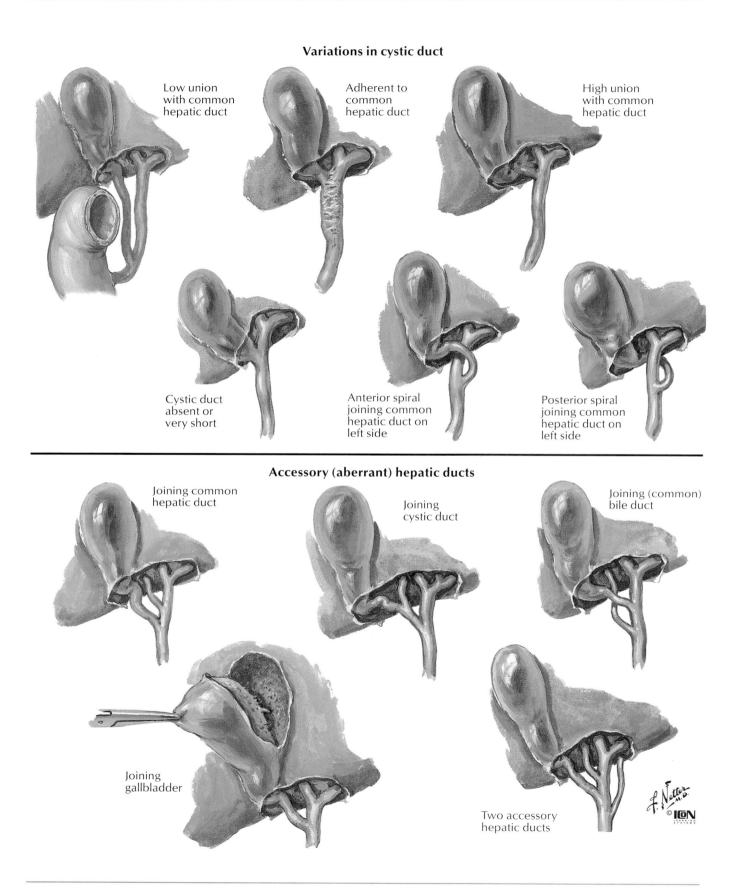

Variations in cystic duct

Low union with common hepatic duct

Adherent to common hepatic duct

High union with common hepatic duct

Cystic duct absent or very short

Anterior spiral joining common hepatic duct on left side

Posterior spiral joining common hepatic duct on left side

Accessory (aberrant) hepatic ducts

Joining common hepatic duct

Joining cystic duct

Joining (common) bile duct

Joining gallbladder

Two accessory hepatic ducts

PLATE 286

ABDOMEN

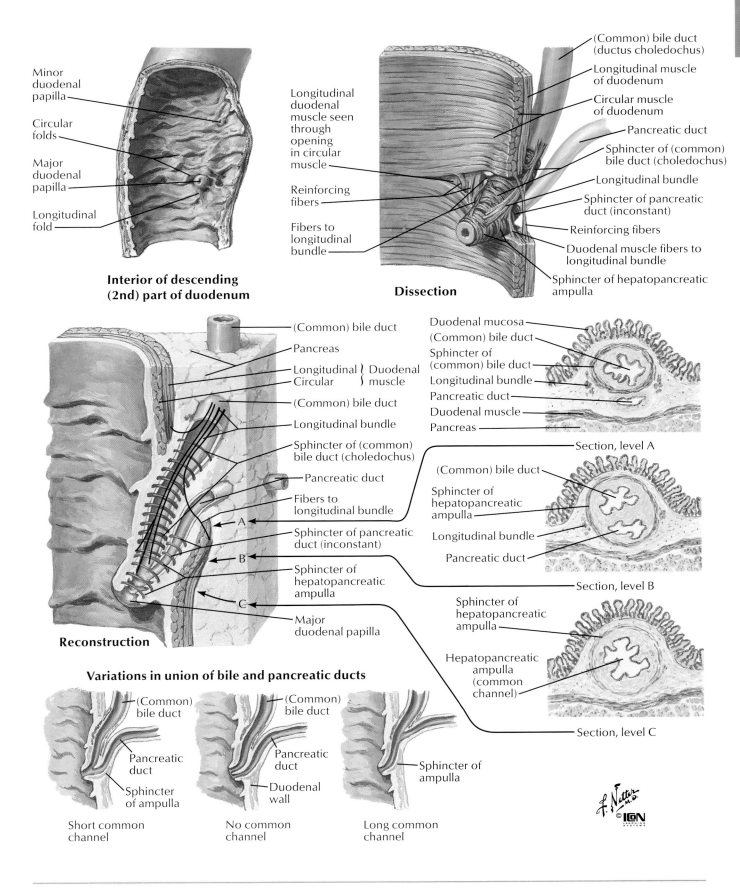

Interior of descending (2nd) part of duodenum

Minor duodenal papilla
Circular folds
Major duodenal papilla
Longitudinal fold

Dissection

(Common) bile duct (ductus choledochus)
Longitudinal muscle of duodenum
Circular muscle of duodenum
Pancreatic duct
Sphincter of (common) bile duct (choledochus)
Longitudinal bundle
Sphincter of pancreatic duct (inconstant)
Reinforcing fibers
Duodenal muscle fibers to longitudinal bundle
Sphincter of hepatopancreatic ampulla

Longitudinal duodenal muscle seen through opening in circular muscle
Reinforcing fibers
Fibers to longitudinal bundle

Reconstruction

(Common) bile duct
Pancreas
Longitudinal } Duodenal
Circular } muscle
(Common) bile duct
Longitudinal bundle
Sphincter of (common) bile duct (choledochus)
Pancreatic duct
Fibers to longitudinal bundle
Sphincter of pancreatic duct (inconstant)
Sphincter of hepatopancreatic ampulla
Major duodenal papilla

A
B
C

Duodenal mucosa
(Common) bile duct
Sphincter of (common) bile duct
Longitudinal bundle
Pancreatic duct
Duodenal muscle
Pancreas

Section, level A

(Common) bile duct
Sphincter of hepatopancreatic ampulla
Longitudinal bundle
Pancreatic duct

Section, level B

Sphincter of hepatopancreatic ampulla
Hepatopancreatic ampulla (common channel)

Section, level C

Variations in union of bile and pancreatic ducts

(Common) bile duct
Pancreatic duct
Sphincter of ampulla

Short common channel

(Common) bile duct
Pancreatic duct
Duodenal wall

No common channel

Sphincter of ampulla

Long common channel

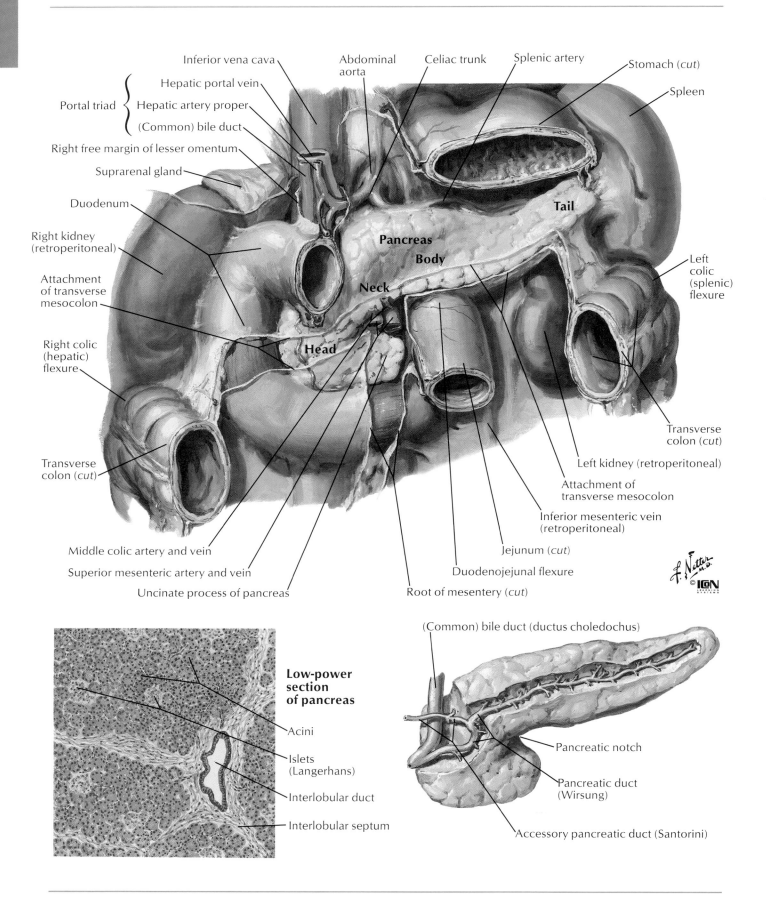

Inferior vena cava

Abdominal aorta

Celiac trunk

Splenic artery

Stomach (*cut*)

Spleen

Portal triad
- Hepatic portal vein
- Hepatic artery proper
- (Common) bile duct

Right free margin of lesser omentum

Suprarenal gland

Duodenum

Right kidney (retroperitoneal)

Attachment of transverse mesocolon

Right colic (hepatic) flexure

Transverse colon (*cut*)

Middle colic artery and vein

Superior mesenteric artery and vein

Uncinate process of pancreas

Tail

Pancreas
Body

Neck

Head

Left colic (splenic) flexure

Transverse colon (*cut*)

Left kidney (retroperitoneal)

Attachment of transverse mesocolon

Inferior mesenteric vein (retroperitoneal)

Jejunum (*cut*)

Duodenojejunal flexure

Root of mesentery (*cut*)

Low-power section of pancreas

Acini

Islets (Langerhans)

Interlobular duct

Interlobular septum

(Common) bile duct (ductus choledochus)

Pancreatic notch

Pancreatic duct (Wirsung)

Accessory pancreatic duct (Santorini)

PLATE 288

ABDOMEN

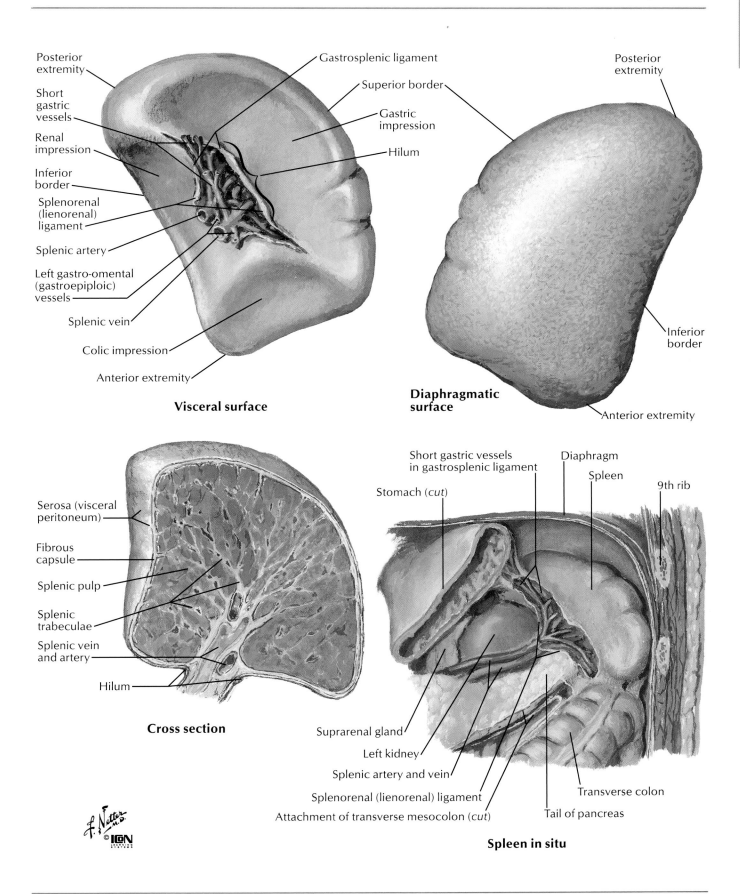

Posterior extremity

Short gastric vessels

Renal impression

Inferior border

Splenorenal (lienorenal) ligament

Splenic artery

Left gastro-omental (gastroepiploic) vessels

Splenic vein

Colic impression

Anterior extremity

Gastrosplenic ligament

Superior border

Gastric impression

Hilum

Visceral surface

Posterior extremity

Inferior border

Anterior extremity

Diaphragmatic surface

Serosa (visceral peritoneum)

Fibrous capsule

Splenic pulp

Splenic trabeculae

Splenic vein and artery

Hilum

Cross section

Short gastric vessels in gastrosplenic ligament

Stomach (*cut*)

Diaphragm

Spleen

9th rib

Suprarenal gland

Left kidney

Splenic artery and vein

Splenorenal (lienorenal) ligament

Attachment of transverse mesocolon (*cut*)

Tail of pancreas

Transverse colon

Spleen in situ

Arteries of Stomach, Liver and Spleen

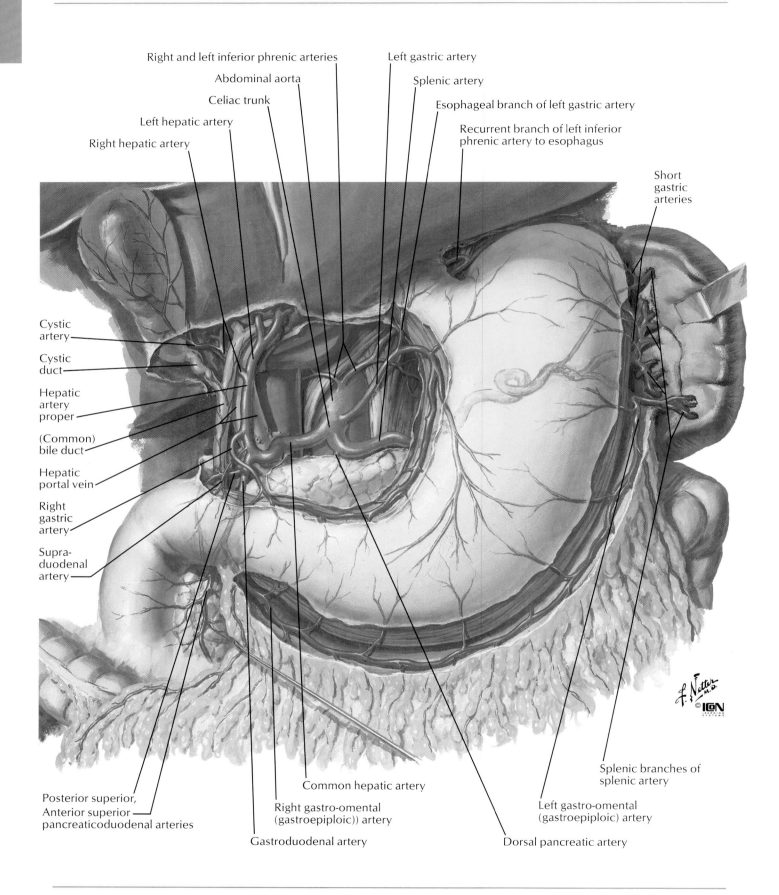

Right and left inferior phrenic arteries

Abdominal aorta

Celiac trunk

Left hepatic artery

Right hepatic artery

Left gastric artery

Splenic artery

Esophageal branch of left gastric artery

Recurrent branch of left inferior phrenic artery to esophagus

Short gastric arteries

Cystic artery

Cystic duct

Hepatic artery proper

(Common) bile duct

Hepatic portal vein

Right gastric artery

Supra-duodenal artery

Posterior superior, Anterior superior pancreaticoduodenal arteries

Gastroduodenal artery

Right gastro-omental (gastroepiploic)) artery

Common hepatic artery

Dorsal pancreatic artery

Left gastro-omental (gastroepiploic) artery

Splenic branches of splenic artery

PLATE 290

ABDOMEN

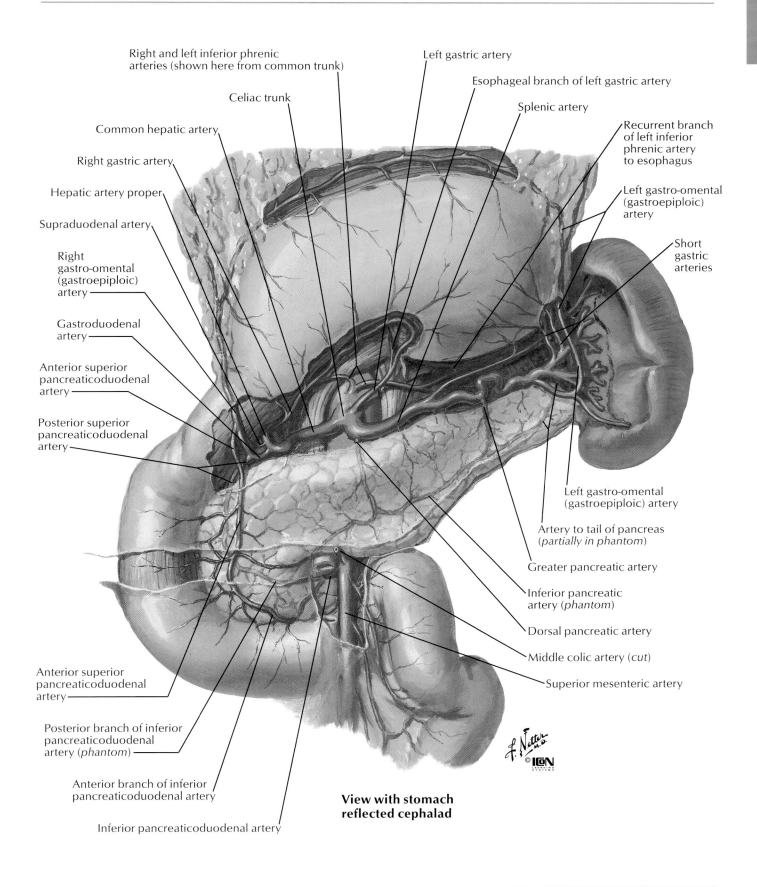

Right and left inferior phrenic arteries (shown here from common trunk)

Celiac trunk

Common hepatic artery

Right gastric artery

Hepatic artery proper

Supraduodenal artery

Right gastro-omental (gastroepiploic) artery

Gastroduodenal artery

Anterior superior pancreaticoduodenal artery

Posterior superior pancreaticoduodenal artery

Anterior superior pancreaticoduodenal artery

Posterior branch of inferior pancreaticoduodenal artery (phantom)

Anterior branch of inferior pancreaticoduodenal artery

Inferior pancreaticoduodenal artery

Left gastric artery

Esophageal branch of left gastric artery

Splenic artery

Recurrent branch of left inferior phrenic artery to esophagus

Left gastro-omental (gastroepiploic) artery

Short gastric arteries

Left gastro-omental (gastroepiploic) artery

Artery to tail of pancreas (partially in phantom)

Greater pancreatic artery

Inferior pancreatic artery (phantom)

Dorsal pancreatic artery

Middle colic artery (cut)

Superior mesenteric artery

View with stomach reflected cephalad

Arteries of Liver, Pancreas, Duodenum and Spleen

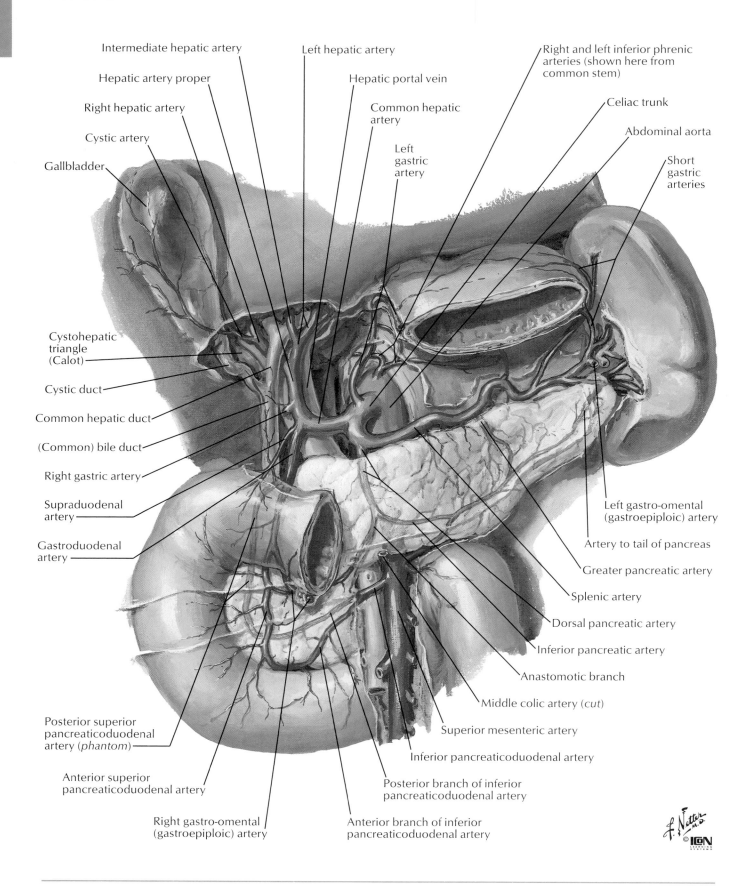

Intermediate hepatic artery

Hepatic artery proper

Right hepatic artery

Cystic artery

Gallbladder

Left hepatic artery

Hepatic portal vein

Common hepatic artery

Left gastric artery

Right and left inferior phrenic arteries (shown here from common stem)

Celiac trunk

Abdominal aorta

Short gastric arteries

Cystohepatic triangle (Calot)

Cystic duct

Common hepatic duct

(Common) bile duct

Right gastric artery

Supraduodenal artery

Gastroduodenal artery

Left gastro-omental (gastroepiploic) artery

Artery to tail of pancreas

Greater pancreatic artery

Splenic artery

Dorsal pancreatic artery

Inferior pancreatic artery

Anastomotic branch

Middle colic artery (cut)

Posterior superior pancreaticoduodenal artery (phantom)

Anterior superior pancreaticoduodenal artery

Right gastro-omental (gastroepiploic) artery

Superior mesenteric artery

Inferior pancreaticoduodenal artery

Posterior branch of inferior pancreaticoduodenal artery

Anterior branch of inferior pancreaticoduodenal artery

PLATE 292

ABDOMEN

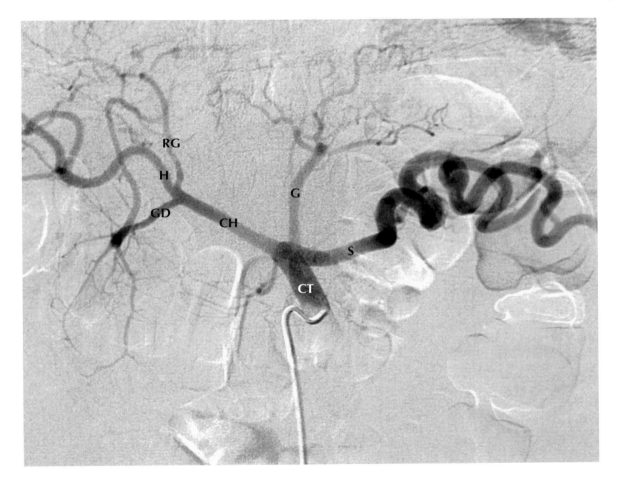

CH	Common hepatic artery
CT	Celiac trunk
G	Left gastric artery
GD	Gastroduodenal artery
H	Hepatic artery proper
RG	Right gastric artery
S	Splenic artery

Duodenum and head of pancreas reflected to left

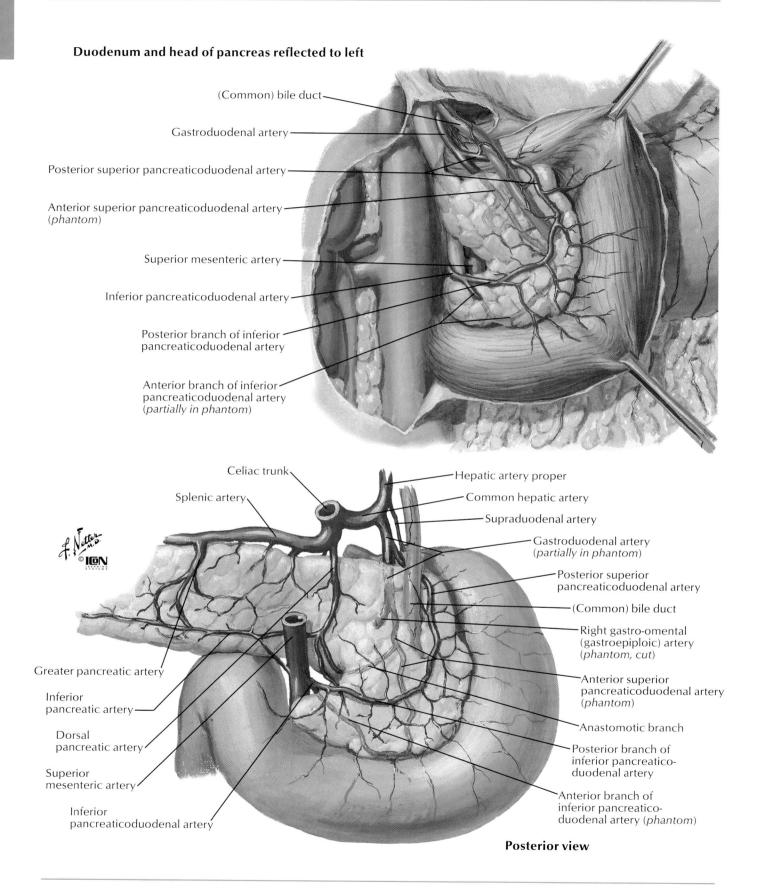

(Common) bile duct

Gastroduodenal artery

Posterior superior pancreaticoduodenal artery

Anterior superior pancreaticoduodenal artery
(*phantom*)

Superior mesenteric artery

Inferior pancreaticoduodenal artery

Posterior branch of inferior
pancreaticoduodenal artery

Anterior branch of inferior
pancreaticoduodenal artery
(*partially in phantom*)

Celiac trunk

Splenic artery

Hepatic artery proper

Common hepatic artery

Supraduodenal artery

Gastroduodenal artery
(*partially in phantom*)

Posterior superior
pancreaticoduodenal artery

(Common) bile duct

Right gastro-omental
(gastroepiploic) artery
(*phantom, cut*)

Anterior superior
pancreaticoduodenal artery
(*phantom*)

Anastomotic branch

Posterior branch of
inferior pancreatico-
duodenal artery

Anterior branch of
inferior pancreatico-
duodenal artery (*phantom*)

Greater pancreatic artery

Inferior
pancreatic artery

Dorsal
pancreatic artery

Superior
mesenteric artery

Inferior
pancreaticoduodenal artery

Posterior view

PLATE 294

ABDOMEN

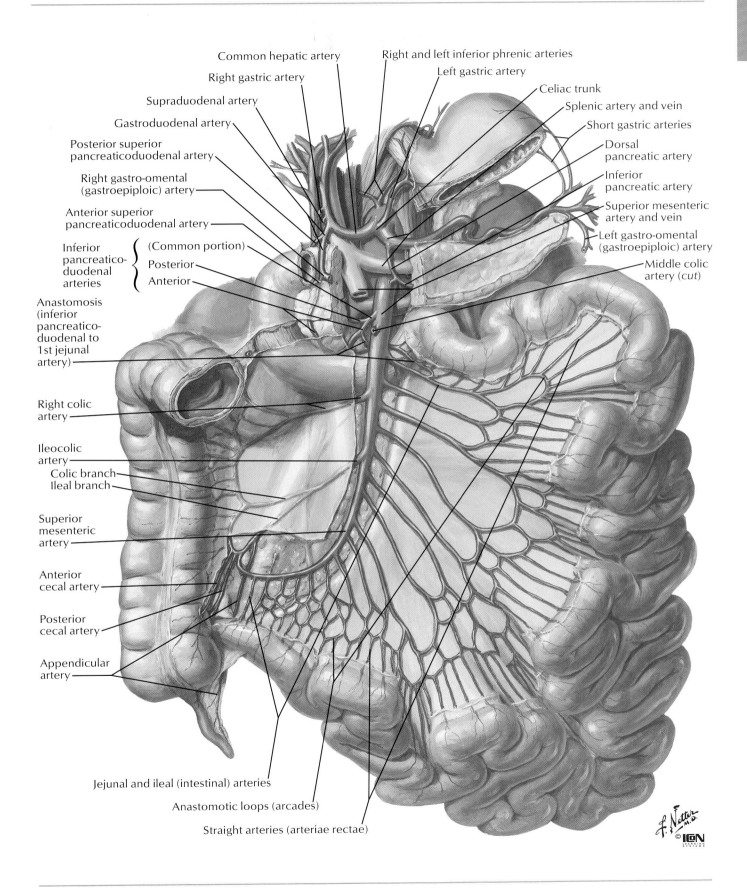

Common hepatic artery

Right and left inferior phrenic arteries

Right gastric artery

Left gastric artery

Supraduodenal artery

Celiac trunk

Gastroduodenal artery

Splenic artery and vein

Short gastric arteries

Posterior superior pancreaticoduodenal artery

Dorsal pancreatic artery

Right gastro-omental (gastroepiploic) artery

Inferior pancreatic artery

Anterior superior pancreaticoduodenal artery

Superior mesenteric artery and vein

Inferior pancreatico-duodenal arteries { (Common portion) Posterior Anterior

Left gastro-omental (gastroepiploic) artery

Middle colic artery (cut)

Anastomosis (inferior pancreatico-duodenal to 1st jejunal artery)

Right colic artery

Ileocolic artery

Colic branch
Ileal branch

Superior mesenteric artery

Anterior cecal artery

Posterior cecal artery

Appendicular artery

Jejunal and ileal (intestinal) arteries

Anastomotic loops (arcades)

Straight arteries (arteriae rectae)

FOR ARTERIES OF RECTUM SEE ALSO PLATE 378

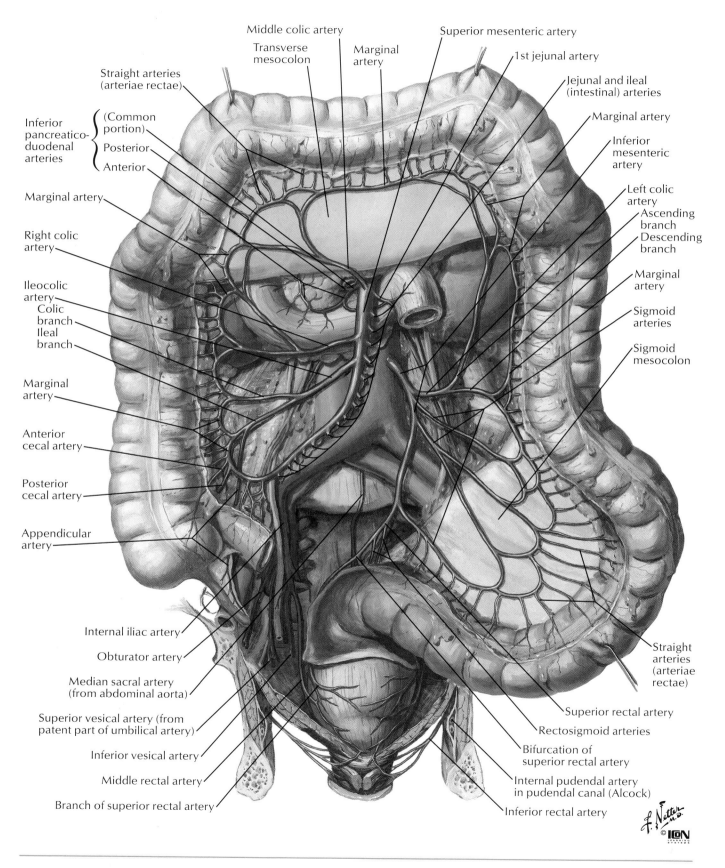

Middle colic artery

Transverse mesocolon

Marginal artery

Superior mesenteric artery

1st jejunal artery

Straight arteries (arteriae rectae)

Inferior pancreatico-duodenal arteries

(Common portion)

Posterior

Anterior

Jejunal and ileal (intestinal) arteries

Marginal artery

Inferior mesenteric artery

Left colic artery

Ascending branch

Descending branch

Marginal artery

Right colic artery

Marginal artery

Sigmoid arteries

Ileocolic artery

Colic branch

Ileal branch

Sigmoid mesocolon

Marginal artery

Anterior cecal artery

Posterior cecal artery

Appendicular artery

Straight arteries (arteriae rectae)

Internal iliac artery

Obturator artery

Median sacral artery (from abdominal aorta)

Superior vesical artery (from patent part of umbilical artery)

Inferior vesical artery

Middle rectal artery

Branch of superior rectal artery

Superior rectal artery

Rectosigmoid arteries

Bifurcation of superior rectal artery

Internal pudendal artery in pudendal canal (Alcock)

Inferior rectal artery

PLATE 296

ABDOMEN

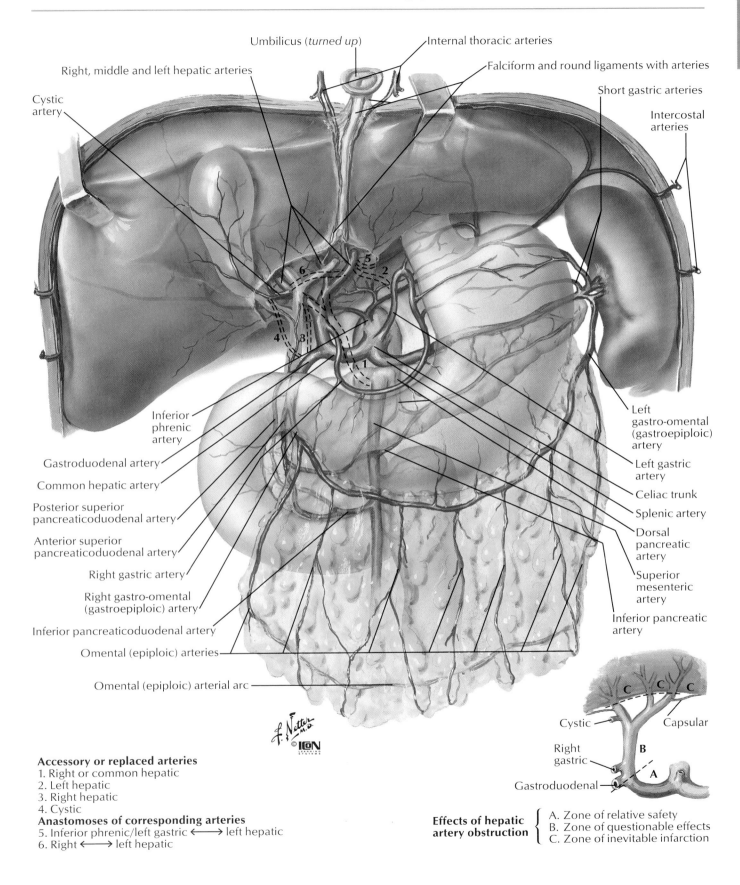

Umbilicus (*turned up*)

Internal thoracic arteries

Right, middle and left hepatic arteries

Falciform and round ligaments with arteries

Short gastric arteries

Cystic artery

Intercostal arteries

Inferior phrenic artery

Gastroduodenal artery

Common hepatic artery

Posterior superior pancreaticoduodenal artery

Anterior superior pancreaticoduodenal artery

Right gastric artery

Right gastro-omental (gastroepiploic) artery

Inferior pancreaticoduodenal artery

Omental (epiploic) arteries

Omental (epiploic) arterial arc

Left gastro-omental (gastroepiploic) artery

Left gastric artery

Celiac trunk

Splenic artery

Dorsal pancreatic artery

Superior mesenteric artery

Inferior pancreatic artery

Accessory or replaced arteries
1. Right or common hepatic
2. Left hepatic
3. Right hepatic
4. Cystic
Anastomoses of corresponding arteries
5. Inferior phrenic/left gastric ⟷ left hepatic
6. Right ⟷ left hepatic

Cystic

Capsular

Right gastric

Gastroduodenal

Effects of hepatic artery obstruction
{ A. Zone of relative safety
B. Zone of questionable effects
C. Zone of inevitable infarction

Variations in Colic Arteries

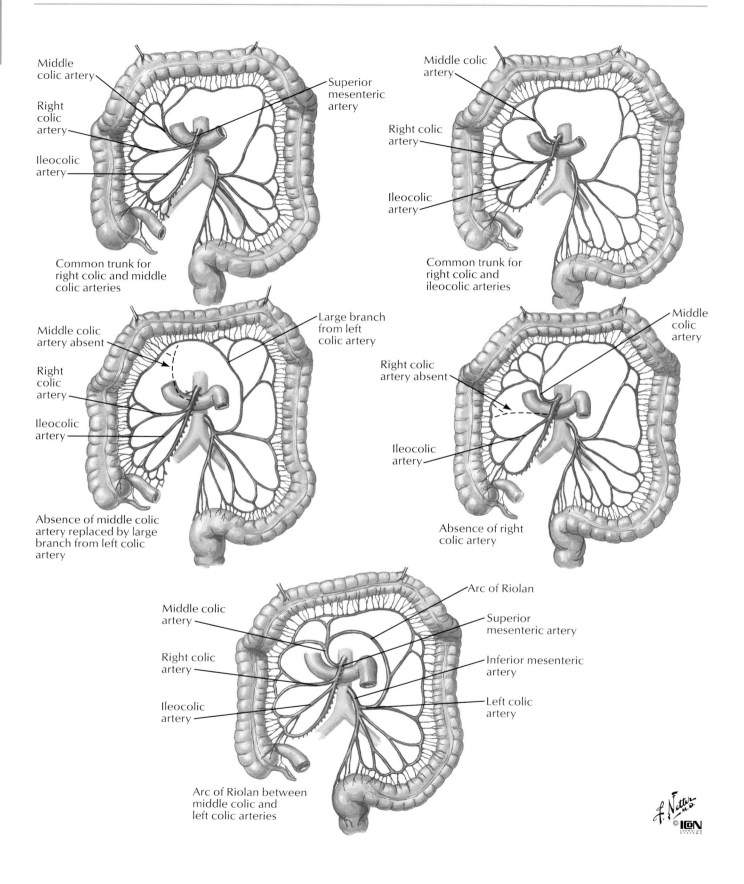

Middle colic artery

Right colic artery

Ileocolic artery

Superior mesenteric artery

Common trunk for right colic and middle colic arteries

Middle colic artery

Right colic artery

Ileocolic artery

Common trunk for right colic and ileocolic arteries

Middle colic artery absent

Right colic artery

Ileocolic artery

Large branch from left colic artery

Absence of middle colic artery replaced by large branch from left colic artery

Right colic artery absent

Ileocolic artery

Middle colic artery

Absence of right colic artery

Middle colic artery

Right colic artery

Ileocolic artery

Arc of Riolan

Superior mesenteric artery

Inferior mesenteric artery

Left colic artery

Arc of Riolan between middle colic and left colic arteries

PLATE 298

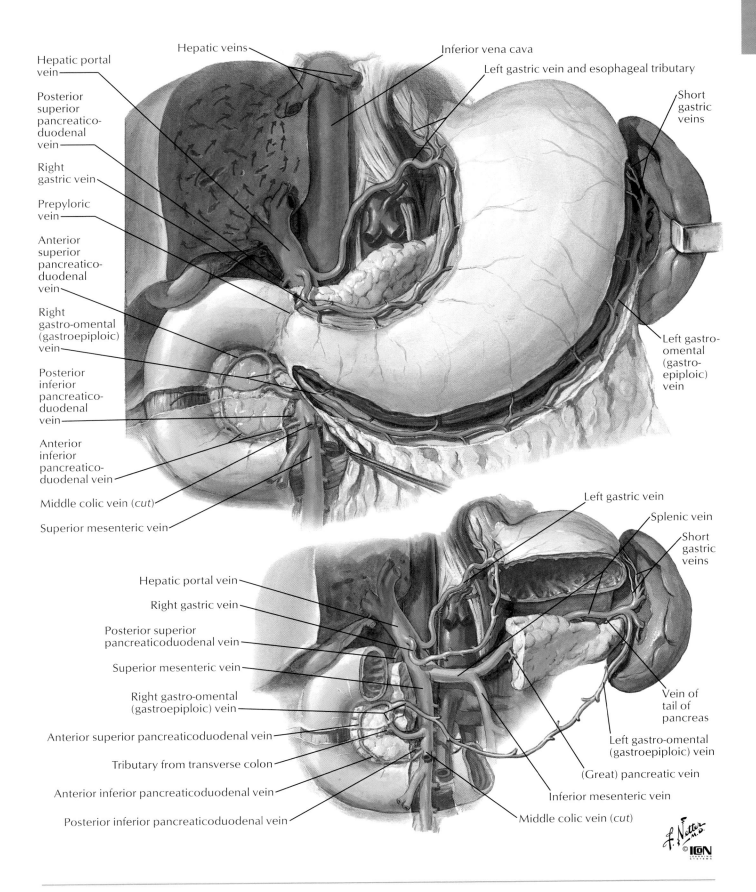

Hepatic veins

Inferior vena cava

Left gastric vein and esophageal tributary

Hepatic portal vein

Posterior superior pancreatico-duodenal vein

Right gastric vein

Prepyloric vein

Anterior superior pancreatico-duodenal vein

Right gastro-omental (gastroepiploic) vein

Posterior inferior pancreatico-duodenal vein

Anterior inferior pancreatico-duodenal vein

Middle colic vein (cut)

Superior mesenteric vein

Short gastric veins

Left gastro-omental (gastro-epiploic) vein

Hepatic portal vein

Right gastric vein

Posterior superior pancreaticoduodenal vein

Superior mesenteric vein

Right gastro-omental (gastroepiploic) vein

Anterior superior pancreaticoduodenal vein

Tributary from transverse colon

Anterior inferior pancreaticoduodenal vein

Posterior inferior pancreaticoduodenal vein

Left gastric vein

Splenic vein

Short gastric veins

Vein of tail of pancreas

Left gastro-omental (gastroepiploic) vein

(Great) pancreatic vein

Inferior mesenteric vein

Middle colic vein (cut)

Veins of Small Intestine

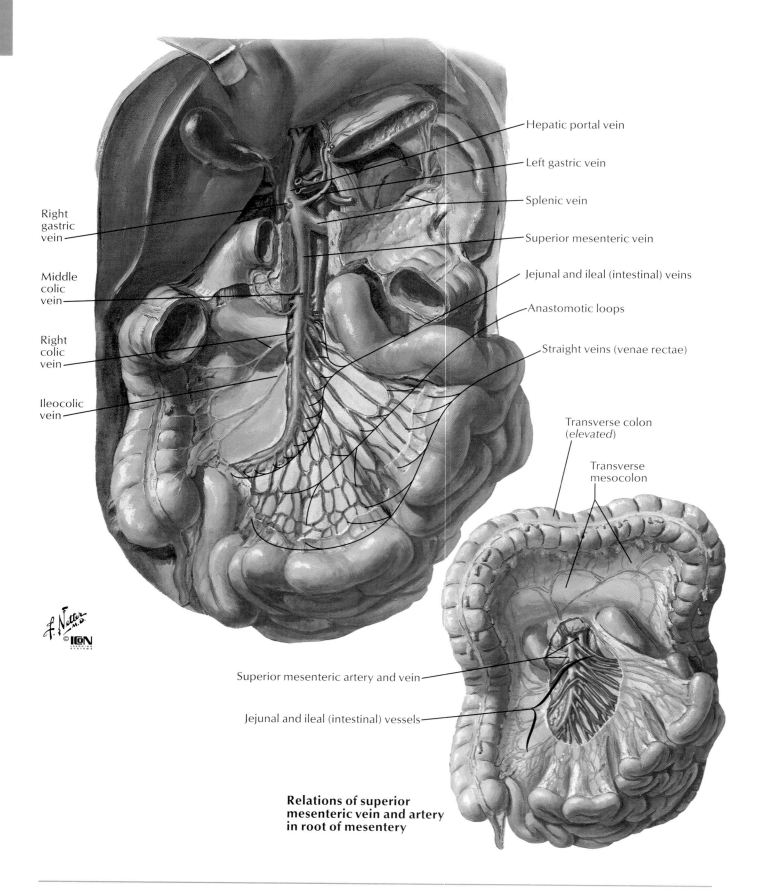

Hepatic portal vein

Left gastric vein

Splenic vein

Superior mesenteric vein

Jejunal and ileal (intestinal) veins

Anastomotic loops

Straight veins (venae rectae)

Right gastric vein

Middle colic vein

Right colic vein

Ileocolic vein

Transverse colon (*elevated*)

Transverse mesocolon

Superior mesenteric artery and vein

Jejunal and ileal (intestinal) vessels

Relations of superior mesenteric vein and artery in root of mesentery

PLATE 300

ABDOMEN

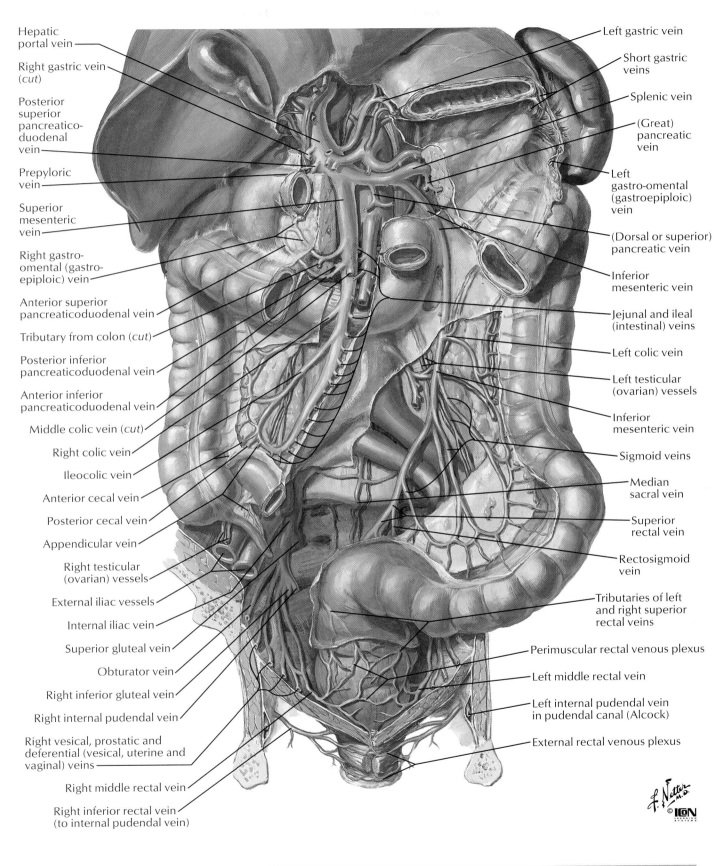

Hepatic portal vein

Right gastric vein (*cut*)

Posterior superior pancreaticoduodenal vein

Prepyloric vein

Superior mesenteric vein

Right gastro-omental (gastro-epiploic) vein

Anterior superior pancreaticoduodenal vein

Tributary from colon (*cut*)

Posterior inferior pancreaticoduodenal vein

Anterior inferior pancreaticoduodenal vein

Middle colic vein (*cut*)

Right colic vein

Ileocolic vein

Anterior cecal vein

Posterior cecal vein

Appendicular vein

Right testicular (ovarian) vessels

External iliac vessels

Internal iliac vein

Superior gluteal vein

Obturator vein

Right inferior gluteal vein

Right internal pudendal vein

Right vesical, prostatic and deferential (vesical, uterine and vaginal) veins

Right middle rectal vein

Right inferior rectal vein (to internal pudendal vein)

Left gastric vein

Short gastric veins

Splenic vein

(Great) pancreatic vein

Left gastro-omental (gastroepiploic) vein

(Dorsal or superior) pancreatic vein

Inferior mesenteric vein

Jejunal and ileal (intestinal) veins

Left colic vein

Left testicular (ovarian) vessels

Inferior mesenteric vein

Sigmoid veins

Median sacral vein

Superior rectal vein

Rectosigmoid vein

Tributaries of left and right superior rectal veins

Perimuscular rectal venous plexus

Left middle rectal vein

Left internal pudendal vein in pudendal canal (Alcock)

External rectal venous plexus

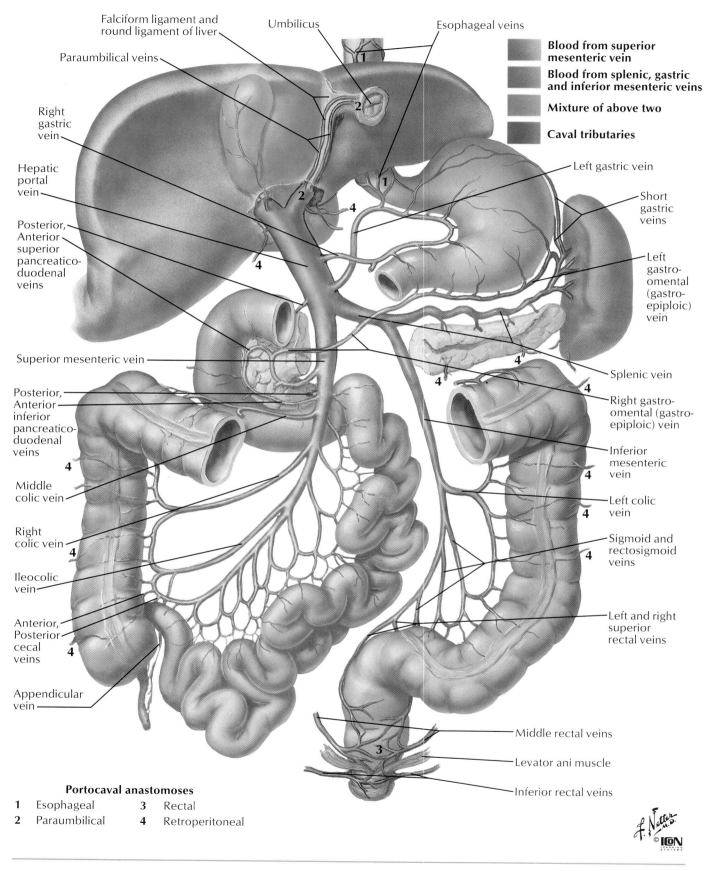

Falciform ligament and round ligament of liver

Umbilicus

Esophageal veins

Blood from superior mesenteric vein

Blood from splenic, gastric and inferior mesenteric veins

Mixture of above two

Caval tributaries

Paraumbilical veins

Right gastric vein

Hepatic portal vein

Posterior, Anterior superior pancreatico-duodenal veins

Superior mesenteric vein

Posterior, Anterior inferior pancreatico-duodenal veins

Middle colic vein

Right colic vein

Ileocolic vein

Anterior, Posterior cecal veins

Appendicular vein

Left gastric vein

Short gastric veins

Left gastro-omental (gastro-epiploic) vein

Splenic vein

Right gastro-omental (gastro-epiploic) vein

Inferior mesenteric vein

Left colic vein

Sigmoid and rectosigmoid veins

Left and right superior rectal veins

Middle rectal veins

Levator ani muscle

Inferior rectal veins

Portocaval anastomoses

1 Esophageal
2 Paraumbilical
3 Rectal
4 Retroperitoneal

F. Netter M.D.

PLATE 302

ABDOMEN

Typical arrangement

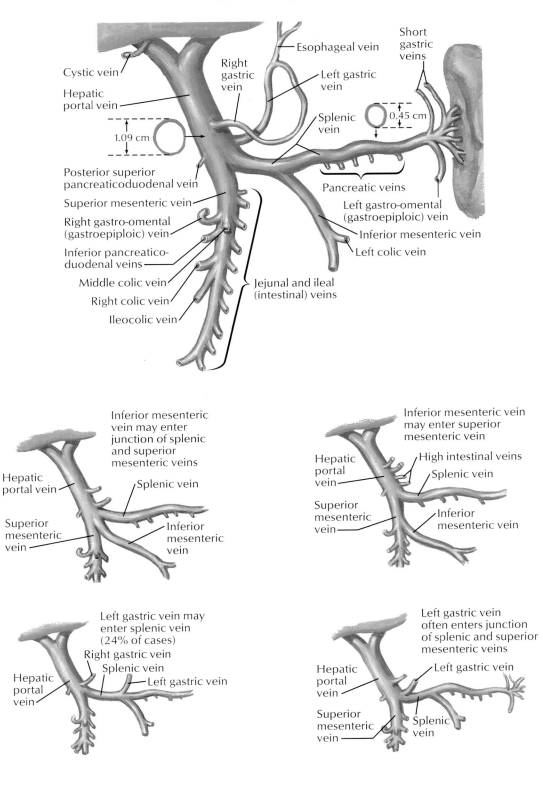

Cystic vein

Hepatic portal vein

1.09 cm

Posterior superior pancreaticoduodenal vein

Superior mesenteric vein

Right gastro-omental (gastroepiploic) vein

Inferior pancreatico-duodenal veins

Middle colic vein

Right colic vein

Ileocolic vein

Right gastric vein

Esophageal vein

Left gastric vein

Splenic vein

Short gastric veins

0.45 cm

Pancreatic veins

Left gastro-omental (gastroepiploic) vein

Inferior mesenteric vein

Left colic vein

Jejunal and ileal (intestinal) veins

Inferior mesenteric vein may enter junction of splenic and superior mesenteric veins

Hepatic portal vein

Superior mesenteric vein

Splenic vein

Inferior mesenteric vein

Inferior mesenteric vein may enter superior mesenteric vein

Hepatic portal vein

Superior mesenteric vein

High intestinal veins

Splenic vein

Inferior mesenteric vein

Left gastric vein may enter splenic vein (24% of cases)

Right gastric vein

Splenic vein

Hepatic portal vein

Left gastric vein

Left gastric vein often enters junction of splenic and superior mesenteric veins

Hepatic portal vein

Superior mesenteric vein

Left gastric vein

Splenic vein

VISCERAL VASCULATURE

PLATE 303

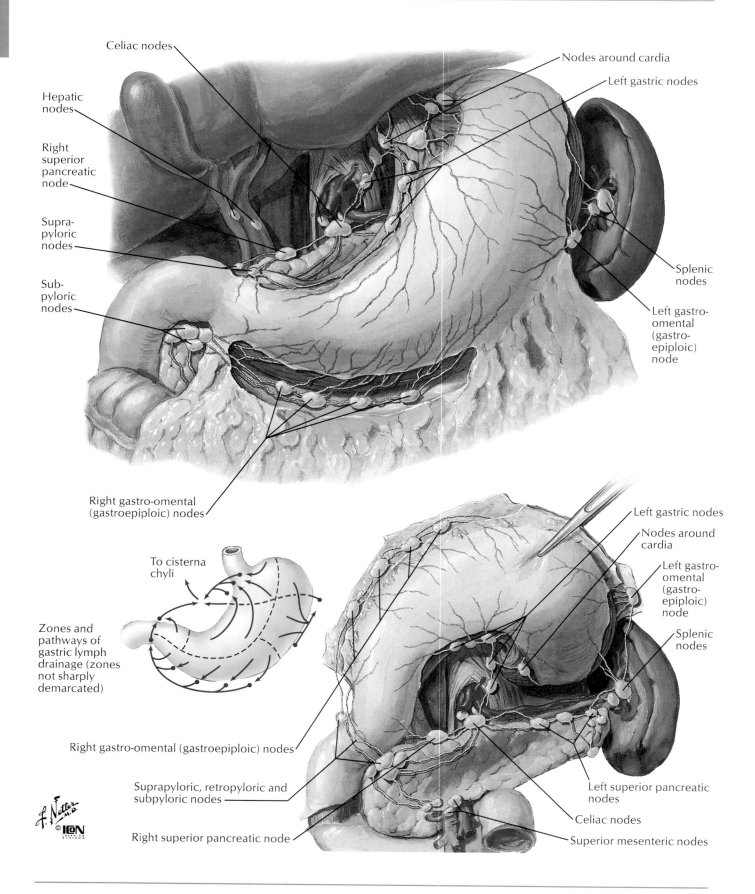

Celiac nodes

Hepatic nodes

Right superior pancreatic node

Supra-pyloric nodes

Sub-pyloric nodes

Nodes around cardia

Left gastric nodes

Splenic nodes

Left gastro-omental (gastro-epiploic) node

Right gastro-omental (gastroepiploic) nodes

To cisterna chyli

Zones and pathways of gastric lymph drainage (zones not sharply demarcated)

Right gastro-omental (gastroepiploic) nodes

Suprapyloric, retropyloric and subpyloric nodes

Right superior pancreatic node

Left gastric nodes

Nodes around cardia

Left gastro-omental (gastro-epiploic) node

Splenic nodes

Left superior pancreatic nodes

Celiac nodes

Superior mesenteric nodes

PLATE 304

ABDOMEN

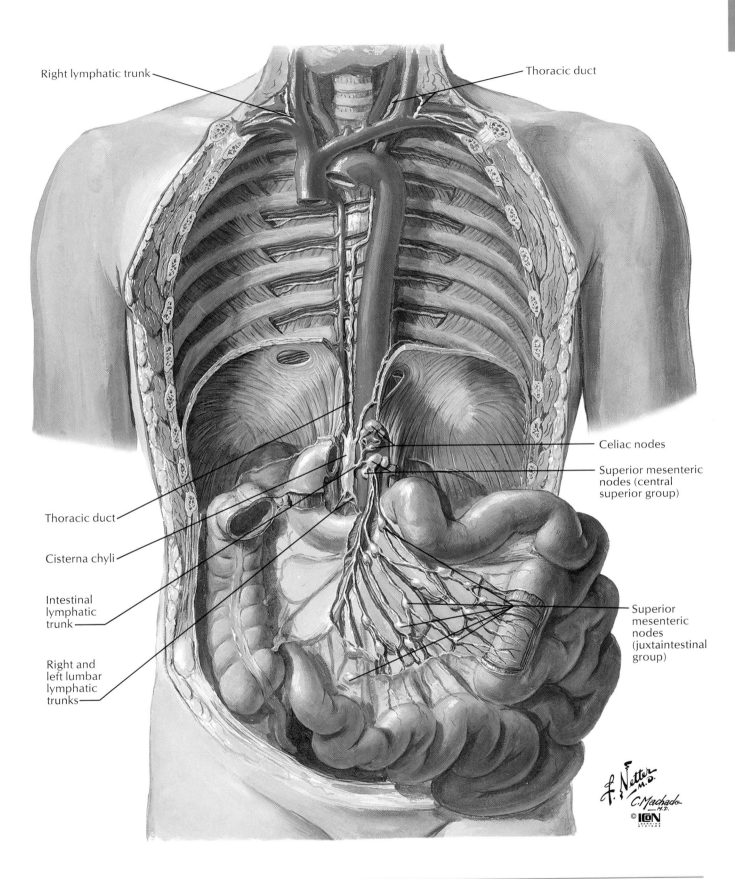

Right lymphatic trunk

Thoracic duct

Thoracic duct

Cisterna chyli

Intestinal lymphatic trunk

Right and left lumbar lymphatic trunks

Celiac nodes

Superior mesenteric nodes (central superior group)

Superior mesenteric nodes (juxtaintestinal group)

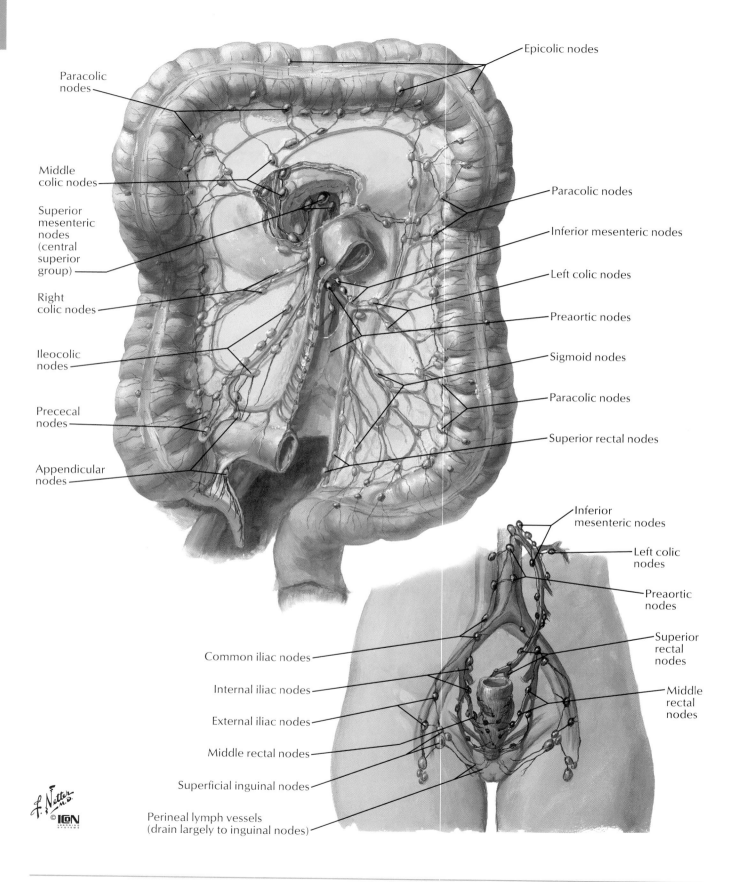

Epicolic nodes

Paracolic nodes

Middle colic nodes

Superior mesenteric nodes (central superior group)

Right colic nodes

Ileocolic nodes

Prececal nodes

Appendicular nodes

Paracolic nodes

Inferior mesenteric nodes

Left colic nodes

Preaortic nodes

Sigmoid nodes

Paracolic nodes

Superior rectal nodes

Inferior mesenteric nodes

Left colic nodes

Preaortic nodes

Superior rectal nodes

Middle rectal nodes

Common iliac nodes

Internal iliac nodes

External iliac nodes

Middle rectal nodes

Superficial inguinal nodes

Perineal lymph vessels (drain largely to inguinal nodes)

PLATE 306

ABDOMEN

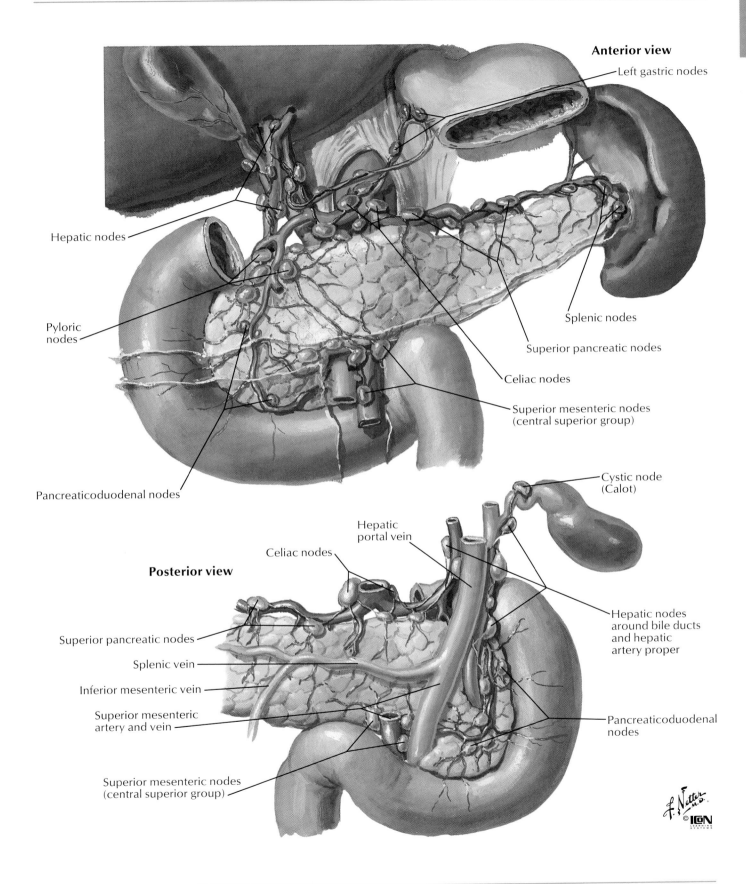

Anterior view

Left gastric nodes

Hepatic nodes

Pyloric nodes

Pancreaticoduodenal nodes

Splenic nodes

Superior pancreatic nodes

Celiac nodes

Superior mesenteric nodes (central superior group)

Cystic node (Calot)

Hepatic portal vein

Celiac nodes

Posterior view

Hepatic nodes around bile ducts and hepatic artery proper

Superior pancreatic nodes

Splenic vein

Inferior mesenteric vein

Superior mesenteric artery and vein

Superior mesenteric nodes (central superior group)

Pancreaticoduodenal nodes

SEE ALSO PLATE 159

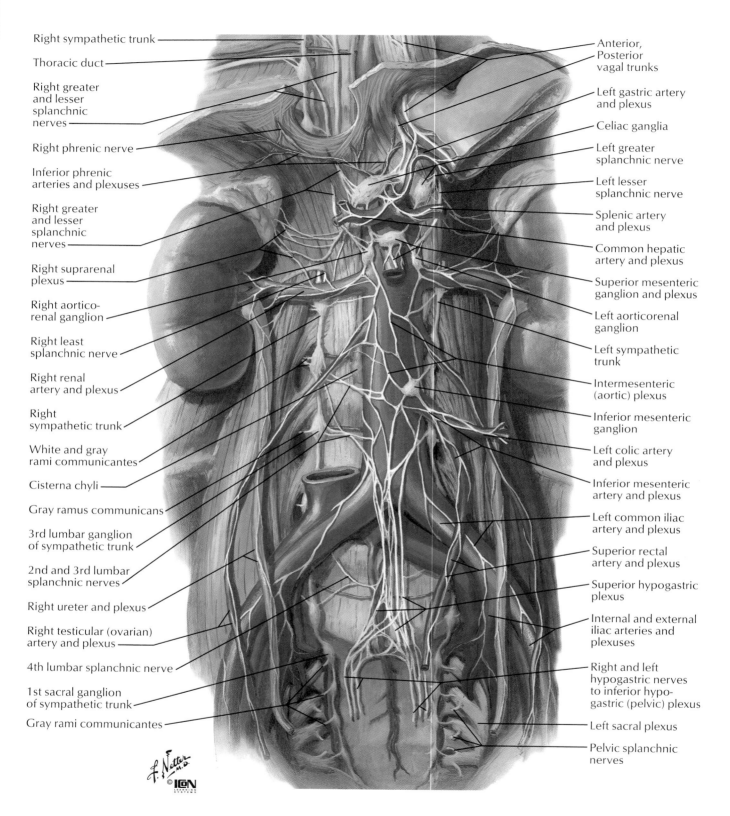

Right sympathetic trunk

Thoracic duct

Right greater and lesser splanchnic nerves

Right phrenic nerve

Inferior phrenic arteries and plexuses

Right greater and lesser splanchnic nerves

Right suprarenal plexus

Right aortico-renal ganglion

Right least splanchnic nerve

Right renal artery and plexus

Right sympathetic trunk

White and gray rami communicantes

Cisterna chyli

Gray ramus communicans

3rd lumbar ganglion of sympathetic trunk

2nd and 3rd lumbar splanchnic nerves

Right ureter and plexus

Right testicular (ovarian) artery and plexus

4th lumbar splanchnic nerve

1st sacral ganglion of sympathetic trunk

Gray rami communicantes

Anterior, Posterior vagal trunks

Left gastric artery and plexus

Celiac ganglia

Left greater splanchnic nerve

Left lesser splanchnic nerve

Splenic artery and plexus

Common hepatic artery and plexus

Superior mesenteric ganglion and plexus

Left aorticorenal ganglion

Left sympathetic trunk

Intermesenteric (aortic) plexus

Inferior mesenteric ganglion

Left colic artery and plexus

Inferior mesenteric artery and plexus

Left common iliac artery and plexus

Superior rectal artery and plexus

Superior hypogastric plexus

Internal and external iliac arteries and plexuses

Right and left hypogastric nerves to inferior hypo-gastric (pelvic) plexus

Left sacral plexus

Pelvic splanchnic nerves

PLATE 308

ABDOMEN

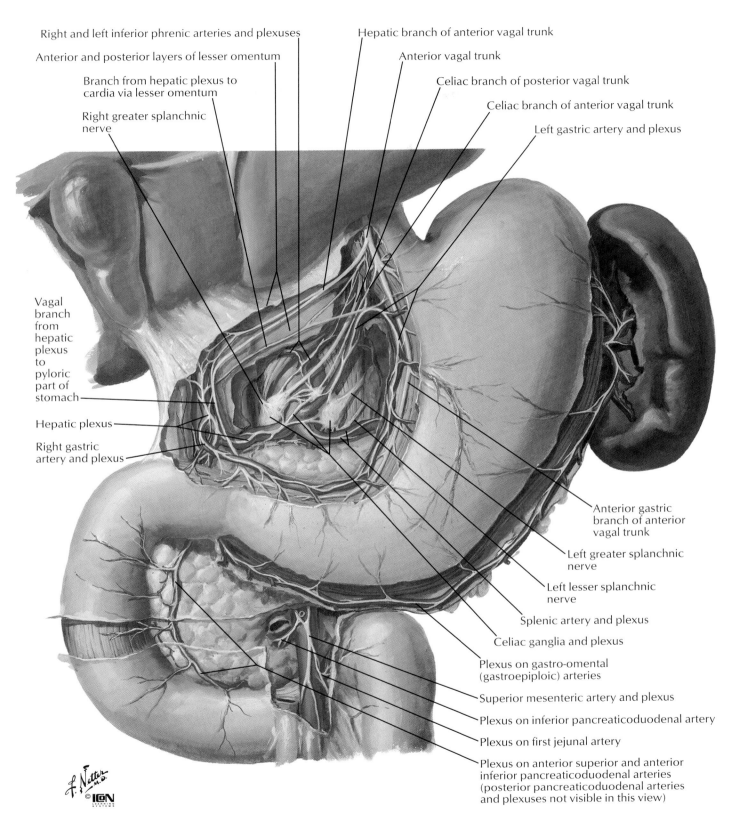

Right and left inferior phrenic arteries and plexuses

Anterior and posterior layers of lesser omentum

Branch from hepatic plexus to cardia via lesser omentum

Right greater splanchnic nerve

Hepatic branch of anterior vagal trunk

Anterior vagal trunk

Celiac branch of posterior vagal trunk

Celiac branch of anterior vagal trunk

Left gastric artery and plexus

Vagal branch from hepatic plexus to pyloric part of stomach

Hepatic plexus

Right gastric artery and plexus

Anterior gastric branch of anterior vagal trunk

Left greater splanchnic nerve

Left lesser splanchnic nerve

Splenic artery and plexus

Celiac ganglia and plexus

Plexus on gastro-omental (gastroepiploic) arteries

Superior mesenteric artery and plexus

Plexus on inferior pancreaticoduodenal artery

Plexus on first jejunal artery

Plexus on anterior superior and anterior inferior pancreaticoduodenal arteries (posterior pancreaticoduodenal arteries and plexuses not visible in this view)

SEE ALSO PLATE 159

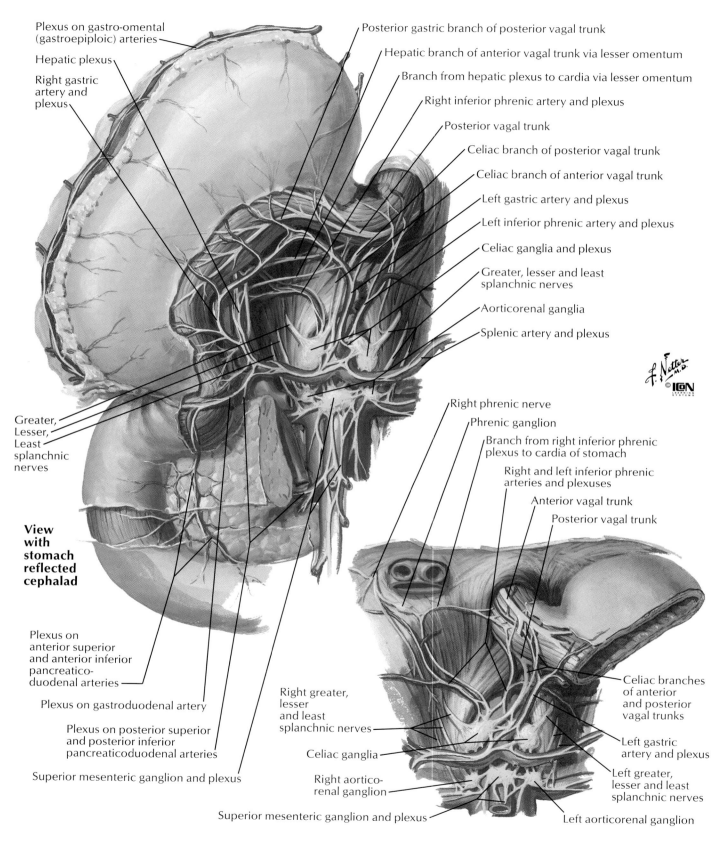

Plexus on gastro-omental (gastroepiploic) arteries

Hepatic plexus

Right gastric artery and plexus

Greater, Lesser, Least splanchnic nerves

View with stomach reflected cephalad

Plexus on anterior superior and anterior inferior pancreatico-duodenal arteries

Plexus on gastroduodenal artery

Plexus on posterior superior and posterior inferior pancreaticoduodenal arteries

Superior mesenteric ganglion and plexus

Posterior gastric branch of posterior vagal trunk

Hepatic branch of anterior vagal trunk via lesser omentum

Branch from hepatic plexus to cardia via lesser omentum

Right inferior phrenic artery and plexus

Posterior vagal trunk

Celiac branch of posterior vagal trunk

Celiac branch of anterior vagal trunk

Left gastric artery and plexus

Left inferior phrenic artery and plexus

Celiac ganglia and plexus

Greater, lesser and least splanchnic nerves

Aorticorenal ganglia

Splenic artery and plexus

Right phrenic nerve

Phrenic ganglion

Branch from right inferior phrenic plexus to cardia of stomach

Right and left inferior phrenic arteries and plexuses

Anterior vagal trunk

Posterior vagal trunk

Right greater, lesser and least splanchnic nerves

Celiac ganglia

Right aortico-renal ganglion

Superior mesenteric ganglion and plexus

Celiac branches of anterior and posterior vagal trunks

Left gastric artery and plexus

Left greater, lesser and least splanchnic nerves

Left aorticorenal ganglion

PLATE 310

ABDOMEN

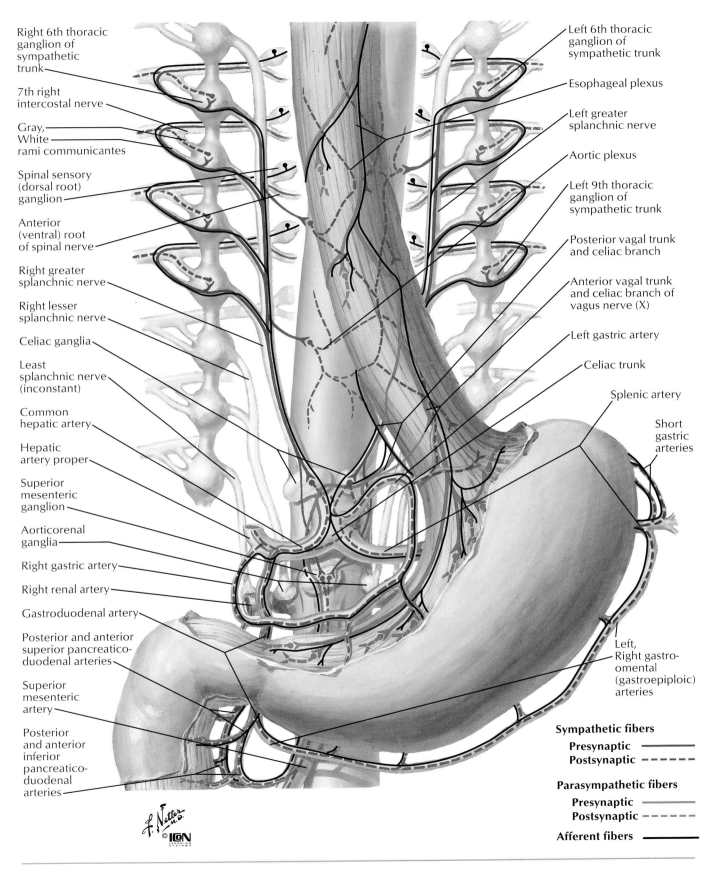

Right 6th thoracic ganglion of sympathetic trunk

7th right intercostal nerve

Gray, White rami communicantes

Spinal sensory (dorsal root) ganglion

Anterior (ventral) root of spinal nerve

Right greater splanchnic nerve

Right lesser splanchnic nerve

Celiac ganglia

Least splanchnic nerve (inconstant)

Common hepatic artery

Hepatic artery proper

Superior mesenteric ganglion

Aorticorenal ganglia

Right gastric artery

Right renal artery

Gastroduodenal artery

Posterior and anterior superior pancreatico-duodenal arteries

Superior mesenteric artery

Posterior and anterior inferior pancreatico-duodenal arteries

Left 6th thoracic ganglion of sympathetic trunk

Esophageal plexus

Left greater splanchnic nerve

Aortic plexus

Left 9th thoracic ganglion of sympathetic trunk

Posterior vagal trunk and celiac branch

Anterior vagal trunk and celiac branch of vagus nerve (X)

Left gastric artery

Celiac trunk

Splenic artery

Short gastric arteries

Left, Right gastro-omental (gastroepiploic) arteries

Sympathetic fibers

Presynaptic ——————

Postsynaptic - - - - - - -

Parasympathetic fibers

Presynaptic ——————

Postsynaptic - - - - - - -

Afferent fibers ——————

INNERVATION

PLATE 311

SEE ALSO PLATE 159

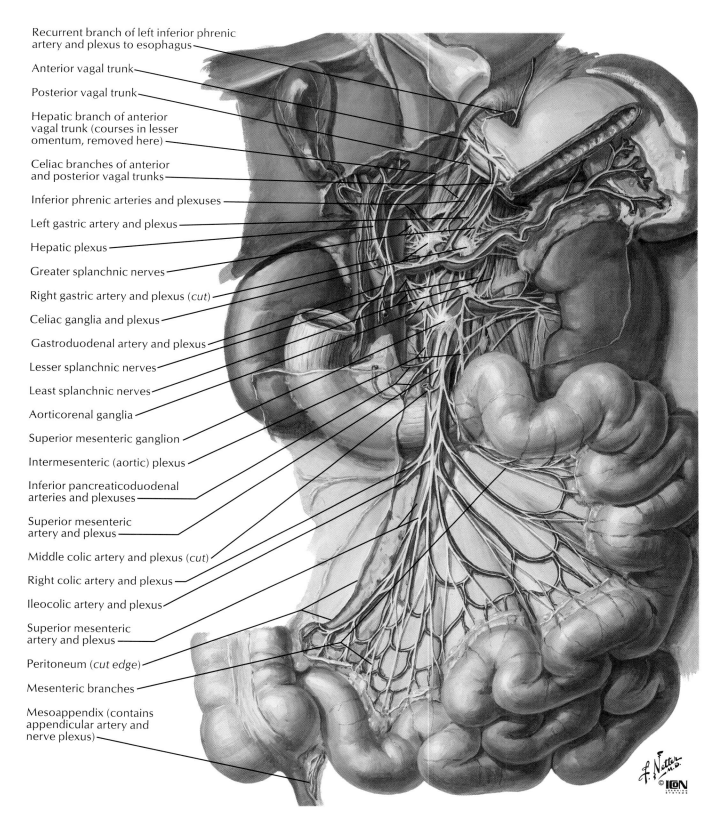

Recurrent branch of left inferior phrenic artery and plexus to esophagus

Anterior vagal trunk

Posterior vagal trunk

Hepatic branch of anterior vagal trunk (courses in lesser omentum, removed here)

Celiac branches of anterior and posterior vagal trunks

Inferior phrenic arteries and plexuses

Left gastric artery and plexus

Hepatic plexus

Greater splanchnic nerves

Right gastric artery and plexus (*cut*)

Celiac ganglia and plexus

Gastroduodenal artery and plexus

Lesser splanchnic nerves

Least splanchnic nerves

Aorticorenal ganglia

Superior mesenteric ganglion

Intermesenteric (aortic) plexus

Inferior pancreaticoduodenal arteries and plexuses

Superior mesenteric artery and plexus

Middle colic artery and plexus (*cut*)

Right colic artery and plexus

Ileocolic artery and plexus

Superior mesenteric artery and plexus

Peritoneum (*cut edge*)

Mesenteric branches

Mesoappendix (contains appendicular artery and nerve plexus)

PLATE 312

ABDOMEN

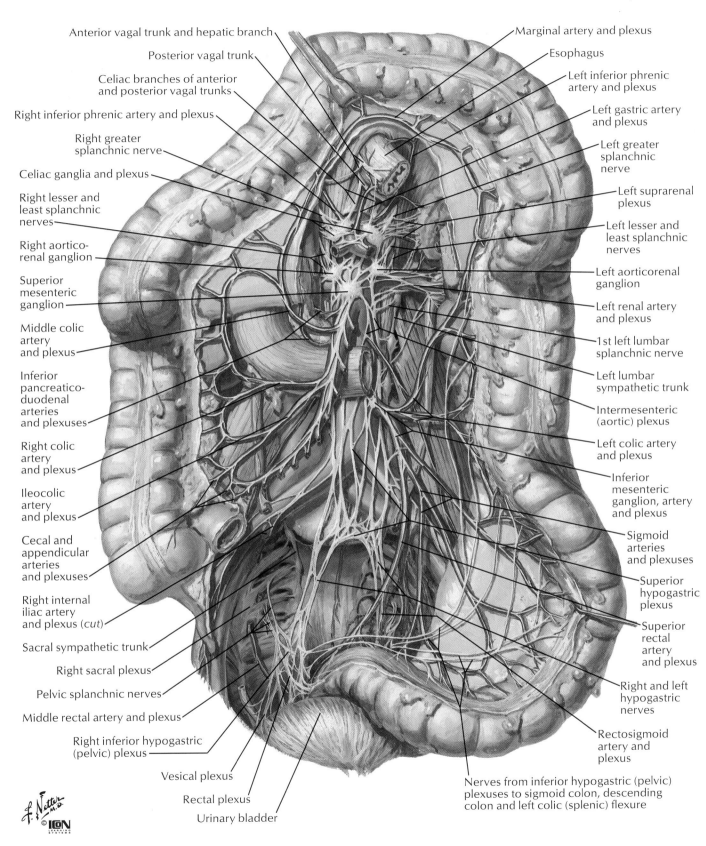

Anterior vagal trunk and hepatic branch

Posterior vagal trunk

Celiac branches of anterior and posterior vagal trunks

Right inferior phrenic artery and plexus

Right greater splanchnic nerve

Celiac ganglia and plexus

Right lesser and least splanchnic nerves

Right aortico-renal ganglion

Superior mesenteric ganglion

Middle colic artery and plexus

Inferior pancreatico-duodenal arteries and plexuses

Right colic artery and plexus

Ileocolic artery and plexus

Cecal and appendicular arteries and plexuses

Right internal iliac artery and plexus (*cut*)

Sacral sympathetic trunk

Right sacral plexus

Pelvic splanchnic nerves

Middle rectal artery and plexus

Right inferior hypogastric (pelvic) plexus

Vesical plexus

Rectal plexus

Urinary bladder

Marginal artery and plexus

Esophagus

Left inferior phrenic artery and plexus

Left gastric artery and plexus

Left greater splanchnic nerve

Left suprarenal plexus

Left lesser and least splanchnic nerves

Left aorticorenal ganglion

Left renal artery and plexus

1st left lumbar splanchnic nerve

Left lumbar sympathetic trunk

Intermesenteric (aortic) plexus

Left colic artery and plexus

Inferior mesenteric ganglion, artery and plexus

Sigmoid arteries and plexuses

Superior hypogastric plexus

Superior rectal artery and plexus

Right and left hypogastric nerves

Rectosigmoid artery and plexus

Nerves from inferior hypogastric (pelvic) plexuses to sigmoid colon, descending colon and left colic (splenic) flexure

f. Netter M.D.
© ICON LEARNING SYSTEMS

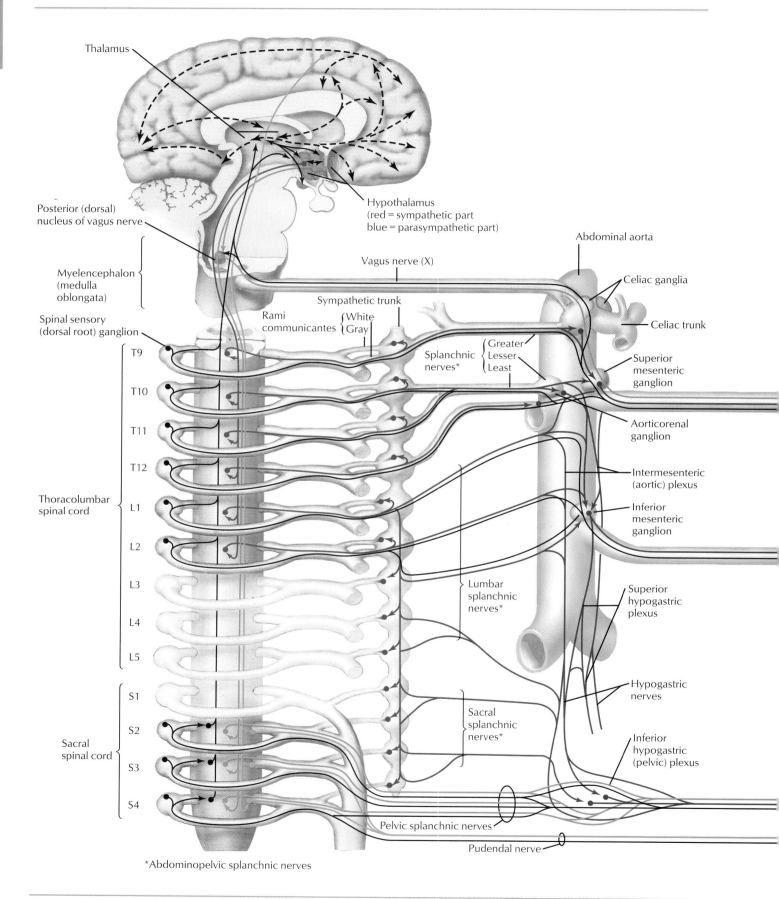

Thalamus

Hypothalamus
(red = sympathetic part
blue = parasympathetic part)

Posterior (dorsal)
nucleus of vagus nerve

Myelencephalon
(medulla
oblongata)

Spinal sensory
(dorsal root) ganglion

Abdominal aorta

Vagus nerve (X)

Sympathetic trunk

Celiac ganglia

Celiac trunk

Rami
communicantes { White
Gray

Splanchnic
nerves*

{ Greater
Lesser
Least

Superior
mesenteric
ganglion

Aorticorenal
ganglion

Intermesenteric
(aortic) plexus

Inferior
mesenteric
ganglion

T9

T10

T11

T12

L1

L2

L3

L4

L5

Thoracolumbar
spinal cord

Lumbar
splanchnic
nerves*

Superior
hypogastric
plexus

S1

S2

S3

S4

Sacral
spinal cord

Sacral
splanchnic
nerves*

Hypogastric
nerves

Inferior
hypogastric
(pelvic) plexus

Pelvic splanchnic nerves

Pudendal nerve

*Abdominopelvic splanchnic nerves

PLATE 314

ABDOMEN

Sympathetic efferents ━━━━━
Parasympathetic efferents ━━━━━
Somatic efferents ━━━━━
Afferents and CNS connections ━━━━━
Indefinite paths ━ ━ ━ ━

Superior mesenteric
artery and plexus

T12, L1

T9 (8)

T9, T10

L1, L2

Inferior mesenteric
and left colic
arteries and plexuses

T10–T12

T10 (11)

T10–T12

L1, L2

Superior rectal artery and nerves

Rectal plexus

Levator
ani muscle

Inferior rectal nerve

External anal
sphincter muscle

Chief segmental sources
of sympathetic fibers
innervating different
regions of intestinal
tract are indicated.
Numerous afferent fibers
are carried centripetally
through approximately
the same sympathetic
splanchnic nerves
that transmit
presynaptic fibers

Autonomic Reflex Pathways: Schema

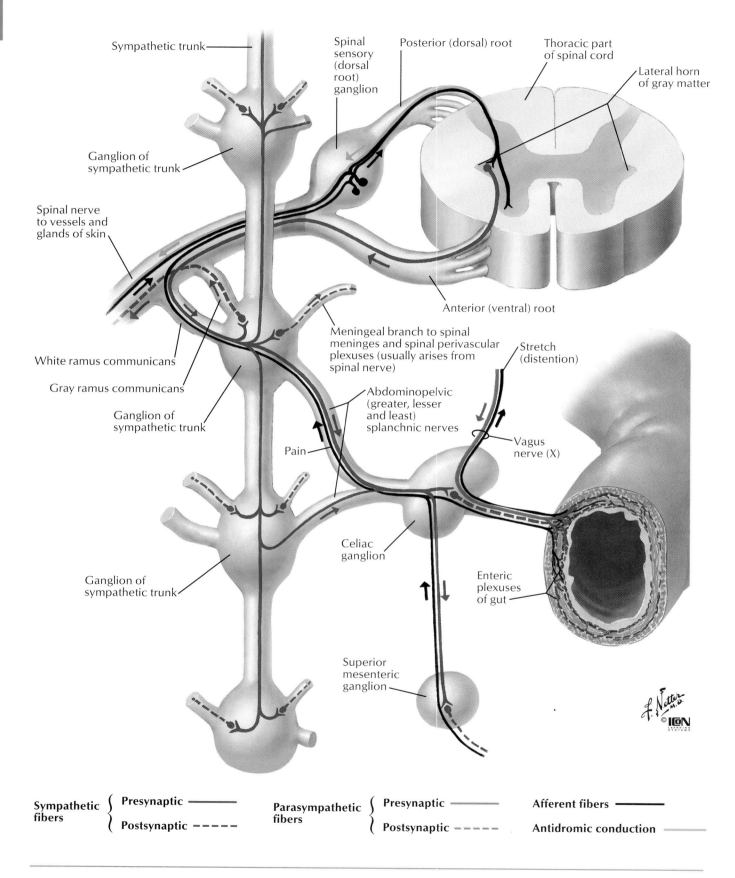

Sympathetic trunk

Ganglion of sympathetic trunk

Spinal nerve to vessels and glands of skin

White ramus communicans

Gray ramus communicans

Ganglion of sympathetic trunk

Ganglion of sympathetic trunk

Spinal sensory (dorsal root) ganglion

Posterior (dorsal) root

Thoracic part of spinal cord

Lateral horn of gray matter

Anterior (ventral) root

Meningeal branch to spinal meninges and spinal perivascular plexuses (usually arises from spinal nerve)

Abdominopelvic (greater, lesser and least) splanchnic nerves

Pain

Celiac ganglion

Superior mesenteric ganglion

Stretch (distention)

Vagus nerve (X)

Enteric plexuses of gut

Sympathetic fibers { Presynaptic ——— Postsynaptic – – – –

Parasympathetic fibers { Presynaptic ——— Postsynaptic – – – –

Afferent fibers ———
Antidromic conduction ———

PLATE 315

ABDOMEN

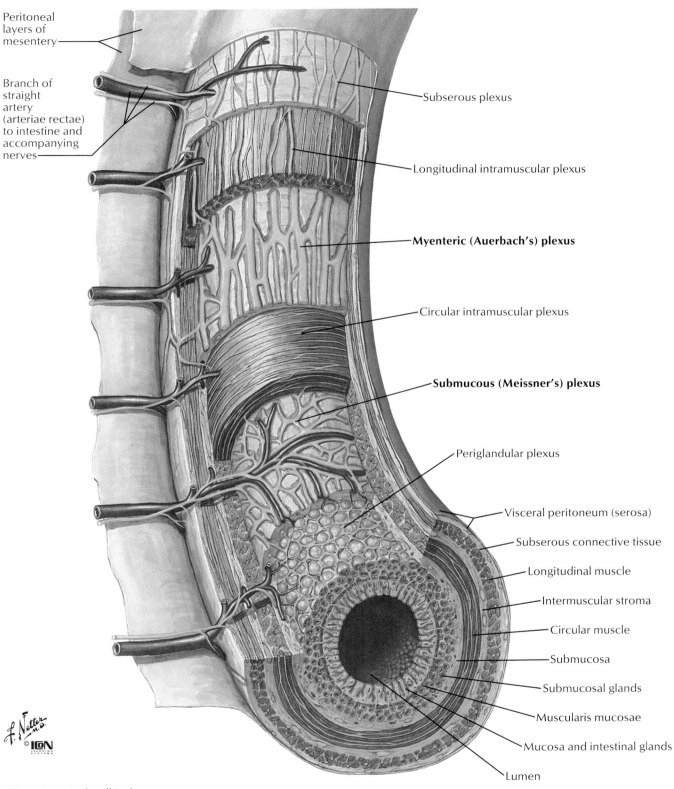

Peritoneal layers of mesentery

Branch of straight artery (arteriae rectae) to intestine and accompanying nerves

Subserous plexus

Longitudinal intramuscular plexus

Myenteric (Auerbach's) plexus

Circular intramuscular plexus

Submucous (Meissner's) plexus

Periglandular plexus

Visceral peritoneum (serosa)

Subserous connective tissue

Longitudinal muscle

Intermuscular stroma

Circular muscle

Submucosa

Submucosal glands

Muscularis mucosae

Mucosa and intestinal glands

Lumen

Note: Intestinal wall is shown much thicker than in actuality

SEE ALSO PLATE 160

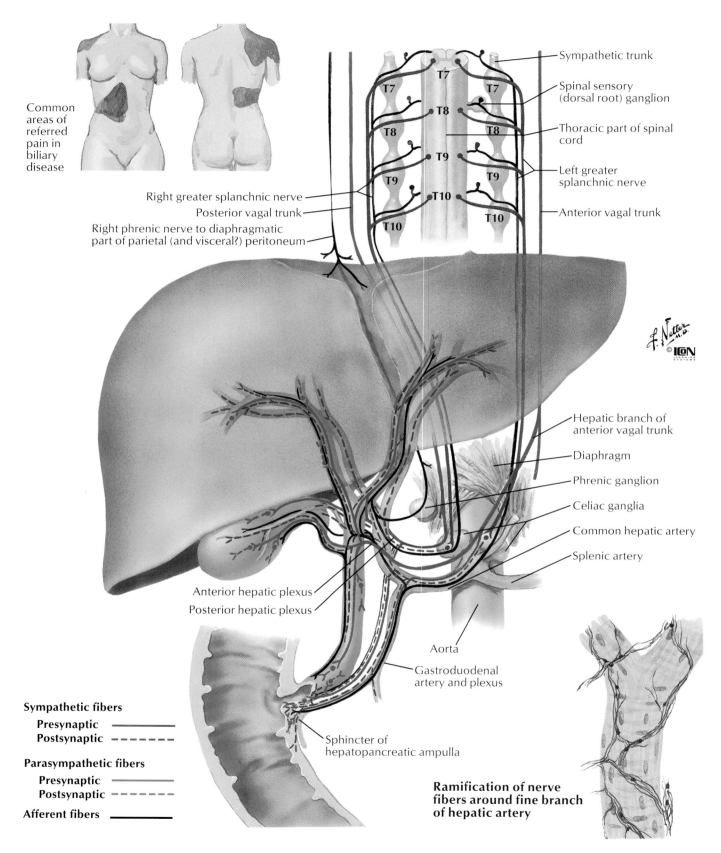

Common areas of referred pain in biliary disease

Sympathetic trunk

Spinal sensory (dorsal root) ganglion

T7

Thoracic part of spinal cord

T8

Left greater splanchnic nerve

Right greater splanchnic nerve

T9

Posterior vagal trunk

Right phrenic nerve to diaphragmatic part of parietal (and visceral?) peritoneum

T10

Anterior vagal trunk

Hepatic branch of anterior vagal trunk

Diaphragm

Phrenic ganglion

Celiac ganglia

Common hepatic artery

Splenic artery

Anterior hepatic plexus

Posterior hepatic plexus

Aorta

Gastroduodenal artery and plexus

Sympathetic fibers
Presynaptic —————
Postsynaptic – – – – –

Parasympathetic fibers
Presynaptic —————
Postsynaptic – – – – –

Afferent fibers ——————

Sphincter of hepatopancreatic ampulla

Ramification of nerve fibers around fine branch of hepatic artery

PLATE 317

ABDOMEN

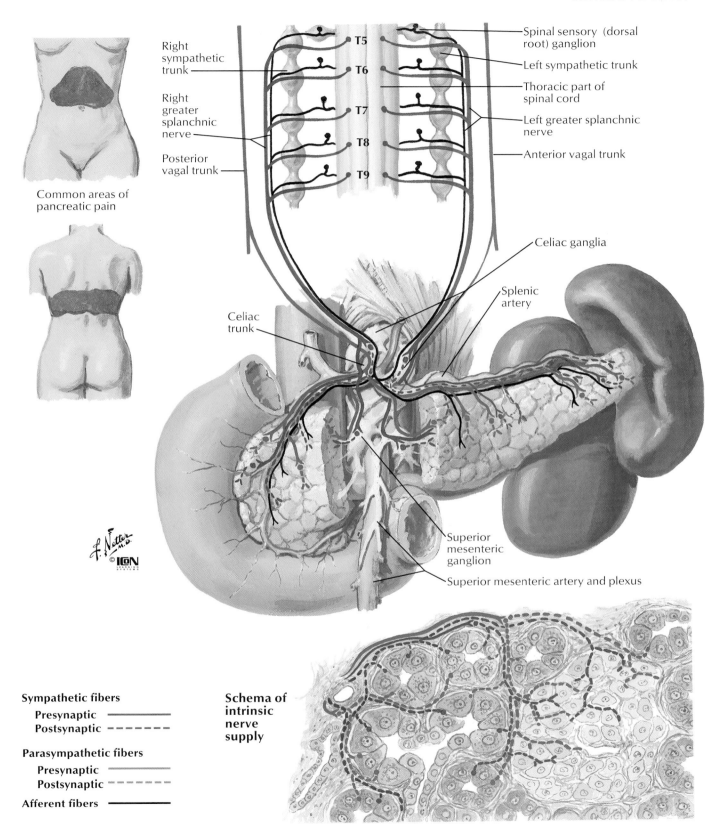

Common areas of pancreatic pain

Right sympathetic trunk

Right greater splanchnic nerve

Posterior vagal trunk

Celiac trunk

T5
T6
T7
T8
T9

Spinal sensory (dorsal root) ganglion

Left sympathetic trunk

Thoracic part of spinal cord

Left greater splanchnic nerve

Anterior vagal trunk

Celiac ganglia

Splenic artery

Superior mesenteric ganglion

Superior mesenteric artery and plexus

Sympathetic fibers
Presynaptic ————
Postsynaptic ------

Parasympathetic fibers
Presynaptic ————
Postsynaptic ------

Afferent fibers ————

Schema of intrinsic nerve supply

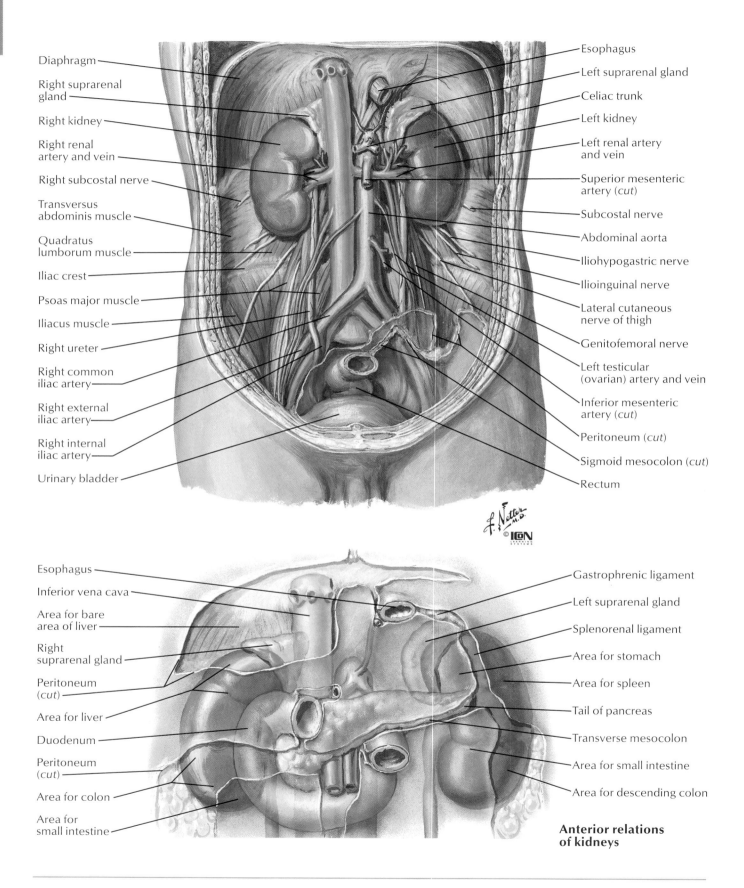

Diaphragm

Right suprarenal gland

Right kidney

Right renal artery and vein

Right subcostal nerve

Transversus abdominis muscle

Quadratus lumborum muscle

Iliac crest

Psoas major muscle

Iliacus muscle

Right ureter

Right common iliac artery

Right external iliac artery

Right internal iliac artery

Urinary bladder

Esophagus

Left suprarenal gland

Celiac trunk

Left kidney

Left renal artery and vein

Superior mesenteric artery (cut)

Subcostal nerve

Abdominal aorta

Iliohypogastric nerve

Ilioinguinal nerve

Lateral cutaneous nerve of thigh

Genitofemoral nerve

Left testicular (ovarian) artery and vein

Inferior mesenteric artery (cut)

Peritoneum (cut)

Sigmoid mesocolon (cut)

Rectum

Esophagus

Inferior vena cava

Area for bare area of liver

Right suprarenal gland

Peritoneum (cut)

Area for liver

Duodenum

Peritoneum (cut)

Area for colon

Area for small intestine

Gastrophrenic ligament

Left suprarenal gland

Splenorenal ligament

Area for stomach

Area for spleen

Tail of pancreas

Transverse mesocolon

Area for small intestine

Area for descending colon

Anterior relations of kidneys

PLATE 319

ABDOMEN

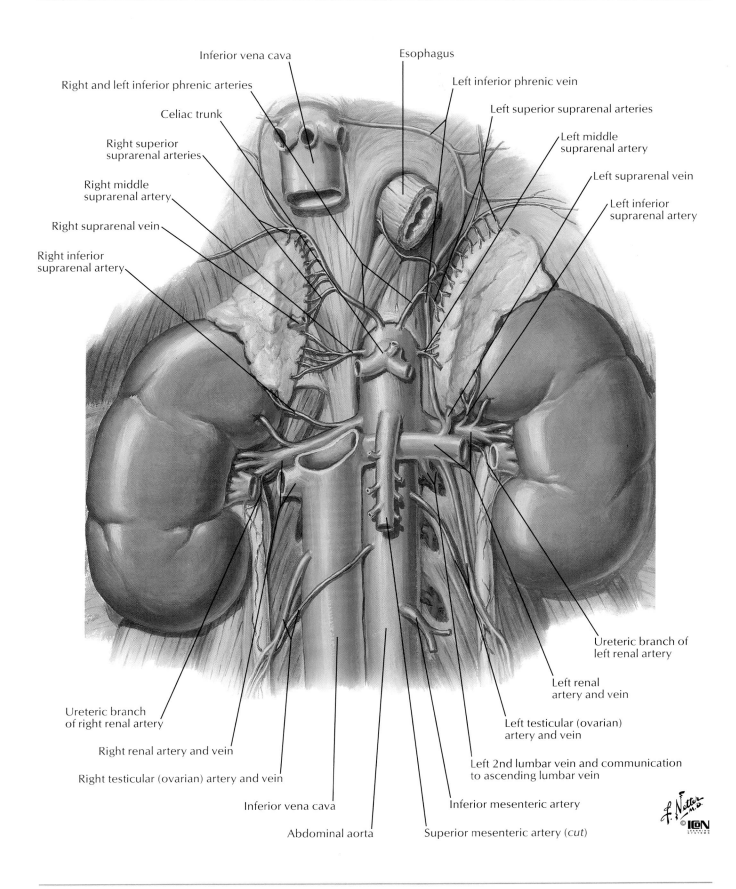

Inferior vena cava

Right and left inferior phrenic arteries

Celiac trunk

Right superior suprarenal arteries

Right middle suprarenal artery

Right suprarenal vein

Right inferior suprarenal artery

Esophagus

Left inferior phrenic vein

Left superior suprarenal arteries

Left middle suprarenal artery

Left suprarenal vein

Left inferior suprarenal artery

Ureteric branch of left renal artery

Left renal artery and vein

Left testicular (ovarian) artery and vein

Left 2nd lumbar vein and communication to ascending lumbar vein

Inferior mesenteric artery

Superior mesenteric artery (*cut*)

Inferior vena cava

Abdominal aorta

Right testicular (ovarian) artery and vein

Right renal artery and vein

Ureteric branch of right renal artery

Intrarenal Arteries and Renal Segments

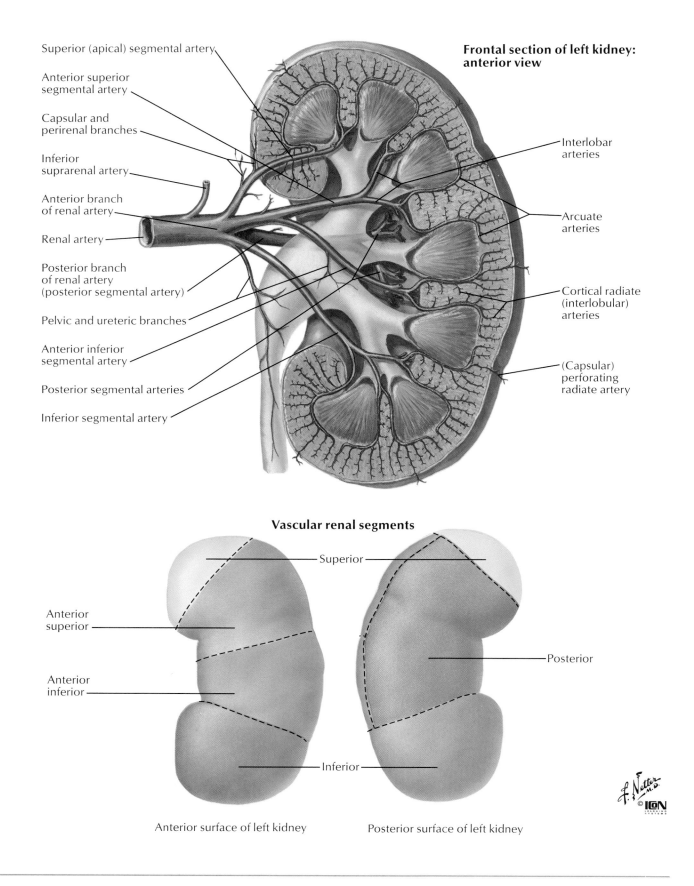

Superior (apical) segmental artery

Anterior superior segmental artery

Capsular and perirenal branches

Inferior suprarenal artery

Anterior branch of renal artery

Renal artery

Posterior branch of renal artery (posterior segmental artery)

Pelvic and ureteric branches

Anterior inferior segmental artery

Posterior segmental arteries

Inferior segmental artery

Frontal section of left kidney: anterior view

Interlobar arteries

Arcuate arteries

Cortical radiate (interlobular) arteries

(Capsular) perforating radiate artery

Vascular renal segments

Superior

Anterior superior

Anterior inferior

Posterior

Inferior

Anterior surface of left kidney

Posterior surface of left kidney

PLATE 323

ABDOMEN

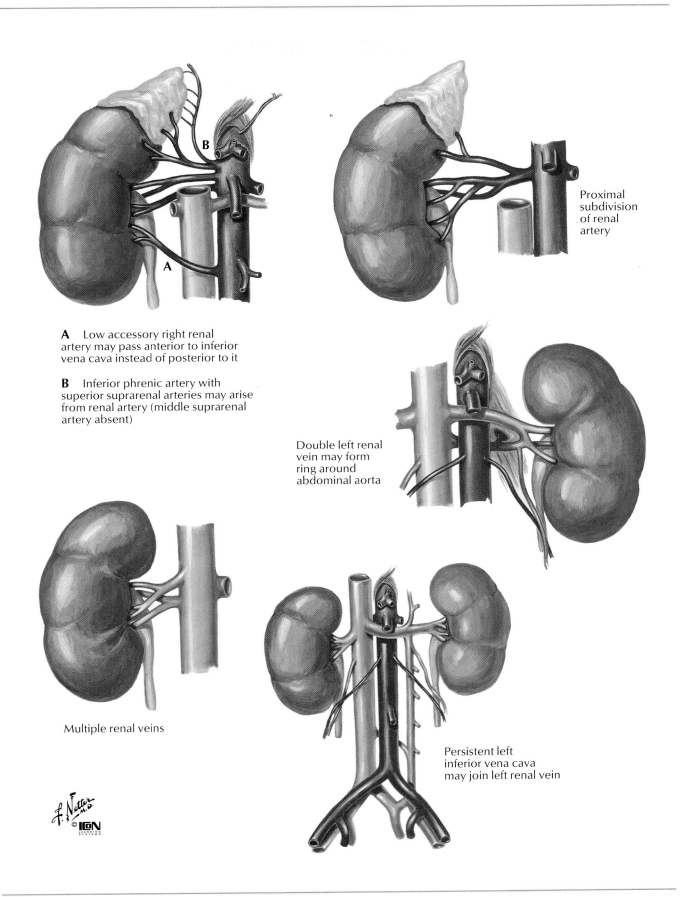

A Low accessory right renal artery may pass anterior to inferior vena cava instead of posterior to it

B Inferior phrenic artery with superior suprarenal arteries may arise from renal artery (middle suprarenal artery absent)

Proximal subdivision of renal artery

Double left renal vein may form ring around abdominal aorta

Multiple renal veins

Persistent left inferior vena cava may join left renal vein

Nephron and Collecting Tubule: Schema

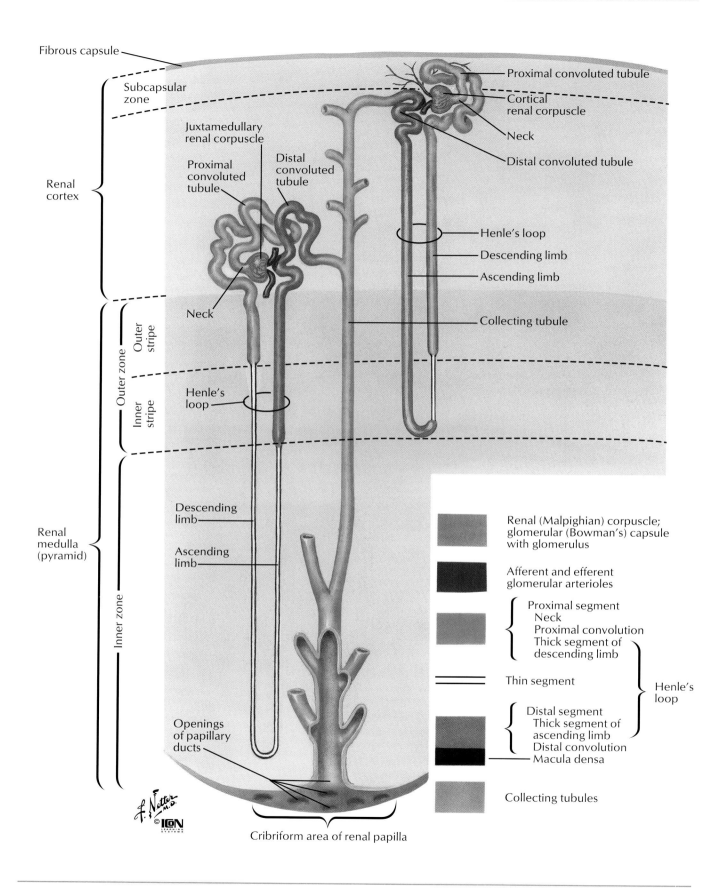

Fibrous capsule

Subcapsular zone

Renal cortex

Juxtamedullary renal corpuscle

Proximal convoluted tubule

Distal convoluted tubule

Neck

Proximal convoluted tubule

Cortical renal corpuscle

Neck

Distal convoluted tubule

Henle's loop

Descending limb

Ascending limb

Collecting tubule

Outer zone

Outer stripe

Inner stripe

Henle's loop

Renal medulla (pyramid)

Inner zone

Descending limb

Ascending limb

Openings of papillary ducts

Renal (Malpighian) corpuscle; glomerular (Bowman's) capsule with glomerulus

Afferent and efferent glomerular arterioles

Proximal segment
Neck
Proximal convolution
Thick segment of descending limb

Thin segment

Henle's loop

Distal segment
Thick segment of ascending limb
Distal convolution
Macula densa

Collecting tubules

Cribriform area of renal papilla

PLATE 325

ABDOMEN

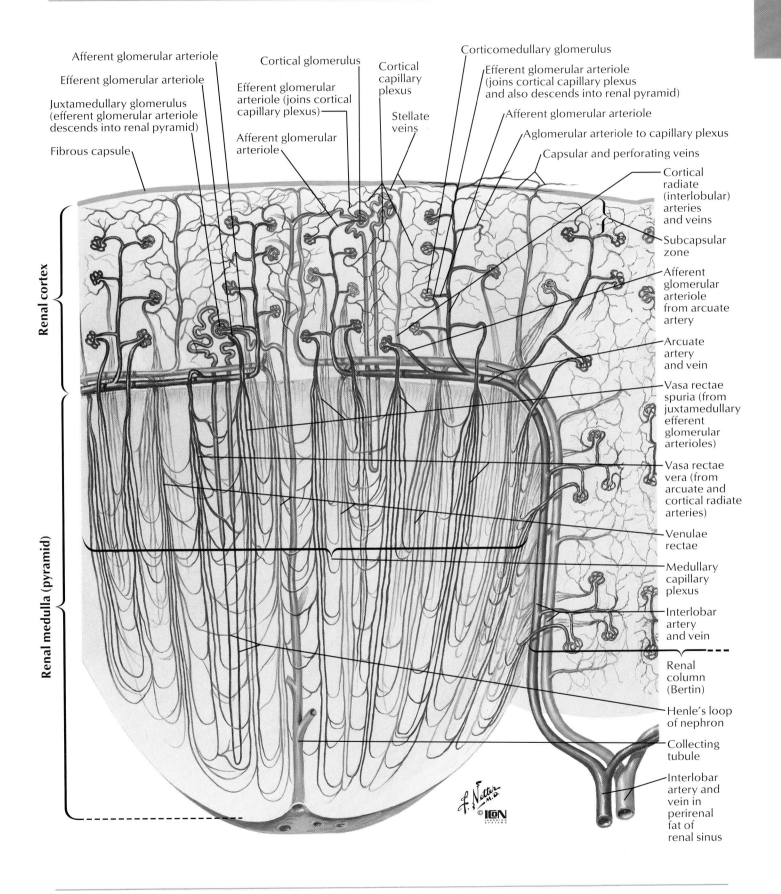

Afferent glomerular arteriole

Efferent glomerular arteriole

Juxtamedullary glomerulus (efferent glomerular arteriole descends into renal pyramid)

Fibrous capsule

Cortical glomerulus

Efferent glomerular arteriole (joins cortical capillary plexus)

Afferent glomerular arteriole

Cortical capillary plexus

Stellate veins

Corticomedullary glomerulus

Efferent glomerular arteriole (joins cortical capillary plexus and also descends into renal pyramid)

Afferent glomerular arteriole

Aglomerular arteriole to capillary plexus

Capsular and perforating veins

Cortical radiate (interlobular) arteries and veins

Subcapsular zone

Afferent glomerular arteriole from arcuate artery

Arcuate artery and vein

Vasa rectae spuria (from juxtamedullary efferent glomerular arterioles)

Vasa rectae vera (from arcuate and cortical radiate arteries)

Venulae rectae

Medullary capillary plexus

Interlobar artery and vein

Renal column (Bertin)

Henle's loop of nephron

Collecting tubule

Interlobar artery and vein in perirenal fat of renal sinus

Renal cortex

Renal medulla (pyramid)

Ureters

SEE ALSO PLATES 349, 350, 354

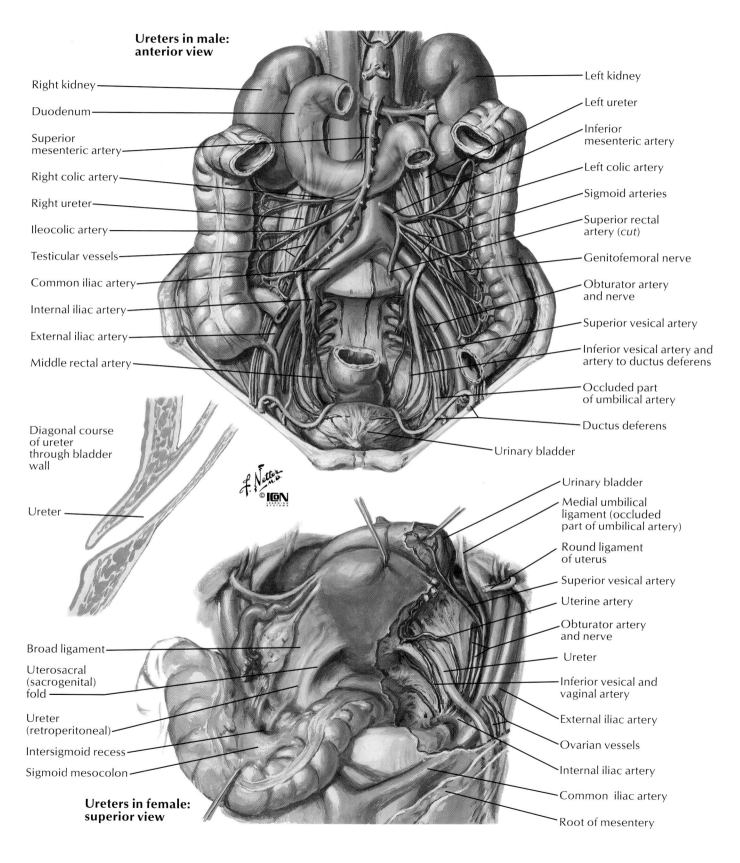

Ureters in male: anterior view

Right kidney

Duodenum

Superior mesenteric artery

Right colic artery

Right ureter

Ileocolic artery

Testicular vessels

Common iliac artery

Internal iliac artery

External iliac artery

Middle rectal artery

Left kidney

Left ureter

Inferior mesenteric artery

Left colic artery

Sigmoid arteries

Superior rectal artery (*cut*)

Genitofemoral nerve

Obturator artery and nerve

Superior vesical artery

Inferior vesical artery and artery to ductus deferens

Occluded part of umbilical artery

Ductus deferens

Urinary bladder

Diagonal course of ureter through bladder wall

Ureter

Urinary bladder

Medial umbilical ligament (occluded part of umbilical artery)

Round ligament of uterus

Superior vesical artery

Uterine artery

Obturator artery and nerve

Ureter

Inferior vesical and vaginal artery

External iliac artery

Ovarian vessels

Internal iliac artery

Common iliac artery

Root of mesentery

Broad ligament

Uterosacral (sacrogenital) fold

Ureter (retroperitoneal)

Intersigmoid recess

Sigmoid mesocolon

Ureters in female: superior view

PLATE 327

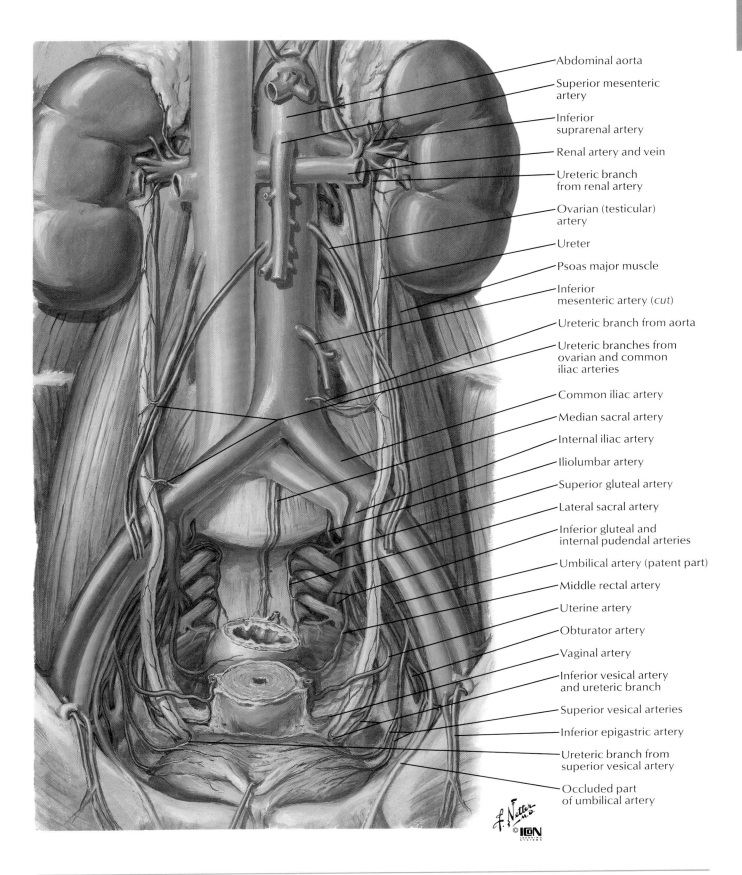

Abdominal aorta

Superior mesenteric artery

Inferior suprarenal artery

Renal artery and vein

Ureteric branch from renal artery

Ovarian (testicular) artery

Ureter

Psoas major muscle

Inferior mesenteric artery (*cut*)

Ureteric branch from aorta

Ureteric branches from ovarian and common iliac arteries

Common iliac artery

Median sacral artery

Internal iliac artery

Iliolumbar artery

Superior gluteal artery

Lateral sacral artery

Inferior gluteal and internal pudendal arteries

Umbilical artery (patent part)

Middle rectal artery

Uterine artery

Obturator artery

Vaginal artery

Inferior vesical artery and ureteric branch

Superior vesical arteries

Inferior epigastric artery

Ureteric branch from superior vesical artery

Occluded part of umbilical artery

SEE ALSO PLATES 386, 388

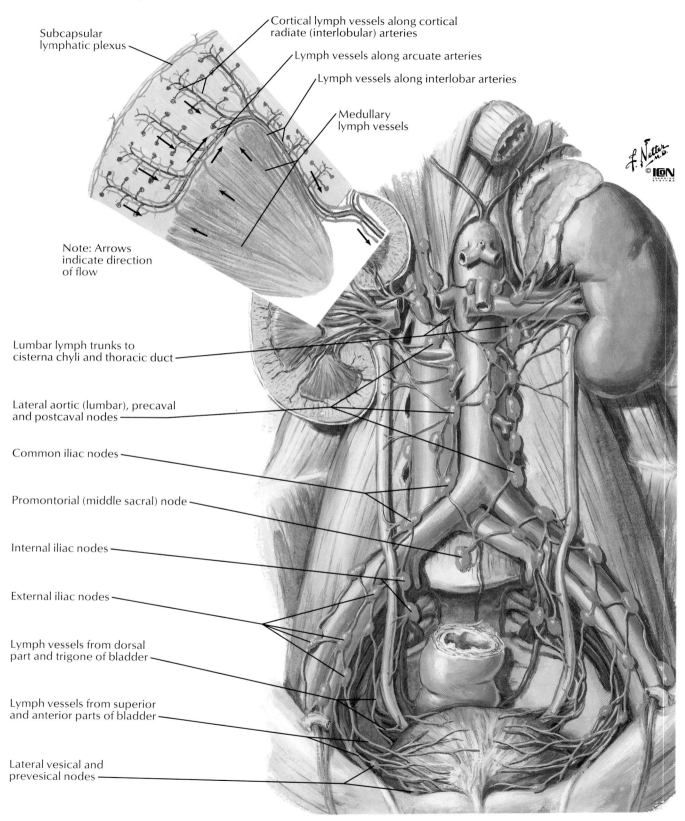

Subcapsular
lymphatic plexus

Cortical lymph vessels along cortical
radiate (interlobular) arteries

Lymph vessels along arcuate arteries

Lymph vessels along interlobar arteries

Medullary
lymph vessels

Note: Arrows
indicate direction
of flow

Lumbar lymph trunks to
cisterna chyli and thoracic duct

Lateral aortic (lumbar), precaval
and postcaval nodes

Common iliac nodes

Promontorial (middle sacral) node

Internal iliac nodes

External iliac nodes

Lymph vessels from dorsal
part and trigone of bladder

Lymph vessels from superior
and anterior parts of bladder

Lateral vesical and
prevesical nodes

PLATE 329

ABDOMEN

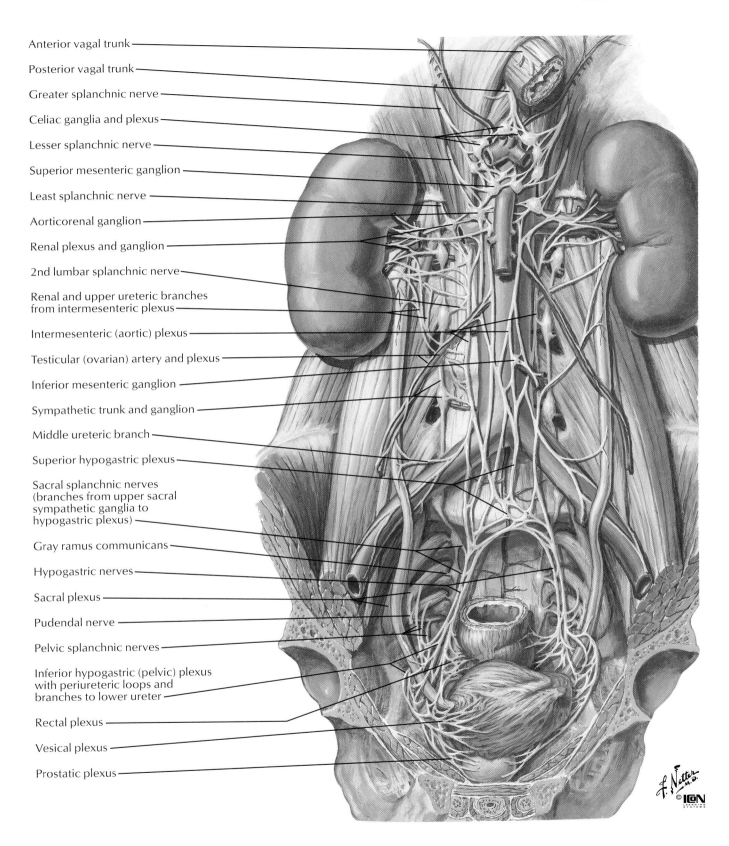

Anterior vagal trunk

Posterior vagal trunk

Greater splanchnic nerve

Celiac ganglia and plexus

Lesser splanchnic nerve

Superior mesenteric ganglion

Least splanchnic nerve

Aorticorenal ganglion

Renal plexus and ganglion

2nd lumbar splanchnic nerve

Renal and upper ureteric branches from intermesenteric plexus

Intermesenteric (aortic) plexus

Testicular (ovarian) artery and plexus

Inferior mesenteric ganglion

Sympathetic trunk and ganglion

Middle ureteric branch

Superior hypogastric plexus

Sacral splanchnic nerves (branches from upper sacral sympathetic ganglia to hypogastric plexus)

Gray ramus communicans

Hypogastric nerves

Sacral plexus

Pudendal nerve

Pelvic splanchnic nerves

Inferior hypogastric (pelvic) plexus with periureteric loops and branches to lower ureter

Rectal plexus

Vesical plexus

Prostatic plexus

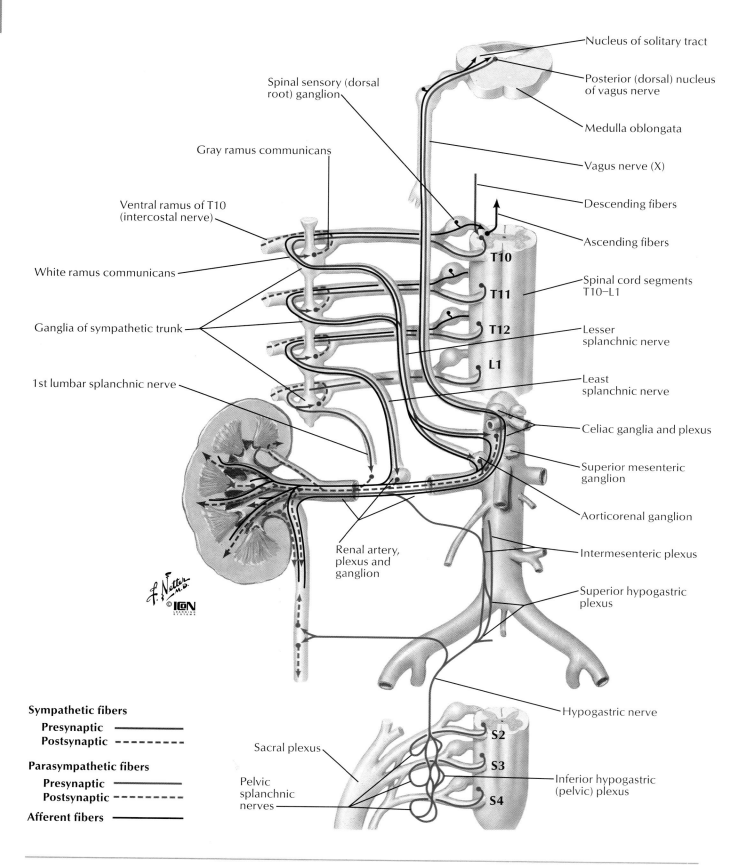

Nucleus of solitary tract

Posterior (dorsal) nucleus of vagus nerve

Medulla oblongata

Vagus nerve (X)

Descending fibers

Ascending fibers

Spinal cord segments T10–L1

Lesser splanchnic nerve

Least splanchnic nerve

Celiac ganglia and plexus

Superior mesenteric ganglion

Aorticorenal ganglion

Intermesenteric plexus

Superior hypogastric plexus

Hypogastric nerve

Inferior hypogastric (pelvic) plexus

Spinal sensory (dorsal root) ganglion

Gray ramus communicans

Ventral ramus of T10 (intercostal nerve)

White ramus communicans

Ganglia of sympathetic trunk

1st lumbar splanchnic nerve

Renal artery, plexus and ganglion

T10

T11

T12

L1

S2

S3

S4

Sacral plexus

Pelvic splanchnic nerves

Sympathetic fibers

Presynaptic ———

Postsynaptic - - - - - -

Parasympathetic fibers

Presynaptic ———

Postsynaptic - - - - - -

Afferent fibers ———

PLATE 331

ABDOMEN

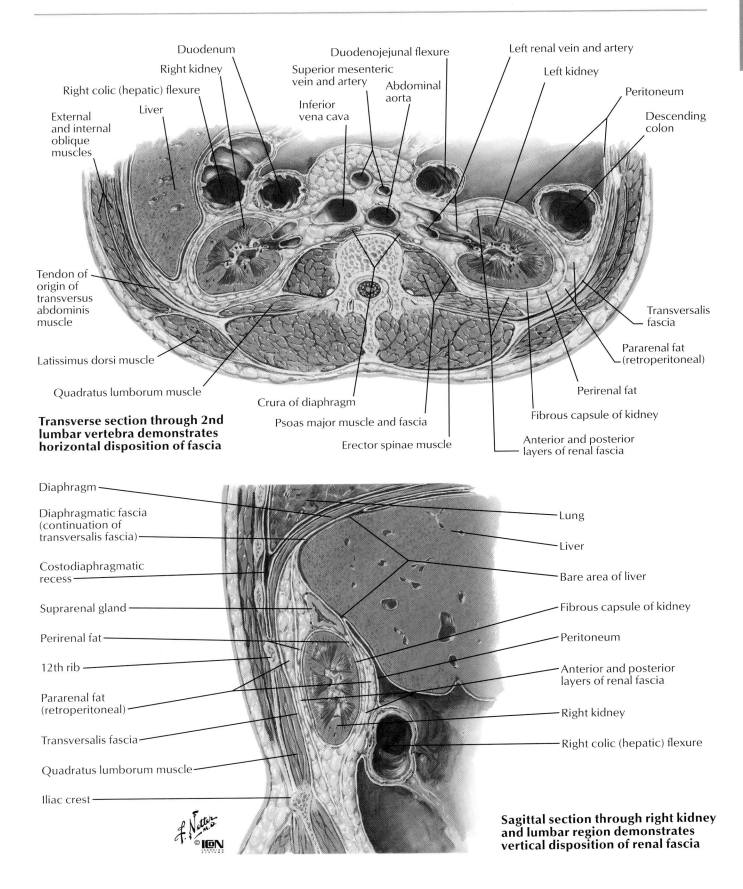

Duodenum

Right kidney

Right colic (hepatic) flexure

Liver

External and internal oblique muscles

Duodenojejunal flexure

Superior mesenteric vein and artery

Inferior vena cava

Abdominal aorta

Left renal vein and artery

Left kidney

Peritoneum

Descending colon

Tendon of origin of transversus abdominis muscle

Latissimus dorsi muscle

Quadratus lumborum muscle

Crura of diaphragm

Psoas major muscle and fascia

Erector spinae muscle

Transversalis fascia

Pararenal fat (retroperitoneal)

Perirenal fat

Fibrous capsule of kidney

Anterior and posterior layers of renal fascia

Transverse section through 2nd lumbar vertebra demonstrates horizontal disposition of fascia

Diaphragm

Diaphragmatic fascia (continuation of transversalis fascia)

Costodiaphragmatic recess

Suprarenal gland

Perirenal fat

12th rib

Pararenal fat (retroperitoneal)

Transversalis fascia

Quadratus lumborum muscle

Iliac crest

Lung

Liver

Bare area of liver

Fibrous capsule of kidney

Peritoneum

Anterior and posterior layers of renal fascia

Right kidney

Right colic (hepatic) flexure

Sagittal section through right kidney and lumbar region demonstrates vertical disposition of renal fascia

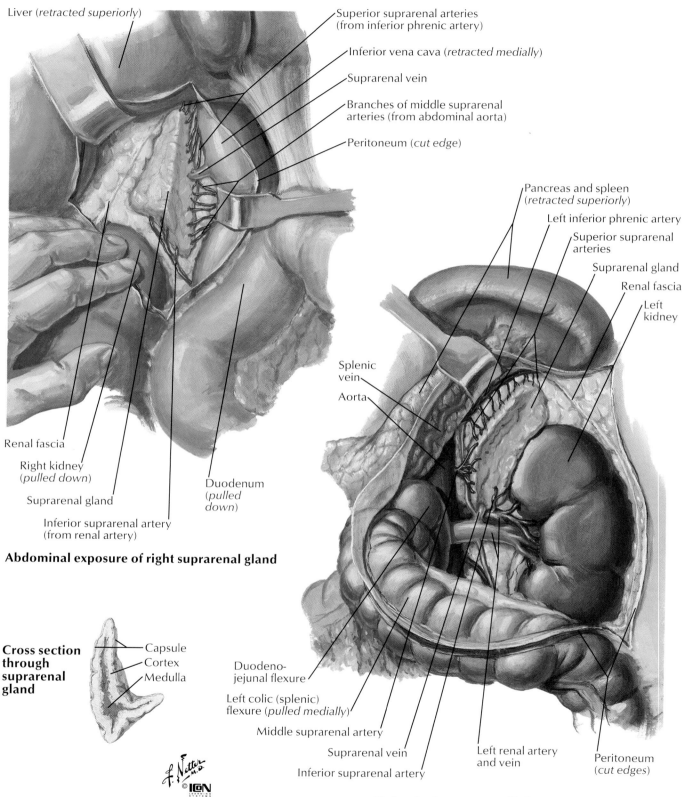

Liver (*retracted superiorly*)

Superior suprarenal arteries
(*from inferior phrenic artery*)

Inferior vena cava (*retracted medially*)

Suprarenal vein

Branches of middle suprarenal
arteries (*from abdominal aorta*)

Peritoneum (*cut edge*)

Pancreas and spleen
(*retracted superiorly*)

Left inferior phrenic artery

Superior suprarenal
arteries

Suprarenal gland

Renal fascia

Left
kidney

Splenic
vein

Aorta

Renal fascia

Right kidney
(*pulled down*)

Suprarenal gland

Inferior suprarenal artery
(*from renal artery*)

Duodenum
(*pulled
down*)

Abdominal exposure of right suprarenal gland

**Cross section
through
suprarenal
gland**

Capsule

Cortex

Medulla

Duodeno-
jejunal flexure

Left colic (splenic)
flexure (*pulled medially*)

Middle suprarenal artery

Suprarenal vein

Inferior suprarenal artery

Left renal artery
and vein

Peritoneum
(*cut edges*)

Abdominal exposure of left suprarenal gland

PLATE 333

ABDOMEN

SEE ALSO PLATES 159, 160

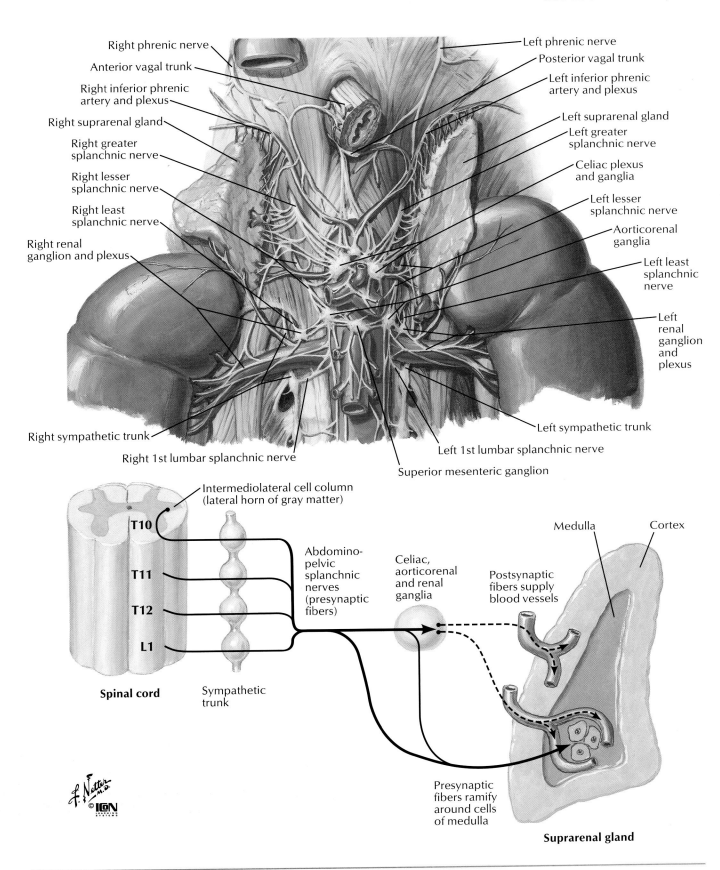

Right phrenic nerve

Anterior vagal trunk

Right inferior phrenic artery and plexus

Right suprarenal gland

Right greater splanchnic nerve

Right lesser splanchnic nerve

Right least splanchnic nerve

Right renal ganglion and plexus

Right sympathetic trunk

Right 1st lumbar splanchnic nerve

Left phrenic nerve

Posterior vagal trunk

Left inferior phrenic artery and plexus

Left suprarenal gland

Left greater splanchnic nerve

Celiac plexus and ganglia

Left lesser splanchnic nerve

Aorticorenal ganglia

Left least splanchnic nerve

Left renal ganglion and plexus

Left sympathetic trunk

Left 1st lumbar splanchnic nerve

Superior mesenteric ganglion

Intermediolateral cell column (lateral horn of gray matter)

T10

T11

T12

L1

Spinal cord

Sympathetic trunk

Abdomino-pelvic splanchnic nerves (presynaptic fibers)

Celiac, aorticorenal and renal ganglia

Postsynaptic fibers supply blood vessels

Medulla

Cortex

Presynaptic fibers ramify around cells of medulla

Suprarenal gland

KIDNEYS AND SUPRARENAL GLANDS

PLATE 334

Sternum

Diaphragm (central tendon)

Inferior diaphragmatic fascia and Parietal peritoneum

Liver

Lesser omentum

Hepatic portal vein and hepatic artery proper in right margin of lesser omentum

Omental bursa (lesser sac)

Stomach

Middle colic artery

Transverse mesocolon

Parietal peritoneum (of anterior abdominal wall)

Transverse colon

Greater omentum

Small intestine

Rectus abdominis muscle

Rectus sheath

Arcuate line

Transversalis fascia

Umbilical prevesical fascia

Median umbilical ligament (urachus)

Fatty layer of subcutaneous tissue (Camper's fascia)

Membranous layer of subcutaneous tissue (Scarpa's fascia)

Urinary bladder

Fundiform ligament of penis

Pubic bone

Suspensory ligament of penis

Retropubic (prevesical) space (cave of Retzius)

Deep (Buck's) fascia of penis

Superficial (dartos) fascia of penis and scrotum

Tunica vaginalis testis

Testis

Puborectalis muscle (thickened medial edge of left levator ani muscle)

Perineal membrane and bulbourethral (Cowper's) gland

T10

T11

T12

L1

L2

L3

L4

L5

S1

S2

Coronary ligament enclosing bare area of liver

Esophagus

Superior recess of omental bursa (lesser sac)

Diaphragm (right crus)

Left gastric artery

Omental (epiploic) foramen (Winslow)

Celiac trunk

Splenic vessels

Renal vessels

Pancreas

Superior mesenteric artery

Inferior (horizontal, or 3rd) part of duodenum

Inferior mesenteric artery

Abdominal aorta

Parietal peritoneum (of posterior abdominal wall)

Mesentery of small intestine

Anterior longitudinal ligament

Vesical fascia

Rectal fascia

Presacral fascia

Rectovesical pouch

Rectum

Rectoprostatic (Denonvilliers') fascia

Levator ani muscle

Prostate

Deep
Superficial
Subcutaneous
} External anal sphincter muscle

Deep and superficial transverse perineal muscles

Bulbospongiosus muscle

Superficial perineal (Colles') fascia

f. Netter M.D.
C. Machado M.D.
© ICN LEARNING SYSTEMS

PLATE 335

ABDOMEN

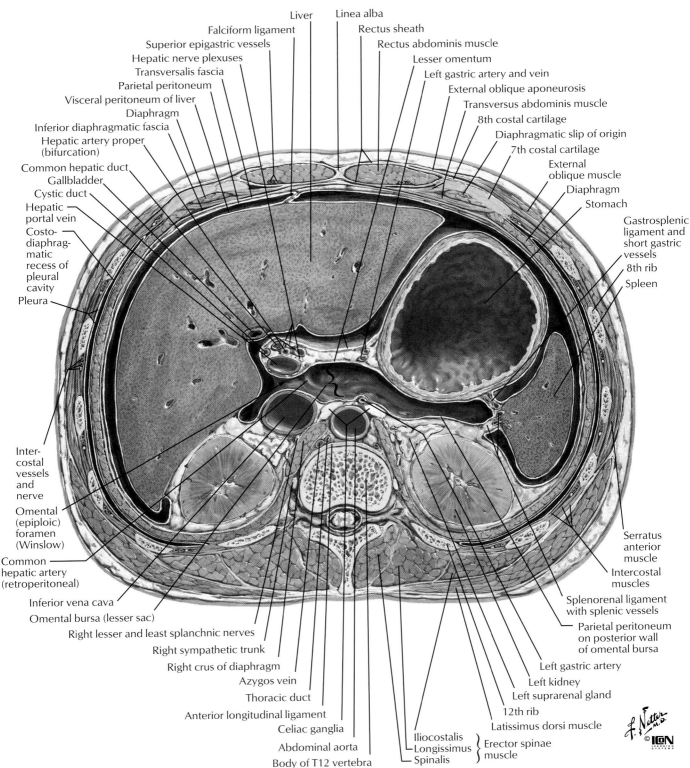

Liver
Linea alba
Falciform ligament
Superior epigastric vessels
Hepatic nerve plexuses
Transversalis fascia
Parietal peritoneum
Visceral peritoneum of liver
Diaphragm
Inferior diaphragmatic fascia
Hepatic artery proper (bifurcation)
Common hepatic duct
Gallbladder
Cystic duct
Hepatic portal vein
Costo-diaphrag-matic recess of pleural cavity
Pleura

Rectus sheath
Rectus abdominis muscle
Lesser omentum
Left gastric artery and vein
External oblique aponeurosis
Transversus abdominis muscle
8th costal cartilage
Diaphragmatic slip of origin
7th costal cartilage
External oblique muscle
Diaphragm
Stomach
Gastrosplenic ligament and short gastric vessels
8th rib
Spleen

Inter-costal vessels and nerve
Omental (epiploic) foramen (Winslow)
Common hepatic artery (retroperitoneal)
Inferior vena cava
Omental bursa (lesser sac)
Right lesser and least splanchnic nerves
Right sympathetic trunk
Right crus of diaphragm
Azygos vein
Thoracic duct
Anterior longitudinal ligament
Celiac ganglia
Abdominal aorta
Body of T12 vertebra

Serratus anterior muscle
Intercostal muscles
Splenorenal ligament with splenic vessels
Parietal peritoneum on posterior wall of omental bursa
Left gastric artery
Left kidney
Left suprarenal gland
12th rib
Latissimus dorsi muscle

Iliocostalis
Longissimus
Spinalis
} Erector spinae muscle

Schematic Cross Section of Abdomen at L3, 4

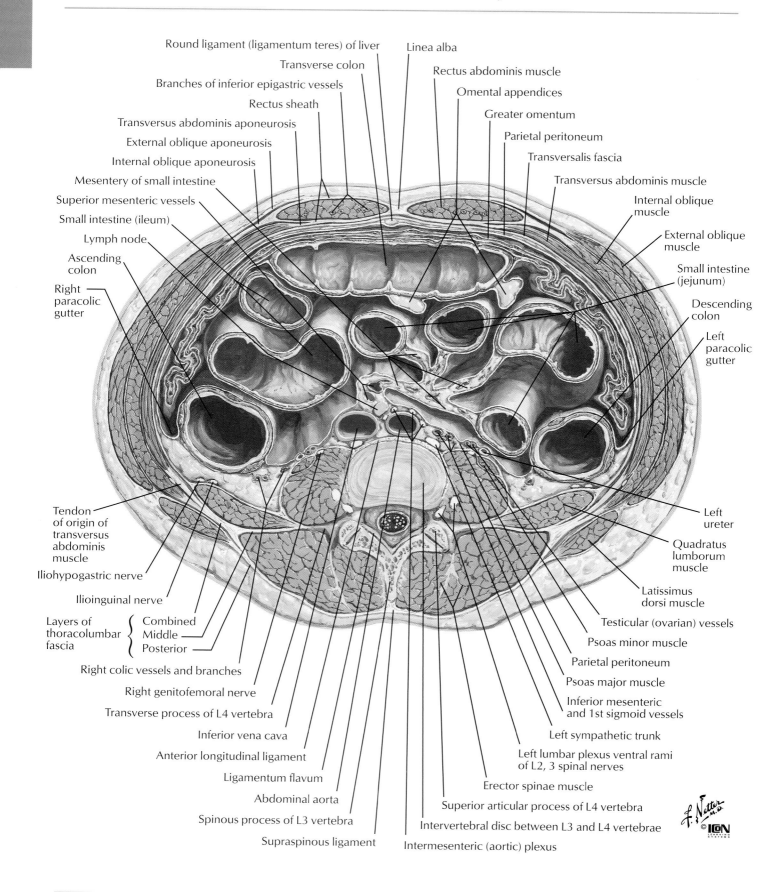

Round ligament (ligamentum teres) of liver

Transverse colon

Branches of inferior epigastric vessels

Rectus sheath

Transversus abdominis aponeurosis

External oblique aponeurosis

Internal oblique aponeurosis

Mesentery of small intestine

Superior mesenteric vessels

Small intestine (ileum)

Lymph node

Ascending colon

Right paracolic gutter

Linea alba

Rectus abdominis muscle

Omental appendices

Greater omentum

Parietal peritoneum

Transversalis fascia

Transversus abdominis muscle

Internal oblique muscle

External oblique muscle

Small intestine (jejunum)

Descending colon

Left paracolic gutter

Tendon of origin of transversus abdominis muscle

Iliohypogastric nerve

Ilioinguinal nerve

Layers of thoracolumbar fascia { Combined Middle Posterior

Right colic vessels and branches

Right genitofemoral nerve

Transverse process of L4 vertebra

Inferior vena cava

Anterior longitudinal ligament

Ligamentum flavum

Abdominal aorta

Spinous process of L3 vertebra

Supraspinous ligament

Left ureter

Quadratus lumborum muscle

Latissimus dorsi muscle

Testicular (ovarian) vessels

Psoas minor muscle

Parietal peritoneum

Psoas major muscle

Inferior mesenteric and 1st sigmoid vessels

Left symphathetic trunk

Left lumbar plexus ventral rami of L2, 3 spinal nerves

Erector spinae muscle

Superior articular process of L4 vertebra

Intervertebral disc between L3 and L4 vertebrae

Intermesenteric (aortic) plexus

PLATE 337

ABDOMEN

Series of abdominal axial CT images from superior (A) to inferior (D)

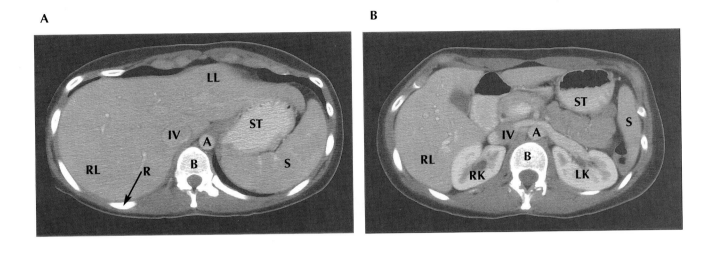

A

B

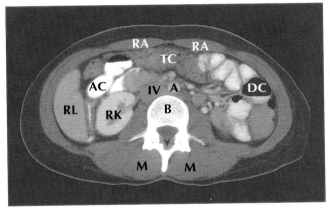

C

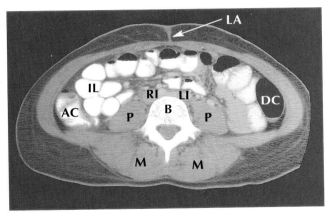

D

A	Aorta	M	Deep back muscles
AC	Ascending colon	P	Psoas muscle
B	Body of vertebra	R	Rib
DC	Descending colon	RA	Rectus abdominis muscle
IL	Ileum	RI	Right common iliac artery
IV	Inferior vena cava	RL	Right lobe of liver
LA	Linea alba	S	Spleen
LI	Left common iliac artery	ST	Stomach
LK	Left kidney	TC	Transverse colon
LL	Left lobe of liver		

Section V
PELVIS AND PERINEUM

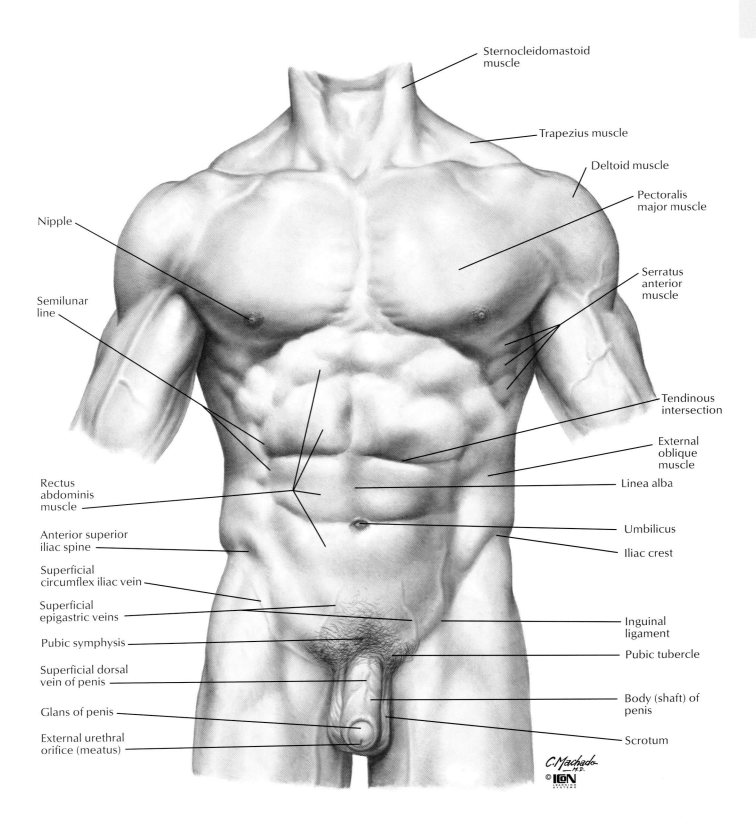

Sternocleidomastoid
muscle

Trapezius muscle

Deltoid muscle

Pectoralis
major muscle

Nipple

Serratus
anterior
muscle

Semilunar
line

Tendinous
intersection

External
oblique
muscle

Rectus
abdominis
muscle

Linea alba

Umbilicus

Anterior superior
iliac spine

Iliac crest

Superficial
circumflex iliac vein

Superficial
epigastric veins

Inguinal
ligament

Pubic symphysis

Pubic tubercle

Superficial dorsal
vein of penis

Body (shaft) of
penis

Glans of penis

Scrotum

External urethral
orifice (meatus)

Bones and Ligaments of Pelvis

SEE ALSO PLATE 468

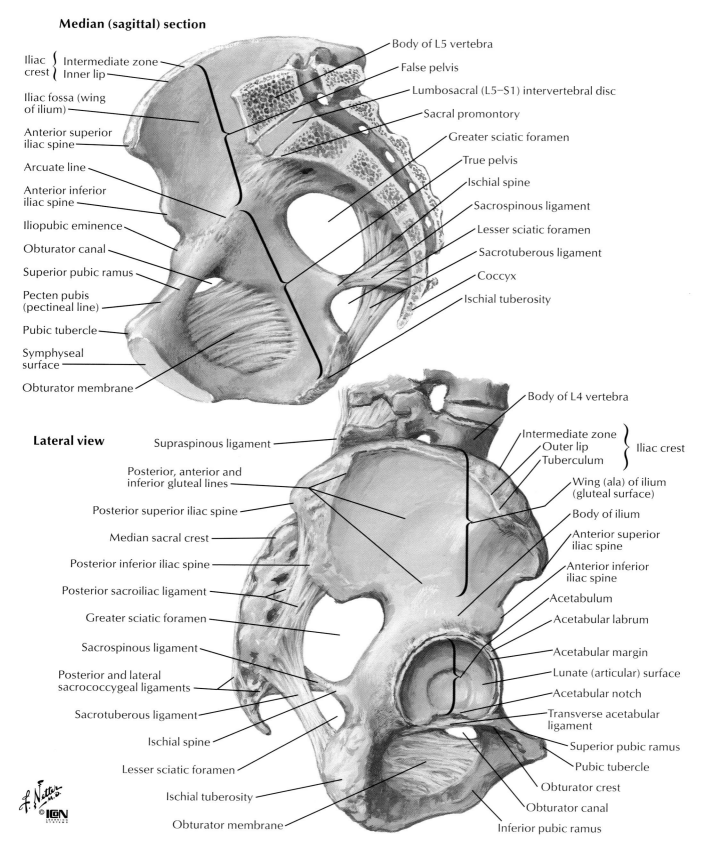

Median (sagittal) section

Iliac crest { Intermediate zone
Iliac crest { Inner lip

Iliac fossa (wing of ilium)

Anterior superior iliac spine

Arcuate line

Anterior inferior iliac spine

Iliopubic eminence

Obturator canal

Superior pubic ramus

Pecten pubis (pectineal line)

Pubic tubercle

Symphyseal surface

Obturator membrane

Body of L5 vertebra

False pelvis

Lumbosacral (L5–S1) intervertebral disc

Sacral promontory

Greater sciatic foramen

True pelvis

Ischial spine

Sacrospinous ligament

Lesser sciatic foramen

Sacrotuberous ligament

Coccyx

Ischial tuberosity

Lateral view

Supraspinous ligament

Posterior, anterior and inferior gluteal lines

Posterior superior iliac spine

Median sacral crest

Posterior inferior iliac spine

Posterior sacroiliac ligament

Greater sciatic foramen

Sacrospinous ligament

Posterior and lateral sacrococcygeal ligaments

Sacrotuberous ligament

Ischial spine

Lesser sciatic foramen

Ischial tuberosity

Obturator membrane

Body of L4 vertebra

Intermediate zone } Iliac crest
Outer lip } Iliac crest
Tuberculum }

Wing (ala) of ilium (gluteal surface)

Body of ilium

Anterior superior iliac spine

Anterior inferior iliac spine

Acetabulum

Acetabular labrum

Acetabular margin

Lunate (articular) surface

Acetabular notch

Transverse acetabular ligament

Superior pubic ramus

Pubic tubercle

Obturator crest

Obturator canal

Inferior pubic ramus

PLATE 340

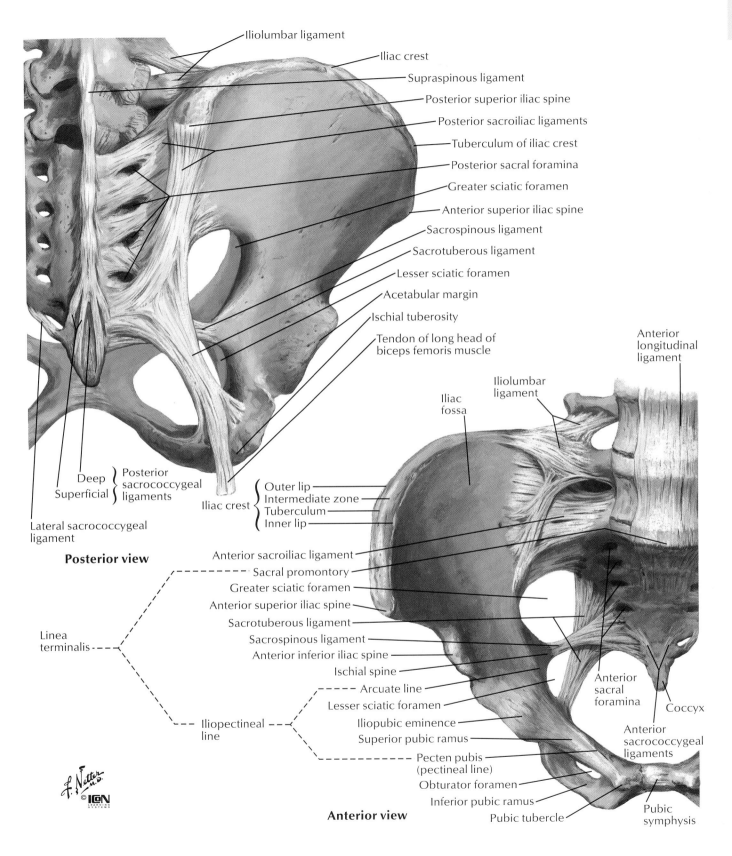

Iliolumbar ligament

Iliac crest

Supraspinous ligament

Posterior superior iliac spine

Posterior sacroiliac ligaments

Tuberculum of iliac crest

Posterior sacral foramina

Greater sciatic foramen

Anterior superior iliac spine

Sacrospinous ligament

Sacrotuberous ligament

Lesser sciatic foramen

Acetabular margin

Ischial tuberosity

Tendon of long head of biceps femoris muscle

Deep / Superficial } Posterior sacrococcygeal ligaments

Iliac crest

Lateral sacrococcygeal ligament

Posterior view

Anterior longitudinal ligament

Iliac fossa

Iliolumbar ligament

Outer lip
Intermediate zone
Tuberculum
Inner lip
} Iliac crest

Anterior sacroiliac ligament

Sacral promontory

Greater sciatic foramen

Anterior superior iliac spine

Sacrotuberous ligament

Sacrospinous ligament

Anterior inferior iliac spine

Ischial spine

Arcuate line

Lesser sciatic foramen

Iliopubic eminence

Superior pubic ramus

Pecten pubis (pectineal line)

Obturator foramen

Inferior pubic ramus

Pubic tubercle

Linea terminalis

Iliopectineal line

Anterior sacral foramina

Coccyx

Anterior sacrococcygeal ligaments

Pubic symphysis

Anterior view

Sex Differences of Pelvis: Measurements

SEE ALSO PLATE 240

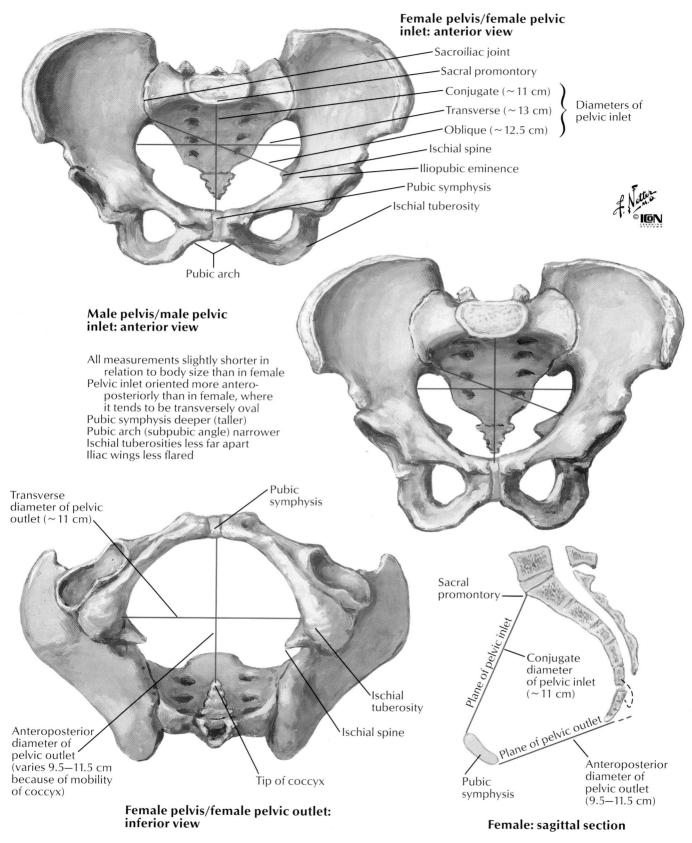

Female pelvis/female pelvic inlet: anterior view

Sacroiliac joint

Sacral promontory

Conjugate (~11 cm)

Transverse (~13 cm) } Diameters of pelvic inlet

Oblique (~12.5 cm)

Ischial spine

Iliopubic eminence

Pubic symphysis

Ischial tuberosity

Pubic arch

Male pelvis/male pelvic inlet: anterior view

All measurements slightly shorter in relation to body size than in female
Pelvic inlet oriented more antero-posteriorly than in female, where it tends to be transversely oval
Pubic symphysis deeper (taller)
Pubic arch (subpubic angle) narrower
Ischial tuberosities less far apart
Iliac wings less flared

Transverse diameter of pelvic outlet (~11 cm)

Pubic symphysis

Anteroposterior diameter of pelvic outlet (varies 9.5–11.5 cm because of mobility of coccyx)

Tip of coccyx

Ischial tuberosity

Ischial spine

Female pelvis/female pelvic outlet: inferior view

Sacral promontory

Plane of pelvic inlet

Conjugate diameter of pelvic inlet (~11 cm)

Plane of pelvic outlet

Pubic symphysis

Anteroposterior diameter of pelvic outlet (9.5–11.5 cm)

Female: sagittal section

PLATE 342

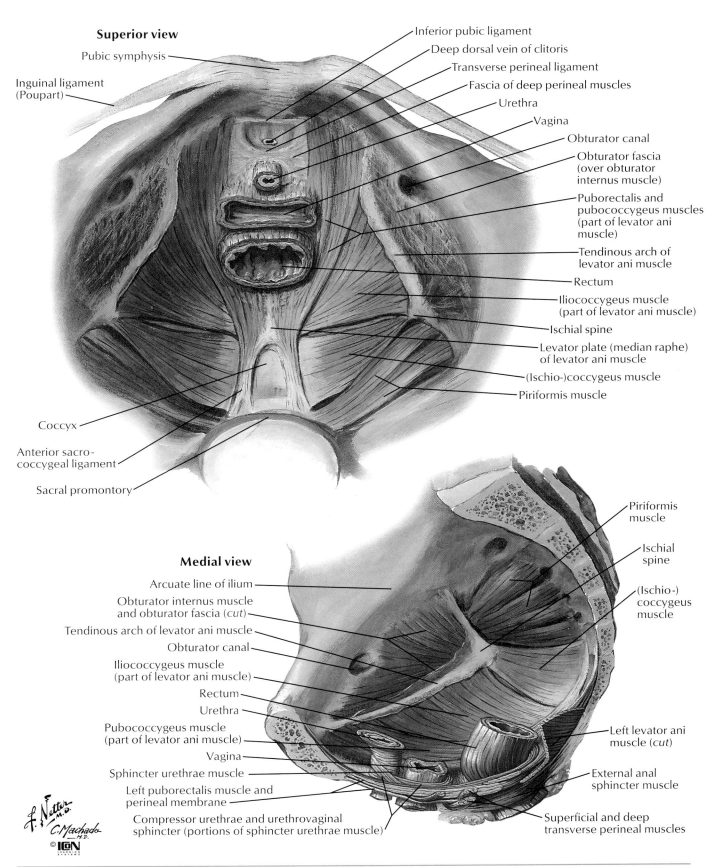

Superior view

Pubic symphysis
Inguinal ligament (Poupart)
Inferior pubic ligament
Deep dorsal vein of clitoris
Transverse perineal ligament
Fascia of deep perineal muscles
Urethra
Vagina
Obturator canal
Obturator fascia (over obturator internus muscle)
Puborectalis and pubococcygeus muscles (part of levator ani muscle)
Tendinous arch of levator ani muscle
Rectum
Iliococcygeus muscle (part of levator ani muscle)
Ischial spine
Levator plate (median raphe) of levator ani muscle
(Ischio-)coccygeus muscle
Piriformis muscle
Coccyx
Anterior sacro-coccygeal ligament
Sacral promontory

Medial view

Arcuate line of ilium
Obturator internus muscle and obturator fascia (cut)
Tendinous arch of levator ani muscle
Obturator canal
Iliococcygeus muscle (part of levator ani muscle)
Rectum
Urethra
Pubococcygeus muscle (part of levator ani muscle)
Vagina
Sphincter urethrae muscle
Left puborectalis muscle and perineal membrane
Compressor urethrae and urethrovaginal sphincter (portions of sphincter urethrae muscle)
Piriformis muscle
Ischial spine
(Ischio-)coccygeus muscle
Left levator ani muscle (cut)
External anal sphincter muscle
Superficial and deep transverse perineal muscles

FOR UROGENITAL DIAPHRAGM SEE PLATE 361

Inferior view

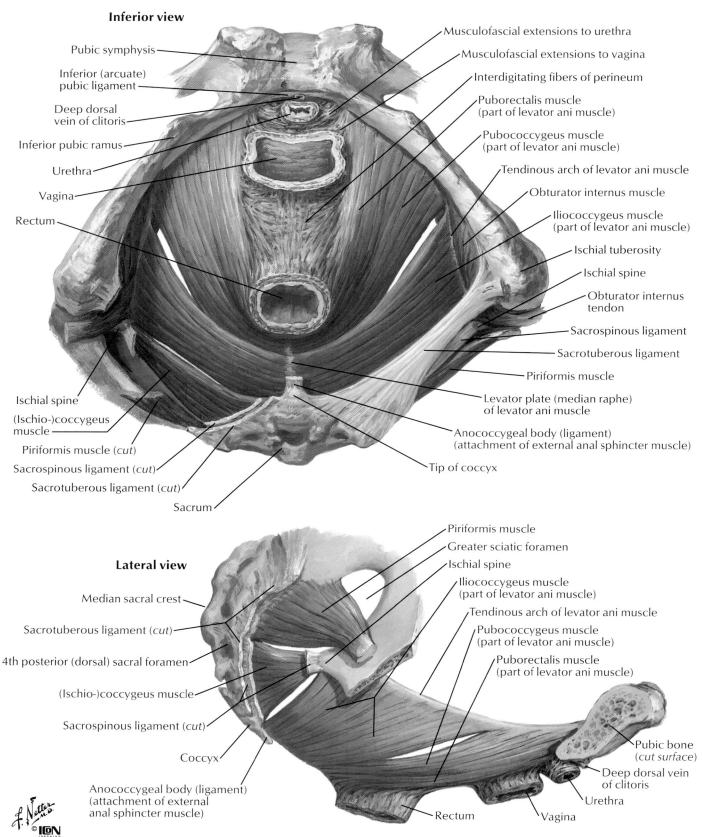

Pubic symphysis

Inferior (arcuate) pubic ligament

Deep dorsal vein of clitoris

Inferior pubic ramus

Urethra

Vagina

Rectum

Ischial spine

(Ischio-)coccygeus muscle

Piriformis muscle (*cut*)

Sacrospinous ligament (*cut*)

Sacrotuberous ligament (*cut*)

Sacrum

Musculofascial extensions to urethra

Musculofascial extensions to vagina

Interdigitating fibers of perineum

Puborectalis muscle (part of levator ani muscle)

Pubococcygeus muscle (part of levator ani muscle)

Tendinous arch of levator ani muscle

Obturator internus muscle

Iliococcygeus muscle (part of levator ani muscle)

Ischial tuberosity

Ischial spine

Obturator internus tendon

Sacrospinous ligament

Sacrotuberous ligament

Piriformis muscle

Levator plate (median raphe) of levator ani muscle

Anococcygeal body (ligament) (attachment of external anal sphincter muscle)

Tip of coccyx

Lateral view

Median sacral crest

Sacrotuberous ligament (*cut*)

4th posterior (dorsal) sacral foramen

(Ischio-)coccygeus muscle

Sacrospinous ligament (*cut*)

Coccyx

Anococcygeal body (ligament) (attachment of external anal sphincter muscle)

Piriformis muscle

Greater sciatic foramen

Ischial spine

Iliococcygeus muscle (part of levator ani muscle)

Tendinous arch of levator ani muscle

Pubococcygeus muscle (part of levator ani muscle)

Puborectalis muscle (part of levator ani muscle)

Pubic bone (*cut surface*)

Deep dorsal vein of clitoris

Urethra

Vagina

Rectum

PLATE 344

PELVIS AND PERINEUM

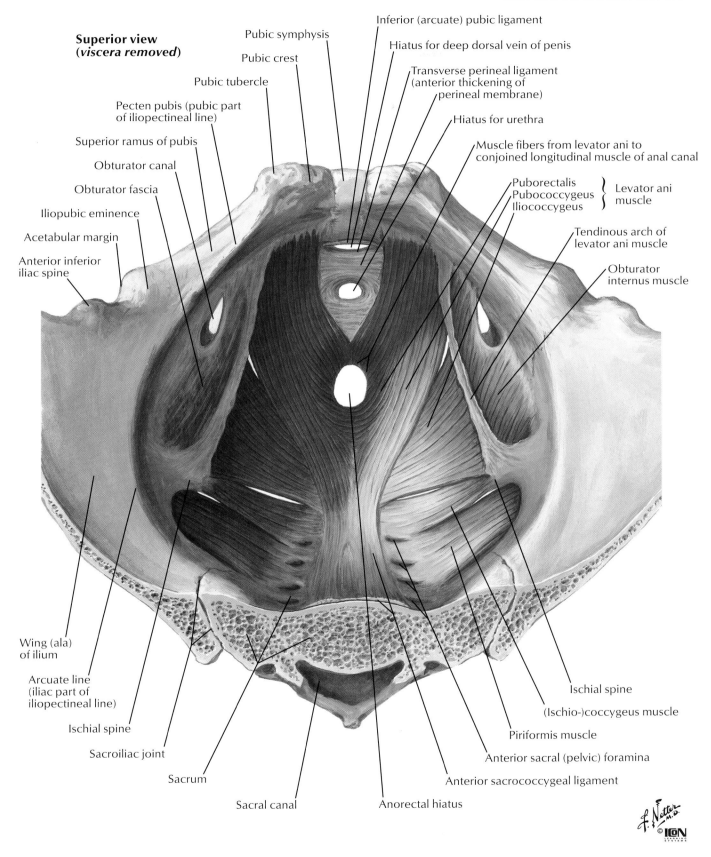

**Superior view
(*viscera removed*)**

Pubic symphysis

Pubic crest

Pubic tubercle

Pecten pubis (pubic part
of iliopectineal line)

Superior ramus of pubis

Obturator canal

Obturator fascia

Iliopubic eminence

Acetabular margin

Anterior inferior
iliac spine

Inferior (arcuate) pubic ligament

Hiatus for deep dorsal vein of penis

Transverse perineal ligament
(anterior thickening of
perineal membrane)

Hiatus for urethra

Muscle fibers from levator ani to
conjoined longitudinal muscle of anal canal

Puborectalis
Pubococcygeus } Levator ani
Iliococcygeus   muscle

Tendinous arch of
levator ani muscle

Obturator
internus muscle

Wing (ala)
of ilium

Arcuate line
(iliac part of
iliopectineal line)

Ischial spine

Sacroiliac joint

Sacrum

Sacral canal

Anorectal hiatus

Anterior sacrococcygeal ligament

Anterior sacral (pelvic) foramina

Piriformis muscle

(Ischio-)coccygeus muscle

Ischial spine

Pelvic Diaphragm: Male (continued)

FOR UROGENITAL DIAPHRAGM SEE PLATE 366

Inferior view

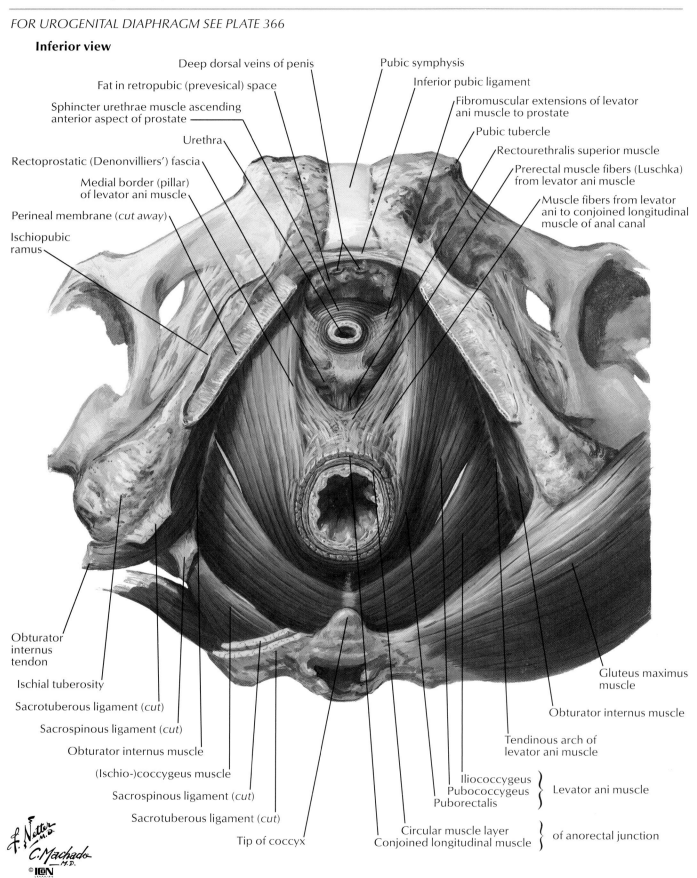

Deep dorsal veins of penis

Fat in retropubic (prevesical) space

Sphincter urethrae muscle ascending
anterior aspect of prostate

Urethra

Rectoprostatic (Denonvilliers') fascia

Medial border (pillar)
of levator ani muscle

Perineal membrane (cut away)

Ischiopubic
ramus

Obturator
internus
tendon

Ischial tuberosity

Sacrotuberous ligament (cut)

Sacrospinous ligament (cut)

Obturator internus muscle

(Ischio-)coccygeus muscle

Sacrospinous ligament (cut)

Sacrotuberous ligament (cut)

Tip of coccyx

Pubic symphysis

Inferior pubic ligament

Fibromuscular extensions of levator
ani muscle to prostate

Pubic tubercle

Rectourethralis superior muscle

Prerectal muscle fibers (Luschka)
from levator ani muscle

Muscle fibers from levator
ani to conjoined longitudinal
muscle of anal canal

Gluteus maximus
muscle

Obturator internus muscle

Tendinous arch of
levator ani muscle

Iliococcygeus }
Pubococcygeus } Levator ani muscle
Puborectalis }

Circular muscle layer }
Conjoined longitudinal muscle } of anorectal junction

PLATE 346

Median (sagittal) section

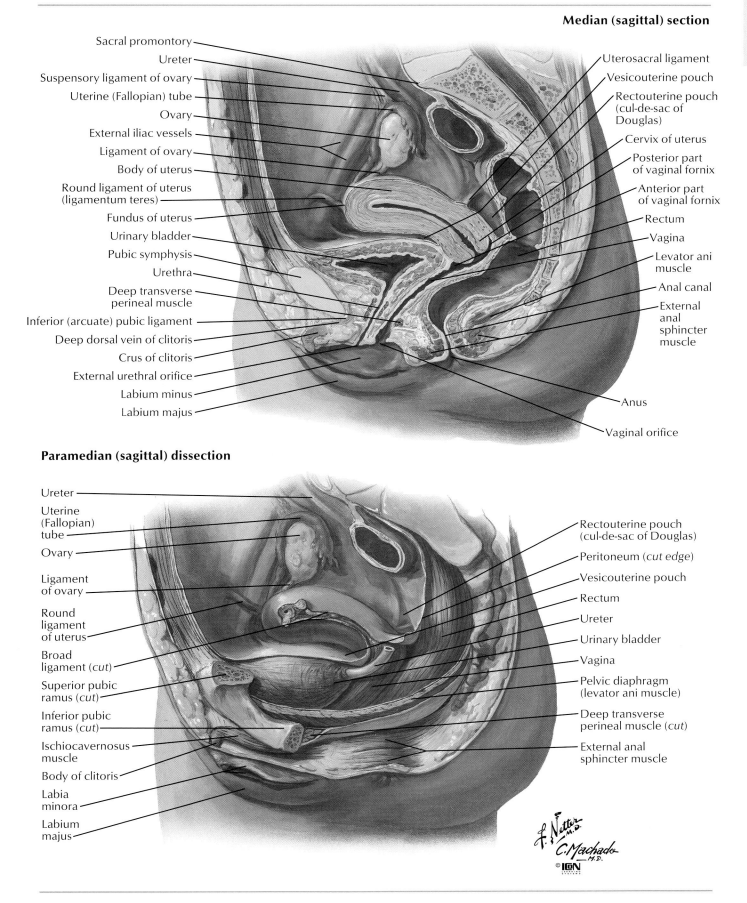

Sacral promontory

Ureter

Suspensory ligament of ovary

Uterine (Fallopian) tube

Ovary

External iliac vessels

Ligament of ovary

Body of uterus

Round ligament of uterus (ligamentum teres)

Fundus of uterus

Urinary bladder

Pubic symphysis

Urethra

Deep transverse perineal muscle

Inferior (arcuate) pubic ligament

Deep dorsal vein of clitoris

Crus of clitoris

External urethral orifice

Labium minus

Labium majus

Uterosacral ligament

Vesicouterine pouch

Rectouterine pouch (cul-de-sac of Douglas)

Cervix of uterus

Posterior part of vaginal fornix

Anterior part of vaginal fornix

Rectum

Vagina

Levator ani muscle

Anal canal

External anal sphincter muscle

Anus

Vaginal orifice

Paramedian (sagittal) dissection

Ureter

Uterine (Fallopian) tube

Ovary

Ligament of ovary

Round ligament of uterus

Broad ligament (cut)

Superior pubic ramus (cut)

Inferior pubic ramus (cut)

Ischiocavernosus muscle

Body of clitoris

Labia minora

Labium majus

Rectouterine pouch (cul-de-sac of Douglas)

Peritoneum (cut edge)

Vesicouterine pouch

Rectum

Ureter

Urinary bladder

Vagina

Pelvic diaphragm (levator ani muscle)

Deep transverse perineal muscle (cut)

External anal sphincter muscle

Pelvic Viscera and Perineum: Male

Paramedian (sagittal) dissection

External iliac vessels

Peritoneum

Rectus abdominis muscle

Anterior layer of rectus sheath

Transversalis fascia

Umbilical prevesical fascia

Subcutaneous tissue { fatty (Camper's) / membranous (Scarpa's) }

Superior pubic ramus (cut)

Fundiform ligament of penis

Suspensory ligament of penis

Areolar tissue and vesical venous plexus in retropubic (prevesical) space

Deep dorsal vein of penis

Corpus cavernosum

Deep (Buck's) fascia of penis

Corpus spongiosum

Superficial (dartos) fascia of penis and scrotum

Septum of scrotum

Ischiocavernosus muscle

Testis

Ductus (vas) deferens

Urinary bladder and fascia

Ureter (cut)

Seminal vesicle

Rectovesical pouch

Rectum

Rectoprostatic (Denonvilliers') fascia

Prostate (covered by fascia)

Ischiopubic ramus (cut)

Pelvic diaphragm (levator ani muscle)

Deep transverse perineal muscle

Perineal body

Deep / Superficial / Subcutaneous } External anal sphincter muscle

Deep perineal (investing or Gallaudet's) fascia

Superficial perineal (Colles') fascia (inferior fascia of superficial perineal space)

Superficial (dartos) fascia of scrotum

External spermatic fascia

Median (sagittal) section

Urachus

Urinary bladder { Apex / Fundus / Body / Trigone / Neck }

Pubic symphysis

Fundiform ligament of penis

Suspensory ligament of penis

Inferior (arcuate) pubic ligament

Transverse perineal ligament (anterior thickening of perineal membrane)

Superficial perineal space

Corpus cavernosum

Corpus spongiosum

Superficial (dartos) fascia of penis and scrotum

Deep (Buck's) fascia of penis

Prepuce

Glans of penis and external urethral meatus

Vesical fascia

Rectovesical pouch

Rectum

Seminal vesicle

Prostate and capsule

Rectoprostatic (Denonvilliers') fascia

Sphincter urethrae muscle

Bulbourethral (Cowper's) gland

Perineal body

Bulbospongiosus muscle

Deep perineal (investing or Gallaudet's) fascia

Superficial perineal (Colles') fascia

Buck's fascia

Septum of scrotum

Navicular fossa

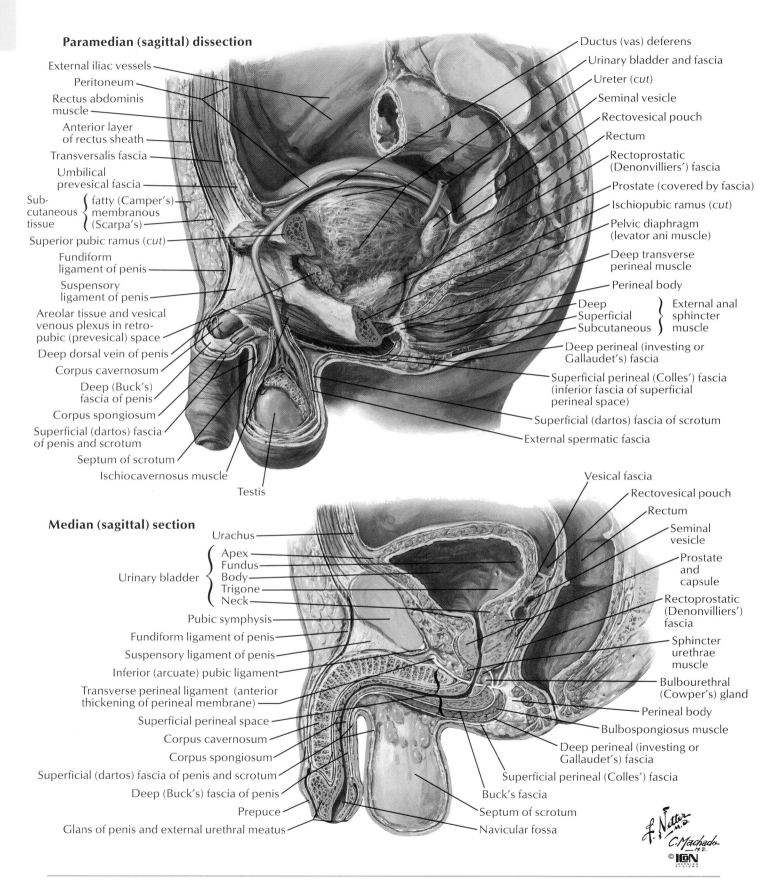

PLATE 348

PELVIS AND PERINEUM

Superior view

Uterus (fundus)
Ligament of ovary
Ovary
Uterine (Fallopian) tube
Round ligament of uterus
Broad (lateral uterine) ligament
Linea terminalis of pelvis
Femoral ring
Deep inguinal ring
Iliopubic tract (covered by peritoneum)
External iliac vessels
Iliac fossa (false pelvis)
Left paracolic gutter

Linea alba
Median umbilical fold and ligament (urachus)

Urinary bladder and transverse vesical fold
Rectus abdominis muscle
Medial umbilical fold and ligament (occluded part of umbilical artery)
Rectouterine pouch (cul-de-sac of Douglas)
Rectum
Inferior epigastric vessels and lateral umbilical fold
Uterosacral fold
Ureteric fold
Suspensory ligament of ovary (contains ovarian vessels)
(Vermiform) appendix
Cecum
Cecal folds
Right paracolic gutter

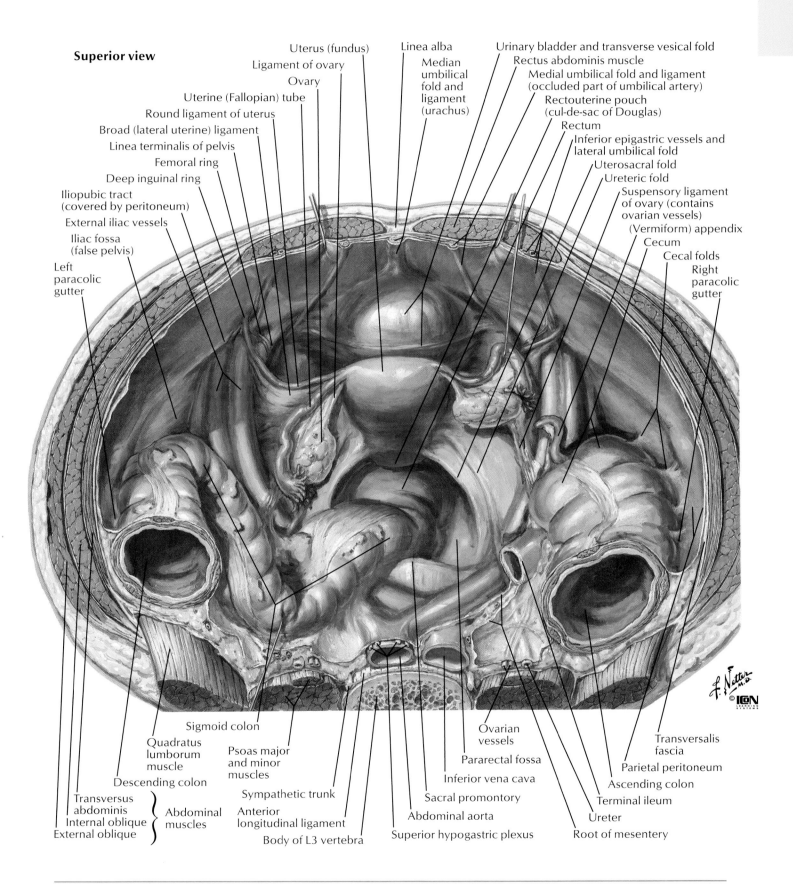

Sigmoid colon
Quadratus lumborum muscle
Descending colon
Transversus abdominis
Internal oblique } Abdominal muscles
External oblique

Psoas major and minor muscles
Sympathetic trunk
Anterior longitudinal ligament
Body of L3 vertebra

Ovarian vessels
Pararectal fossa
Inferior vena cava
Sacral promontory
Abdominal aorta
Superior hypogastric plexus

Transversalis fascia
Parietal peritoneum
Ascending colon
Terminal ileum
Ureter
Root of mesentery

Pelvic Contents: Male

Superior view

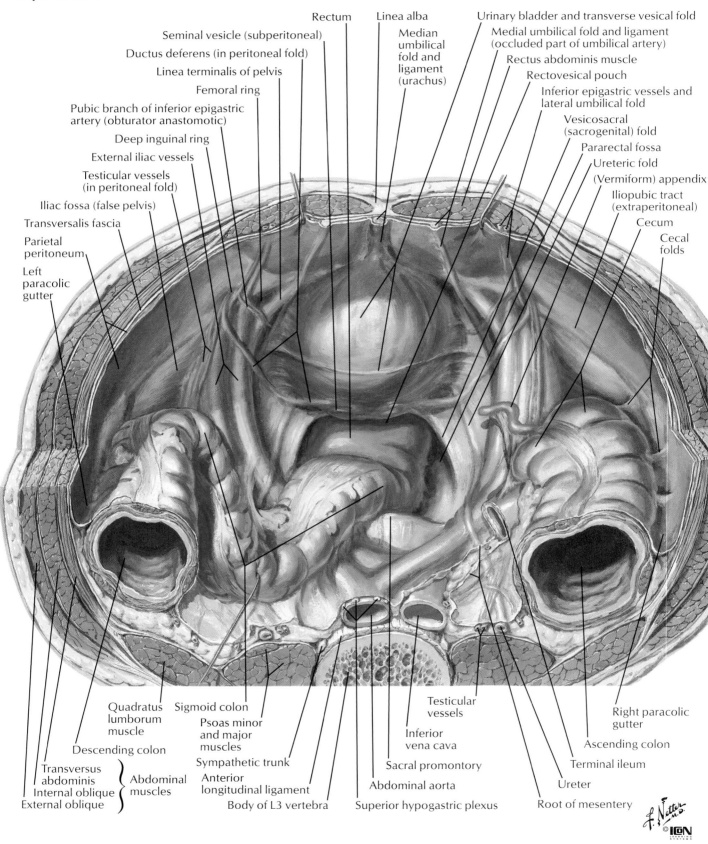

Rectum

Linea alba

Urinary bladder and transverse vesical fold

Seminal vesicle (subperitoneal)

Ductus deferens (in peritoneal fold)

Linea terminalis of pelvis

Femoral ring

Pubic branch of inferior epigastric artery (obturator anastomotic)

Deep inguinal ring

External iliac vessels

Testicular vessels (in peritoneal fold)

Iliac fossa (false pelvis)

Transversalis fascia

Parietal peritoneum

Left paracolic gutter

Median umbilical fold and ligament (urachus)

Medial umbilical fold and ligament (occluded part of umbilical artery)

Rectus abdominis muscle

Rectovesical pouch

Inferior epigastric vessels and lateral umbilical fold

Vesicosacral (sacrogenital) fold

Pararectal fossa

Ureteric fold

(Vermiform) appendix

Iliopubic tract (extraperitoneal)

Cecum

Cecal folds

Quadratus lumborum muscle

Sigmoid colon

Psoas minor and major muscles

Descending colon

Transversus abdominis
Internal oblique
External oblique } Abdominal muscles

Anterior longitudinal ligament

Body of L3 vertebra

Sympathetic trunk

Testicular vessels

Inferior vena cava

Sacral promontory

Abdominal aorta

Superior hypogastric plexus

Right paracolic gutter

Ascending colon

Terminal ileum

Ureter

Root of mesentery

PLATE 350

PELVIS AND PERINEUM

Female: superior view (peritoneum and loose areolar tissue removed)

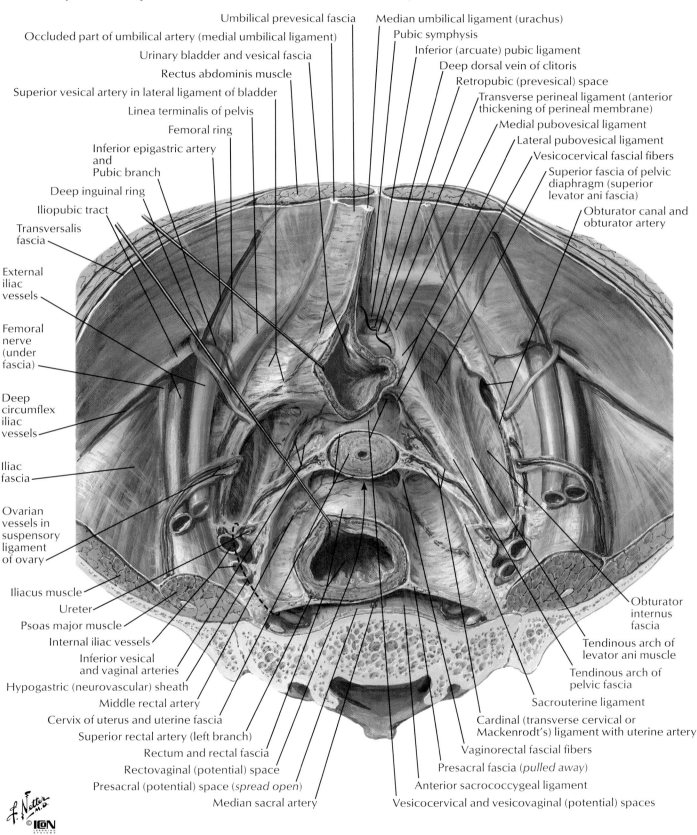

Umbilical prevesical fascia

Occluded part of umbilical artery (medial umbilical ligament)

Urinary bladder and vesical fascia

Rectus abdominis muscle

Superior vesical artery in lateral ligament of bladder

Linea terminalis of pelvis

Femoral ring

Inferior epigastric artery and Pubic branch

Deep inguinal ring

Iliopubic tract

Transversalis fascia

External iliac vessels

Femoral nerve (under fascia)

Deep circumflex iliac vessels

Iliac fascia

Ovarian vessels in suspensory ligament of ovary

Iliacus muscle

Ureter

Psoas major muscle

Internal iliac vessels

Inferior vesical and vaginal arteries

Hypogastric (neurovascular) sheath

Middle rectal artery

Cervix of uterus and uterine fascia

Superior rectal artery (left branch)

Rectum and rectal fascia

Rectovaginal (potential) space

Presacral (potential) space (spread open)

Median sacral artery

Median umbilical ligament (urachus)

Pubic symphysis

Inferior (arcuate) pubic ligament

Deep dorsal vein of clitoris

Retropubic (prevesical) space

Transverse perineal ligament (anterior thickening of perineal membrane)

Medial pubovesical ligament

Lateral pubovesical ligament

Vesicocervical fascial fibers

Superior fascia of pelvic diaphragm (superior levator ani fascia)

Obturator canal and obturator artery

Obturator internus fascia

Tendinous arch of levator ani muscle

Tendinous arch of pelvic fascia

Sacrouterine ligament

Cardinal (transverse cervical or Mackenrodt's) ligament with uterine artery

Vaginorectal fascial fibers

Presacral fascia (pulled away)

Anterior sacrococcygeal ligament

Vesicocervical and vesicovaginal (potential) spaces

Female: midsagittal section

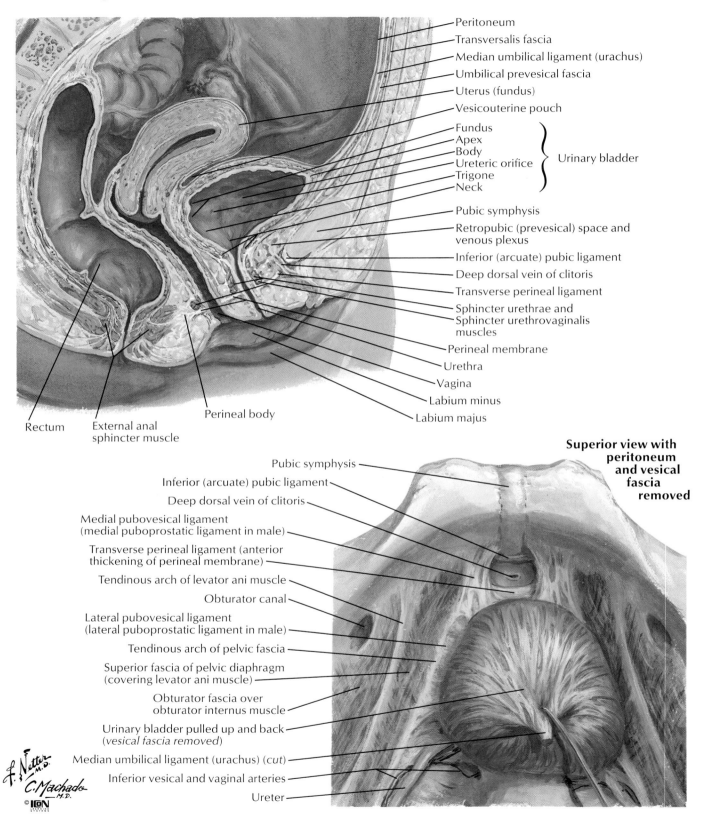

Peritoneum
Transversalis fascia
Median umbilical ligament (urachus)
Umbilical prevesical fascia
Uterus (fundus)
Vesicouterine pouch
Fundus
Apex
Body
Ureteric orifice
Trigone
Neck
} Urinary bladder
Pubic symphysis
Retropubic (prevesical) space and venous plexus
Inferior (arcuate) pubic ligament
Deep dorsal vein of clitoris
Transverse perineal ligament
Sphincter urethrae and Sphincter urethrovaginalis muscles
Perineal membrane
Urethra
Vagina
Labium minus
Labium majus

Rectum
External anal sphincter muscle
Perineal body

Superior view with peritoneum and vesical fascia removed

Pubic symphysis
Inferior (arcuate) pubic ligament
Deep dorsal vein of clitoris
Medial pubovesical ligament (medial puboprostatic ligament in male)
Transverse perineal ligament (anterior thickening of perineal membrane)
Tendinous arch of levator ani muscle
Obturator canal
Lateral pubovesical ligament (lateral puboprostatic ligament in male)
Tendinous arch of pelvic fascia
Superior fascia of pelvic diaphragm (covering levator ani muscle)
Obturator fascia over obturator internus muscle
Urinary bladder pulled up and back (vesical fascia removed)
Median umbilical ligament (urachus) (cut)
Inferior vesical and vaginal arteries
Ureter

PLATE 352

PELVIS AND PERINEUM

Urinary Bladder: Female and Male

SEE ALSO PLATES 329, 347, 348, 352, 380, 382, 383, 397

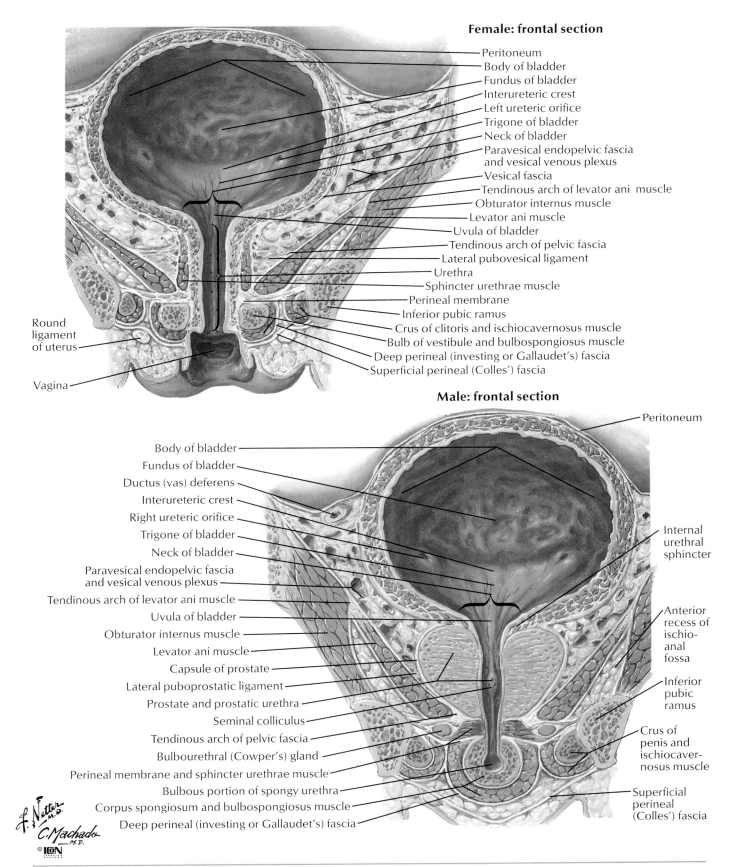

Female: frontal section

- Peritoneum
- Body of bladder
- Fundus of bladder
- Interureteric crest
- Left ureteric orifice
- Trigone of bladder
- Neck of bladder
- Paravesical endopelvic fascia and vesical venous plexus
- Vesical fascia
- Tendinous arch of levator ani muscle
- Obturator internus muscle
- Levator ani muscle
- Uvula of bladder
- Tendinous arch of pelvic fascia
- Lateral pubovesical ligament
- Urethra
- Sphincter urethrae muscle
- Perineal membrane
- Inferior pubic ramus
- Crus of clitoris and ischiocavernosus muscle
- Bulb of vestibule and bulbospongiosus muscle
- Deep perineal (investing or Gallaudet's) fascia
- Superficial perineal (Colles') fascia

Round ligament of uterus

Vagina

Male: frontal section

- Body of bladder
- Fundus of bladder
- Ductus (vas) deferens
- Interureteric crest
- Right ureteric orifice
- Trigone of bladder
- Neck of bladder
- Paravesical endopelvic fascia and vesical venous plexus
- Tendinous arch of levator ani muscle
- Uvula of bladder
- Obturator internus muscle
- Levator ani muscle
- Capsule of prostate
- Lateral puboprostatic ligament
- Prostate and prostatic urethra
- Seminal colliculus
- Tendinous arch of pelvic fascia
- Bulbourethral (Cowper's) gland
- Perineal membrane and sphincter urethrae muscle
- Bulbous portion of spongy urethra
- Corpus spongiosum and bulbospongiosus muscle
- Deep perineal (investing or Gallaudet's) fascia

- Peritoneum
- Internal urethral sphincter
- Anterior recess of ischio-anal fossa
- Inferior pubic ramus
- Crus of penis and ischiocavernosus muscle
- Superficial perineal (Colles') fascia

Pelvic Viscera: Female

Superior view with peritoneum intact

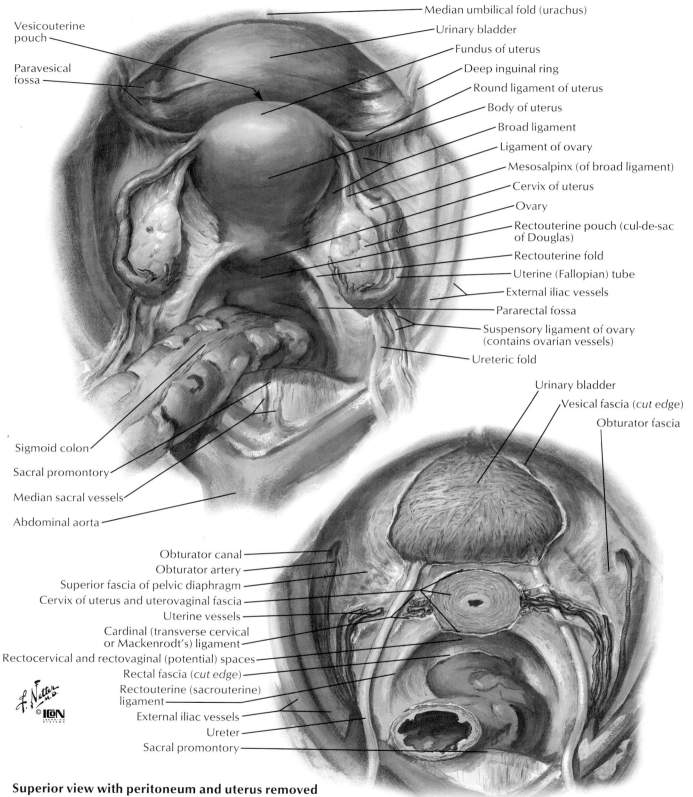

Median umbilical fold (urachus)

Urinary bladder

Fundus of uterus

Deep inguinal ring

Round ligament of uterus

Body of uterus

Broad ligament

Ligament of ovary

Mesosalpinx (of broad ligament)

Cervix of uterus

Ovary

Rectouterine pouch (cul-de-sac of Douglas)

Rectouterine fold

Uterine (Fallopian) tube

External iliac vessels

Pararectal fossa

Suspensory ligament of ovary (contains ovarian vessels)

Ureteric fold

Vesicouterine pouch

Paravesical fossa

Sigmoid colon

Sacral promontory

Median sacral vessels

Abdominal aorta

Urinary bladder

Vesical fascia (*cut edge*)

Obturator fascia

Obturator canal

Obturator artery

Superior fascia of pelvic diaphragm

Cervix of uterus and uterovaginal fascia

Uterine vessels

Cardinal (transverse cervical or Mackenrodt's) ligament

Rectocervical and rectovaginal (potential) spaces

Rectal fascia (*cut edge*)

Rectouterine (sacrouterine) ligament

External iliac vessels

Ureter

Sacral promontory

Superior view with peritoneum and uterus removed

PLATE 354

PELVIS AND PERINEUM

SEE ALSO PLATES 380, 382, 384, 386, 392, 394, 395

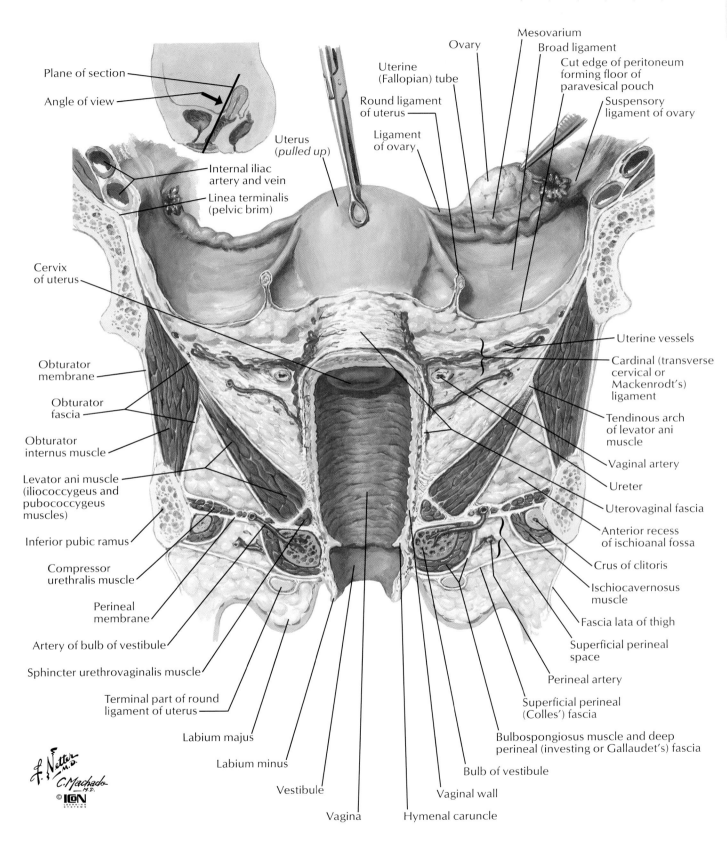

Plane of section

Angle of view

Uterus (*pulled up*)

Internal iliac artery and vein

Linea terminalis (pelvic brim)

Mesovarium

Ovary

Broad ligament

Uterine (Fallopian) tube

Cut edge of peritoneum forming floor of paravesical pouch

Round ligament of uterus

Suspensory ligament of ovary

Ligament of ovary

Cervix of uterus

Uterine vessels

Cardinal (transverse cervical or Mackenrodt's) ligament

Obturator membrane

Obturator fascia

Tendinous arch of levator ani muscle

Obturator internus muscle

Vaginal artery

Levator ani muscle (iliococcygeus and pubococcygeus muscles)

Ureter

Uterovaginal fascia

Inferior pubic ramus

Anterior recess of ischioanal fossa

Compressor urethralis muscle

Crus of clitoris

Ischiocavernosus muscle

Perineal membrane

Fascia lata of thigh

Artery of bulb of vestibule

Superficial perineal space

Sphincter urethrovaginalis muscle

Perineal artery

Terminal part of round ligament of uterus

Superficial perineal (Colles') fascia

Labium majus

Bulbospongiosus muscle and deep perineal (investing or Gallaudet's) fascia

Labium minus

Bulb of vestibule

Vestibule

Vaginal wall

Vagina

Hymenal caruncle

Uterus and Adnexa

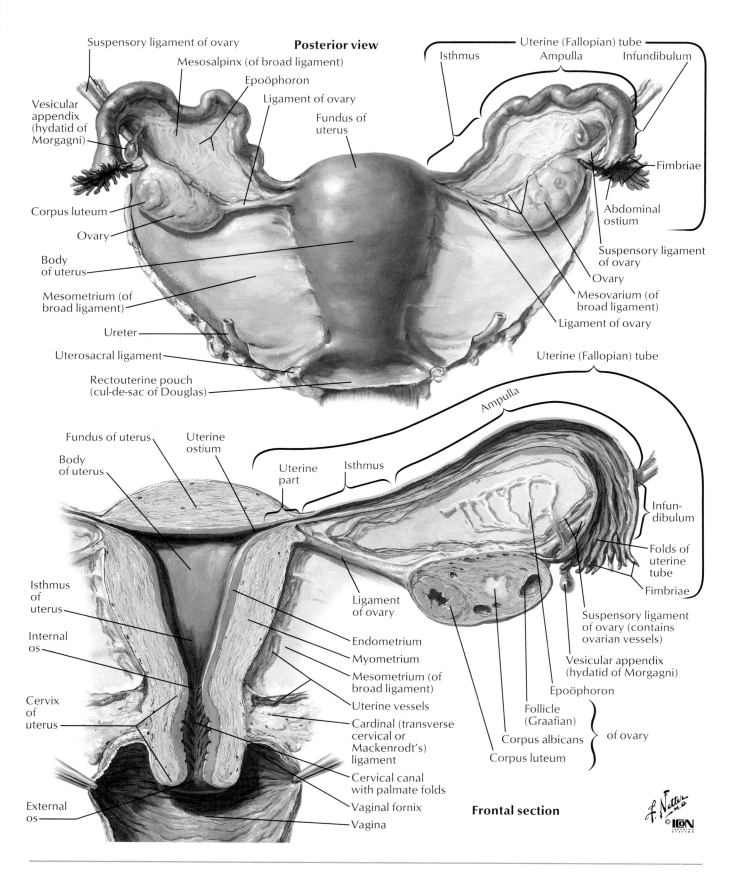

Posterior view

Suspensory ligament of ovary

Mesosalpinx (of broad ligament)

Epoöphoron

Ligament of ovary

Fundus of uterus

Vesicular appendix (hydatid of Morgagni)

Corpus luteum

Ovary

Body of uterus

Mesometrium (of broad ligament)

Ureter

Uterosacral ligament

Rectouterine pouch (cul-de-sac of Douglas)

Isthmus

Uterine (Fallopian) tube

Ampulla

Infundibulum

Fimbriae

Abdominal ostium

Suspensory ligament of ovary

Ovary

Mesovarium (of broad ligament)

Ligament of ovary

Uterine (Fallopian) tube

Ampulla

Fundus of uterus

Uterine ostium

Body of uterus

Uterine part

Isthmus

Isthmus of uterus

Internal os

Cervix of uterus

External os

Ligament of ovary

Endometrium

Myometrium

Mesometrium (of broad ligament)

Uterine vessels

Cardinal (transverse cervical or Mackenrodt's) ligament

Cervical canal with palmate folds

Vaginal fornix

Vagina

Infundibulum

Folds of uterine tube

Fimbriae

Suspensory ligament of ovary (contains ovarian vessels)

Vesicular appendix (hydatid of Morgagni)

Epoöphoron

Follicle (Graafian)

Corpus albicans

Corpus luteum

of ovary

Frontal section

PLATE 356

PELVIS AND PERINEUM

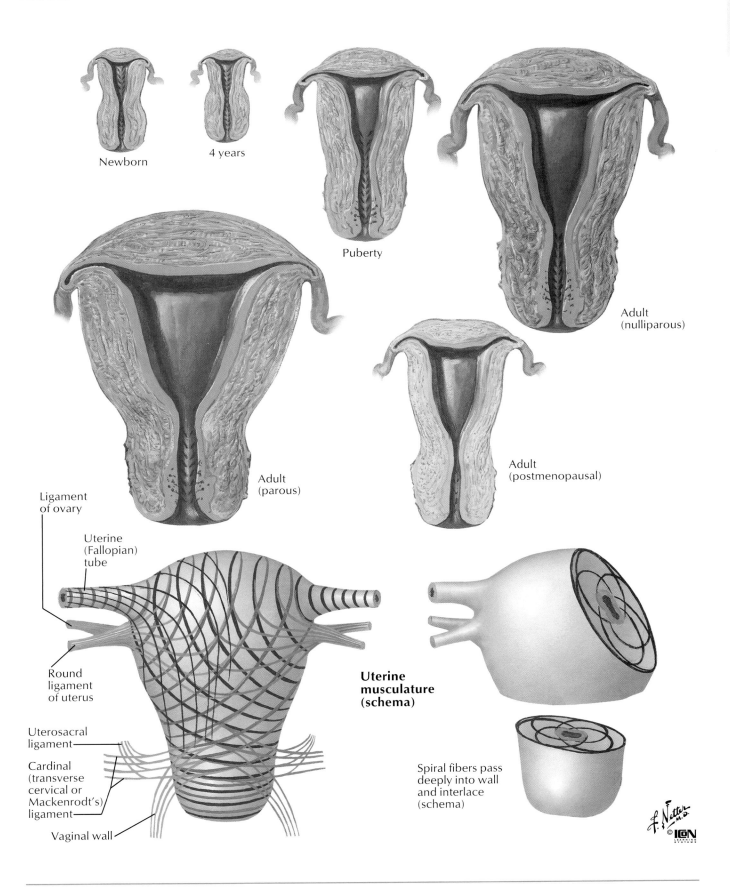

Newborn

4 years

Puberty

Adult
(nulliparous)

Adult
(parous)

Adult
(postmenopausal)

Ligament
of ovary

Uterine
(Fallopian)
tube

Round
ligament
of uterus

Uterosacral
ligament

Cardinal
(transverse
cervical or
Mackenrodt's)
ligament

Vaginal wall

**Uterine
musculature
(schema)**

Spiral fibers pass
deeply into wall
and interlace
(schema)

Uterus: Variations in Position

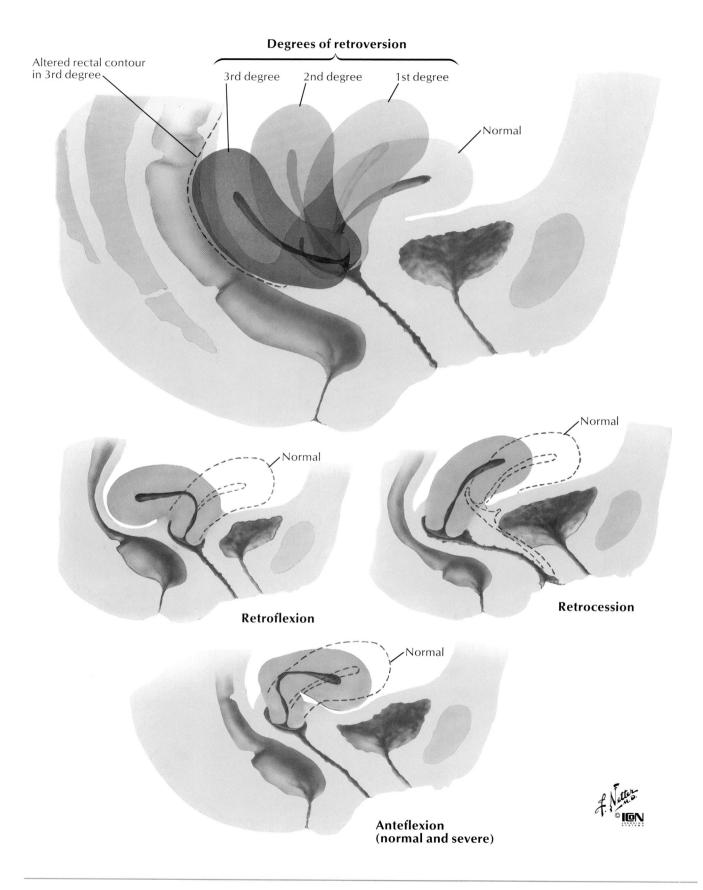

Degrees of retroversion

Altered rectal contour in 3rd degree

3rd degree   2nd degree   1st degree

Normal

Normal

Retroflexion

Normal

Retrocession

Normal

Anteflexion
(normal and severe)

PLATE 358

PELVIS AND PERINEUM

Perineum and External Genitalia (Pudendum or Vulva)

SEE ALSO PLATES 384, 386, 387, 393

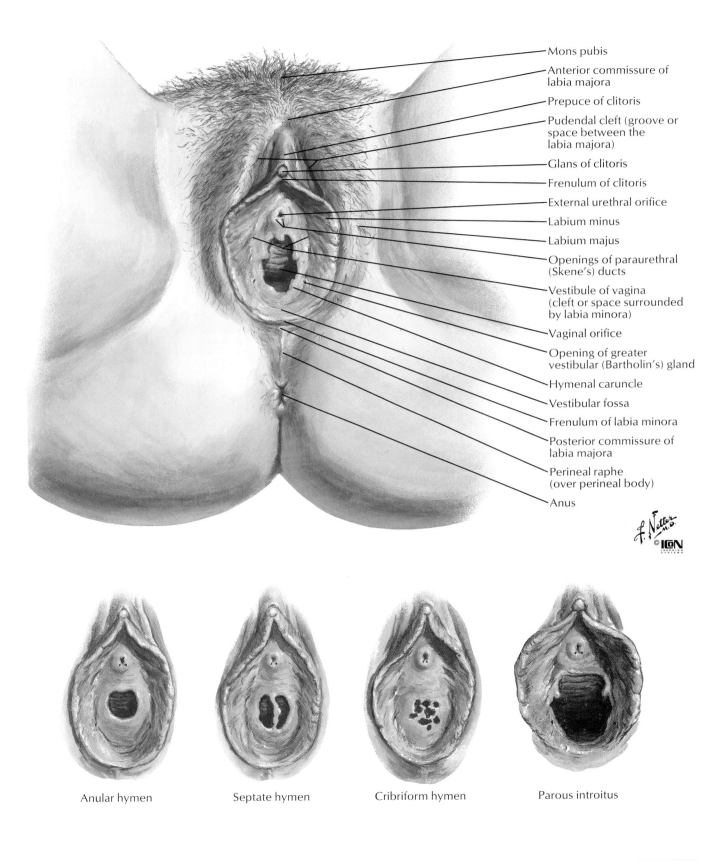

Mons pubis

Anterior commissure of labia majora

Prepuce of clitoris

Pudendal cleft (groove or space between the labia majora)

Glans of clitoris

Frenulum of clitoris

External urethral orifice

Labium minus

Labium majus

Openings of paraurethral (Skene's) ducts

Vestibule of vagina (cleft or space surrounded by labia minora)

Vaginal orifice

Opening of greater vestibular (Bartholin's) gland

Hymenal caruncle

Vestibular fossa

Frenulum of labia minora

Posterior commissure of labia majora

Perineal raphe (over perineal body)

Anus

| Anular hymen | Septate hymen | Cribriform hymen | Parous introitus |

FEMALE STRUCTURES

PLATE 359

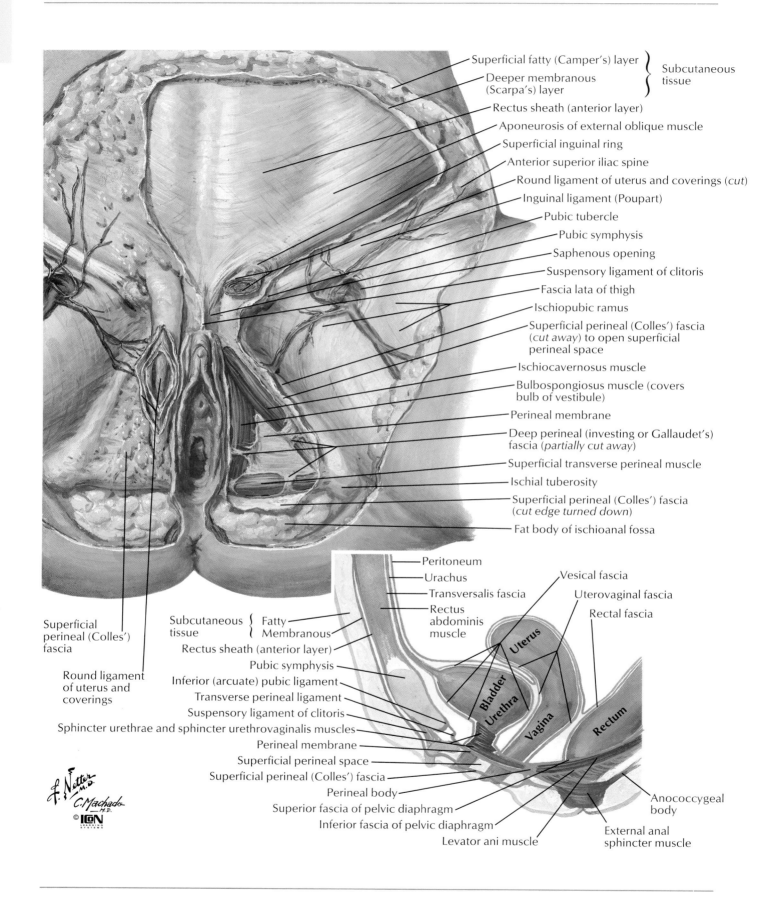

Superficial fatty (Camper's) layer ⎫
Deeper membranous (Scarpa's) layer ⎬ Subcutaneous tissue
Rectus sheath (anterior layer)
Aponeurosis of external oblique muscle
Superficial inguinal ring
Anterior superior iliac spine
Round ligament of uterus and coverings (cut)
Inguinal ligament (Poupart)
Pubic tubercle
Pubic symphysis
Saphenous opening
Suspensory ligament of clitoris
Fascia lata of thigh
Ischiopubic ramus
Superficial perineal (Colles') fascia (cut away) to open superficial perineal space
Ischiocavernosus muscle
Bulbospongiosus muscle (covers bulb of vestibule)
Perineal membrane
Deep perineal (investing or Gallaudet's) fascia (partially cut away)
Superficial transverse perineal muscle
Ischial tuberosity
Superficial perineal (Colles') fascia (cut edge turned down)
Fat body of ischioanal fossa

Superficial perineal (Colles') fascia

Round ligament of uterus and coverings

Subcutaneous tissue ⎰ Fatty
⎱ Membranous
Rectus sheath (anterior layer)
Pubic symphysis
Inferior (arcuate) pubic ligament
Transverse perineal ligament
Suspensory ligament of clitoris
Sphincter urethrae and sphincter urethrovaginalis muscles
Perineal membrane
Superficial perineal space
Superficial perineal (Colles') fascia
Perineal body
Superior fascia of pelvic diaphragm
Inferior fascia of pelvic diaphragm
Levator ani muscle

Peritoneum
Urachus
Transversalis fascia
Rectus abdominis muscle
Vesical fascia
Uterovaginal fascia
Rectal fascia

Uterus
Bladder
Urethra
Vagina
Rectum

Anococcygeal body

External anal sphincter muscle

PLATE 360

PELVIS AND PERINEUM

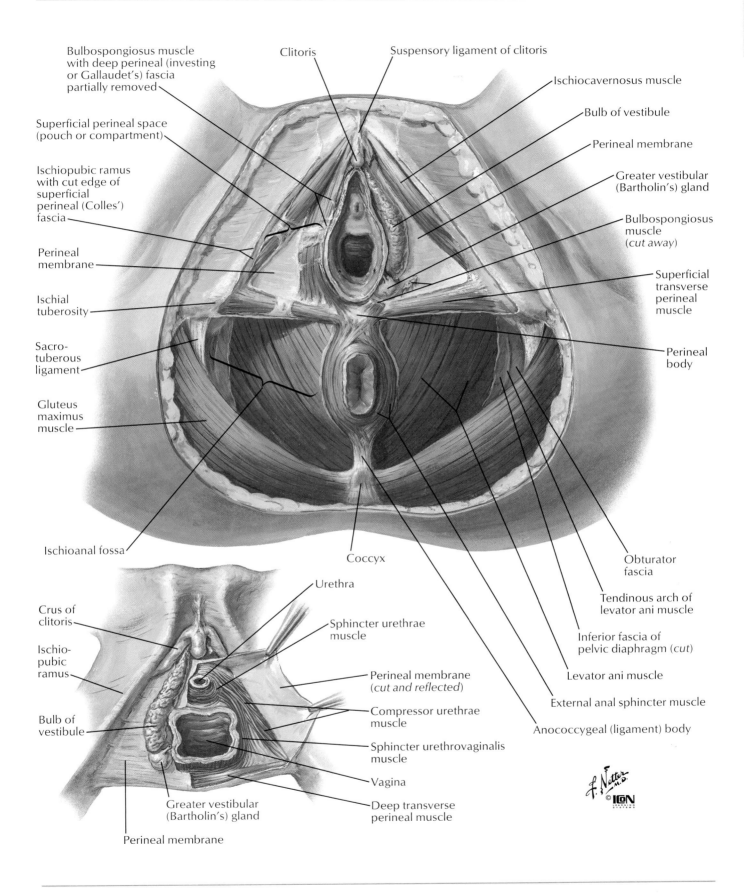

Bulbospongiosus muscle with deep perineal (investing or Gallaudet's) fascia partially removed

Clitoris

Suspensory ligament of clitoris

Ischiocavernosus muscle

Bulb of vestibule

Perineal membrane

Superficial perineal space (pouch or compartment)

Greater vestibular (Bartholin's) gland

Ischiopubic ramus with cut edge of superficial perineal (Colles') fascia

Bulbospongiosus muscle (*cut away*)

Perineal membrane

Superficial transverse perineal muscle

Ischial tuberosity

Sacro-tuberous ligament

Perineal body

Gluteus maximus muscle

Ischioanal fossa

Coccyx

Obturator fascia

Tendinous arch of levator ani muscle

Crus of clitoris

Urethra

Sphincter urethrae muscle

Inferior fascia of pelvic diaphragm (*cut*)

Ischio-pubic ramus

Perineal membrane (*cut and reflected*)

Levator ani muscle

Compressor urethrae muscle

External anal sphincter muscle

Bulb of vestibule

Sphincter urethrovaginalis muscle

Anococcygeal (ligament) body

Vagina

Greater vestibular (Bartholin's) gland

Deep transverse perineal muscle

Perineal membrane

SEE ALSO PLATES 347, 352

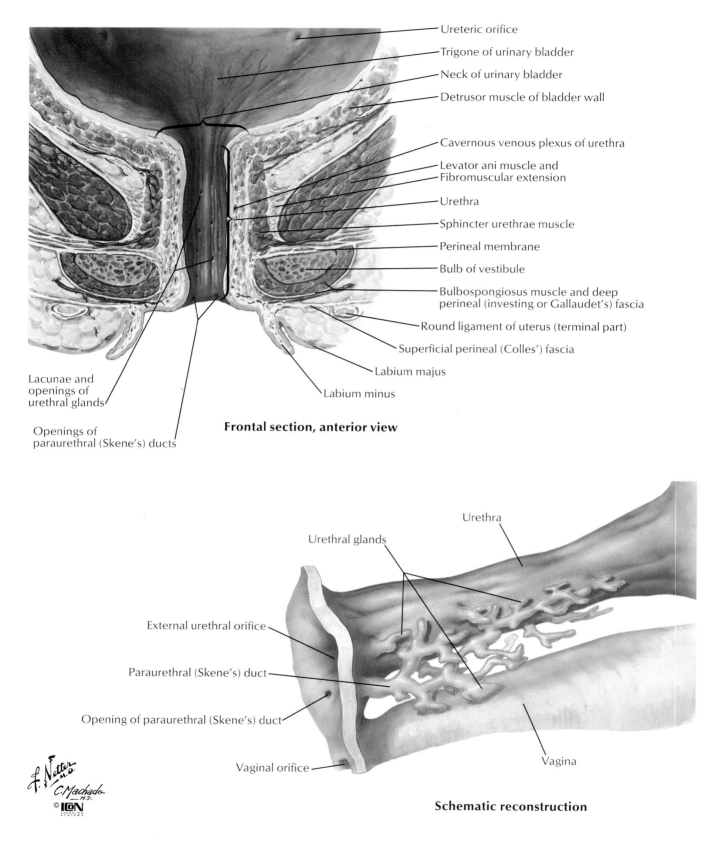

Ureteric orifice

Trigone of urinary bladder

Neck of urinary bladder

Detrusor muscle of bladder wall

Cavernous venous plexus of urethra

Levator ani muscle and
Fibromuscular extension

Urethra

Sphincter urethrae muscle

Perineal membrane

Bulb of vestibule

Bulbospongiosus muscle and deep
perineal (investing or Gallaudet's) fascia

Round ligament of uterus (terminal part)

Superficial perineal (Colles') fascia

Labium majus

Labium minus

Lacunae and
openings of
urethral glands

Openings of
paraurethral (Skene's) ducts

Frontal section, anterior view

Urethra

Urethral glands

External urethral orifice

Paraurethral (Skene's) duct

Opening of paraurethral (Skene's) duct

Vaginal orifice

Vagina

Schematic reconstruction

PLATE 362

PELVIS AND PERINEUM

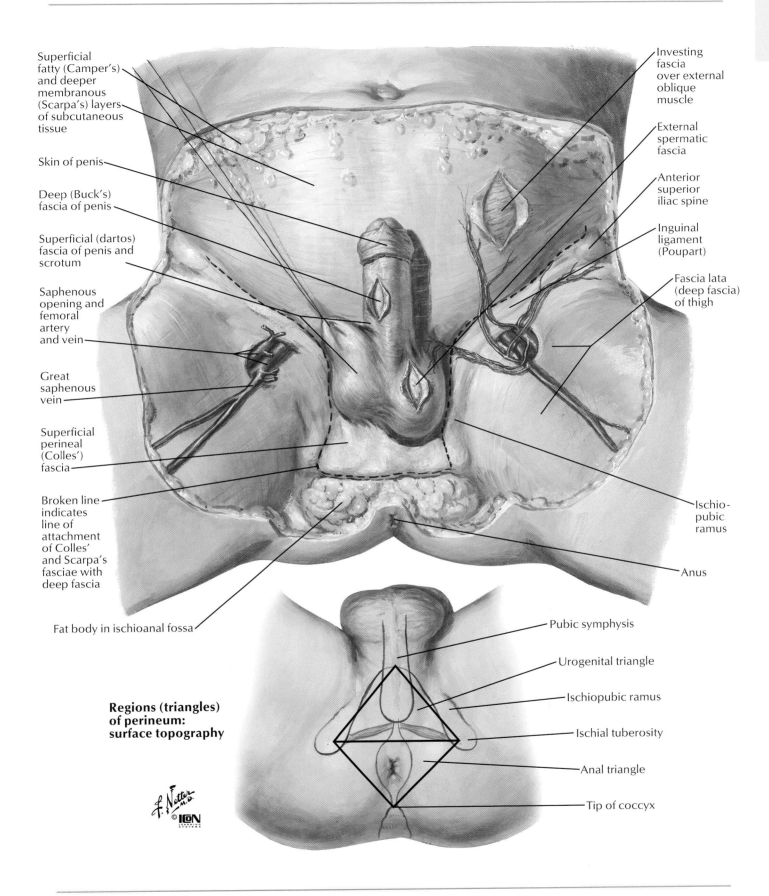

Superficial fatty (Camper's) and deeper membranous (Scarpa's) layers of subcutaneous tissue

Skin of penis

Deep (Buck's) fascia of penis

Superficial (dartos) fascia of penis and scrotum

Saphenous opening and femoral artery and vein

Great saphenous vein

Superficial perineal (Colles') fascia

Broken line indicates line of attachment of Colles' and Scarpa's fasciae with deep fascia

Fat body in ischioanal fossa

Investing fascia over external oblique muscle

External spermatic fascia

Anterior superior iliac spine

Inguinal ligament (Poupart)

Fascia lata (deep fascia) of thigh

Ischio-pubic ramus

Anus

Regions (triangles) of perineum: surface topography

Pubic symphysis

Urogenital triangle

Ischiopubic ramus

Ischial tuberosity

Anal triangle

Tip of coccyx

MALE STRUCTURES

PLATE 363

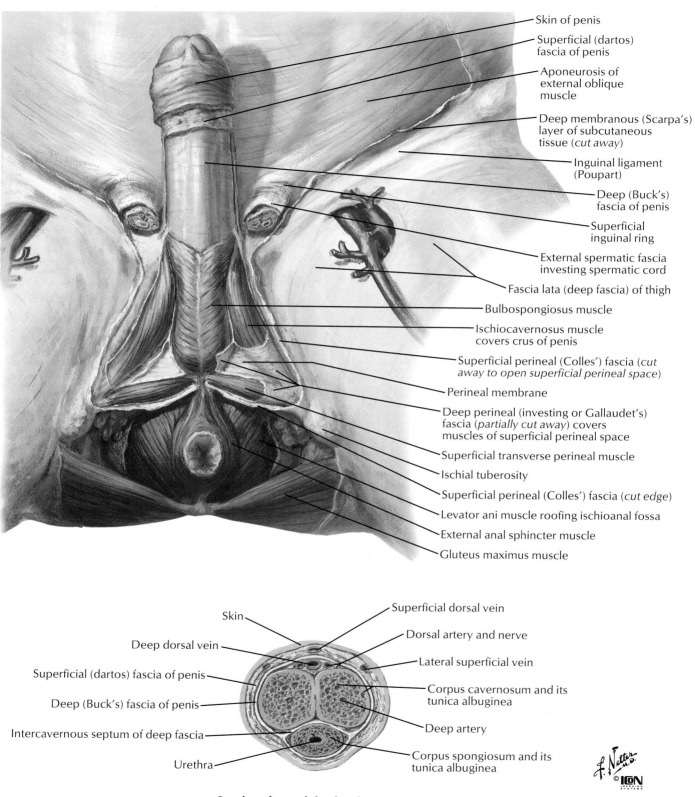

Skin of penis

Superficial (dartos) fascia of penis

Aponeurosis of external oblique muscle

Deep membranous (Scarpa's) layer of subcutaneous tissue (cut away)

Inguinal ligament (Poupart)

Deep (Buck's) fascia of penis

Superficial inguinal ring

External spermatic fascia investing spermatic cord

Fascia lata (deep fascia) of thigh

Bulbospongiosus muscle

Ischiocavernosus muscle covers crus of penis

Superficial perineal (Colles') fascia (cut away to open superficial perineal space)

Perineal membrane

Deep perineal (investing or Gallaudet's) fascia (partially cut away) covers muscles of superficial perineal space

Superficial transverse perineal muscle

Ischial tuberosity

Superficial perineal (Colles') fascia (cut edge)

Levator ani muscle roofing ischioanal fossa

External anal sphincter muscle

Gluteus maximus muscle

Skin

Superficial dorsal vein

Deep dorsal vein

Dorsal artery and nerve

Superficial (dartos) fascia of penis

Lateral superficial vein

Deep (Buck's) fascia of penis

Corpus cavernosum and its tunica albuginea

Intercavernous septum of deep fascia

Deep artery

Urethra

Corpus spongiosum and its tunica albuginea

Section through body of penis

PLATE 364

PELVIS AND PERINEUM

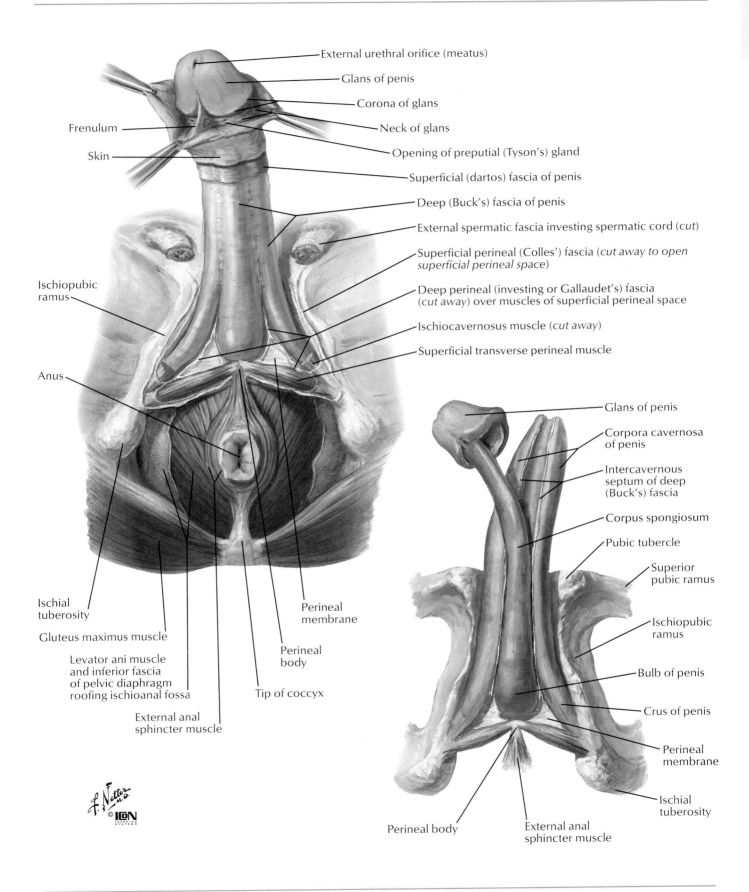

External urethral orifice (meatus)

Glans of penis

Corona of glans

Frenulum

Neck of glans

Skin

Opening of preputial (Tyson's) gland

Superficial (dartos) fascia of penis

Deep (Buck's) fascia of penis

External spermatic fascia investing spermatic cord (*cut*)

Superficial perineal (Colles') fascia (*cut away to open superficial perineal space*)

Ischiopubic ramus

Deep perineal (investing or Gallaudet's) fascia (*cut away*) over muscles of superficial perineal space

Ischiocavernosus muscle (*cut away*)

Superficial transverse perineal muscle

Anus

Glans of penis

Corpora cavernosa of penis

Intercavernous septum of deep (Buck's) fascia

Corpus spongiosum

Pubic tubercle

Superior pubic ramus

Ischial tuberosity

Ischiopubic ramus

Gluteus maximus muscle

Perineal membrane

Bulb of penis

Levator ani muscle and inferior fascia of pelvic diaphragm roofing ischioanal fossa

Perineal body

Crus of penis

External anal sphincter muscle

Tip of coccyx

Perineal membrane

Perineal body

External anal sphincter muscle

Ischial tuberosity

Perineal Spaces

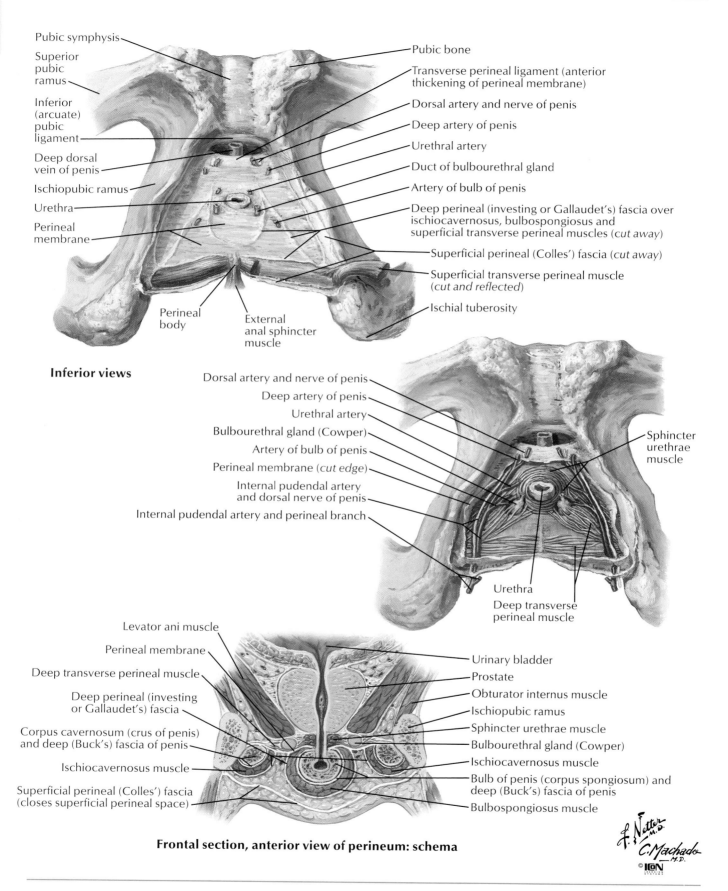

Pubic symphysis

Superior pubic ramus

Inferior (arcuate) pubic ligament

Deep dorsal vein of penis

Ischiopubic ramus

Urethra

Perineal membrane

Perineal body

External anal sphincter muscle

Pubic bone

Transverse perineal ligament (anterior thickening of perineal membrane)

Dorsal artery and nerve of penis

Deep artery of penis

Urethral artery

Duct of bulbourethral gland

Artery of bulb of penis

Deep perineal (investing or Gallaudet's) fascia over ischiocavernosus, bulbospongiosus and superficial transverse perineal muscles (*cut away*)

Superficial perineal (Colles') fascia (*cut away*)

Superficial transverse perineal muscle (*cut and reflected*)

Ischial tuberosity

Inferior views

Dorsal artery and nerve of penis

Deep artery of penis

Urethral artery

Bulbourethral gland (Cowper)

Artery of bulb of penis

Perineal membrane (*cut edge*)

Internal pudendal artery and dorsal nerve of penis

Internal pudendal artery and perineal branch

Sphincter urethrae muscle

Urethra

Deep transverse perineal muscle

Levator ani muscle

Perineal membrane

Deep transverse perineal muscle

Deep perineal (investing or Gallaudet's) fascia

Corpus cavernosum (crus of penis) and deep (Buck's) fascia of penis

Ischiocavernosus muscle

Superficial perineal (Colles') fascia (closes superficial perineal space)

Urinary bladder

Prostate

Obturator internus muscle

Ischiopubic ramus

Sphincter urethrae muscle

Bulbourethral gland (Cowper)

Ischiocavernosus muscle

Bulb of penis (corpus spongiosum) and deep (Buck's) fascia of penis

Bulbospongiosus muscle

Frontal section, anterior view of perineum: schema

PLATE 366

PELVIS AND PERINEUM

SEE ALSO PLATES 348, 350, 353, 383, 390

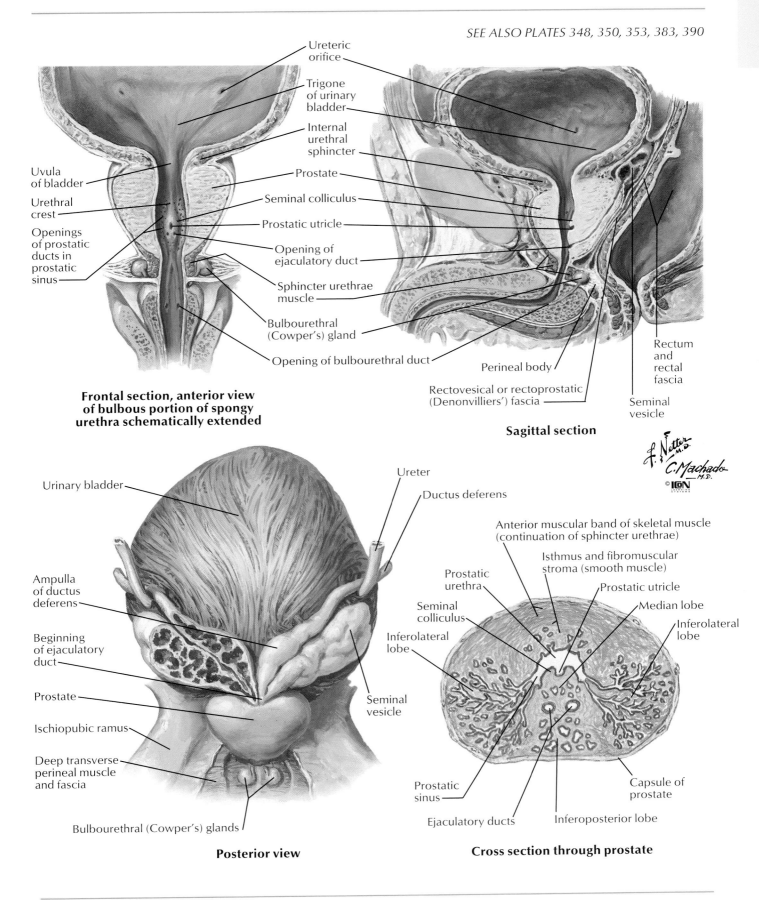

Ureteric orifice

Trigone of urinary bladder

Internal urethral sphincter

Uvula of bladder

Urethral crest

Openings of prostatic ducts in prostatic sinus

Prostate

Seminal colliculus

Prostatic utricle

Opening of ejaculatory duct

Sphincter urethrae muscle

Bulbourethral (Cowper's) gland

Opening of bulbourethral duct

Rectum and rectal fascia

Rectovesical or rectoprostatic (Denonvilliers') fascia

Perineal body

Seminal vesicle

Frontal section, anterior view of bulbous portion of spongy urethra schematically extended

Sagittal section

Urinary bladder

Ureter

Ductus deferens

Ampulla of ductus deferens

Beginning of ejaculatory duct

Prostate

Ischiopubic ramus

Deep transverse perineal muscle and fascia

Bulbourethral (Cowper's) glands

Seminal vesicle

Posterior view

Anterior muscular band of skeletal muscle (continuation of sphincter urethrae)

Isthmus and fibromuscular stroma (smooth muscle)

Prostatic urethra

Prostatic utricle

Seminal colliculus

Median lobe

Inferolateral lobe

Inferolateral lobe

Prostatic sinus

Ejaculatory ducts

Inferoposterior lobe

Capsule of prostate

Cross section through prostate

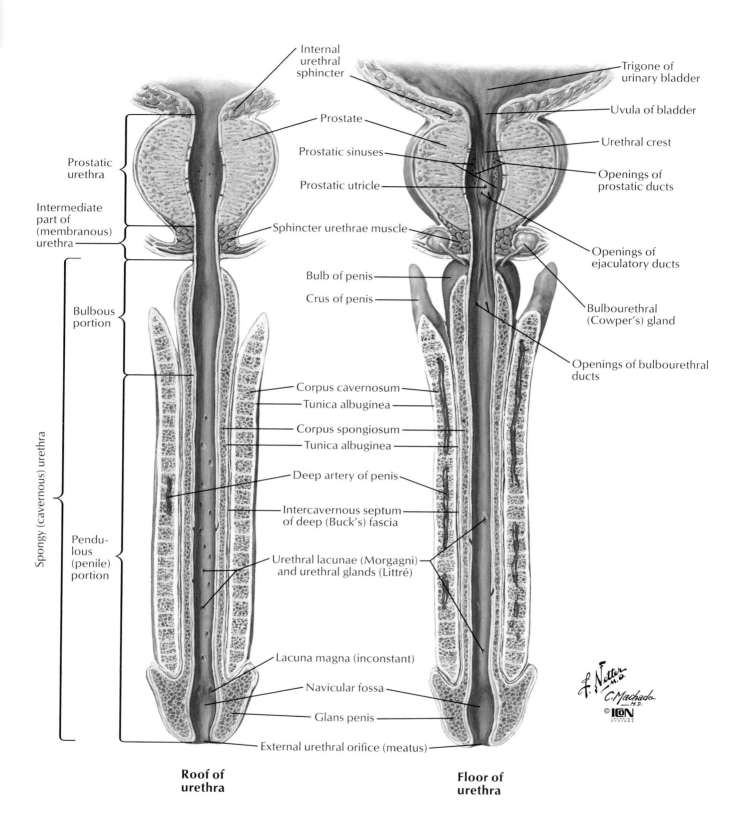

Internal urethral sphincter

Trigone of urinary bladder

Prostate

Uvula of bladder

Prostatic sinuses

Urethral crest

Prostatic utricle

Openings of prostatic ducts

Sphincter urethrae muscle

Openings of ejaculatory ducts

Bulb of penis

Crus of penis

Bulbourethral (Cowper's) gland

Openings of bulbourethral ducts

Corpus cavernosum

Tunica albuginea

Corpus spongiosum

Tunica albuginea

Deep artery of penis

Intercavernous septum of deep (Buck's) fascia

Urethral lacunae (Morgagni) and urethral glands (Littré)

Lacuna magna (inconstant)

Navicular fossa

Glans penis

External urethral orifice (meatus)

Prostatic urethra

Intermediate part of (membranous) urethra

Bulbous portion

Spongy (cavernous) urethra

Pendu-lous (penile) portion

Roof of urethra

Floor of urethra

PLATE 368

PELVIS AND PERINEUM

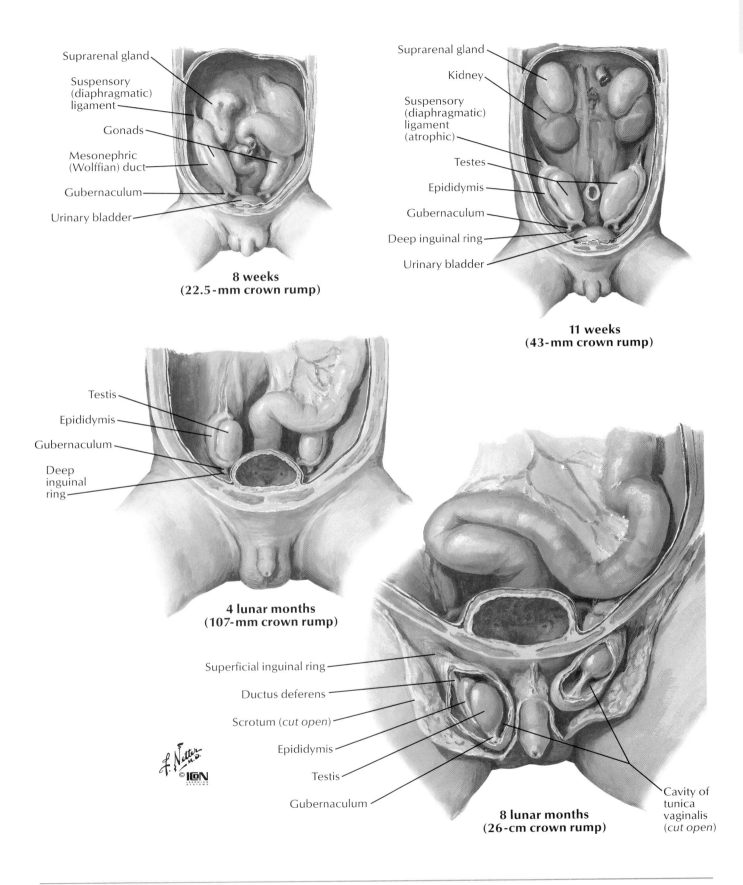

Suprarenal gland
Suspensory (diaphragmatic) ligament
Gonads
Mesonephric (Wolffian) duct
Gubernaculum
Urinary bladder

8 weeks
(22.5-mm crown rump)

Suprarenal gland
Kidney
Suspensory (diaphragmatic) ligament (atrophic)
Testes
Epididymis
Gubernaculum
Deep inguinal ring
Urinary bladder

11 weeks
(43-mm crown rump)

Testis
Epididymis
Gubernaculum
Deep inguinal ring

4 lunar months
(107-mm crown rump)

Superficial inguinal ring
Ductus deferens
Scrotum (*cut open*)
Epididymis
Testis
Gubernaculum

Cavity of tunica vaginalis (*cut open*)

8 lunar months
(26-cm crown rump)

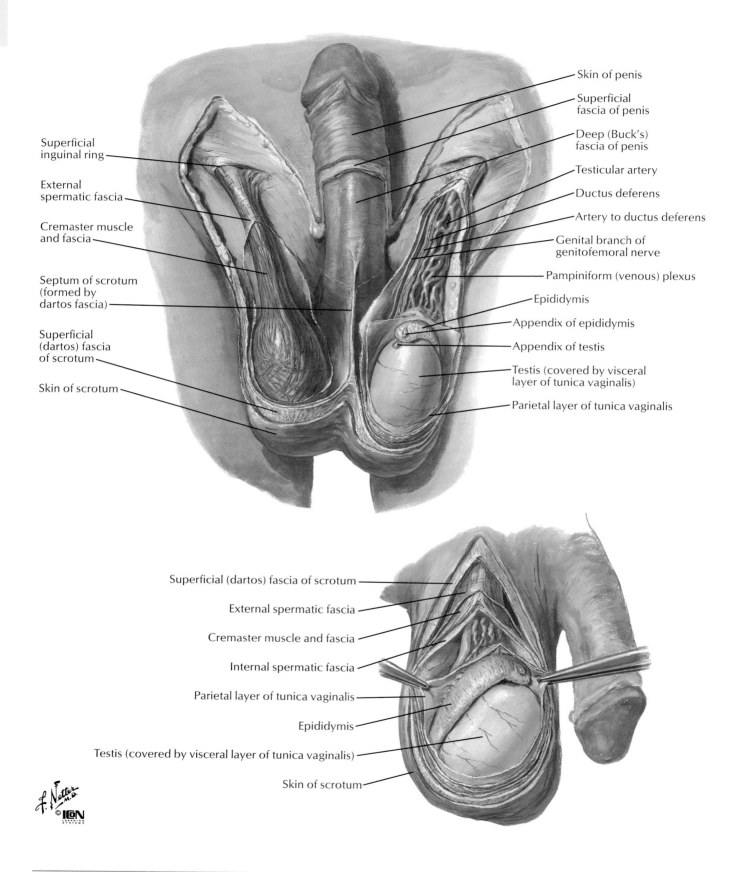

Skin of penis

Superficial fascia of penis

Deep (Buck's) fascia of penis

Testicular artery

Ductus deferens

Artery to ductus deferens

Genital branch of genitofemoral nerve

Pampiniform (venous) plexus

Epididymis

Appendix of epididymis

Appendix of testis

Testis (covered by visceral layer of tunica vaginalis)

Parietal layer of tunica vaginalis

Superficial inguinal ring

External spermatic fascia

Cremaster muscle and fascia

Septum of scrotum (formed by dartos fascia)

Superficial (dartos) fascia of scrotum

Skin of scrotum

Superficial (dartos) fascia of scrotum

External spermatic fascia

Cremaster muscle and fascia

Internal spermatic fascia

Parietal layer of tunica vaginalis

Epididymis

Testis (covered by visceral layer of tunica vaginalis)

Skin of scrotum

PLATE 370

PELVIS AND PERINEUM

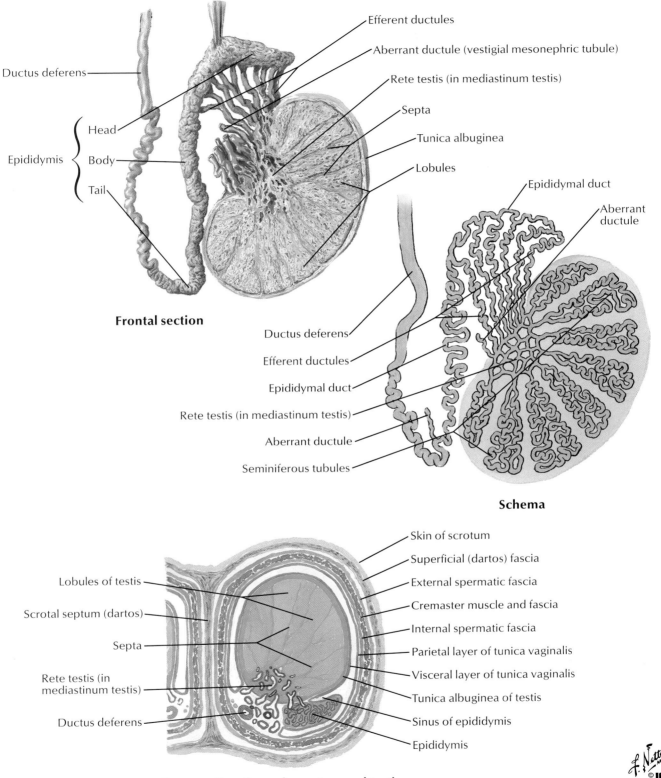

Frontal section

Ductus deferens

Epididymis
{
Head
Body
Tail
}

Efferent ductules

Aberrant ductule (vestigial mesonephric tubule)

Rete testis (in mediastinum testis)

Septa

Tunica albuginea

Lobules

Schema

Epididymal duct

Aberrant ductule

Ductus deferens

Efferent ductules

Epididymal duct

Rete testis (in mediastinum testis)

Aberrant ductule

Seminiferous tubules

Cross section through scrotum and testis

Lobules of testis

Scrotal septum (dartos)

Septa

Rete testis (in mediastinum testis)

Ductus deferens

Skin of scrotum

Superficial (dartos) fascia

External spermatic fascia

Cremaster muscle and fascia

Internal spermatic fascia

Parietal layer of tunica vaginalis

Visceral layer of tunica vaginalis

Tunica albuginea of testis

Sinus of epididymis

Epididymis

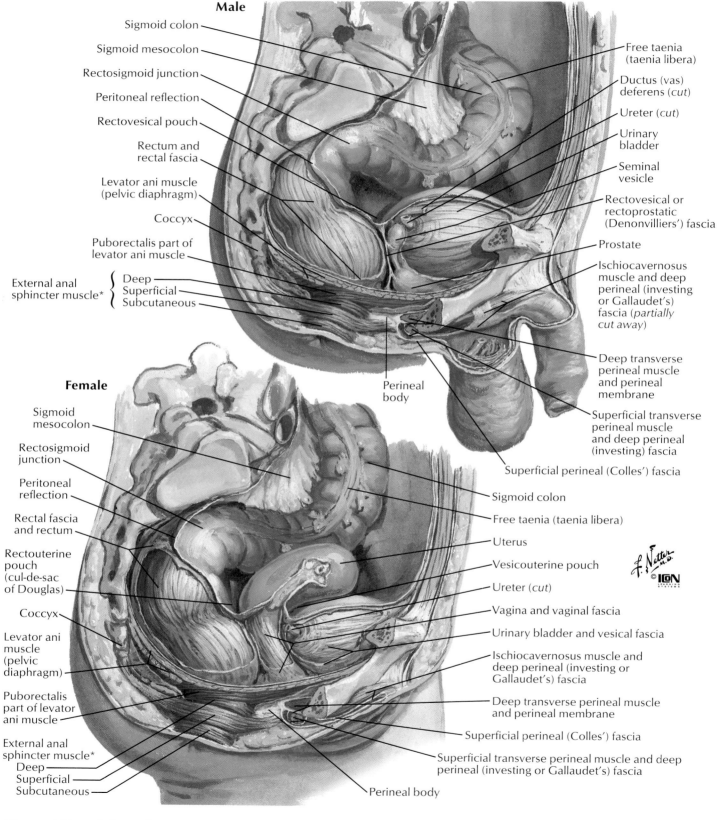

Male

Sigmoid colon

Sigmoid mesocolon

Rectosigmoid junction

Peritoneal reflection

Rectovesical pouch

Rectum and rectal fascia

Levator ani muscle (pelvic diaphragm)

Coccyx

Puborectalis part of levator ani muscle

External anal sphincter muscle*
{ Deep
Superficial
Subcutaneous

Free taenia (taenia libera)

Ductus (vas) deferens (*cut*)

Ureter (*cut*)

Urinary bladder

Seminal vesicle

Rectovesical or rectoprostatic (Denonvilliers') fascia

Prostate

Ischiocavernosus muscle and deep perineal (investing or Gallaudet's) fascia (*partially cut away*)

Deep transverse perineal muscle and perineal membrane

Superficial transverse perineal muscle and deep perineal (investing) fascia

Superficial perineal (Colles') fascia

Perineal body

Female

Sigmoid mesocolon

Rectosigmoid junction

Peritoneal reflection

Rectal fascia and rectum

Rectouterine pouch (cul-de-sac of Douglas)

Coccyx

Levator ani muscle (pelvic diaphragm)

Puborectalis part of levator ani muscle

External anal sphincter muscle*
Deep
Superficial
Subcutaneous

Sigmoid colon

Free taenia (taenia libera)

Uterus

Vesicouterine pouch

Ureter (*cut*)

Vagina and vaginal fascia

Urinary bladder and vesical fascia

Ischiocavernosus muscle and deep perineal (investing or Gallaudet's) fascia

Deep transverse perineal muscle and perineal membrane

Superficial perineal (Colles') fascia

Superficial transverse perineal muscle and deep perineal (investing or Gallaudet's) fascia

Perineal body

*Parts variable and often indistinct

PLATE 372

PELVIS AND PERINEUM

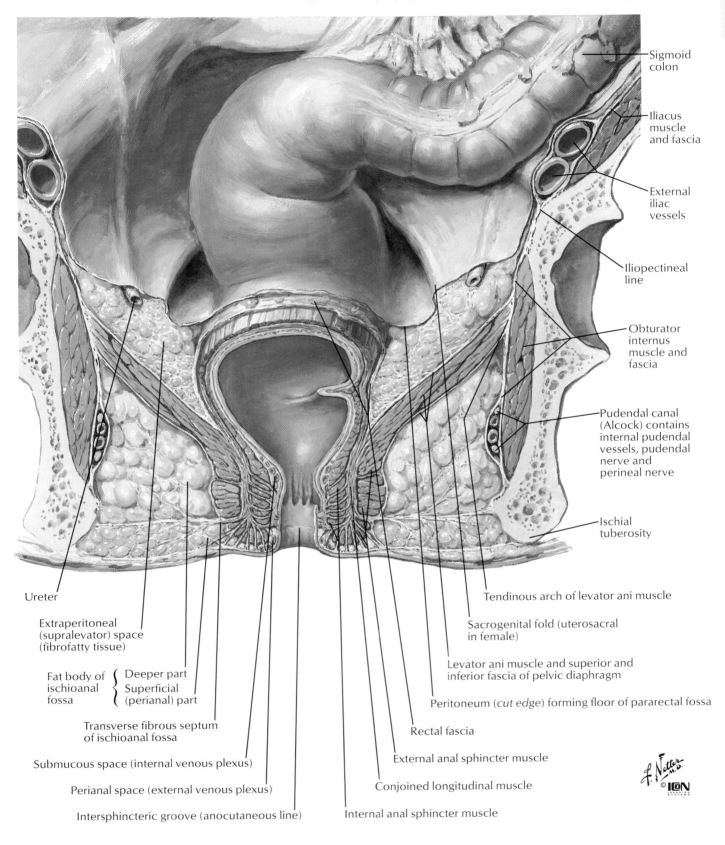

Sigmoid colon

Iliacus muscle and fascia

External iliac vessels

Iliopectineal line

Obturator internus muscle and fascia

Pudendal canal (Alcock) contains internal pudendal vessels, pudendal nerve and perineal nerve

Ischial tuberosity

Tendinous arch of levator ani muscle

Sacrogenital fold (uterosacral in female)

Levator ani muscle and superior and inferior fascia of pelvic diaphragm

Peritoneum (*cut edge*) forming floor of pararectal fossa

Rectal fascia

External anal sphincter muscle

Conjoined longitudinal muscle

Internal anal sphincter muscle

Ureter

Extraperitoneal (supralevator) space (fibrofatty tissue)

Fat body of ischioanal fossa { Deeper part / Superficial (perianal) part

Transverse fibrous septum of ischioanal fossa

Submucous space (internal venous plexus)

Perianal space (external venous plexus)

Intersphincteric groove (anocutaneous line)

Rectum and Anal Canal

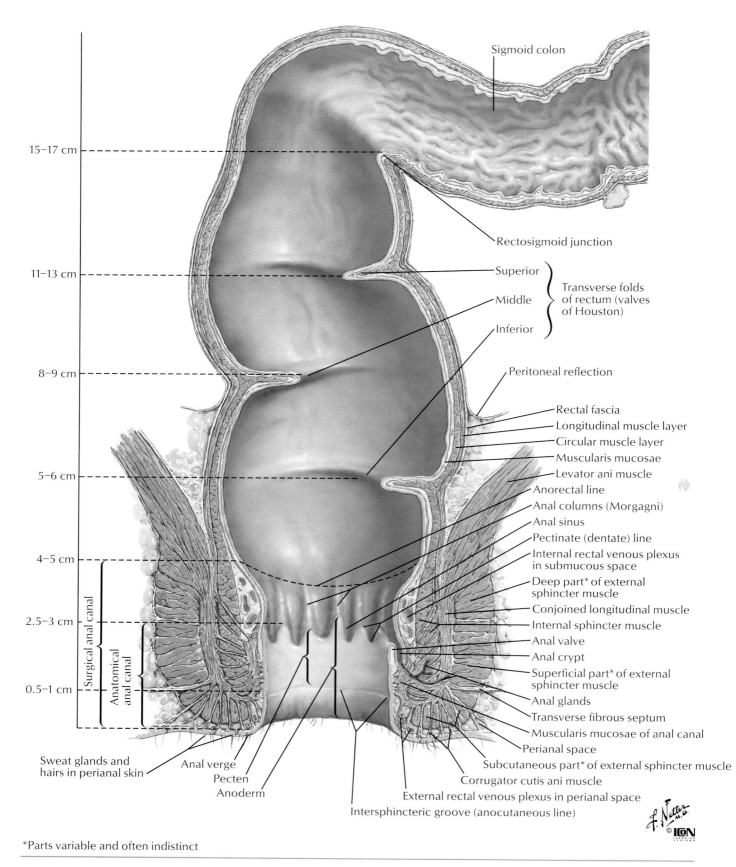

Sigmoid colon

Rectosigmoid junction

Superior
Middle
Inferior
} Transverse folds of rectum (valves of Houston)

Peritoneal reflection

Rectal fascia
Longitudinal muscle layer
Circular muscle layer
Muscularis mucosae
Levator ani muscle
Anorectal line
Anal columns (Morgagni)
Anal sinus
Pectinate (dentate) line
Internal rectal venous plexus in submucous space
Deep part* of external sphincter muscle
Conjoined longitudinal muscle
Internal sphincter muscle
Anal valve
Anal crypt
Superficial part* of external sphincter muscle
Anal glands
Transverse fibrous septum
Muscularis mucosae of anal canal
Perianal space
Subcutaneous part* of external sphincter muscle
Corrugator cutis ani muscle
External rectal venous plexus in perianal space

15–17 cm
11–13 cm
8–9 cm
5–6 cm
4–5 cm
2.5–3 cm
0.5–1 cm

Surgical anal canal
Anatomical anal canal

Sweat glands and hairs in perianal skin
Anal verge
Pecten
Anoderm
Intersphincteric groove (anocutaneous line)

*Parts variable and often indistinct

PLATE 374

PELVIS AND PERINEUM

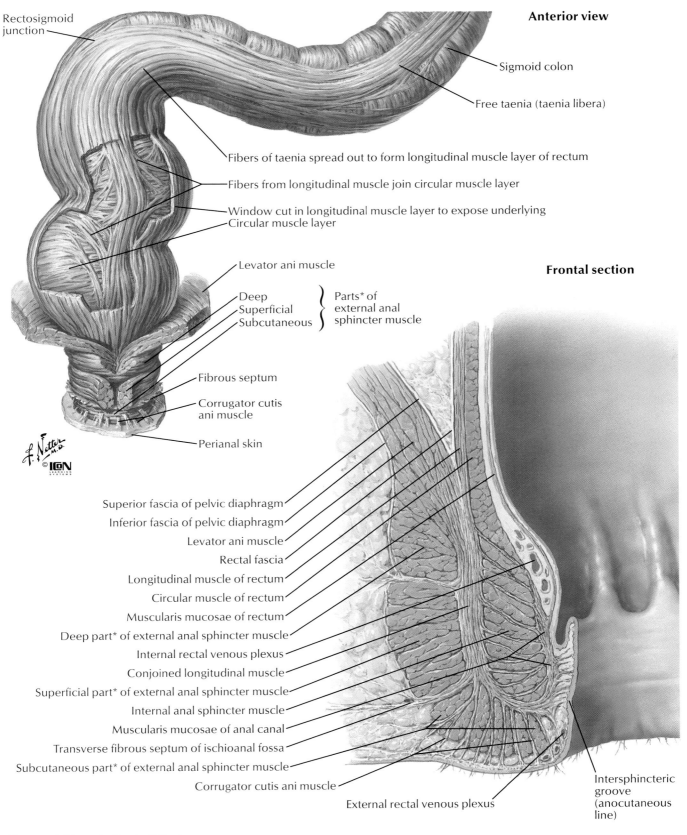

Anterior view

Rectosigmoid junction

Sigmoid colon

Free taenia (taenia libera)

Fibers of taenia spread out to form longitudinal muscle layer of rectum

Fibers from longitudinal muscle join circular muscle layer

Window cut in longitudinal muscle layer to expose underlying
Circular muscle layer

Levator ani muscle

Frontal section

Deep
Superficial
Subcutaneous

Parts* of external anal sphincter muscle

Fibrous septum

Corrugator cutis ani muscle

Perianal skin

Superior fascia of pelvic diaphragm
Inferior fascia of pelvic diaphragm
Levator ani muscle
Rectal fascia
Longitudinal muscle of rectum
Circular muscle of rectum
Muscularis mucosae of rectum
Deep part* of external anal sphincter muscle
Internal rectal venous plexus
Conjoined longitudinal muscle
Superficial part* of external anal sphincter muscle
Internal anal sphincter muscle
Muscularis mucosae of anal canal
Transverse fibrous septum of ischioanal fossa
Subcutaneous part* of external anal sphincter muscle
Corrugator cutis ani muscle

External rectal venous plexus

Intersphincteric groove (anocutaneous line)

*Parts variable and often indistinct

RECTUM

PLATE 375

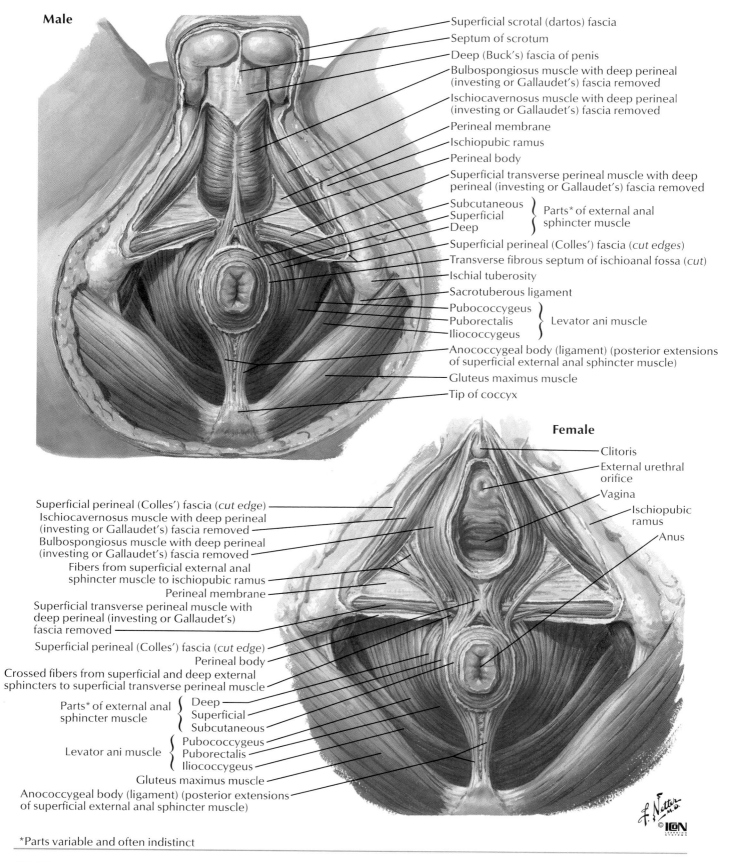

Male

Superficial scrotal (dartos) fascia
Septum of scrotum
Deep (Buck's) fascia of penis
Bulbospongiosus muscle with deep perineal (investing or Gallaudet's) fascia removed
Ischiocavernosus muscle with deep perineal (investing or Gallaudet's) fascia removed
Perineal membrane
Ischiopubic ramus
Perineal body
Superficial transverse perineal muscle with deep perineal (investing or Gallaudet's) fascia removed
Subcutaneous
Superficial   } Parts* of external anal
Deep   sphincter muscle
Superficial perineal (Colles') fascia (cut edges)
Transverse fibrous septum of ischioanal fossa (cut)
Ischial tuberosity
Sacrotuberous ligament
Pubococcygeus
Puborectalis   } Levator ani muscle
Iliococcygeus
Anococcygeal body (ligament) (posterior extensions of superficial external anal sphincter muscle)
Gluteus maximus muscle
Tip of coccyx

Female

Clitoris
External urethral orifice
Vagina
Ischiopubic ramus
Anus

Superficial perineal (Colles') fascia (cut edge)
Ischiocavernosus muscle with deep perineal (investing or Gallaudet's) fascia removed
Bulbospongiosus muscle with deep perineal (investing or Gallaudet's) fascia removed
Fibers from superficial external anal sphincter muscle to ischiopubic ramus
Perineal membrane
Superficial transverse perineal muscle with deep perineal (investing or Gallaudet's) fascia removed
Superficial perineal (Colles') fascia (cut edge)
Perineal body
Crossed fibers from superficial and deep external sphincters to superficial transverse perineal muscle
Parts* of external anal sphincter muscle { Deep / Superficial / Subcutaneous
Levator ani muscle { Pubococcygeus / Puborectalis / Iliococcygeus
Gluteus maximus muscle
Anococcygeal body (ligament) (posterior extensions of superficial external anal sphincter muscle)

*Parts variable and often indistinct

PLATE 376   **PELVIS AND PERINEUM**

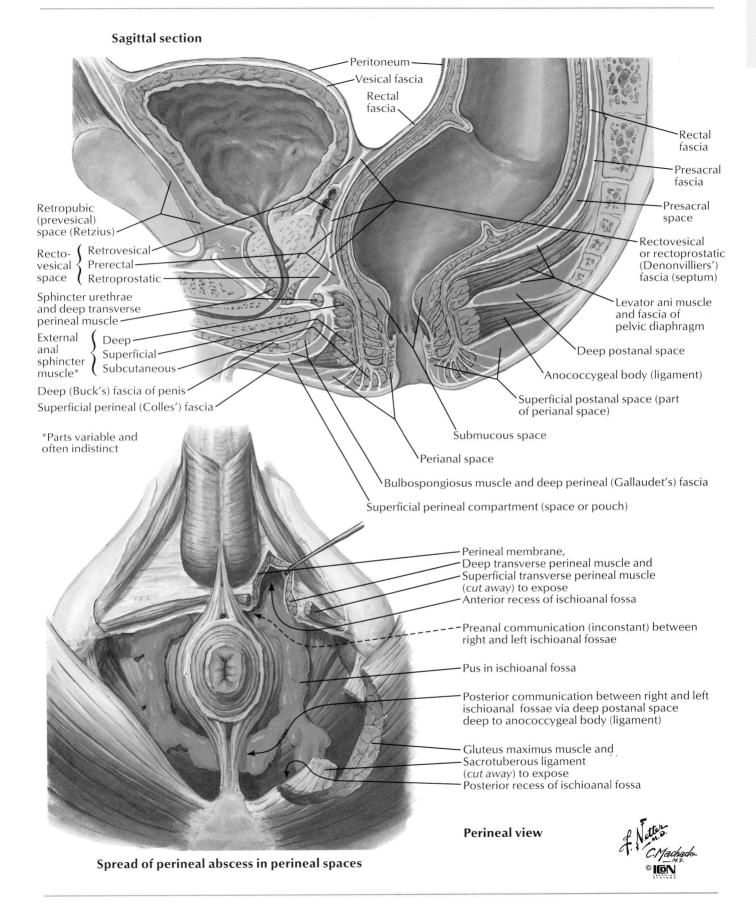

Sagittal section

Peritoneum

Vesical fascia

Rectal fascia

Rectal fascia

Presacral fascia

Presacral space

Retropubic (prevesical) space (Retzius)

Rectovesical or rectoprostatic (Denonvilliers') fascia (septum)

Recto-vesical space {
Retrovesical
Prerectal
Retroprostatic
}

Levator ani muscle and fascia of pelvic diaphragm

Sphincter urethrae and deep transverse perineal muscle

Deep postanal space

External anal sphincter muscle* {
Deep
Superficial
Subcutaneous
}

Anococcygeal body (ligament)

Superficial postanal space (part of perianal space)

Deep (Buck's) fascia of penis

Superficial perineal (Colles') fascia

Submucous space

*Parts variable and often indistinct

Perianal space

Bulbospongiosus muscle and deep perineal (Gallaudet's) fascia

Superficial perineal compartment (space or pouch)

Perineal membrane,
Deep transverse perineal muscle and
Superficial transverse perineal muscle
(*cut away*) to expose
Anterior recess of ischioanal fossa

Preanal communication (inconstant) between right and left ischioanal fossae

Pus in ischioanal fossa

Posterior communication between right and left ischioanal fossae via deep postanal space deep to anococcygeal body (ligament)

Gluteus maximus muscle and
Sacrotuberous ligament
(*cut away*) to expose
Posterior recess of ischioanal fossa

Perineal view

Spread of perineal abscess in perineal spaces

Arteries of Rectum and Anal Canal

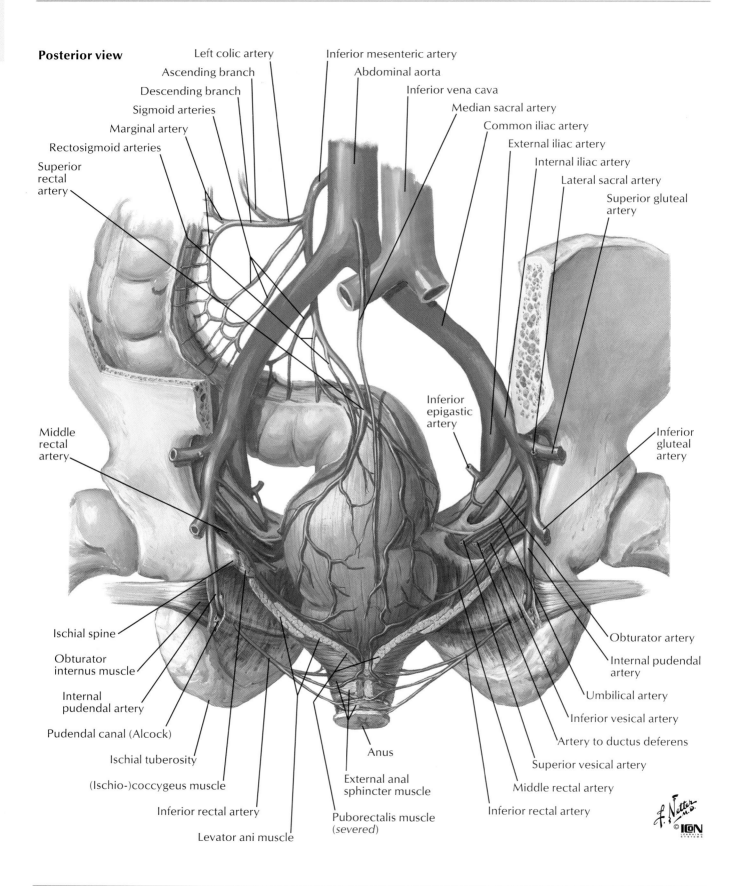

Posterior view

Left colic artery
Ascending branch
Descending branch
Sigmoid arteries
Marginal artery
Rectosigmoid arteries
Superior rectal artery

Inferior mesenteric artery
Abdominal aorta
Inferior vena cava
Median sacral artery
Common iliac artery
External iliac artery
Internal iliac artery
Lateral sacral artery
Superior gluteal artery

Middle rectal artery

Inferior epigastic artery

Inferior gluteal artery

Ischial spine
Obturator internus muscle
Internal pudendal artery
Pudendal canal (Alcock)
Ischial tuberosity
(Ischio-)coccygeus muscle
Inferior rectal artery
Levator ani muscle

Anus
External anal sphincter muscle
Puborectalis muscle (*severed*)

Obturator artery
Internal pudendal artery
Umbilical artery
Inferior vesical artery
Artery to ductus deferens
Superior vesical artery
Middle rectal artery
Inferior rectal artery

PLATE 378

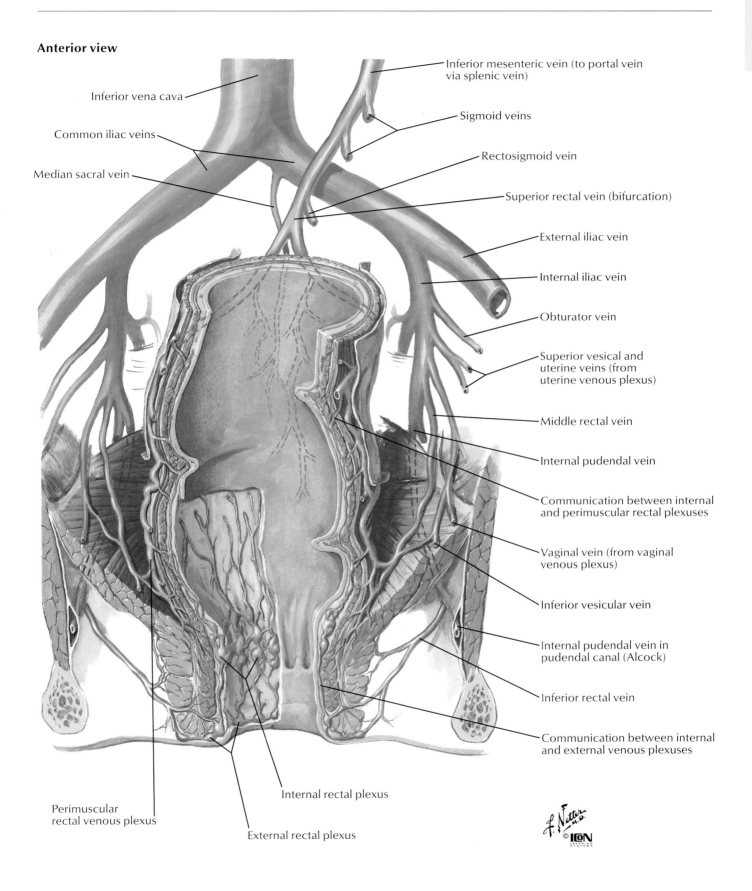

Anterior view

Inferior vena cava

Common iliac veins

Median sacral vein

Inferior mesenteric vein (to portal vein via splenic vein)

Sigmoid veins

Rectosigmoid vein

Superior rectal vein (bifurcation)

External iliac vein

Internal iliac vein

Obturator vein

Superior vesical and uterine veins (from uterine venous plexus)

Middle rectal vein

Internal pudendal vein

Communication between internal and perimuscular rectal plexuses

Vaginal vein (from vaginal venous plexus)

Inferior vesicular vein

Internal pudendal vein in pudendal canal (Alcock)

Inferior rectal vein

Communication between internal and external venous plexuses

Internal rectal plexus

Perimuscular rectal venous plexus

External rectal plexus

Arteries and Veins of Pelvic Organs: Female

Anterior view

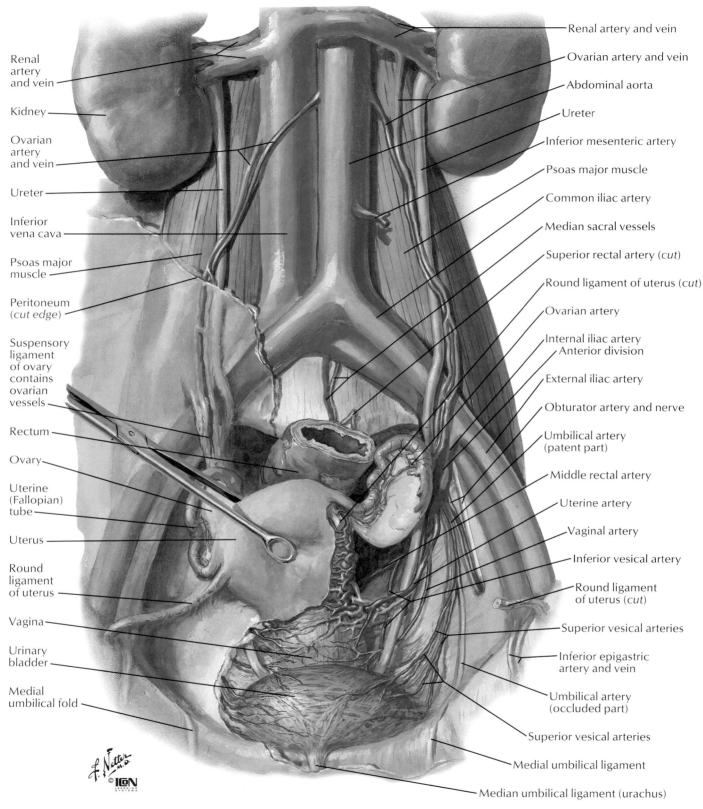

Renal artery and vein

Renal artery and vein

Ovarian artery and vein

Kidney

Abdominal aorta

Ovarian artery and vein

Ureter

Ureter

Inferior mesenteric artery

Inferior vena cava

Psoas major muscle

Psoas major muscle

Common iliac artery

Peritoneum (*cut edge*)

Median sacral vessels

Superior rectal artery (*cut*)

Suspensory ligament of ovary contains ovarian vessels

Round ligament of uterus (*cut*)

Ovarian artery

Rectum

Internal iliac artery
Anterior division

Ovary

External iliac artery

Uterine (Fallopian) tube

Obturator artery and nerve

Umbilical artery (patent part)

Uterus

Middle rectal artery

Round ligament of uterus

Uterine artery

Vaginal artery

Vagina

Inferior vesical artery

Urinary bladder

Round ligament of uterus (*cut*)

Medial umbilical fold

Superior vesical arteries

Inferior epigastric artery and vein

Umbilical artery (occluded part)

Superior vesical arteries

Medial umbilical ligament

Median umbilical ligament (urachus)

PLATE 380

PELVIS AND PERINEUM

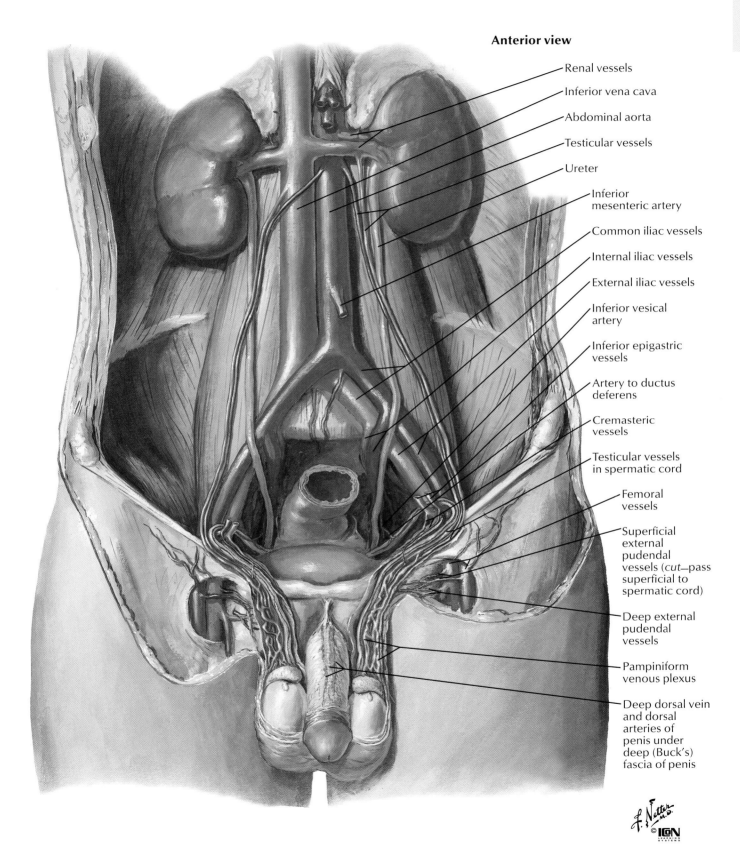

Anterior view

Renal vessels

Inferior vena cava

Abdominal aorta

Testicular vessels

Ureter

Inferior mesenteric artery

Common iliac vessels

Internal iliac vessels

External iliac vessels

Inferior vesical artery

Inferior epigastric vessels

Artery to ductus deferens

Cremasteric vessels

Testicular vessels in spermatic cord

Femoral vessels

Superficial external pudendal vessels (*cut*–pass superficial to spermatic cord)

Deep external pudendal vessels

Pampiniform venous plexus

Deep dorsal vein and dorsal arteries of penis under deep (Buck's) fascia of penis

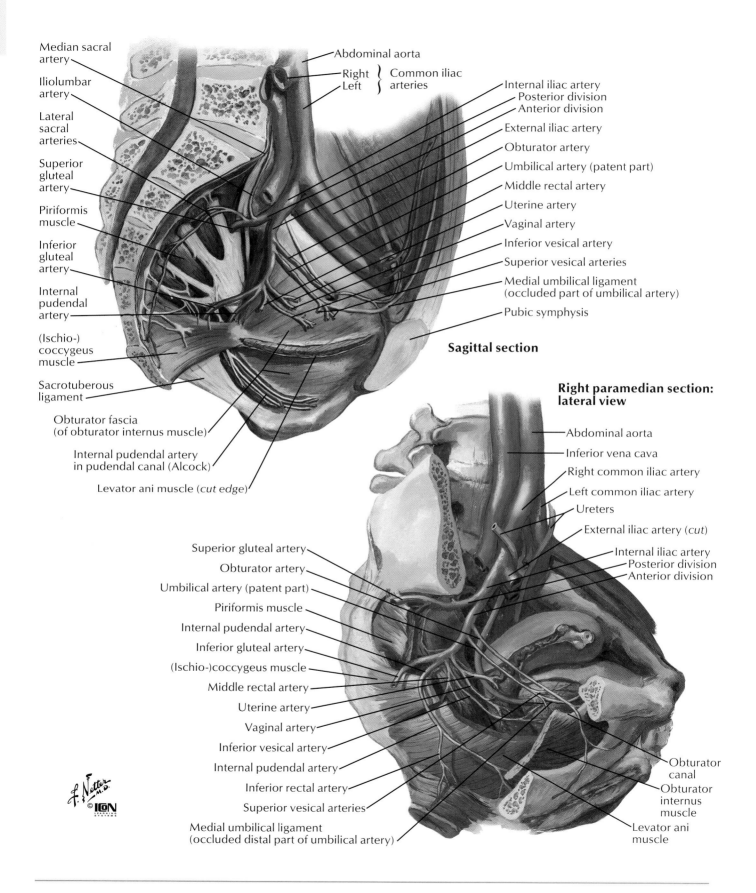

Median sacral artery

Iliolumbar artery

Lateral sacral arteries

Superior gluteal artery

Piriformis muscle

Inferior gluteal artery

Internal pudendal artery

(Ischio-)coccygeus muscle

Sacrotuberous ligament

Obturator fascia (of obturator internus muscle)

Internal pudendal artery in pudendal canal (Alcock)

Levator ani muscle (*cut edge*)

Abdominal aorta

Right } Common iliac
Left } arteries

Internal iliac artery
Posterior division
Anterior division

External iliac artery

Obturator artery

Umbilical artery (patent part)

Middle rectal artery

Uterine artery

Vaginal artery

Inferior vesical artery

Superior vesical arteries

Medial umbilical ligament (occluded part of umbilical artery)

Pubic symphysis

Sagittal section

Right paramedian section: lateral view

Abdominal aorta

Inferior vena cava

Right common iliac artery

Left common iliac artery

Ureters

External iliac artery (*cut*)

Internal iliac artery
Posterior division
Anterior division

Superior gluteal artery

Obturator artery

Umbilical artery (patent part)

Piriformis muscle

Internal pudendal artery

Inferior gluteal artery

(Ischio-)coccygeus muscle

Middle rectal artery

Uterine artery

Vaginal artery

Inferior vesical artery

Internal pudendal artery

Inferior rectal artery

Superior vesical arteries

Medial umbilical ligament (occluded distal part of umbilical artery)

Obturator canal

Obturator internus muscle

Levator ani muscle

PLATE 382

PELVIS AND PERINEUM

Left paramedian section: lateral view

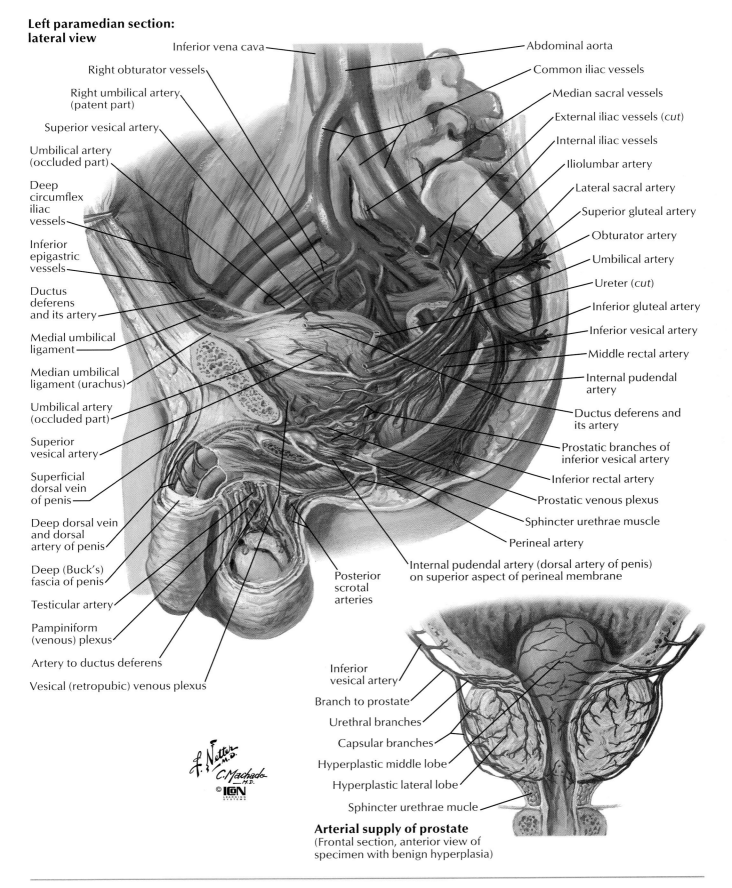

Inferior vena cava

Right obturator vessels

Right umbilical artery (patent part)

Superior vesical artery

Umbilical artery (occluded part)

Deep circumflex iliac vessels

Inferior epigastric vessels

Ductus deferens and its artery

Medial umbilical ligament

Median umbilical ligament (urachus)

Umbilical artery (occluded part)

Superior vesical artery

Superficial dorsal vein of penis

Deep dorsal vein and dorsal artery of penis

Deep (Buck's) fascia of penis

Testicular artery

Pampiniform (venous) plexus

Artery to ductus deferens

Vesical (retropubic) venous plexus

Posterior scrotal arteries

Abdominal aorta

Common iliac vessels

Median sacral vessels

External iliac vessels (cut)

Internal iliac vessels

Iliolumbar artery

Lateral sacral artery

Superior gluteal artery

Obturator artery

Umbilical artery

Ureter (cut)

Inferior gluteal artery

Inferior vesical artery

Middle rectal artery

Internal pudendal artery

Ductus deferens and its artery

Prostatic branches of inferior vesical artery

Inferior rectal artery

Prostatic venous plexus

Sphincter urethrae muscle

Perineal artery

Internal pudendal artery (dorsal artery of penis) on superior aspect of perineal membrane

Inferior vesical artery

Branch to prostate

Urethral branches

Capsular branches

Hyperplastic middle lobe

Hyperplastic lateral lobe

Sphincter urethrae mucle

Arterial supply of prostate
(Frontal section, anterior view of specimen with benign hyperplasia)

Arteries and Veins of Perineum and Uterus

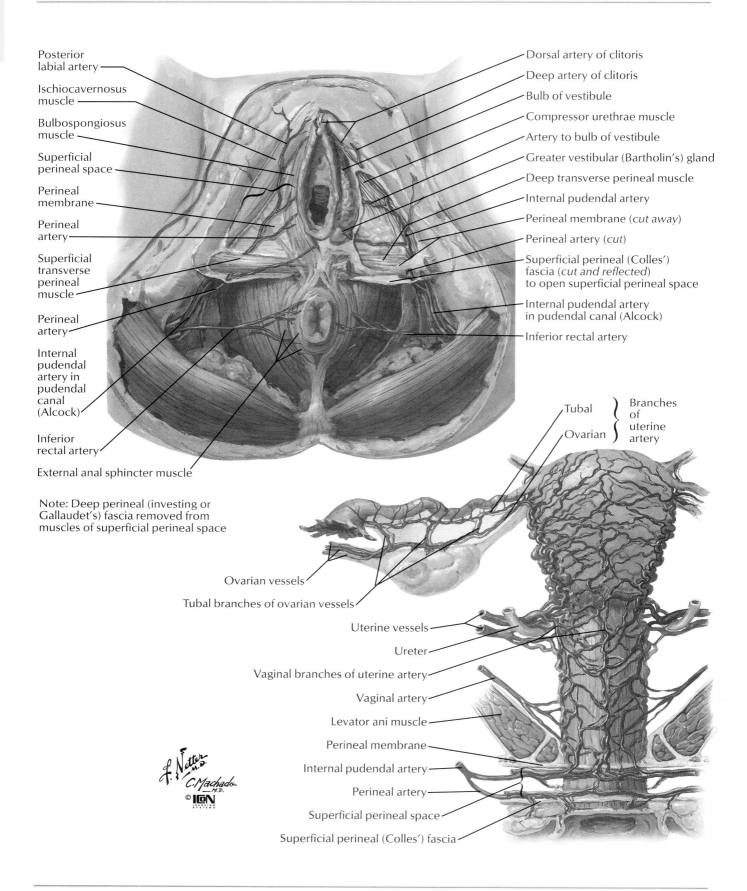

Posterior labial artery

Ischiocavernosus muscle

Bulbospongiosus muscle

Superficial perineal space

Perineal membrane

Perineal artery

Superficial transverse perineal muscle

Perineal artery

Internal pudendal artery in pudendal canal (Alcock)

Inferior rectal artery

External anal sphincter muscle

Note: Deep perineal (investing or Gallaudet's) fascia removed from muscles of superficial perineal space

Dorsal artery of clitoris

Deep artery of clitoris

Bulb of vestibule

Compressor urethrae muscle

Artery to bulb of vestibule

Greater vestibular (Bartholin's) gland

Deep transverse perineal muscle

Internal pudendal artery

Perineal membrane (cut away)

Perineal artery (cut)

Superficial perineal (Colles') fascia (cut and reflected) to open superficial perineal space

Internal pudendal artery in pudendal canal (Alcock)

Inferior rectal artery

Tubal } Branches of uterine artery
Ovarian }

Ovarian vessels

Tubal branches of ovarian vessels

Uterine vessels

Ureter

Vaginal branches of uterine artery

Vaginal artery

Levator ani muscle

Perineal membrane

Internal pudendal artery

Perineal artery

Superficial perineal space

Superficial perineal (Colles') fascia

PLATE 384

PELVIS AND PERINEUM

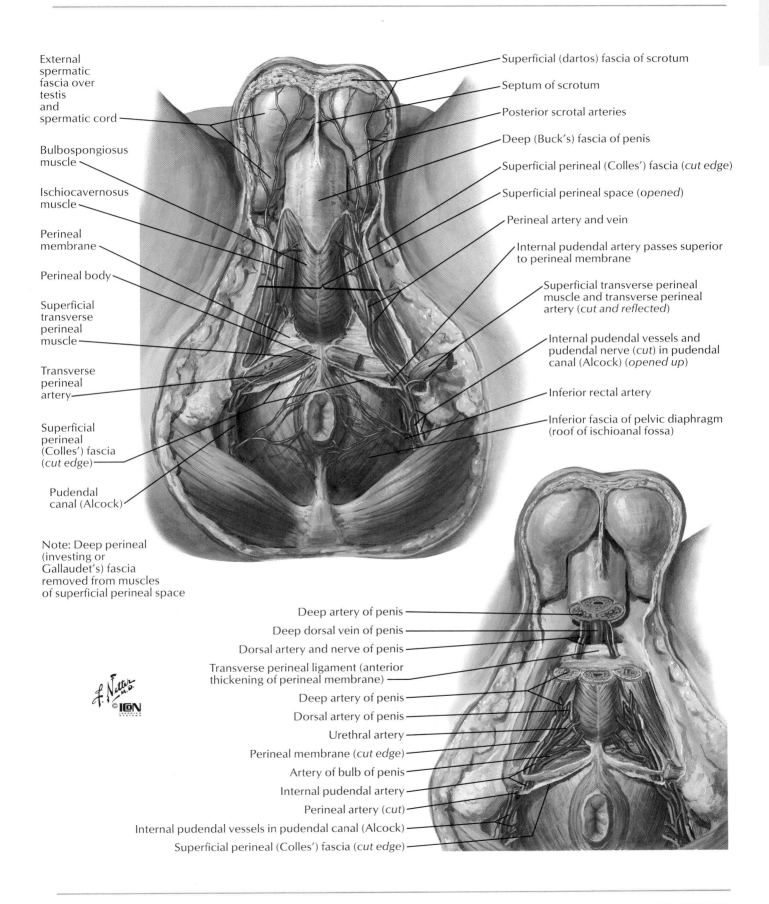

External spermatic fascia over testis and spermatic cord

Bulbospongiosus muscle

Ischiocavernosus muscle

Perineal membrane

Perineal body

Superficial transverse perineal muscle

Transverse perineal artery

Superficial perineal (Colles') fascia (cut edge)

Pudendal canal (Alcock)

Note: Deep perineal (investing or Gallaudet's) fascia removed from muscles of superficial perineal space

Superficial (dartos) fascia of scrotum

Septum of scrotum

Posterior scrotal arteries

Deep (Buck's) fascia of penis

Superficial perineal (Colles') fascia (cut edge)

Superficial perineal space (opened)

Perineal artery and vein

Internal pudendal artery passes superior to perineal membrane

Superficial transverse perineal muscle and transverse perineal artery (cut and reflected)

Internal pudendal vessels and pudendal nerve (cut) in pudendal canal (Alcock) (opened up)

Inferior rectal artery

Inferior fascia of pelvic diaphragm (roof of ischioanal fossa)

Deep artery of penis

Deep dorsal vein of penis

Dorsal artery and nerve of penis

Transverse perineal ligament (anterior thickening of perineal membrane)

Deep artery of penis

Dorsal artery of penis

Urethral artery

Perineal membrane (cut edge)

Artery of bulb of penis

Internal pudendal artery

Perineal artery (cut)

Internal pudendal vessels in pudendal canal (Alcock)

Superficial perineal (Colles') fascia (cut edge)

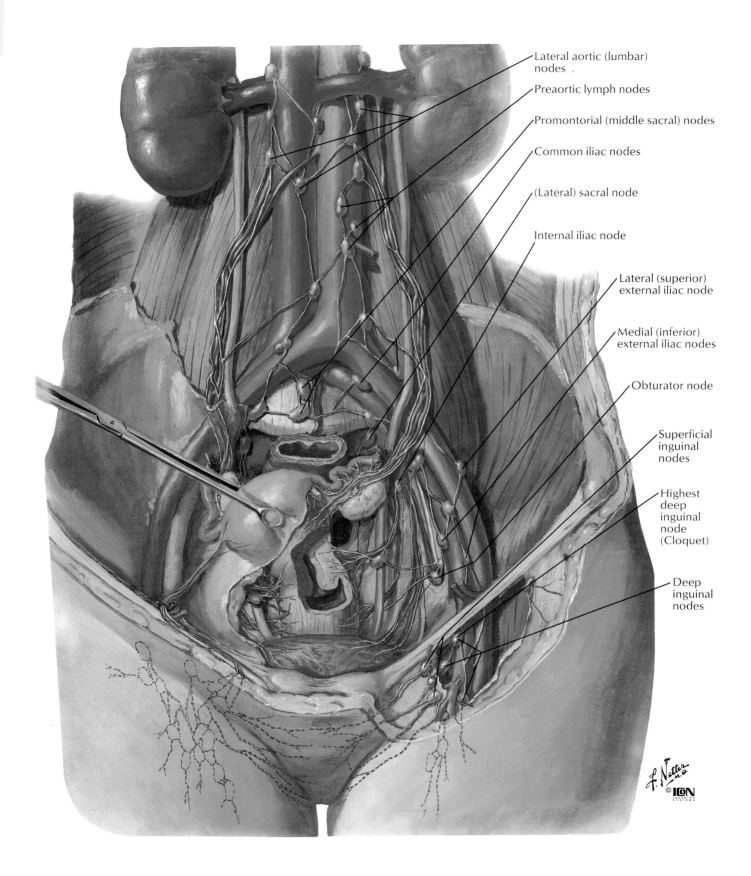

Lateral aortic (lumbar) nodes

Preaortic lymph nodes

Promontorial (middle sacral) nodes

Common iliac nodes

(Lateral) sacral node

Internal iliac node

Lateral (superior) external iliac node

Medial (inferior) external iliac nodes

Obturator node

Superficial inguinal nodes

Highest deep inguinal node (Cloquet)

Deep inguinal nodes

PLATE 386

PELVIS AND PERINEUM

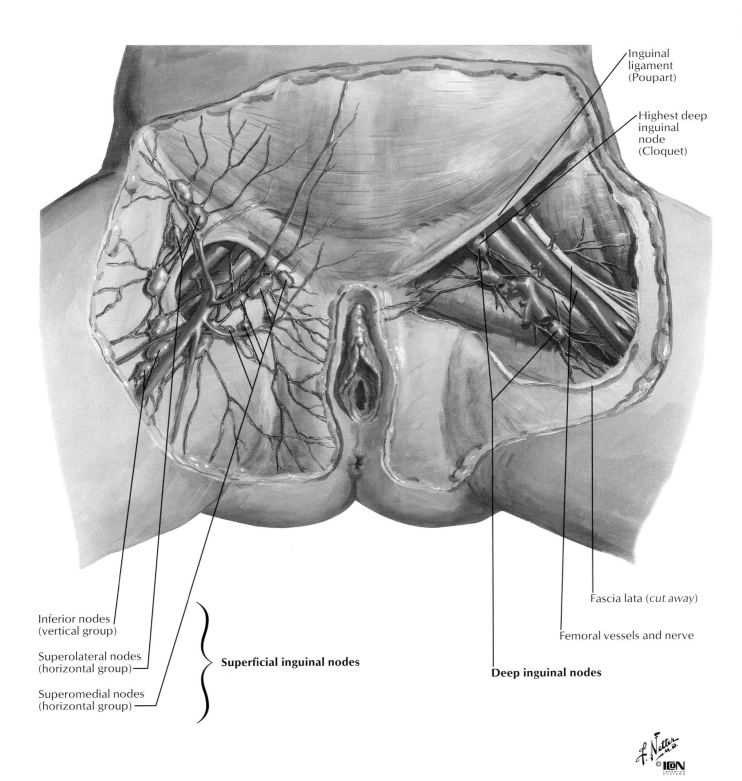

Inguinal
ligament
(Poupart)

Highest deep
inguinal
node
(Cloquet)

Fascia lata (*cut away*)

Femoral vessels and nerve

Deep inguinal nodes

Inferior nodes
(vertical group)

Superolateral nodes
(horizontal group)

Superomedial nodes
(horizontal group)

Superficial inguinal nodes

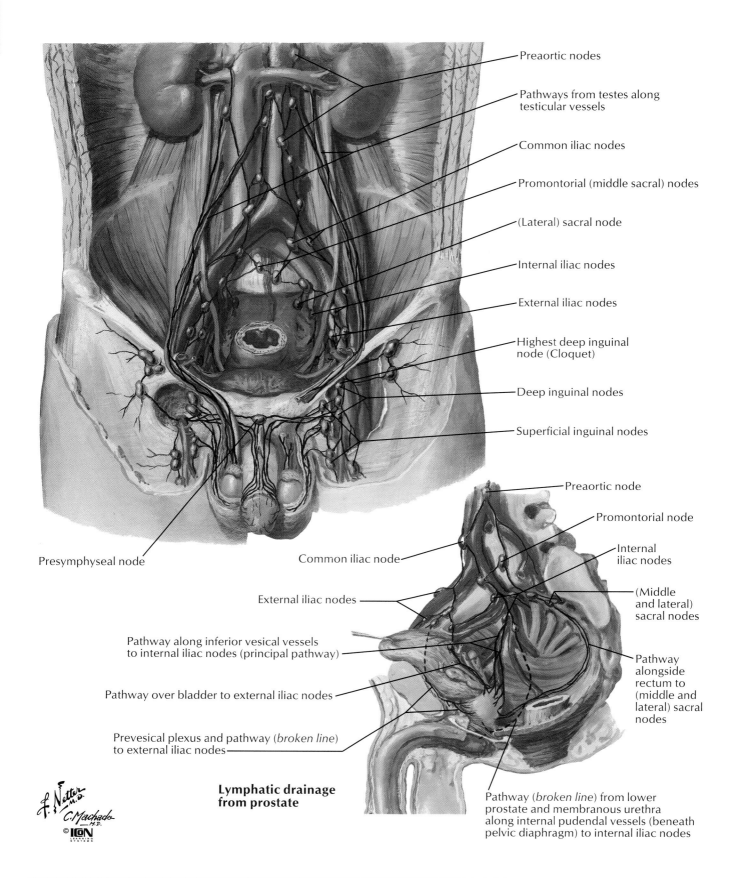

Preaortic nodes

Pathways from testes along testicular vessels

Common iliac nodes

Promontorial (middle sacral) nodes

(Lateral) sacral node

Internal iliac nodes

External iliac nodes

Highest deep inguinal node (Cloquet)

Deep inguinal nodes

Superficial inguinal nodes

Presymphyseal node

Preaortic node

Promontorial node

Internal iliac nodes

Common iliac node

(Middle and lateral) sacral nodes

External iliac nodes

Pathway along inferior vesical vessels to internal iliac nodes (principal pathway)

Pathway over bladder to external iliac nodes

Pathway alongside rectum to (middle and lateral) sacral nodes

Prevesical plexus and pathway (*broken line*) to external iliac nodes

Lymphatic drainage from prostate

Pathway (*broken line*) from lower prostate and membranous urethra along internal pudendal vessels (beneath pelvic diaphragm) to internal iliac nodes

PLATE 388

PELVIS AND PERINEUM

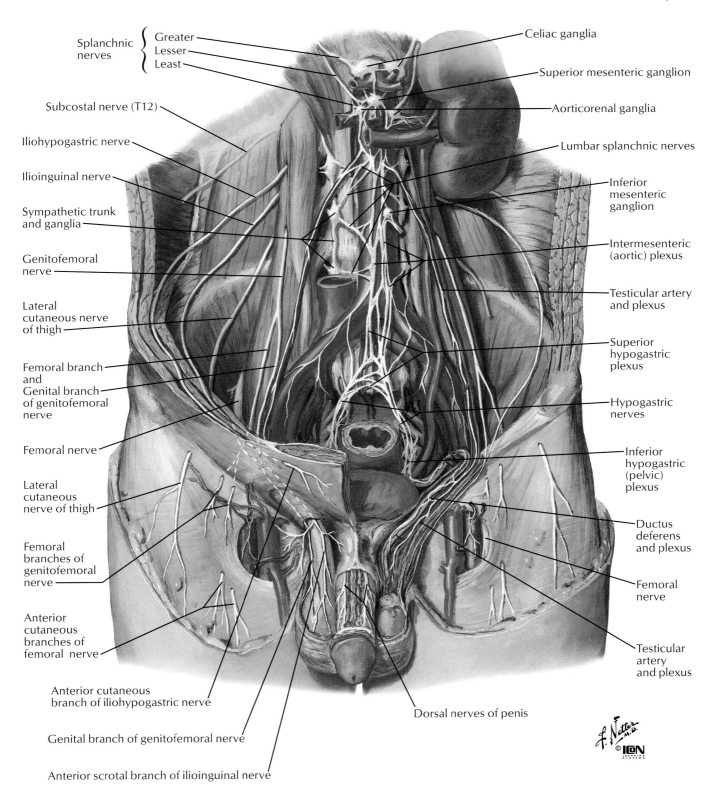

Splanchnic nerves { Greater / Lesser / Least }

Celiac ganglia

Subcostal nerve (T12)

Superior mesenteric ganglion

Iliohypogastric nerve

Aorticorenal ganglia

Ilioinguinal nerve

Lumbar splanchnic nerves

Sympathetic trunk and ganglia

Inferior mesenteric ganglion

Genitofemoral nerve

Intermesenteric (aortic) plexus

Lateral cutaneous nerve of thigh

Testicular artery and plexus

Femoral branch and Genital branch of genitofemoral nerve

Superior hypogastric plexus

Femoral nerve

Hypogastric nerves

Lateral cutaneous nerve of thigh

Inferior hypogastric (pelvic) plexus

Femoral branches of genitofemoral nerve

Ductus deferens and plexus

Anterior cutaneous branches of femoral nerve

Femoral nerve

Anterior cutaneous branch of iliohypogastric nerve

Testicular artery and plexus

Genital branch of genitofemoral nerve

Dorsal nerves of penis

Anterior scrotal branch of ilioinguinal nerve

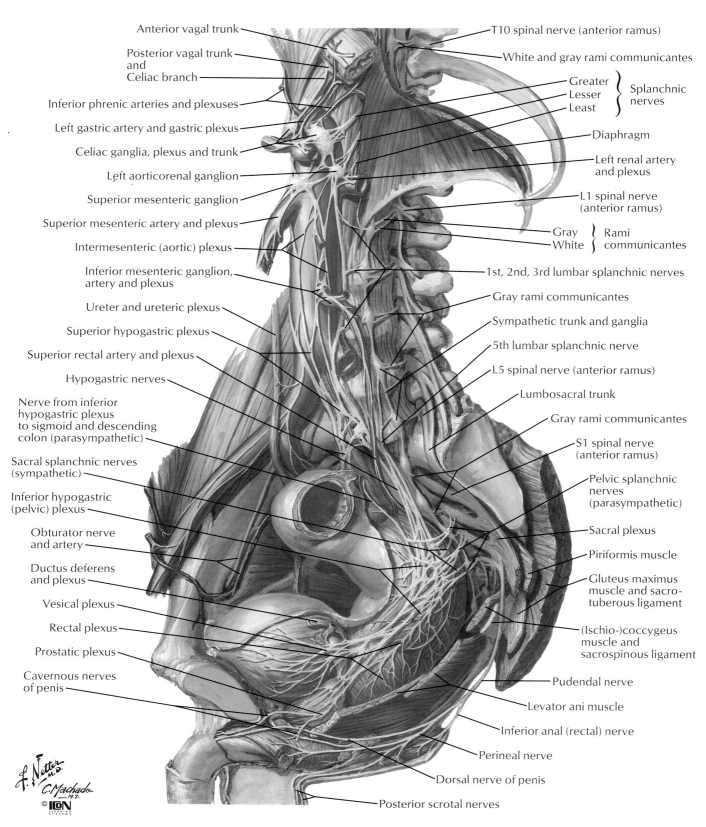

Anterior vagal trunk

Posterior vagal trunk and Celiac branch

Inferior phrenic arteries and plexuses

Left gastric artery and gastric plexus

Celiac ganglia, plexus and trunk

Left aorticorenal ganglion

Superior mesenteric ganglion

Superior mesenteric artery and plexus

Intermesenteric (aortic) plexus

Inferior mesenteric ganglion, artery and plexus

Ureter and ureteric plexus

Superior hypogastric plexus

Superior rectal artery and plexus

Hypogastric nerves

Nerve from inferior hypogastric plexus to sigmoid and descending colon (parasympathetic)

Sacral splanchnic nerves (sympathetic)

Inferior hypogastric (pelvic) plexus

Obturator nerve and artery

Ductus deferens and plexus

Vesical plexus

Rectal plexus

Prostatic plexus

Cavernous nerves of penis

T10 spinal nerve (anterior ramus)

White and gray rami communicantes

Greater
Lesser   } Splanchnic
Least   nerves

Diaphragm

Left renal artery and plexus

L1 spinal nerve (anterior ramus)

Gray   } Rami
White } communicantes

1st, 2nd, 3rd lumbar splanchnic nerves

Gray rami communicantes

Sympathetic trunk and ganglia

5th lumbar splanchnic nerve

L5 spinal nerve (anterior ramus)

Lumbosacral trunk

Gray rami communicantes

S1 spinal nerve (anterior ramus)

Pelvic splanchnic nerves (parasympathetic)

Sacral plexus

Piriformis muscle

Gluteus maximus muscle and sacro-tuberous ligament

(Ischio-)coccygeus muscle and sacrospinous ligament

Pudendal nerve

Levator ani muscle

Inferior anal (rectal) nerve

Perineal nerve

Dorsal nerve of penis

Posterior scrotal nerves

PLATE 390

PELVIS AND PERINEUM

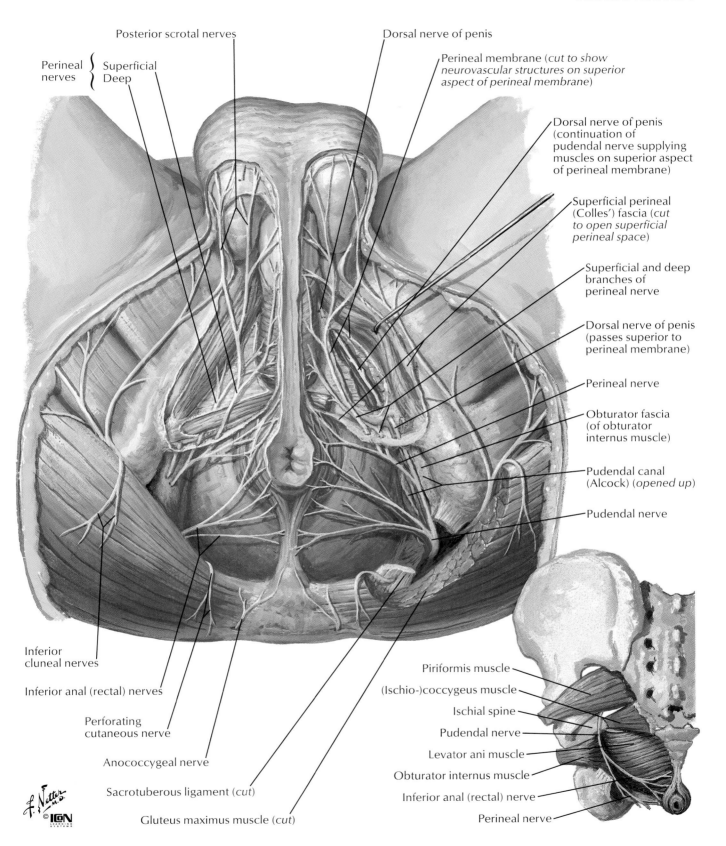

Posterior scrotal nerves

Dorsal nerve of penis

Perineal nerves { Superficial / Deep }

Perineal membrane (*cut to show neurovascular structures on superior aspect of perineal membrane*)

Dorsal nerve of penis (continuation of pudendal nerve supplying muscles on superior aspect of perineal membrane)

Superficial perineal (Colles') fascia (*cut to open superficial perineal space*)

Superficial and deep branches of perineal nerve

Dorsal nerve of penis (passes superior to perineal membrane)

Perineal nerve

Obturator fascia (of obturator internus muscle)

Pudendal canal (Alcock) (*opened up*)

Pudendal nerve

Inferior cluneal nerves

Inferior anal (rectal) nerves

Perforating cutaneous nerve

Anococcygeal nerve

Sacrotuberous ligament (*cut*)

Gluteus maximus muscle (*cut*)

Piriformis muscle

(Ischio-)coccygeus muscle

Ischial spine

Pudendal nerve

Levator ani muscle

Obturator internus muscle

Inferior anal (rectal) nerve

Perineal nerve

SEE ALSO PLATES 159, 308

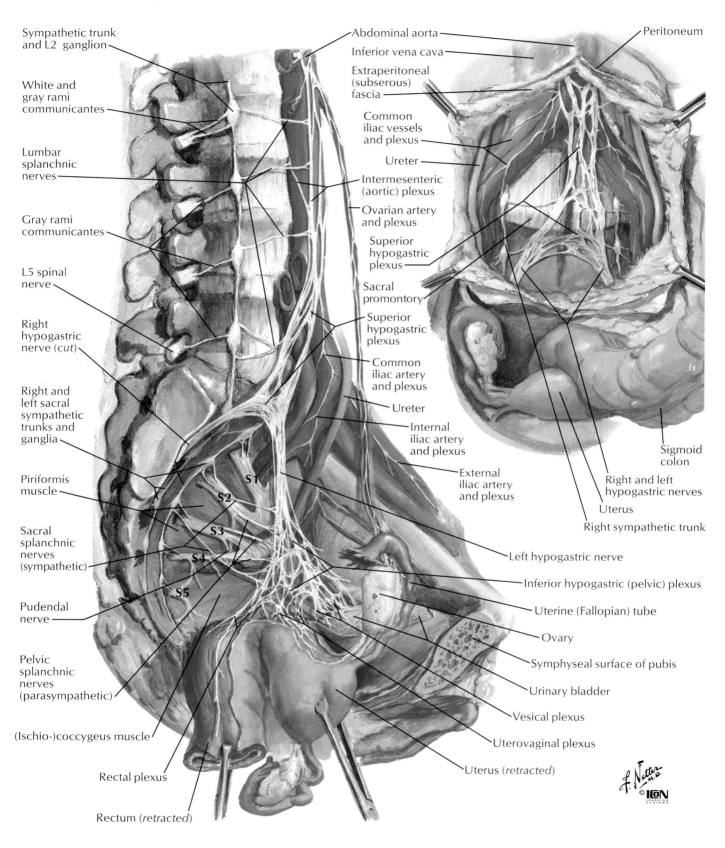

Sympathetic trunk and L2 ganglion

White and gray rami communicantes

Lumbar splanchnic nerves

Gray rami communicantes

L5 spinal nerve

Right hypogastric nerve (*cut*)

Right and left sacral sympathetic trunks and ganglia

Piriformis muscle

Sacral splanchnic nerves (sympathetic)

Pudendal nerve

Pelvic splanchnic nerves (parasympathetic)

(Ischio-)coccygeus muscle

Rectal plexus

Rectum (*retracted*)

S1
S2
S3
S4
S5

Abdominal aorta

Inferior vena cava

Extraperitoneal (subserous) fascia

Common iliac vessels and plexus

Ureter

Intermesenteric (aortic) plexus

Ovarian artery and plexus

Superior hypogastric plexus

Sacral promontory

Superior hypogastric plexus

Common iliac artery and plexus

Ureter

Internal iliac artery and plexus

External iliac artery and plexus

Peritoneum

Sigmoid colon

Right and left hypogastric nerves

Uterus

Right sympathetic trunk

Left hypogastric nerve

Inferior hypogastric (pelvic) plexus

Uterine (Fallopian) tube

Ovary

Symphyseal surface of pubis

Urinary bladder

Vesical plexus

Uterovaginal plexus

Uterus (*retracted*)

PLATE 392

PELVIS AND PERINEUM

SEE ALSO PLATE 395

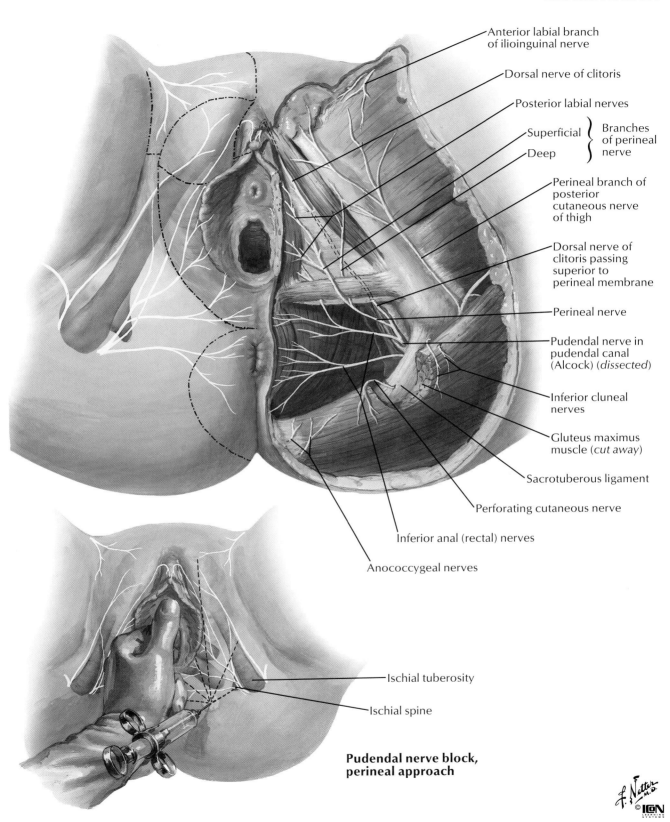

Anterior labial branch
of ilioinguinal nerve

Dorsal nerve of clitoris

Posterior labial nerves

Superficial } Branches
of perineal
Deep } nerve

Perineal branch of
posterior
cutaneous nerve
of thigh

Dorsal nerve of
clitoris passing
superior to
perineal membrane

Perineal nerve

Pudendal nerve in
pudendal canal
(Alcock) (*dissected*)

Inferior cluneal
nerves

Gluteus maximus
muscle (*cut away*)

Sacrotuberous ligament

Perforating cutaneous nerve

Inferior anal (rectal) nerves

Anococcygeal nerves

Ischial tuberosity

Ischial spine

**Pudendal nerve block,
perineal approach**

Neuropathways in Parturition

SEE ALSO PLATE 159

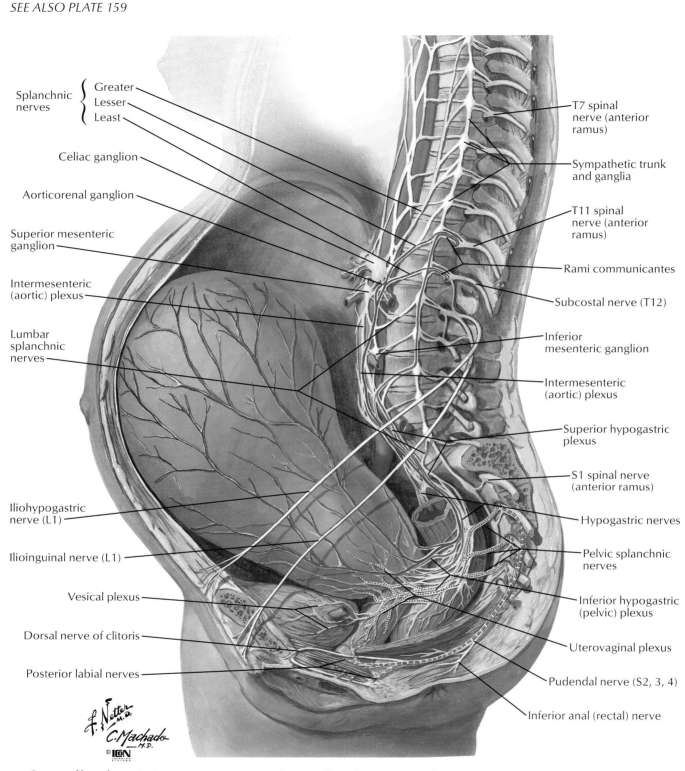

Splanchnic nerves
- Greater
- Lesser
- Least

Celiac ganglion

Aorticorenal ganglion

Superior mesenteric ganglion

Intermesenteric (aortic) plexus

Lumbar splanchnic nerves

Iliohypogastric nerve (L1)

Ilioinguinal nerve (L1)

Vesical plexus

Dorsal nerve of clitoris

Posterior labial nerves

T7 spinal nerve (anterior ramus)

Sympathetic trunk and ganglia

T11 spinal nerve (anterior ramus)

Rami communicantes

Subcostal nerve (T12)

Inferior mesenteric ganglion

Intermesenteric (aortic) plexus

Superior hypogastric plexus

S1 spinal nerve (anterior ramus)

Hypogastric nerves

Pelvic splanchnic nerves

Inferior hypogastric (pelvic) plexus

Uterovaginal plexus

Pudendal nerve (S2, 3, 4)

Inferior anal (rectal) nerve

—————— Sensory fibers from uterine body and fundus accompany sympathetic fibers via hypogastric plexuses to T11, 12 (L1?)

—————— Motor fibers to uterine body and fundus (sympathetic)

············ Sensory fibers from cervix and upper vagina accompany pelvic splanchnic nerves (parasympathetic) to S2, 3, 4

············ Motor fibers to lower uterine segment, cervix and upper vagina (parasympathetic)

– – – – Sensory fibers from lower vagina and perineum accompany somatic fibers via pudendal nerve to S2, 3, 4

– – – – Motor fibers to lower vagina and perineum via pudendal nerve (somatic)

PLATE 394

PELVIS AND PERINEUM

SEE ALSO PLATE 160

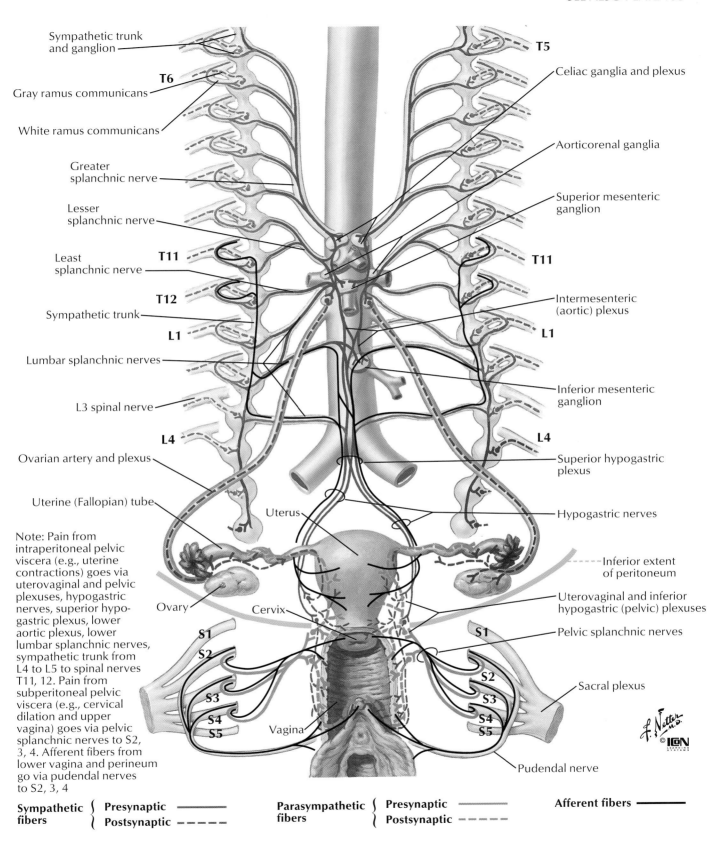

Sympathetic trunk and ganglion

T6

Gray ramus communicans

White ramus communicans

Greater splanchnic nerve

Lesser splanchnic nerve

Least splanchnic nerve

T11

T12

Sympathetic trunk

L1

Lumbar splanchnic nerves

L3 spinal nerve

L4

Ovarian artery and plexus

Uterine (Fallopian) tube

Note: Pain from intraperitoneal pelvic viscera (e.g., uterine contractions) goes via uterovaginal and pelvic plexuses, hypogastric nerves, superior hypogastric plexus, lower aortic plexus, lower lumbar splanchnic nerves, sympathetic trunk from L4 to L5 to spinal nerves T11, 12. Pain from subperitoneal pelvic viscera (e.g., cervical dilation and upper vagina) goes via pelvic splanchnic nerves to S2, 3, 4. Afferent fibers from lower vagina and perineum go via pudendal nerves to S2, 3, 4

Ovary

Cervix

Uterus

S1

S2

S3

S4

S5

Vagina

T5

Celiac ganglia and plexus

Aorticorenal ganglia

Superior mesenteric ganglion

T11

Intermesenteric (aortic) plexus

L1

Inferior mesenteric ganglion

L4

Superior hypogastric plexus

Hypogastric nerves

Inferior extent of peritoneum

Uterovaginal and inferior hypogastric (pelvic) plexuses

Pelvic splanchnic nerves

S1

S2

S3

S4

S5

Sacral plexus

Pudendal nerve

| Sympathetic fibers | Presynaptic —— | Parasympathetic fibers | Presynaptic —— | Afferent fibers —— |
| | Postsynaptic – – – | | Postsynaptic – – – | |

SEE ALSO PLATE 160

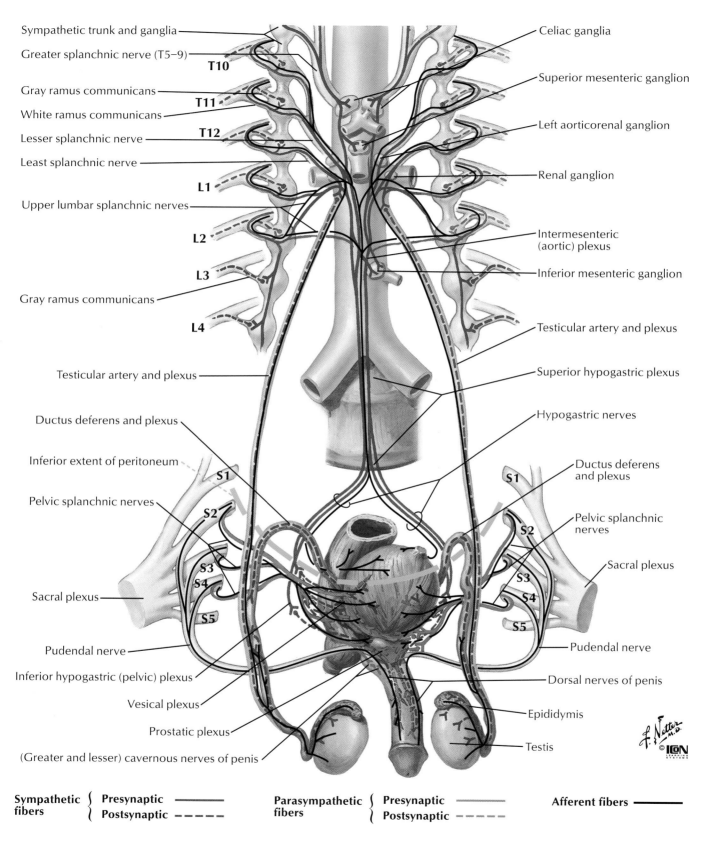

Sympathetic trunk and ganglia

Greater splanchnic nerve (T5–9)

T10

Gray ramus communicans

T11

White ramus communicans

Lesser splanchnic nerve

T12

Least splanchnic nerve

L1

Upper lumbar splanchnic nerves

L2

L3

Gray ramus communicans

L4

Testicular artery and plexus

Ductus deferens and plexus

Inferior extent of peritoneum

S1

Pelvic splanchnic nerves

S2

S3

S4

Sacral plexus

S5

Pudendal nerve

Inferior hypogastric (pelvic) plexus

Vesical plexus

Prostatic plexus

(Greater and lesser) cavernous nerves of penis

Celiac ganglia

Superior mesenteric ganglion

Left aorticorenal ganglion

Renal ganglion

Intermesenteric (aortic) plexus

Inferior mesenteric ganglion

Testicular artery and plexus

Superior hypogastric plexus

Hypogastric nerves

Ductus deferens and plexus

S1

Pelvic splanchnic nerves

S2

Sacral plexus

S3

S4

S5

Pudendal nerve

Dorsal nerves of penis

Epididymis

Testis

| Sympathetic fibers | Presynaptic —— Postsynaptic ----- | Parasympathetic fibers | Presynaptic —— Postsynaptic ----- | Afferent fibers —— |

PLATE 396

PELVIS AND PERINEUM

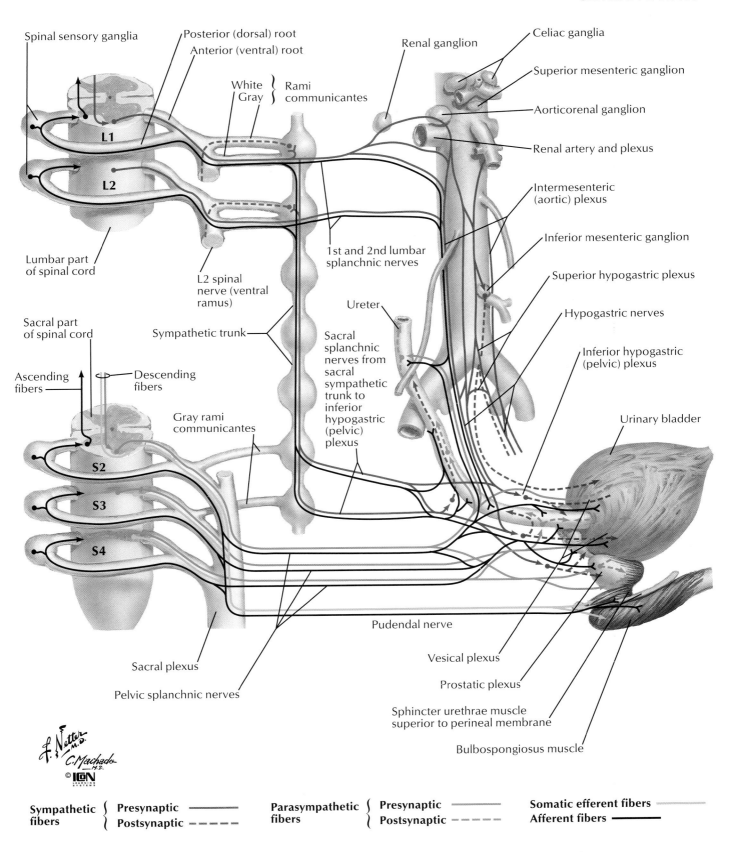

Spinal sensory ganglia

Posterior (dorsal) root

Anterior (ventral) root

White } Rami
Gray } communicantes

Renal ganglion

Celiac ganglia

Superior mesenteric ganglion

Aorticorenal ganglion

Renal artery and plexus

Intermesenteric (aortic) plexus

Inferior mesenteric ganglion

Superior hypogastric plexus

Hypogastric nerves

Inferior hypogastric (pelvic) plexus

Urinary bladder

L1

L2

Lumbar part of spinal cord

L2 spinal nerve (ventral ramus)

1st and 2nd lumbar splanchnic nerves

Ureter

Sacral splanchnic nerves from sacral sympathetic trunk to inferior hypogastric (pelvic) plexus

Sympathetic trunk

Sacral part of spinal cord

Ascending fibers

Descending fibers

Gray rami communicantes

S2

S3

S4

Sacral plexus

Pelvic splanchnic nerves

Pudendal nerve

Vesical plexus

Prostatic plexus

Sphincter urethrae muscle superior to perineal membrane

Bulbospongiosus muscle

Sympathetic fibers {	Presynaptic ———	Parasympathetic fibers {	Presynaptic ———	**Somatic efferent fibers** -----
	Postsynaptic -----		Postsynaptic -----	**Afferent fibers** ———

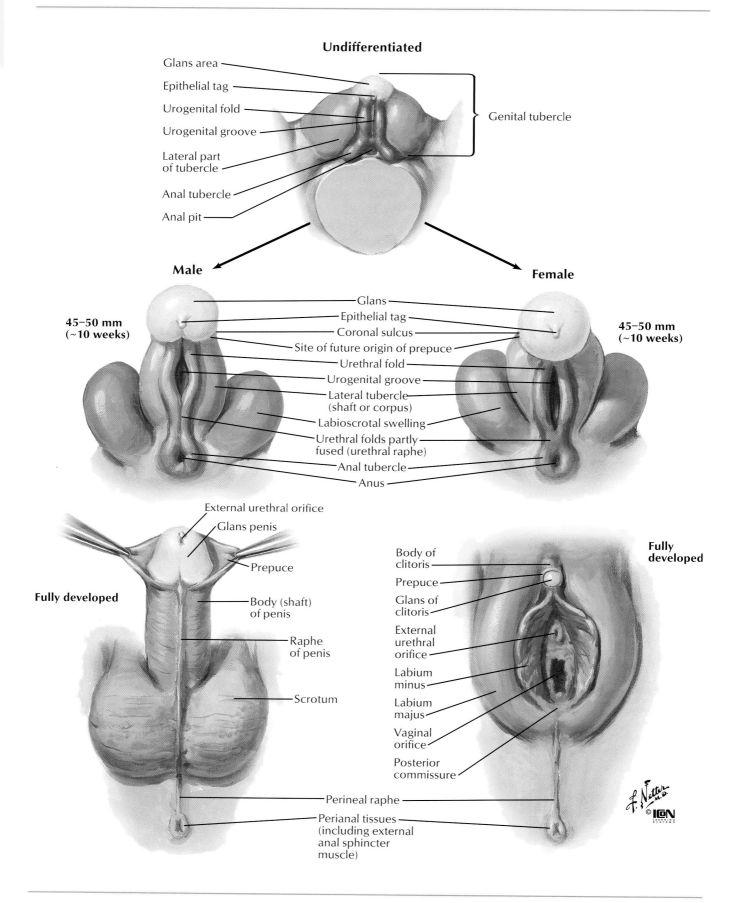

Undifferentiated

Glans area

Epithelial tag

Urogenital fold

Urogenital groove

Lateral part of tubercle

Anal tubercle

Anal pit

Genital tubercle

Male

Female

45–50 mm (~10 weeks)

45–50 mm (~10 weeks)

Glans

Epithelial tag

Coronal sulcus

Site of future origin of prepuce

Urethral fold

Urogenital groove

Lateral tubercle (shaft or corpus)

Labioscrotal swelling

Urethral folds partly fused (urethral raphe)

Anal tubercle

Anus

External urethral orifice

Glans penis

Prepuce

Fully developed

Body (shaft) of penis

Raphe of penis

Scrotum

Fully developed

Body of clitoris

Prepuce

Glans of clitoris

External urethral orifice

Labium minus

Labium majus

Vaginal orifice

Posterior commissure

Perineal raphe

Perianal tissues (including external anal sphincter muscle)

PLATE 398

PELVIS AND PERINEUM

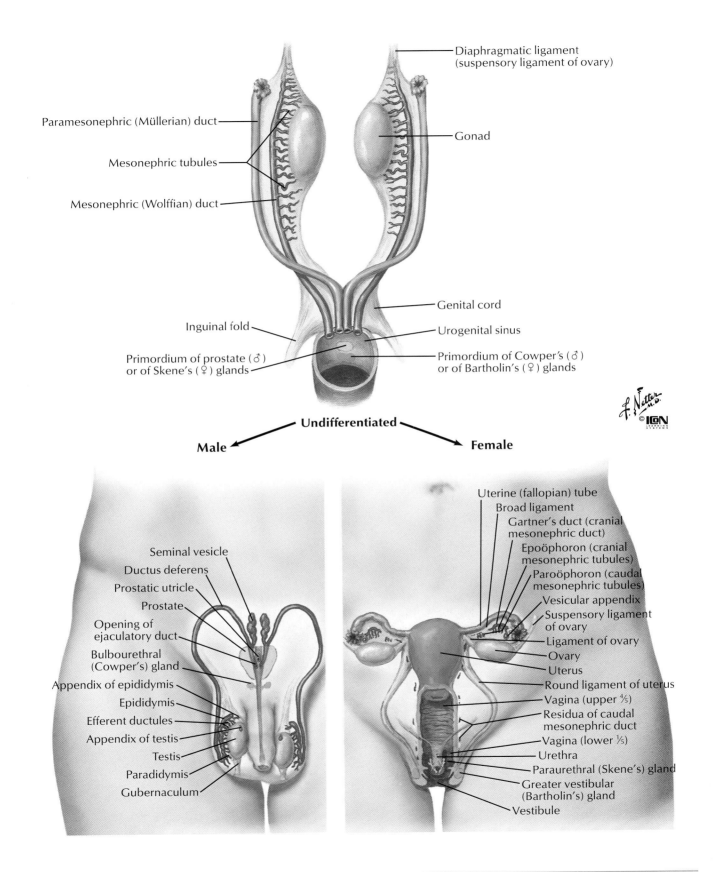

Diaphragmatic ligament
(suspensory ligament of ovary)

Paramesonephric (Müllerian) duct

Mesonephric tubules

Mesonephric (Wolffian) duct

Gonad

Genital cord

Inguinal fold

Urogenital sinus

Primordium of prostate (♂)
or of Skene's (♀) glands

Primordium of Cowper's (♂)
or of Bartholin's (♀) glands

Undifferentiated

Male

Female

Seminal vesicle

Ductus deferens

Prostatic utricle

Prostate

Opening of
ejaculatory duct

Bulbourethral
(Cowper's) gland

Appendix of epididymis

Epididymis

Efferent ductules

Appendix of testis

Testis

Paradidymis

Gubernaculum

Uterine (fallopian) tube

Broad ligament

Gartner's duct (cranial
mesonephric duct)

Epoöphoron (cranial
mesonephric tubules)

Paroöphoron (caudal
mesonephric tubules)

Vesicular appendix

Suspensory ligament
of ovary

Ligament of ovary

Ovary

Uterus

Round ligament of uterus

Vagina (upper ⅘)

Residua of caudal
mesonephric duct

Vagina (lower ⅕)

Urethra

Paraurethral (Skene's) gland

Greater vestibular
(Bartholin's) gland

Vestibule

Pelvic Scans: Sagittal MR Images

Median (A) and paramedian (B) sagittal MR images of female pelvis

A

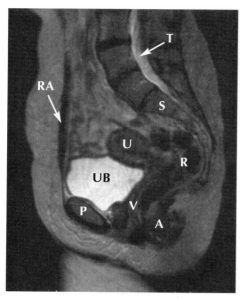

B

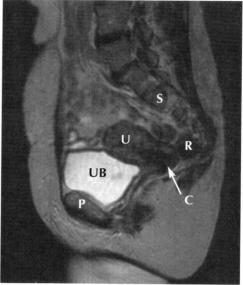

A	Anal canal	**S**	Sacrum
C	External os of cervix	**T**	Thecal sac
P	Pubic symphysis	**U**	Uterus
R	Rectum	**UB**	Urinary bladder
RA	Rectus abdominis muscle	**V**	Vagina

Median (C) and paramedian (D) sagittal MR images of male pelvis

C

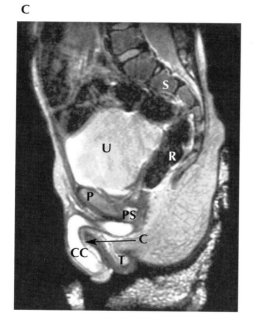

D

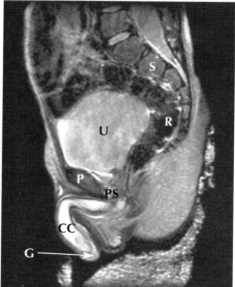

C	Corpus spongiosum	**R**	Rectum
CC	Corpus cavernosum	**S**	Sacrum
G	Glans of penis	**T**	Testis
P	Pubic symphysis	**U**	Urinary bladder
PS	Prostate		

PLATE 400

PELVIS AND PERINEUM

Section VI
UPPER LIMB

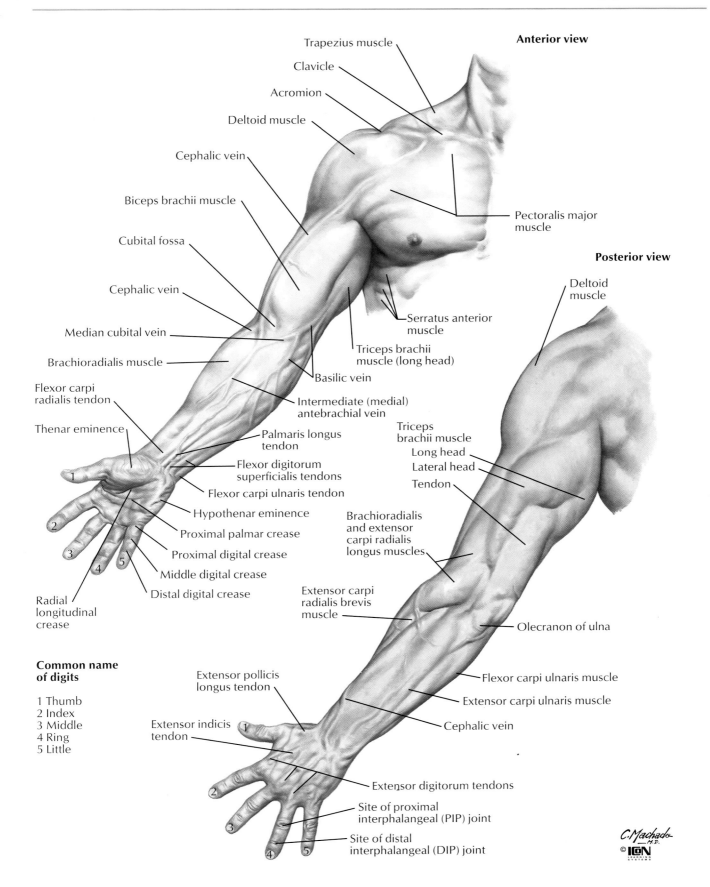

Anterior view

Trapezius muscle

Clavicle

Acromion

Deltoid muscle

Cephalic vein

Biceps brachii muscle

Cubital fossa

Cephalic vein

Median cubital vein

Brachioradialis muscle

Flexor carpi radialis tendon

Thenar eminence

Palmaris longus tendon

Flexor digitorum superficialis tendons

Flexor carpi ulnaris tendon

Hypothenar eminence

Proximal palmar crease

Proximal digital crease

Middle digital crease

Distal digital crease

Radial longitudinal crease

Pectoralis major muscle

Posterior view

Deltoid muscle

Serratus anterior muscle

Triceps brachii muscle (long head)

Basilic vein

Intermediate (medial) antebrachial vein

Triceps brachii muscle

Long head

Lateral head

Tendon

Brachioradialis and extensor carpi radialis longus muscles

Extensor carpi radialis brevis muscle

Olecranon of ulna

Flexor carpi ulnaris muscle

Extensor carpi ulnaris muscle

Cephalic vein

Common name of digits

1 Thumb
2 Index
3 Middle
4 Ring
5 Little

Extensor pollicis longus tendon

Extensor indicis tendon

Extensor digitorum tendons

Site of proximal interphalangeal (PIP) joint

Site of distal interphalangeal (DIP) joint

C. Machado
M.D.
© ICON
LEARNING
SYSTEMS

SURFACE ANATOMY

PLATE 401

Clavicle and Sternoclavicular Joint

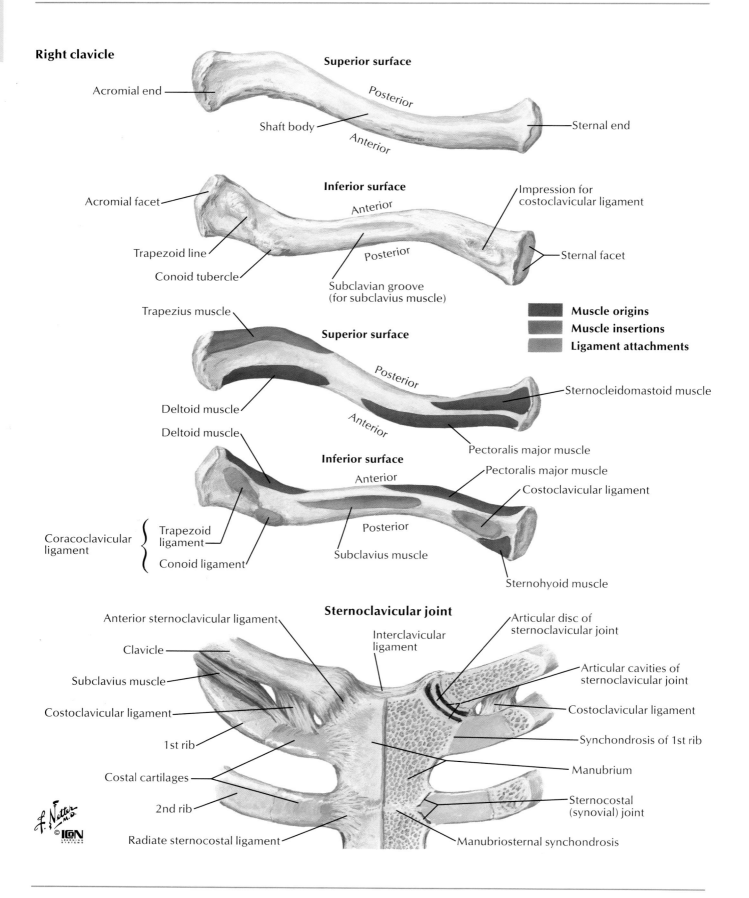

Right clavicle

Superior surface

Acromial end

Posterior

Shaft body

Anterior

Sternal end

Inferior surface

Acromial facet

Anterior

Impression for costoclavicular ligament

Trapezoid line

Posterior

Conoid tubercle

Subclavian groove (for subclavius muscle)

Sternal facet

Muscle origins
Muscle insertions
Ligament attachments

Trapezius muscle

Superior surface

Posterior

Anterior

Sternocleidomastoid muscle

Deltoid muscle

Pectoralis major muscle

Deltoid muscle

Inferior surface

Anterior

Pectoralis major muscle

Costoclavicular ligament

Coracoclavicular ligament

Trapezoid ligament

Posterior

Conoid ligament

Subclavius muscle

Sternohyoid muscle

Sternoclavicular joint

Anterior sternoclavicular ligament

Interclavicular ligament

Articular disc of sternoclavicular joint

Clavicle

Subclavius muscle

Articular cavities of sternoclavicular joint

Costoclavicular ligament

Costoclavicular ligament

1st rib

Synchondrosis of 1st rib

Costal cartilages

Manubrium

2nd rib

Sternocostal (synovial) joint

Radiate sternocostal ligament

Manubriosternal synchondrosis

PLATE 402

UPPER LIMB

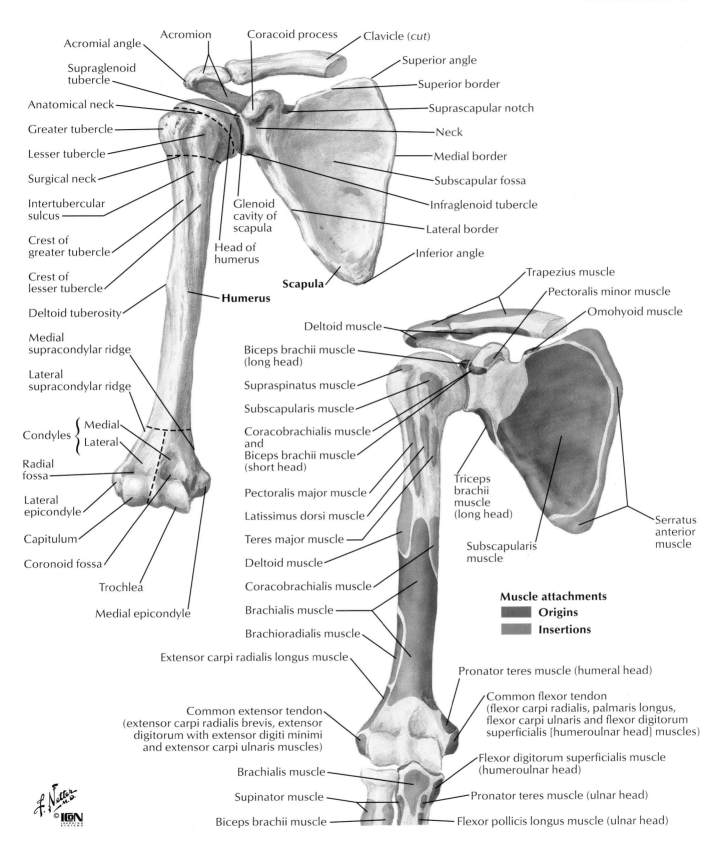

Acromial angle
Acromion
Coracoid process
Clavicle (*cut*)
Supraglenoid tubercle
Anatomical neck
Greater tubercle
Lesser tubercle
Surgical neck
Intertubercular sulcus
Crest of greater tubercle
Crest of lesser tubercle
Deltoid tuberosity
Medial supracondylar ridge
Lateral supracondylar ridge
Condyles { Medial / Lateral
Radial fossa
Lateral epicondyle
Capitulum
Coronoid fossa
Trochlea
Medial epicondyle

Superior angle
Superior border
Suprascapular notch
Neck
Medial border
Subscapular fossa
Infraglenoid tubercle
Lateral border
Inferior angle

Glenoid cavity of scapula
Head of humerus

Scapula
Humerus

Trapezius muscle
Pectoralis minor muscle
Omohyoid muscle
Deltoid muscle
Biceps brachii muscle (long head)
Supraspinatus muscle
Subscapularis muscle
Coracobrachialis muscle and Biceps brachii muscle (short head)
Pectoralis major muscle
Latissimus dorsi muscle
Teres major muscle
Deltoid muscle
Coracobrachialis muscle
Brachialis muscle
Brachioradialis muscle
Extensor carpi radialis longus muscle

Triceps brachii muscle (long head)
Subscapularis muscle
Serratus anterior muscle

Muscle attachments
■ **Origins**
■ **Insertions**

Pronator teres muscle (humeral head)
Common flexor tendon (flexor carpi radialis, palmaris longus, flexor carpi ulnaris and flexor digitorum superficialis [humeroulnar head] muscles)

Common extensor tendon (extensor carpi radialis brevis, extensor digitorum with extensor digiti minimi and extensor carpi ulnaris muscles)
Brachialis muscle
Supinator muscle
Biceps brachii muscle

Flexor digitorum superficialis muscle (humeroulnar head)
Pronator teres muscle (ulnar head)
Flexor pollicis longus muscle (ulnar head)

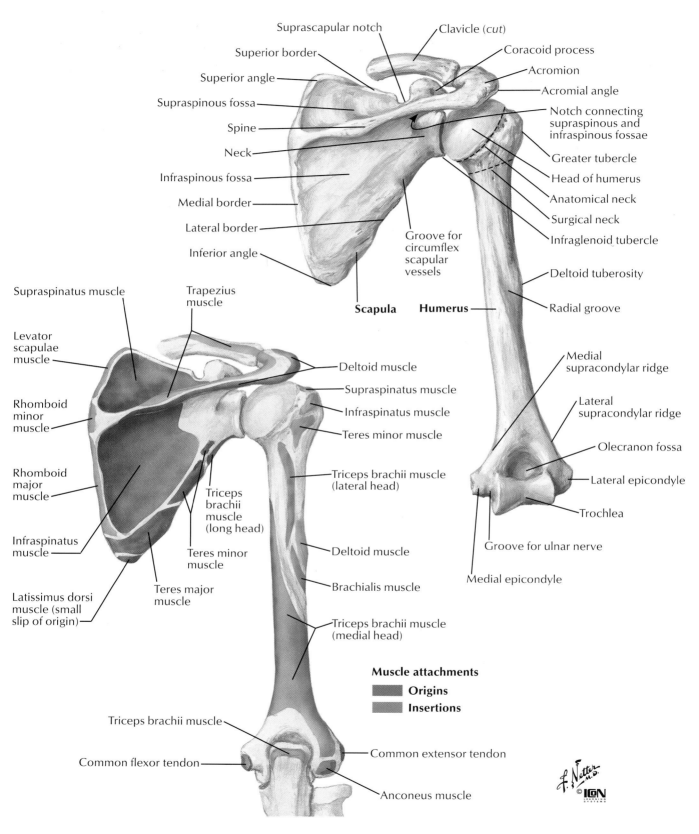

Suprascapular notch

Clavicle (*cut*)

Superior border

Coracoid process

Superior angle

Acromion

Supraspinous fossa

Acromial angle

Spine

Notch connecting supraspinous and infraspinous fossae

Neck

Greater tubercle

Infraspinous fossa

Head of humerus

Medial border

Anatomical neck

Lateral border

Surgical neck

Inferior angle

Infraglenoid tubercle

Groove for circumflex scapular vessels

Deltoid tuberosity

Scapula   **Humerus**

Radial groove

Supraspinatus muscle

Trapezius muscle

Levator scapulae muscle

Deltoid muscle

Supraspinatus muscle

Medial supracondylar ridge

Rhomboid minor muscle

Infraspinatus muscle

Lateral supracondylar ridge

Teres minor muscle

Olecranon fossa

Rhomboid major muscle

Triceps brachii muscle (lateral head)

Triceps brachii muscle (long head)

Lateral epicondyle

Infraspinatus muscle

Trochlea

Teres minor muscle

Deltoid muscle

Groove for ulnar nerve

Latissimus dorsi muscle (small slip of origin)

Teres major muscle

Brachialis muscle

Medial epicondyle

Triceps brachii muscle (medial head)

Muscle attachments

■ **Origins**

■ **Insertions**

Triceps brachii muscle

Common extensor tendon

Common flexor tendon

Anconeus muscle

PLATE 404

UPPER LIMB

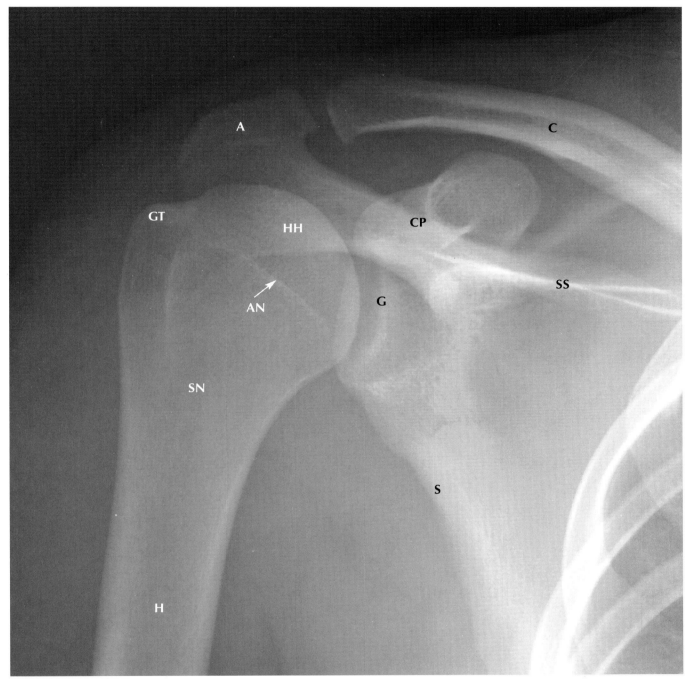

A	Acromion
AN	Anatomical neck of humerus
C	Clavicle
CP	Coracoid process
G	Glenoid cavity of scapula
GT	Greater tubercle
H	Humerus
HH	Head of humerus
S	Scapula (lateral border)
SN	Surgical neck of humerus
SS	Spine of scapula

Shoulder (Glenohumeral) Joint

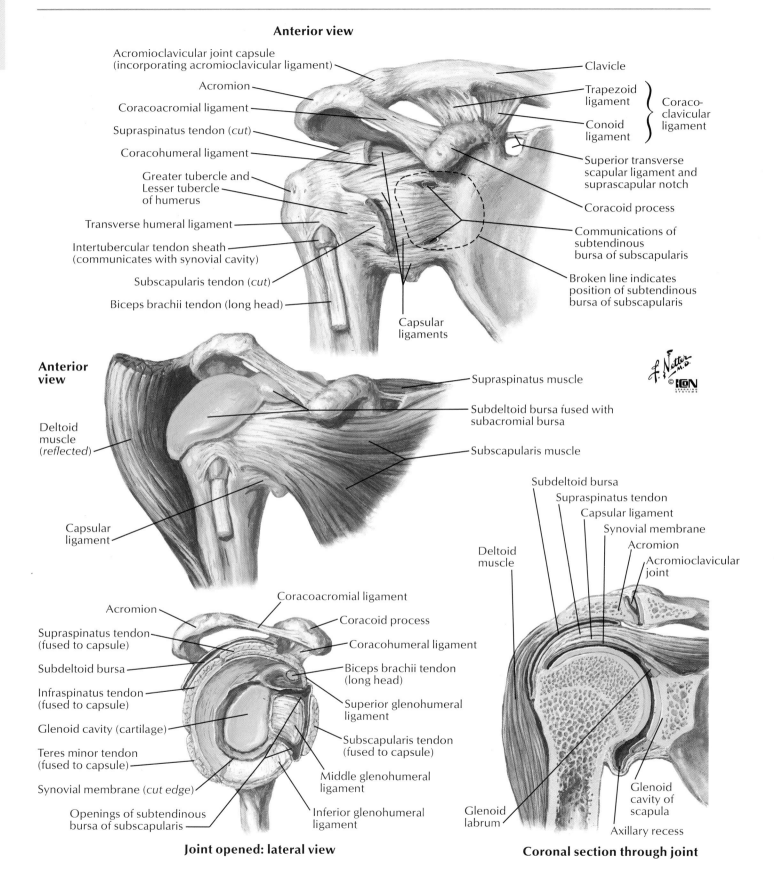

Anterior view

Acromioclavicular joint capsule (incorporating acromioclavicular ligament)

Acromion

Coracoacromial ligament

Supraspinatus tendon (*cut*)

Coracohumeral ligament

Greater tubercle and Lesser tubercle of humerus

Transverse humeral ligament

Intertubercular tendon sheath (communicates with synovial cavity)

Subscapularis tendon (*cut*)

Biceps brachii tendon (long head)

Capsular ligaments

Clavicle

Trapezoid ligament

Conoid ligament

Coraco-clavicular ligament

Superior transverse scapular ligament and suprascapular notch

Coracoid process

Communications of subtendinous bursa of subscapularis

Broken line indicates position of subtendinous bursa of subscapularis

Anterior view

Deltoid muscle (*reflected*)

Capsular ligament

Supraspinatus muscle

Subdeltoid bursa fused with subacromial bursa

Subscapularis muscle

Subdeltoid bursa

Supraspinatus tendon

Capsular ligament

Synovial membrane

Acromion

Acromioclavicular joint

Deltoid muscle

Glenoid labrum

Glenoid cavity of scapula

Axillary recess

Coronal section through joint

Acromion

Coracoacromial ligament

Coracoid process

Supraspinatus tendon (fused to capsule)

Coracohumeral ligament

Subdeltoid bursa

Biceps brachii tendon (long head)

Infraspinatus tendon (fused to capsule)

Superior glenohumeral ligament

Glenoid cavity (cartilage)

Subscapularis tendon (fused to capsule)

Teres minor tendon (fused to capsule)

Synovial membrane (*cut edge*)

Middle glenohumeral ligament

Openings of subtendinous bursa of subscapularis

Inferior glenohumeral ligament

Joint opened: lateral view

PLATE 406

UPPER LIMB

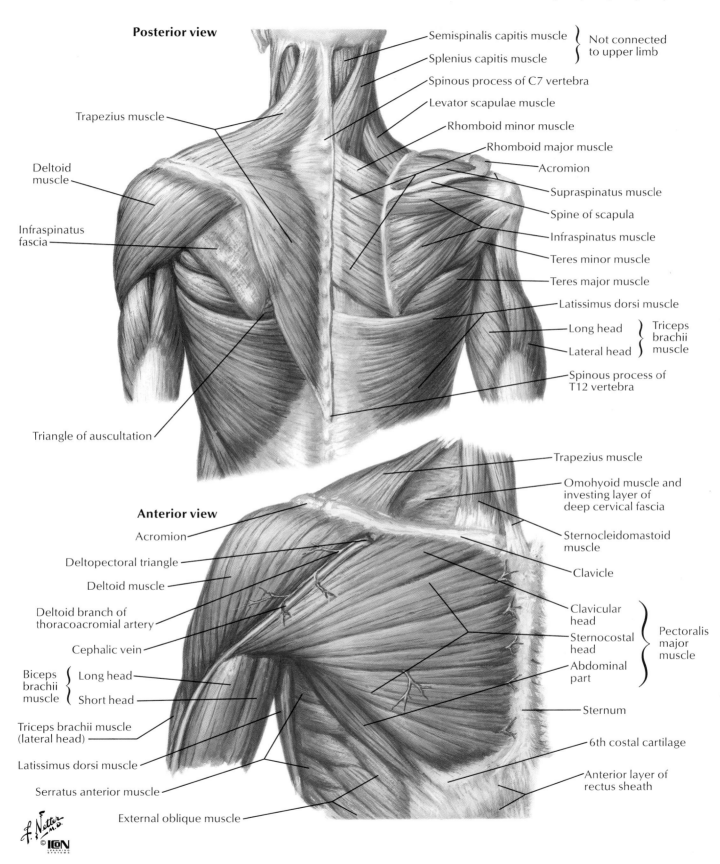

Posterior view

Semispinalis capitis muscle } Not connected to upper limb

Splenius capitis muscle

Spinous process of C7 vertebra

Levator scapulae muscle

Rhomboid minor muscle

Trapezius muscle

Rhomboid major muscle

Acromion

Deltoid muscle

Supraspinatus muscle

Spine of scapula

Infraspinatus fascia

Infraspinatus muscle

Teres minor muscle

Teres major muscle

Latissimus dorsi muscle

Long head } Triceps brachii muscle

Lateral head

Spinous process of T12 vertebra

Triangle of auscultation

Anterior view

Trapezius muscle

Omohyoid muscle and investing layer of deep cervical fascia

Sternocleidomastoid muscle

Acromion

Deltopectoral triangle

Clavicle

Deltoid muscle

Clavicular head

Deltoid branch of thoracoacromial artery

Sternocostal head } Pectoralis major muscle

Cephalic vein

Biceps brachii muscle { Long head

Short head

Abdominal part

Sternum

Triceps brachii muscle (lateral head)

6th costal cartilage

Latissimus dorsi muscle

Anterior layer of rectus sheath

Serratus anterior muscle

External oblique muscle

Muscles of Rotator Cuff

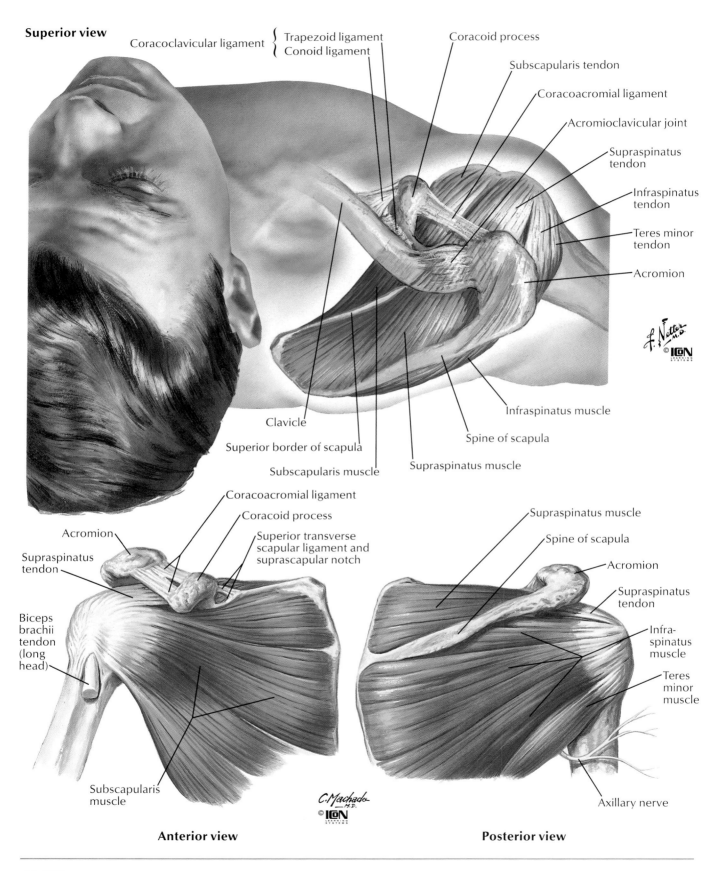

Superior view

Coracoclavicular ligament { Trapezoid ligament
Conoid ligament

Coracoid process

Subscapularis tendon

Coracoacromial ligament

Acromioclavicular joint

Supraspinatus tendon

Infraspinatus tendon

Teres minor tendon

Acromion

Infraspinatus muscle

Spine of scapula

Supraspinatus muscle

Subscapularis muscle

Subscapularis muscle

Superior border of scapula

Clavicle

Coracoacromial ligament

Coracoid process

Superior transverse scapular ligament and suprascapular notch

Acromion

Supraspinatus tendon

Biceps brachii tendon (long head)

Supraspinatus muscle

Spine of scapula

Acromion

Supraspinatus tendon

Infra-spinatus muscle

Teres minor muscle

Axillary nerve

Anterior view

Posterior view

PLATE 408

UPPER LIMB

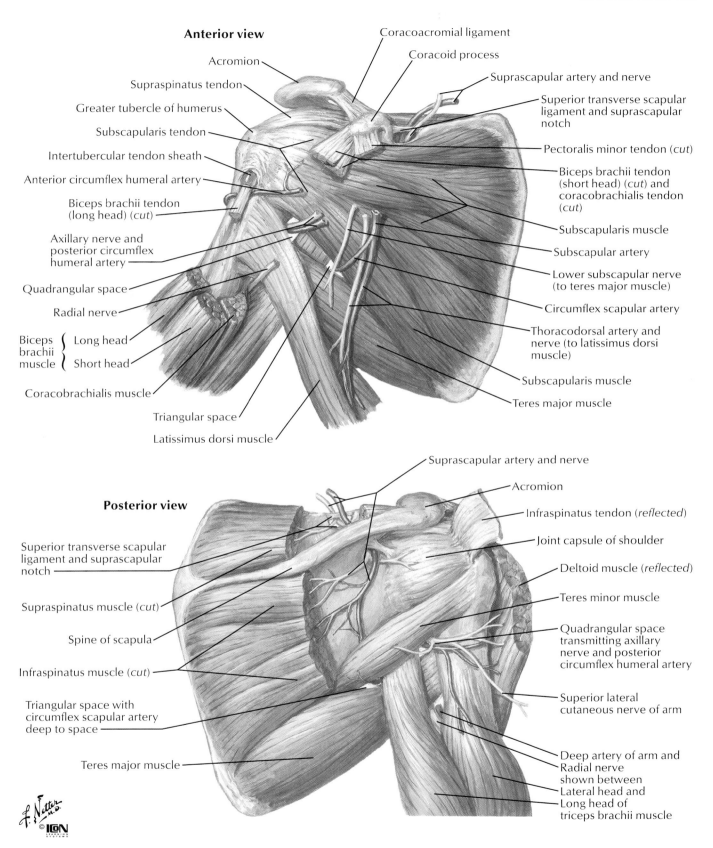

Anterior view

Coracoacromial ligament

Coracoid process

Acromion

Suprascapular artery and nerve

Supraspinatus tendon

Superior transverse scapular ligament and suprascapular notch

Greater tubercle of humerus

Subscapularis tendon

Pectoralis minor tendon (*cut*)

Intertubercular tendon sheath

Biceps brachii tendon (short head) (*cut*) and coracobrachialis tendon (*cut*)

Anterior circumflex humeral artery

Biceps brachii tendon (long head) (*cut*)

Subscapularis muscle

Axillary nerve and posterior circumflex humeral artery

Subscapular artery

Lower subscapular nerve (to teres major muscle)

Quadrangular space

Circumflex scapular artery

Radial nerve

Thoracodorsal artery and nerve (to latissimus dorsi muscle)

Biceps brachii muscle { Long head / Short head }

Subscapularis muscle

Coracobrachialis muscle

Teres major muscle

Triangular space

Latissimus dorsi muscle

Posterior view

Suprascapular artery and nerve

Acromion

Infraspinatus tendon (*reflected*)

Superior transverse scapular ligament and suprascapular notch

Joint capsule of shoulder

Supraspinatus muscle (*cut*)

Deltoid muscle (*reflected*)

Teres minor muscle

Spine of scapula

Quadrangular space transmitting axillary nerve and posterior circumflex humeral artery

Infraspinatus muscle (*cut*)

Triangular space with circumflex scapular artery deep to space

Superior lateral cutaneous nerve of arm

Teres major muscle

Deep artery of arm and Radial nerve shown between Lateral head and Long head of triceps brachii muscle

Axillary Artery and Anastomoses Around Scapula

SEE ALSO PLATES 29, 417

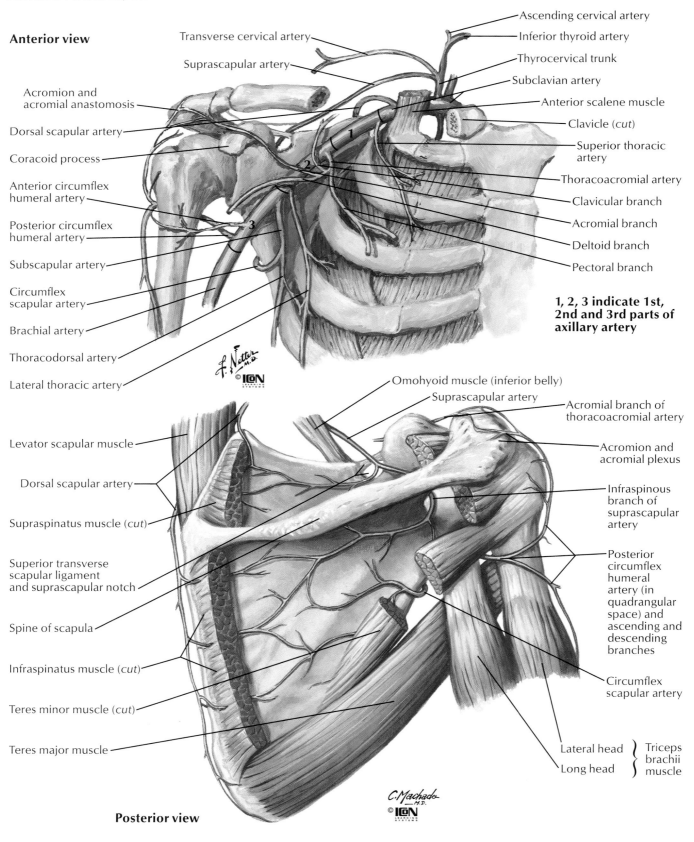

Anterior view

Transverse cervical artery

Suprascapular artery

Ascending cervical artery

Inferior thyroid artery

Thyrocervical trunk

Subclavian artery

Anterior scalene muscle

Clavicle (*cut*)

Superior thoracic artery

Thoracoacromial artery

Clavicular branch

Acromial branch

Deltoid branch

Pectoral branch

Acromion and acromial anastomosis

Dorsal scapular artery

Coracoid process

Anterior circumflex humeral artery

Posterior circumflex humeral artery

Subscapular artery

Circumflex scapular artery

Brachial artery

Thoracodorsal artery

Lateral thoracic artery

1, 2, 3 indicate 1st, 2nd and 3rd parts of axillary artery

Omohyoid muscle (inferior belly)

Suprascapular artery

Acromial branch of thoracoacromial artery

Acromion and acromial plexus

Infraspinous branch of suprascapular artery

Posterior circumflex humeral artery (in quadrangular space) and ascending and descending branches

Circumflex scapular artery

Levator scapular muscle

Dorsal scapular artery

Supraspinatus muscle (*cut*)

Superior transverse scapular ligament and suprascapular notch

Spine of scapula

Infraspinatus muscle (*cut*)

Teres minor muscle (*cut*)

Teres major muscle

Lateral head ⎱ Triceps
Long head ⎰ brachii muscle

Posterior view

PLATE 410

UPPER LIMB

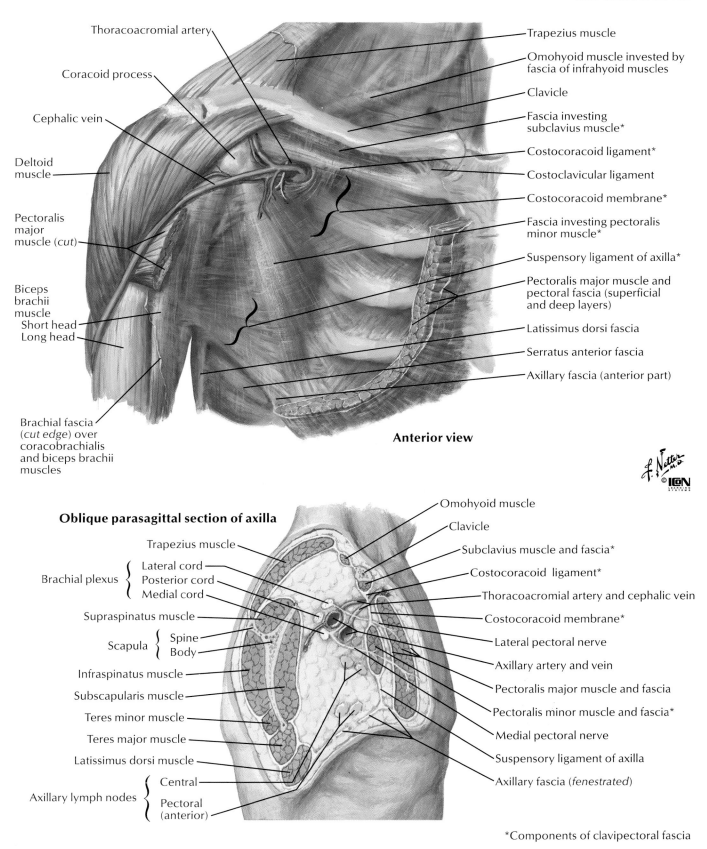

Thoracoacromial artery

Coracoid process

Cephalic vein

Deltoid muscle

Pectoralis major muscle (*cut*)

Biceps brachii muscle
Short head
Long head

Brachial fascia (*cut edge*) over coracobrachialis and biceps brachii muscles

Trapezius muscle

Omohyoid muscle invested by fascia of infrahyoid muscles

Clavicle

Fascia investing subclavius muscle*

Costocoracoid ligament*

Costoclavicular ligament

Costocoracoid membrane*

Fascia investing pectoralis minor muscle*

Suspensory ligament of axilla*

Pectoralis major muscle and pectoral fascia (superficial and deep layers)

Latissimus dorsi fascia

Serratus anterior fascia

Axillary fascia (anterior part)

Anterior view

Oblique parasagittal section of axilla

Brachial plexus
{
Lateral cord
Posterior cord
Medial cord
}

Supraspinatus muscle

Scapula
{
Spine
Body
}

Infraspinatus muscle

Subscapularis muscle

Teres minor muscle

Teres major muscle

Latissimus dorsi muscle

Axillary lymph nodes
{
Central
Pectoral (anterior)
}

Omohyoid muscle

Clavicle

Subclavius muscle and fascia*

Costocoracoid ligament*

Thoracoacromial artery and cephalic vein

Costocoracoid membrane*

Lateral pectoral nerve

Axillary artery and vein

Pectoralis major muscle and fascia

Pectoralis minor muscle and fascia*

Medial pectoral nerve

Suspensory ligament of axilla

Axillary fascia (*fenestrated*)

*Components of clavipectoral fascia

Axilla (Dissection): Anterior View

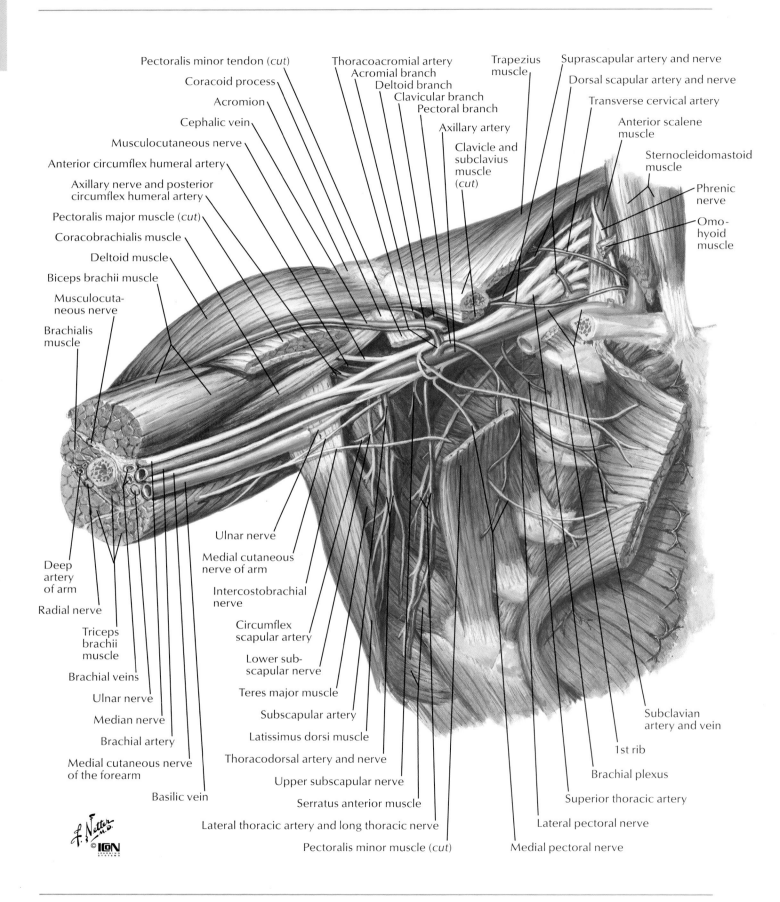

Pectoralis minor tendon (*cut*)
Coracoid process
Acromion
Cephalic vein
Musculocutaneous nerve
Anterior circumflex humeral artery
Axillary nerve and posterior circumflex humeral artery
Pectoralis major muscle (*cut*)
Coracobrachialis muscle
Deltoid muscle
Biceps brachii muscle
Musculocutaneous nerve
Brachialis muscle

Thoracoacromial artery
Acromial branch
Deltoid branch
Clavicular branch
Pectoral branch
Axillary artery
Clavicle and subclavius muscle (*cut*)

Trapezius muscle
Suprascapular artery and nerve
Dorsal scapular artery and nerve
Transverse cervical artery
Anterior scalene muscle
Sternocleidomastoid muscle
Phrenic nerve
Omo-hyoid muscle

Deep artery of arm
Radial nerve
Triceps brachii muscle
Brachial veins
Ulnar nerve
Median nerve
Brachial artery
Medial cutaneous nerve of the forearm
Basilic vein

Ulnar nerve
Medial cutaneous nerve of arm
Intercostobrachial nerve
Circumflex scapular artery
Lower sub-scapular nerve
Teres major muscle
Subscapular artery
Latissimus dorsi muscle
Thoracodorsal artery and nerve
Upper subscapular nerve
Serratus anterior muscle
Lateral thoracic artery and long thoracic nerve
Pectoralis minor muscle (*cut*)

Subclavian artery and vein
1st rib
Brachial plexus
Superior thoracic artery
Lateral pectoral nerve
Medial pectoral nerve

PLATE 412

UPPER LIMB

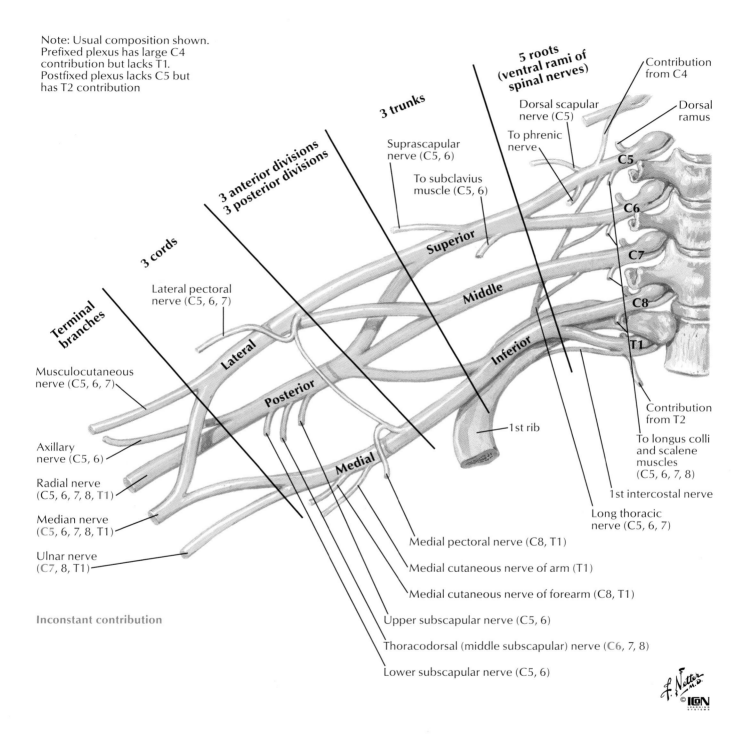

Note: Usual composition shown. Prefixed plexus has large C4 contribution but lacks T1. Postfixed plexus lacks C5 but has T2 contribution

5 roots (ventral rami of spinal nerves)

Contribution from C4

Dorsal scapular nerve (C5)

To phrenic nerve

Dorsal ramus

3 trunks

Suprascapular nerve (C5, 6)

To subclavius muscle (C5, 6)

C5

C6

C7

C8

T1

3 anterior divisions
3 posterior divisions

Superior

Middle

Inferior

3 cords

Lateral pectoral nerve (C5, 6, 7)

Lateral

Superior

Middle

Inferior

1st rib

Contribution from T2

Terminal branches

Posterior

To longus colli and scalene muscles (C5, 6, 7, 8)

Musculocutaneous nerve (C5, 6, 7)

1st intercostal nerve

Axillary nerve (C5, 6)

Medial

Long thoracic nerve (C5, 6, 7)

Radial nerve (C5, 6, 7, 8, T1)

Median nerve (C5, 6, 7, 8, T1)

Ulnar nerve (C7, 8, T1)

Medial pectoral nerve (C8, T1)

Medial cutaneous nerve of arm (T1)

Medial cutaneous nerve of forearm (C8, T1)

Inconstant contribution

Upper subscapular nerve (C5, 6)

Thoracodorsal (middle subscapular) nerve (C6, 7, 8)

Lower subscapular nerve (C5, 6)

F. Netter M.D.
© ICON

Muscles of Arm: Anterior Views

SEE ALSO PLATE 457

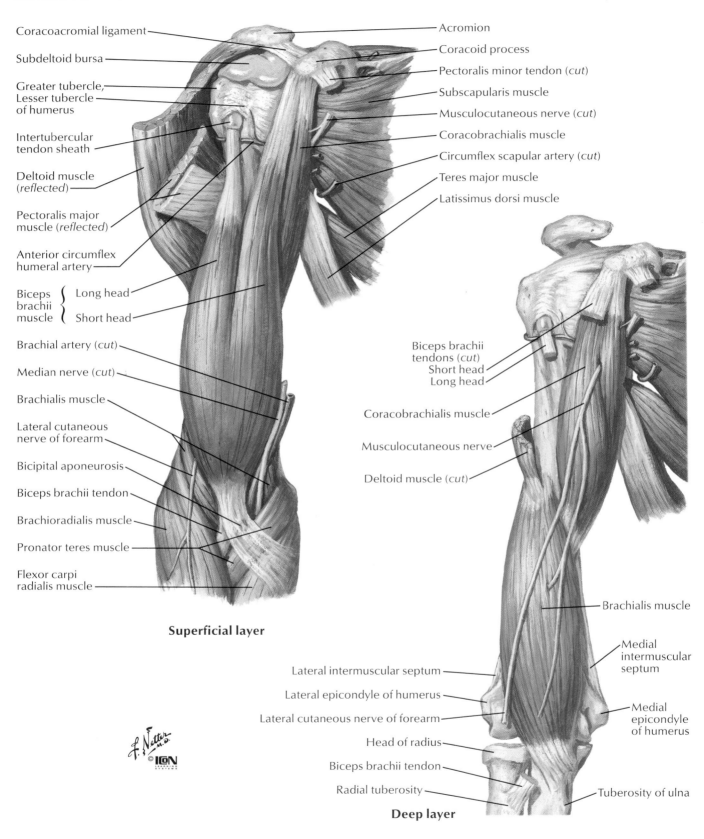

Coracoacromial ligament

Subdeltoid bursa

Greater tubercle,
Lesser tubercle
of humerus

Intertubercular
tendon sheath

Deltoid muscle
(reflected)

Pectoralis major
muscle (reflected)

Anterior circumflex
humeral artery

Biceps brachii muscle { Long head

Short head

Brachial artery (cut)

Median nerve (cut)

Brachialis muscle

Lateral cutaneous
nerve of forearm

Bicipital aponeurosis

Biceps brachii tendon

Brachioradialis muscle

Pronator teres muscle

Flexor carpi
radialis muscle

Acromion

Coracoid process

Pectoralis minor tendon (cut)

Subscapularis muscle

Musculocutaneous nerve (cut)

Coracobrachialis muscle

Circumflex scapular artery (cut)

Teres major muscle

Latissimus dorsi muscle

Superficial layer

Biceps brachii
tendons (cut)
Short head
Long head

Coracobrachialis muscle

Musculocutaneous nerve

Deltoid muscle (cut)

Brachialis muscle

Medial
intermuscular
septum

Lateral intermuscular septum

Lateral epicondyle of humerus

Lateral cutaneous nerve of forearm

Head of radius

Biceps brachii tendon

Radial tuberosity

Medial
epicondyle
of humerus

Tuberosity of ulna

Deep layer

PLATE 414

UPPER LIMB

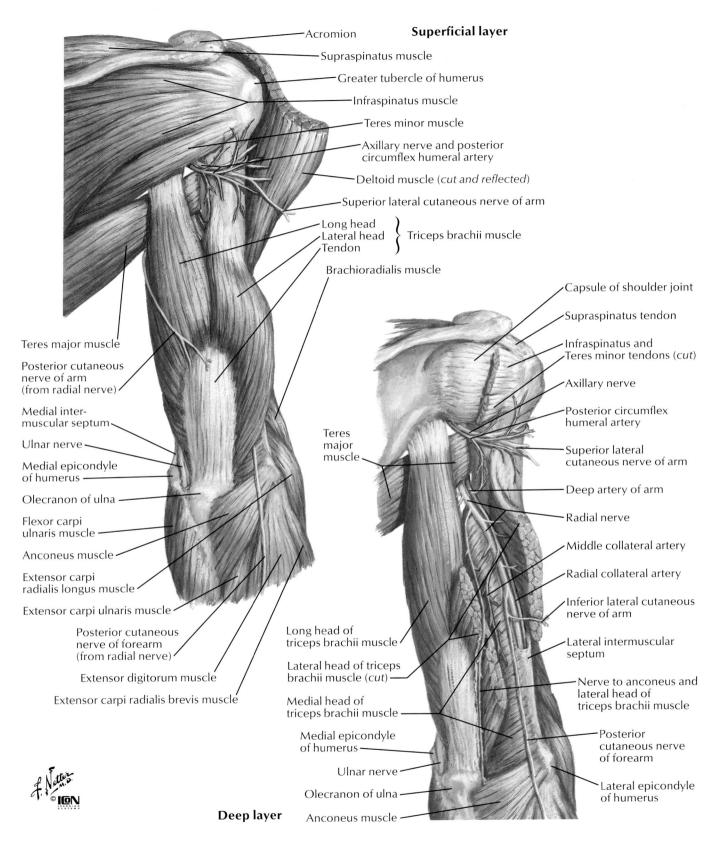

Superficial layer

Acromion

Supraspinatus muscle

Greater tubercle of humerus

Infraspinatus muscle

Teres minor muscle

Axillary nerve and posterior circumflex humeral artery

Deltoid muscle (*cut and reflected*)

Superior lateral cutaneous nerve of arm

Long head
Lateral head } Triceps brachii muscle
Tendon

Brachioradialis muscle

Capsule of shoulder joint

Supraspinatus tendon

Infraspinatus and Teres minor tendons (*cut*)

Axillary nerve

Posterior circumflex humeral artery

Superior lateral cutaneous nerve of arm

Deep artery of arm

Radial nerve

Middle collateral artery

Radial collateral artery

Inferior lateral cutaneous nerve of arm

Lateral intermuscular septum

Nerve to anconeus and lateral head of triceps brachii muscle

Posterior cutaneous nerve of forearm

Lateral epicondyle of humerus

Teres major muscle

Posterior cutaneous nerve of arm (from radial nerve)

Medial inter-muscular septum

Ulnar nerve

Medial epicondyle of humerus

Olecranon of ulna

Flexor carpi ulnaris muscle

Anconeus muscle

Extensor carpi radialis longus muscle

Extensor carpi ulnaris muscle

Posterior cutaneous nerve of forearm (from radial nerve)

Extensor digitorum muscle

Extensor carpi radialis brevis muscle

Teres major muscle

Long head of triceps brachii muscle

Lateral head of triceps brachii muscle (*cut*)

Medial head of triceps brachii muscle

Medial epicondyle of humerus

Ulnar nerve

Olecranon of ulna

Deep layer

Anconeus muscle

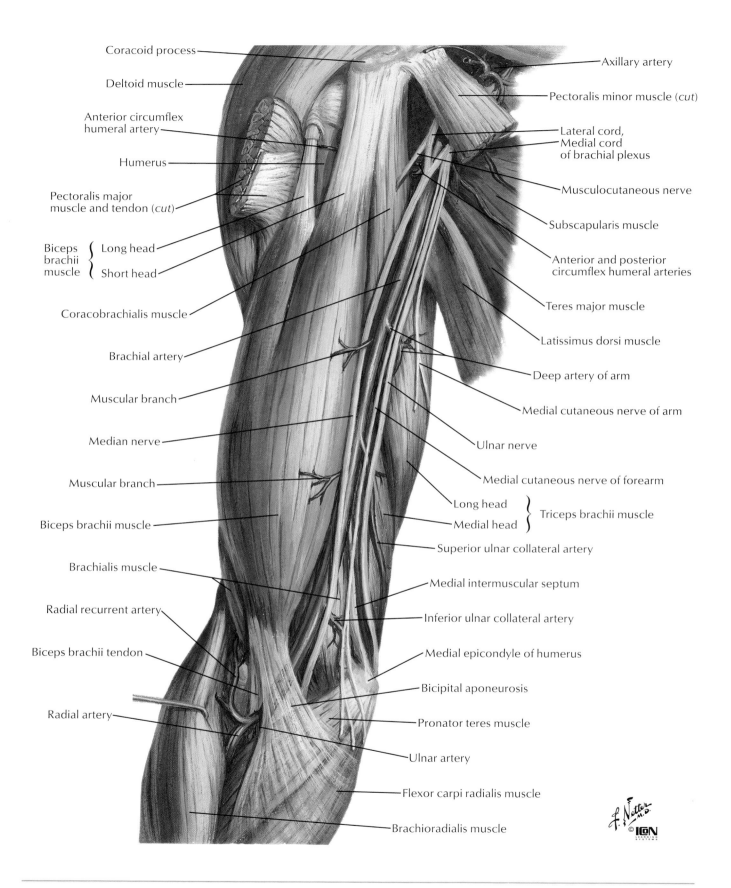

Coracoid process

Deltoid muscle

Anterior circumflex humeral artery

Humerus

Pectoralis major muscle and tendon (cut)

Biceps brachii muscle { Long head / Short head }

Coracobrachialis muscle

Brachial artery

Muscular branch

Median nerve

Muscular branch

Biceps brachii muscle

Brachialis muscle

Radial recurrent artery

Biceps brachii tendon

Radial artery

Axillary artery

Pectoralis minor muscle (cut)

Lateral cord, Medial cord of brachial plexus

Musculocutaneous nerve

Subscapularis muscle

Anterior and posterior circumflex humeral arteries

Teres major muscle

Latissimus dorsi muscle

Deep artery of arm

Medial cutaneous nerve of arm

Ulnar nerve

Medial cutaneous nerve of forearm

Long head / Medial head } Triceps brachii muscle

Superior ulnar collateral artery

Medial intermuscular septum

Inferior ulnar collateral artery

Medial epicondyle of humerus

Bicipital aponeurosis

Pronator teres muscle

Ulnar artery

Flexor carpi radialis muscle

Brachioradialis muscle

PLATE 416

UPPER LIMB

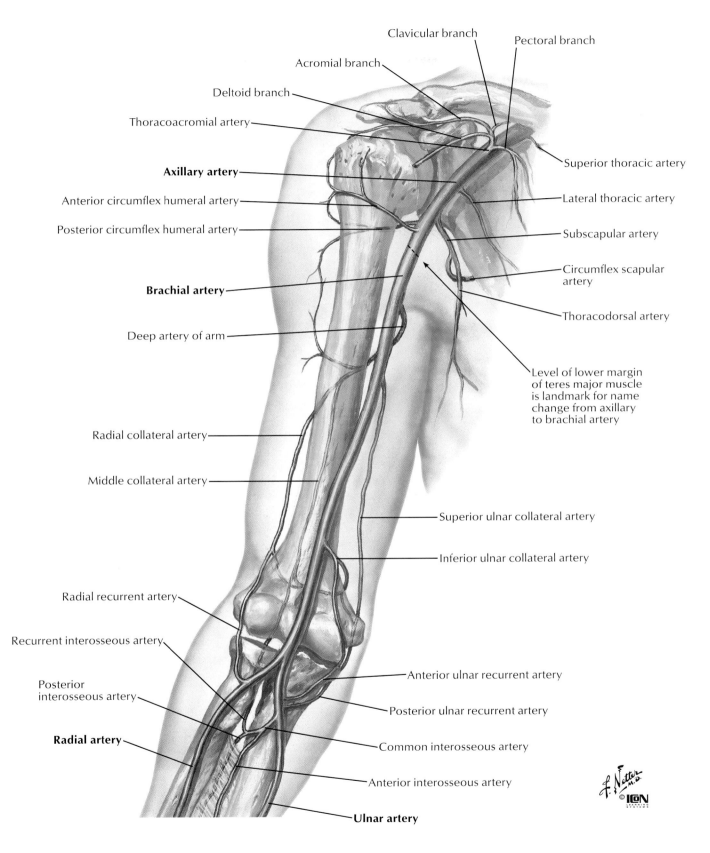

Clavicular branch

Pectoral branch

Acromial branch

Deltoid branch

Thoracoacromial artery

Axillary artery

Anterior circumflex humeral artery

Posterior circumflex humeral artery

Brachial artery

Deep artery of arm

Radial collateral artery

Middle collateral artery

Radial recurrent artery

Recurrent interosseous artery

Posterior interosseous artery

Radial artery

Superior thoracic artery

Lateral thoracic artery

Subscapular artery

Circumflex scapular artery

Thoracodorsal artery

Level of lower margin of teres major muscle is landmark for name change from axillary to brachial artery

Superior ulnar collateral artery

Inferior ulnar collateral artery

Anterior ulnar recurrent artery

Posterior ulnar recurrent artery

Common interosseous artery

Anterior interosseous artery

Ulnar artery

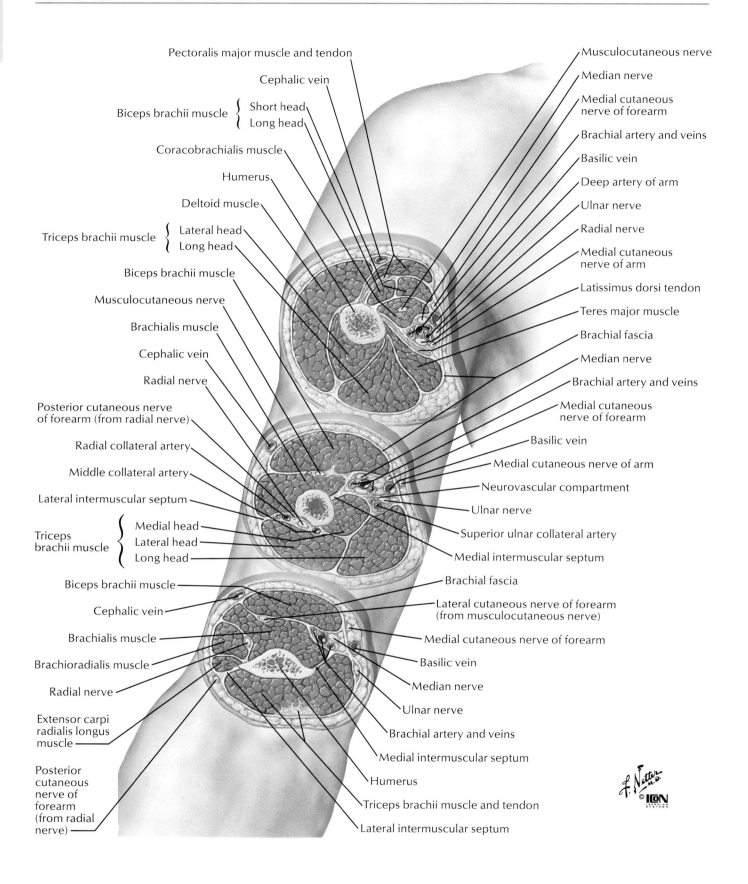

Pectoralis major muscle and tendon

Cephalic vein

Biceps brachii muscle { Short head / Long head

Coracobrachialis muscle

Humerus

Deltoid muscle

Triceps brachii muscle { Lateral head / Long head

Biceps brachii muscle

Musculocutaneous nerve

Brachialis muscle

Cephalic vein

Radial nerve

Posterior cutaneous nerve of forearm (from radial nerve)

Radial collateral artery

Middle collateral artery

Lateral intermuscular septum

Triceps brachii muscle { Medial head / Lateral head / Long head

Biceps brachii muscle

Cephalic vein

Brachialis muscle

Brachioradialis muscle

Radial nerve

Extensor carpi radialis longus muscle

Posterior cutaneous nerve of forearm (from radial nerve)

Musculocutaneous nerve

Median nerve

Medial cutaneous nerve of forearm

Brachial artery and veins

Basilic vein

Deep artery of arm

Ulnar nerve

Radial nerve

Medial cutaneous nerve of arm

Latissimus dorsi tendon

Teres major muscle

Brachial fascia

Median nerve

Brachial artery and veins

Medial cutaneous nerve of forearm

Basilic vein

Medial cutaneous nerve of arm

Neurovascular compartment

Ulnar nerve

Superior ulnar collateral artery

Medial intermuscular septum

Brachial fascia

Lateral cutaneous nerve of forearm (from musculocutaneous nerve)

Medial cutaneous nerve of forearm

Basilic vein

Median nerve

Ulnar nerve

Brachial artery and veins

Medial intermuscular septum

Humerus

Triceps brachii muscle and tendon

Lateral intermuscular septum

PLATE 418

UPPER LIMB

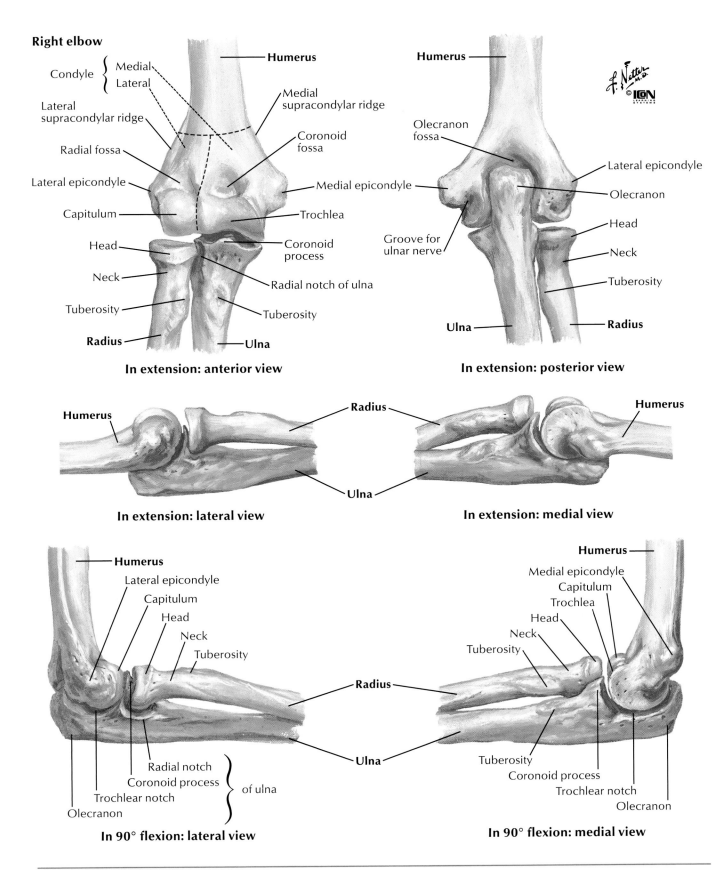

Right elbow

Condyle { Medial
         Lateral

Lateral supracondylar ridge

Radial fossa

Lateral epicondyle

Capitulum

Head

Neck

Tuberosity

Radius

Humerus

Medial supracondylar ridge

Coronoid fossa

Medial epicondyle

Trochlea

Coronoid process

Radial notch of ulna

Tuberosity

Ulna

In extension: anterior view

Humerus

Olecranon fossa

Groove for ulnar nerve

Lateral epicondyle

Olecranon

Head

Neck

Tuberosity

Radius

Ulna

In extension: posterior view

Humerus

Radius

Ulna

In extension: lateral view

Radius

Ulna

Humerus

In extension: medial view

Humerus

Lateral epicondyle

Capitulum

Head

Neck

Tuberosity

Radius

Radial notch
Coronoid process } of ulna
Trochlear notch

Olecranon

Ulna

In 90° flexion: lateral view

Humerus

Medial epicondyle

Capitulum

Trochlea

Head

Neck

Tuberosity

Tuberosity

Coronoid process

Trochlear notch

Olecranon

Radius

Ulna

In 90° flexion: medial view

Elbow: Radiographs

SEE ALSO PLATE 419

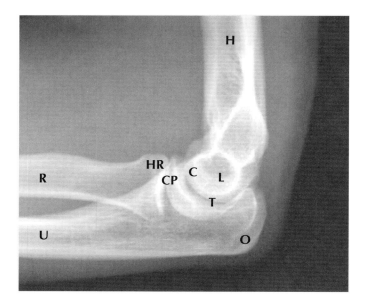

Lateral radiograph

C	Capitulum
CP	Coronoid process of ulna
H	Humerus
HR	Head of radius
L	Lateral epicondyle
O	Olecranon
R	Radius
T	Trochlear notch
U	Ulna

Anteroposterior radiograph

C	Capitulum
CP	Coronoid process of ulna
H	Humerus
HR	Head of radius
L	Lateral epicondyle
M	Medial of epicondyle
NR	Neck of radius
O	Olecranon
OF	Olecranon fossa
R	Radius
T	Trochlea of humerus
RT	Radial tuberosity
U	Ulna

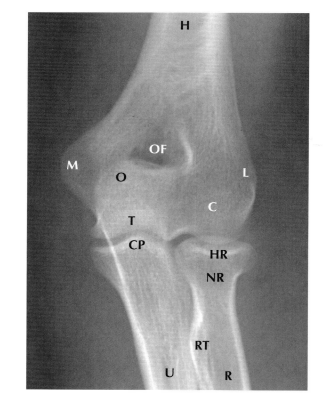

PLATE 420   **UPPER LIMB**

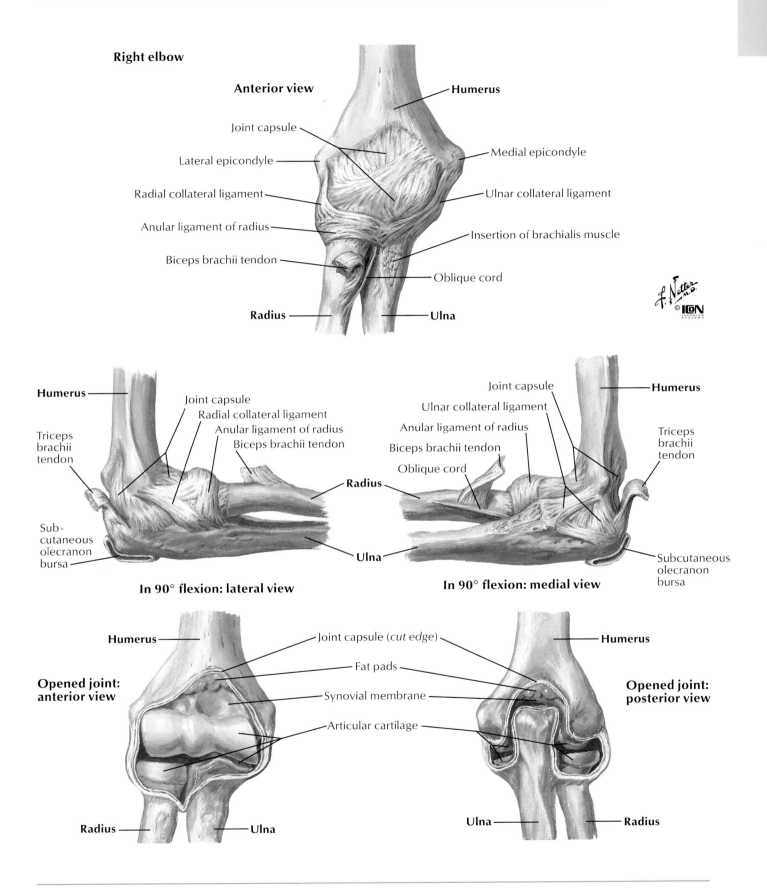

Right elbow

Anterior view

Joint capsule

Lateral epicondyle

Radial collateral ligament

Anular ligament of radius

Biceps brachii tendon

Radius

Humerus

Medial epicondyle

Ulnar collateral ligament

Insertion of brachialis muscle

Oblique cord

Ulna

Humerus

Triceps brachii tendon

Sub-cutaneous olecranon bursa

Joint capsule
Radial collateral ligament
Anular ligament of radius
Biceps brachii tendon

Radius

Ulna

In 90° flexion: lateral view

Joint capsule
Ulnar collateral ligament
Anular ligament of radius
Biceps brachii tendon
Oblique cord

Radius

Humerus

Triceps brachii tendon

Subcutaneous olecranon bursa

In 90° flexion: medial view

Humerus

Opened joint: anterior view

Joint capsule (*cut edge*)

Fat pads

Synovial membrane

Articular cartilage

Radius   **Ulna**

Humerus

Opened joint: posterior view

Ulna   **Radius**

Bones of Forearm

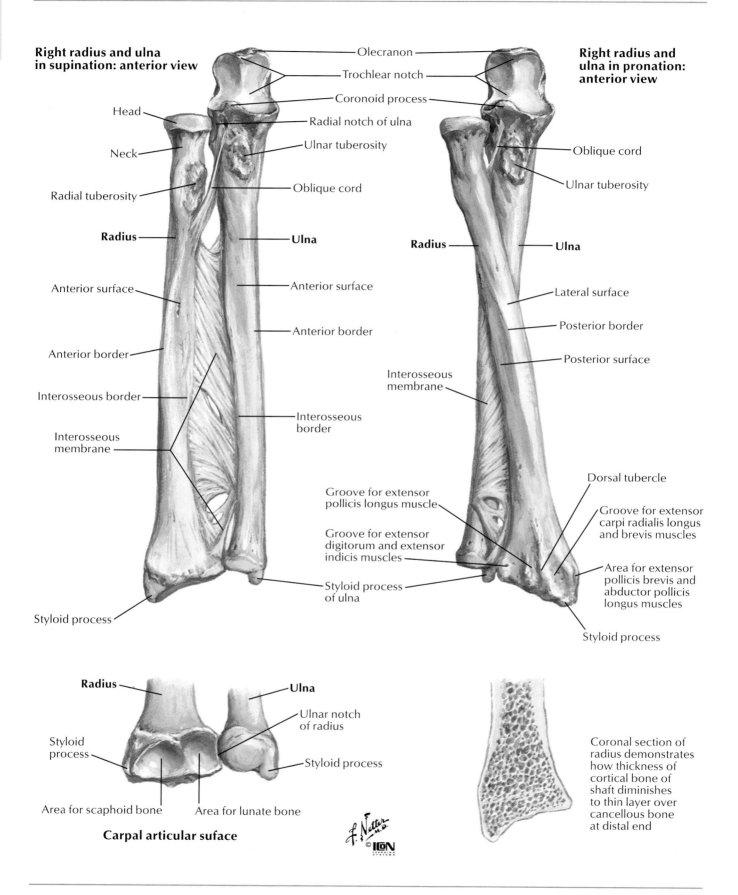

Right radius and ulna in supination: anterior view

Head

Neck

Radial tuberosity

Radius

Anterior surface

Anterior border

Interosseous border

Interosseous membrane

Styloid process

Olecranon

Trochlear notch

Coronoid process

Radial notch of ulna

Ulnar tuberosity

Oblique cord

Ulna

Anterior surface

Anterior border

Interosseous border

Groove for extensor pollicis longus muscle

Groove for extensor digitorum and extensor indicis muscles

Styloid process of ulna

Right radius and ulna in pronation: anterior view

Oblique cord

Ulnar tuberosity

Radius   **Ulna**

Lateral surface

Posterior border

Posterior surface

Interosseous membrane

Dorsal tubercle

Groove for extensor carpi radialis longus and brevis muscles

Area for extensor pollicis brevis and abductor pollicis longus muscles

Styloid process

Radius   **Ulna**

Styloid process

Ulnar notch of radius

Styloid process

Area for scaphoid bone   Area for lunate bone

Carpal articular suface

Coronal section of radius demonstrates how thickness of cortical bone of shaft diminishes to thin layer over cancellous bone at distal end

PLATE 422

UPPER LIMB

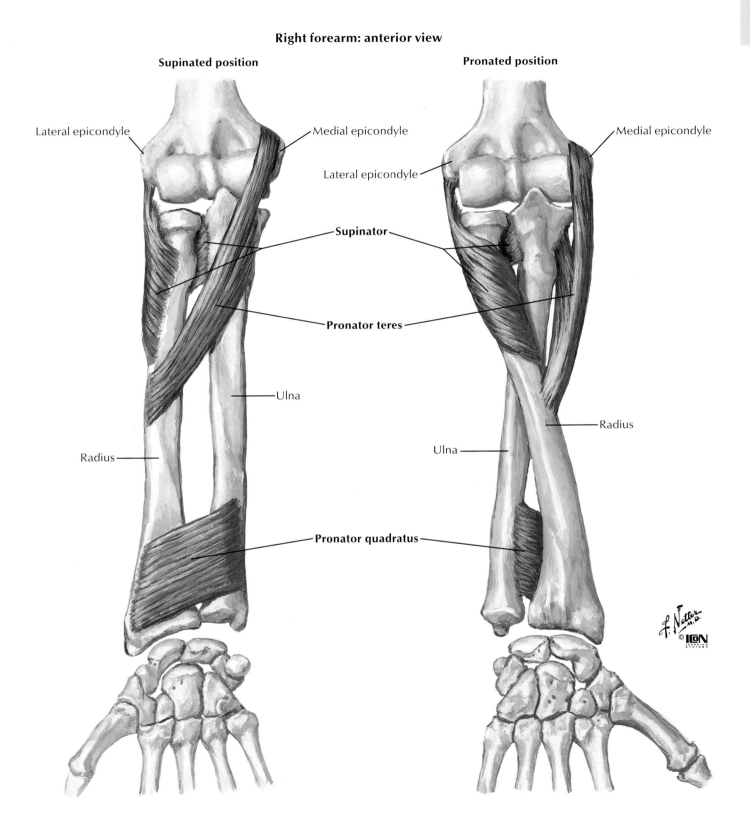

Right forearm: anterior view

Supinated position

Pronated position

Lateral epicondyle

Medial epicondyle

Medial epicondyle

Lateral epicondyle

Supinator

Pronator teres

Ulna

Radius

Radius

Ulna

Pronator quadratus

Individual Muscles of Forearm: Extensors of Wrist and Digits

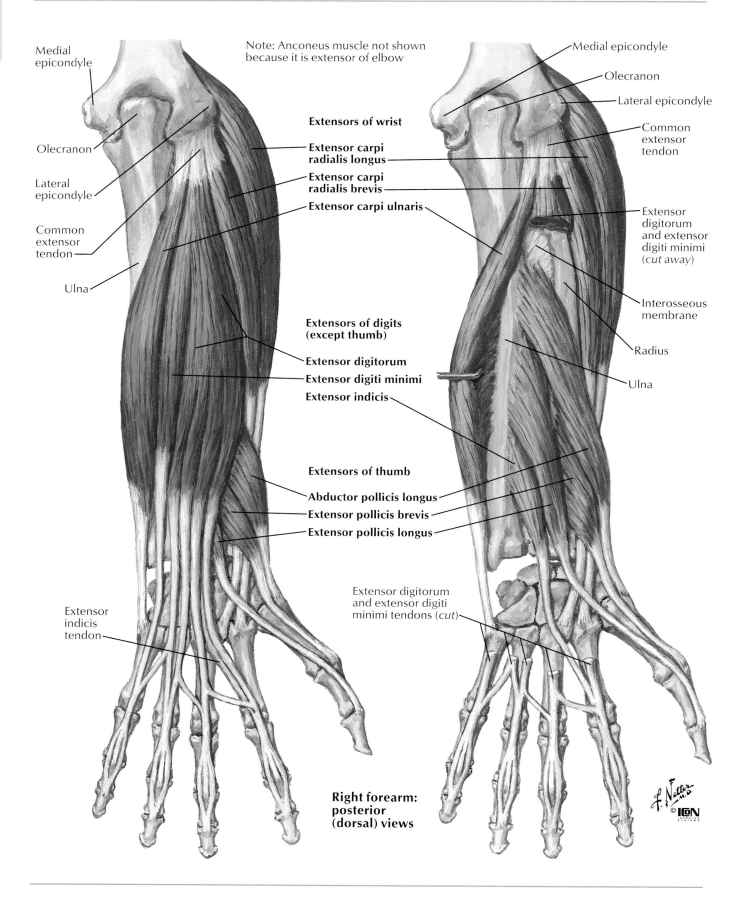

Note: Anconeus muscle not shown because it is extensor of elbow

Medial epicondyle

Olecranon

Lateral epicondyle

Common extensor tendon

Ulna

Extensors of wrist

Extensor carpi radialis longus

Extensor carpi radialis brevis

Extensor carpi ulnaris

Extensors of digits (except thumb)

Extensor digitorum

Extensor digiti minimi

Extensor indicis

Extensors of thumb

Abductor pollicis longus

Extensor pollicis brevis

Extensor pollicis longus

Extensor indicis tendon

Medial epicondyle

Olecranon

Lateral epicondyle

Common extensor tendon

Extensor digitorum and extensor digiti minimi (cut away)

Interosseous membrane

Radius

Ulna

Extensor digitorum and extensor digiti minimi tendons (cut)

Right forearm: posterior (dorsal) views

PLATE 424

UPPER LIMB

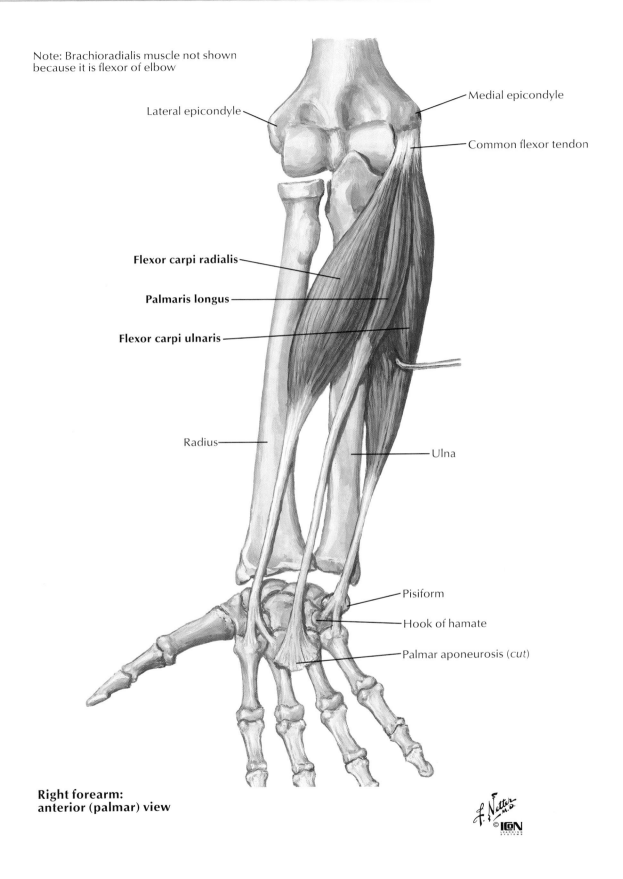

Note: Brachioradialis muscle not shown
because it is flexor of elbow

Lateral epicondyle

Medial epicondyle

Common flexor tendon

Flexor carpi radialis

Palmaris longus

Flexor carpi ulnaris

Radius

Ulna

Pisiform

Hook of hamate

Palmar aponeurosis (*cut*)

**Right forearm:
anterior (palmar) view**

Individual Muscles of Forearm: Flexors of Digits

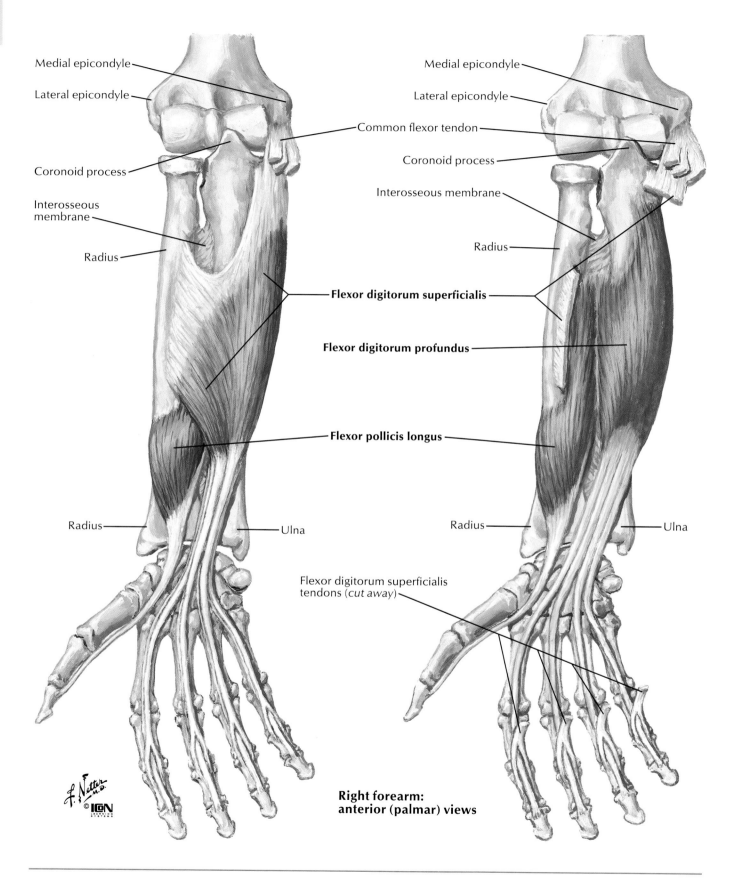

Medial epicondyle

Lateral epicondyle

Coronoid process

Interosseous membrane

Radius

Medial epicondyle

Lateral epicondyle

Common flexor tendon

Coronoid process

Interosseous membrane

Radius

Flexor digitorum superficialis

Flexor digitorum profundus

Flexor pollicis longus

Radius

Ulna

Radius

Ulna

Flexor digitorum superficialis tendons (*cut away*)

Right forearm: anterior (palmar) views

PLATE 426

UPPER LIMB

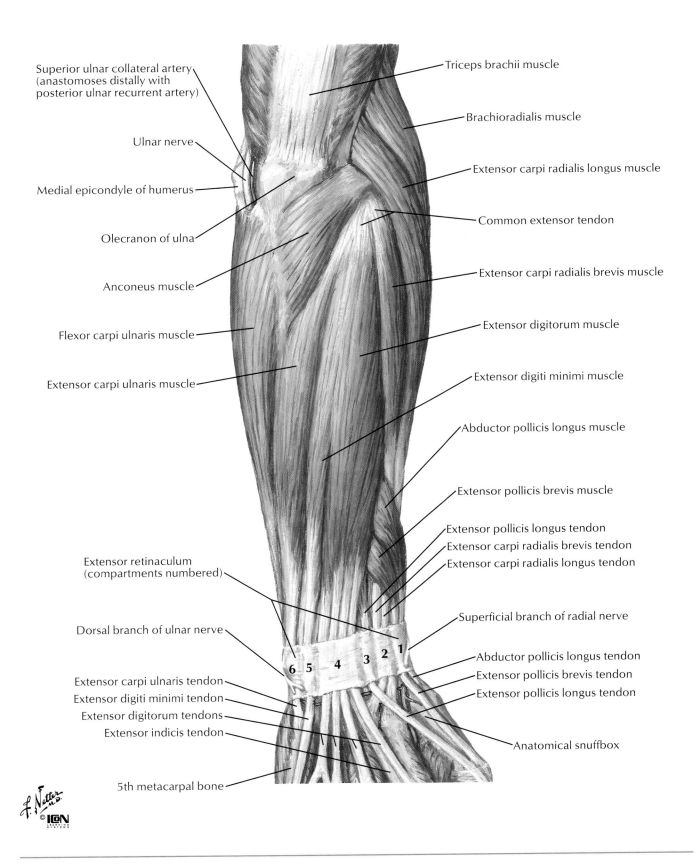

Superior ulnar collateral artery (anastomoses distally with posterior ulnar recurrent artery)

Ulnar nerve

Medial epicondyle of humerus

Olecranon of ulna

Anconeus muscle

Flexor carpi ulnaris muscle

Extensor carpi ulnaris muscle

Extensor retinaculum (compartments numbered)

Dorsal branch of ulnar nerve

Extensor carpi ulnaris tendon

Extensor digiti minimi tendon

Extensor digitorum tendons

Extensor indicis tendon

5th metacarpal bone

Triceps brachii muscle

Brachioradialis muscle

Extensor carpi radialis longus muscle

Common extensor tendon

Extensor carpi radialis brevis muscle

Extensor digitorum muscle

Extensor digiti minimi muscle

Abductor pollicis longus muscle

Extensor pollicis brevis muscle

Extensor pollicis longus tendon

Extensor carpi radialis brevis tendon

Extensor carpi radialis longus tendon

Superficial branch of radial nerve

Abductor pollicis longus tendon

Extensor pollicis brevis tendon

Extensor pollicis longus tendon

Anatomical snuffbox

6 5 4 3 2 1

SEE ALSO PLATES 453, 461

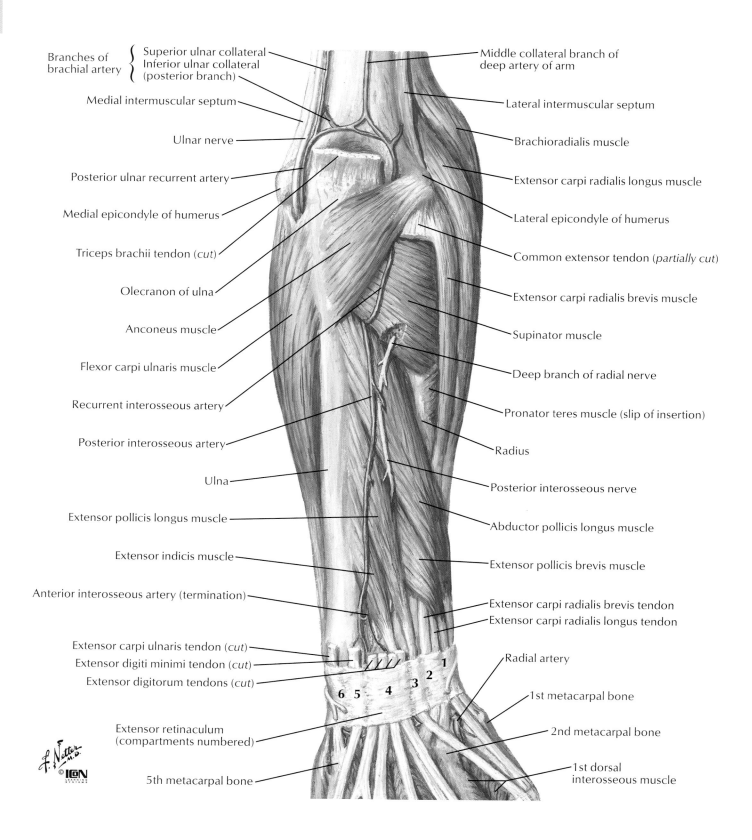

Branches of brachial artery {
Superior ulnar collateral
Inferior ulnar collateral (posterior branch)

Medial intermuscular septum

Ulnar nerve

Posterior ulnar recurrent artery

Medial epicondyle of humerus

Triceps brachii tendon (cut)

Olecranon of ulna

Anconeus muscle

Flexor carpi ulnaris muscle

Recurrent interosseous artery

Posterior interosseous artery

Ulna

Extensor pollicis longus muscle

Extensor indicis muscle

Anterior interosseous artery (termination)

Extensor carpi ulnaris tendon (cut)

Extensor digiti minimi tendon (cut)

Extensor digitorum tendons (cut)

Extensor retinaculum (compartments numbered)

5th metacarpal bone

Middle collateral branch of deep artery of arm

Lateral intermuscular septum

Brachioradialis muscle

Extensor carpi radialis longus muscle

Lateral epicondyle of humerus

Common extensor tendon (partially cut)

Extensor carpi radialis brevis muscle

Supinator muscle

Deep branch of radial nerve

Pronator teres muscle (slip of insertion)

Radius

Posterior interosseous nerve

Abductor pollicis longus muscle

Extensor pollicis brevis muscle

Extensor carpi radialis brevis tendon

Extensor carpi radialis longus tendon

Radial artery

1st metacarpal bone

2nd metacarpal bone

1st dorsal interosseous muscle

PLATE 428

UPPER LIMB

SEE ALSO PLATES 458, 459

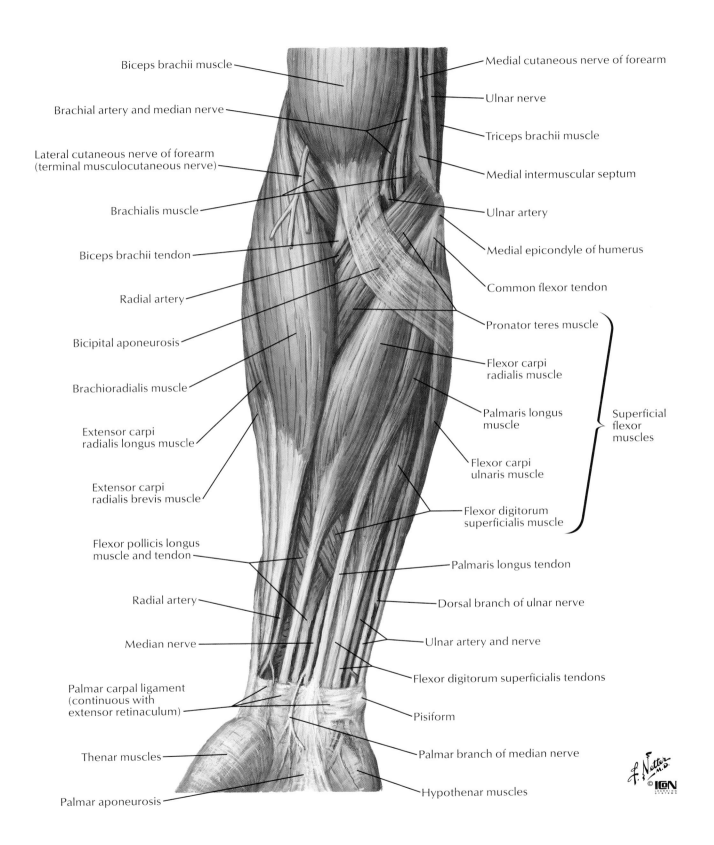

Biceps brachii muscle

Brachial artery and median nerve

Lateral cutaneous nerve of forearm
(terminal musculocutaneous nerve)

Brachialis muscle

Biceps brachii tendon

Radial artery

Bicipital aponeurosis

Brachioradialis muscle

Extensor carpi
radialis longus muscle

Extensor carpi
radialis brevis muscle

Flexor pollicis longus
muscle and tendon

Radial artery

Median nerve

Palmar carpal ligament
(continuous with
extensor retinaculum)

Thenar muscles

Palmar aponeurosis

Medial cutaneous nerve of forearm

Ulnar nerve

Triceps brachii muscle

Medial intermuscular septum

Ulnar artery

Medial epicondyle of humerus

Common flexor tendon

Pronator teres muscle

Flexor carpi
radialis muscle

Palmaris longus
muscle

Flexor carpi
ulnaris muscle

Flexor digitorum
superficialis muscle

Superficial
flexor
muscles

Palmaris longus tendon

Dorsal branch of ulnar nerve

Ulnar artery and nerve

Flexor digitorum superficialis tendons

Pisiform

Palmar branch of median nerve

Hypothenar muscles

ELBOW AND FOREARM

PLATE 429

SEE ALSO PLATES 458, 459

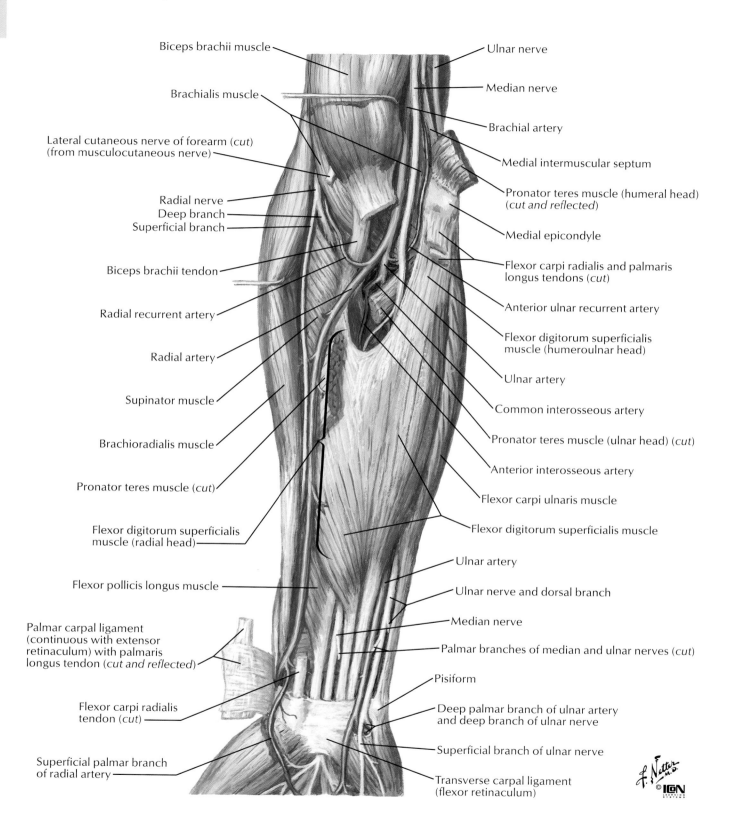

Biceps brachii muscle

Brachialis muscle

Lateral cutaneous nerve of forearm (*cut*)
(from musculocutaneous nerve)

Radial nerve
Deep branch
Superficial branch

Biceps brachii tendon

Radial recurrent artery

Radial artery

Supinator muscle

Brachioradialis muscle

Pronator teres muscle (*cut*)

Flexor digitorum superficialis
muscle (radial head)

Flexor pollicis longus muscle

Palmar carpal ligament
(continuous with extensor
retinaculum) with palmaris
longus tendon (*cut and reflected*)

Flexor carpi radialis
tendon (*cut*)

Superficial palmar branch
of radial artery

Ulnar nerve

Median nerve

Brachial artery

Medial intermuscular septum

Pronator teres muscle (humeral head)
(*cut and reflected*)

Medial epicondyle

Flexor carpi radialis and palmaris
longus tendons (*cut*)

Anterior ulnar recurrent artery

Flexor digitorum superficialis
muscle (humeroulnar head)

Ulnar artery

Common interosseous artery

Pronator teres muscle (ulnar head) (*cut*)

Anterior interosseous artery

Flexor carpi ulnaris muscle

Flexor digitorum superficialis muscle

Ulnar artery

Ulnar nerve and dorsal branch

Median nerve

Palmar branches of median and ulnar nerves (*cut*)

Pisiform

Deep palmar branch of ulnar artery
and deep branch of ulnar nerve

Superficial branch of ulnar nerve

Transverse carpal ligament
(flexor retinaculum)

PLATE 430

UPPER LIMB

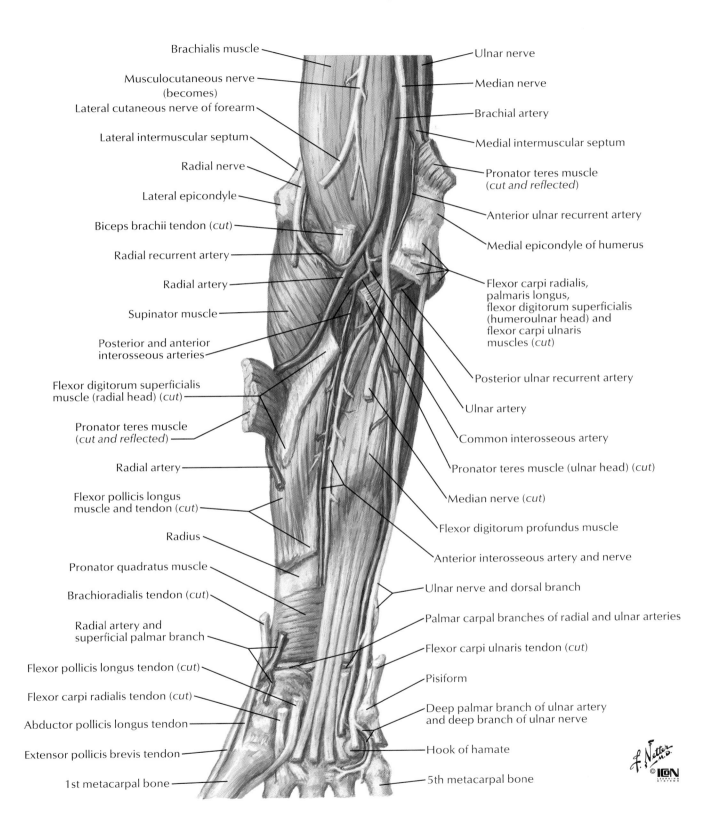

Brachialis muscle

Musculocutaneous nerve (becomes)

Lateral cutaneous nerve of forearm

Lateral intermuscular septum

Radial nerve

Lateral epicondyle

Biceps brachii tendon (*cut*)

Radial recurrent artery

Radial artery

Supinator muscle

Posterior and anterior interosseous arteries

Flexor digitorum superficialis muscle (radial head) (*cut*)

Pronator teres muscle (*cut and reflected*)

Radial artery

Flexor pollicis longus muscle and tendon (*cut*)

Radius

Pronator quadratus muscle

Brachioradialis tendon (*cut*)

Radial artery and superficial palmar branch

Flexor pollicis longus tendon (*cut*)

Flexor carpi radialis tendon (*cut*)

Abductor pollicis longus tendon

Extensor pollicis brevis tendon

1st metacarpal bone

Ulnar nerve

Median nerve

Brachial artery

Medial intermuscular septum

Pronator teres muscle (*cut and reflected*)

Anterior ulnar recurrent artery

Medial epicondyle of humerus

Flexor carpi radialis, palmaris longus, flexor digitorum superficialis (humeroulnar head) and flexor carpi ulnaris muscles (*cut*)

Posterior ulnar recurrent artery

Ulnar artery

Common interosseous artery

Pronator teres muscle (ulnar head) (*cut*)

Median nerve (*cut*)

Flexor digitorum profundus muscle

Anterior interosseous artery and nerve

Ulnar nerve and dorsal branch

Palmar carpal branches of radial and ulnar arteries

Flexor carpi ulnaris tendon (*cut*)

Pisiform

Deep palmar branch of ulnar artery and deep branch of ulnar nerve

Hook of hamate

5th metacarpal bone

Forearm: Serial Cross Sections

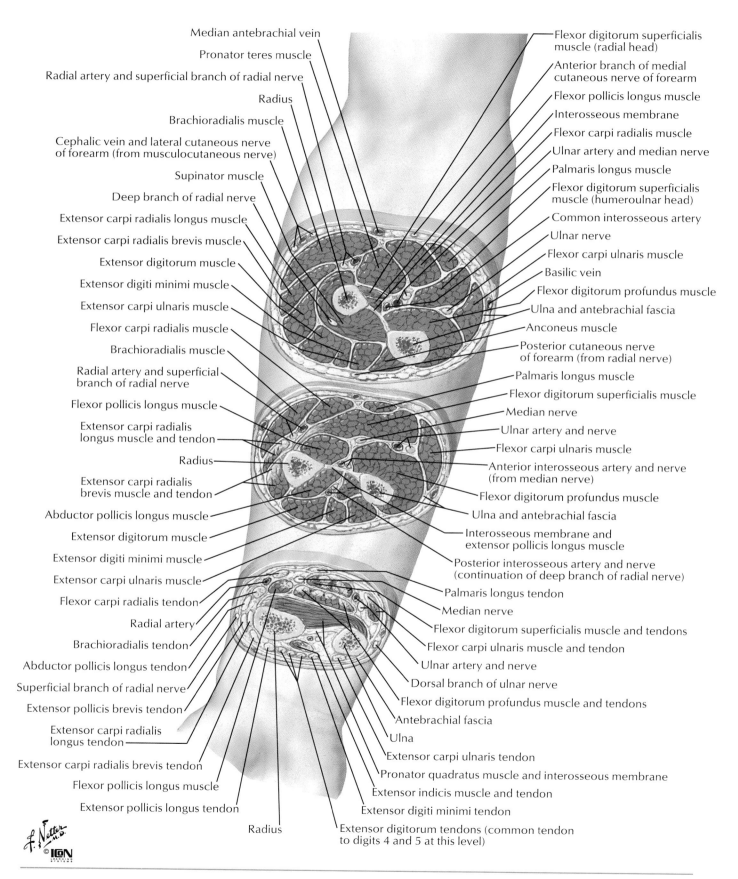

Median antebrachial vein
Pronator teres muscle
Radial artery and superficial branch of radial nerve
Radius
Brachioradialis muscle
Cephalic vein and lateral cutaneous nerve of forearm (from musculocutaneous nerve)
Supinator muscle
Deep branch of radial nerve
Extensor carpi radialis longus muscle
Extensor carpi radialis brevis muscle
Extensor digitorum muscle
Extensor digiti minimi muscle
Extensor carpi ulnaris muscle
Flexor carpi radialis muscle
Brachioradialis muscle
Radial artery and superficial branch of radial nerve
Flexor pollicis longus muscle
Extensor carpi radialis longus muscle and tendon
Radius
Extensor carpi radialis brevis muscle and tendon
Abductor pollicis longus muscle
Extensor digitorum muscle
Extensor digiti minimi muscle
Extensor carpi ulnaris muscle
Flexor carpi radialis tendon
Radial artery
Brachioradialis tendon
Abductor pollicis longus tendon
Superficial branch of radial nerve
Extensor pollicis brevis tendon
Extensor carpi radialis longus tendon
Extensor carpi radialis brevis tendon
Flexor pollicis longus muscle
Extensor pollicis longus tendon
Radius

Flexor digitorum superficialis muscle (radial head)
Anterior branch of medial cutaneous nerve of forearm
Flexor pollicis longus muscle
Interosseous membrane
Flexor carpi radialis muscle
Ulnar artery and median nerve
Palmaris longus muscle
Flexor digitorum superficialis muscle (humeroulnar head)
Common interosseous artery
Ulnar nerve
Flexor carpi ulnaris muscle
Basilic vein
Flexor digitorum profundus muscle
Ulna and antebrachial fascia
Anconeus muscle
Posterior cutaneous nerve of forearm (from radial nerve)
Palmaris longus muscle
Flexor digitorum superficialis muscle
Median nerve
Ulnar artery and nerve
Flexor carpi ulnaris muscle
Anterior interosseous artery and nerve (from median nerve)
Flexor digitorum profundus muscle
Ulna and antebrachial fascia
Interosseous membrane and extensor pollicis longus muscle
Posterior interosseous artery and nerve (continuation of deep branch of radial nerve)
Palmaris longus tendon
Median nerve
Flexor digitorum superficialis muscle and tendons
Flexor carpi ulnaris muscle and tendon
Ulnar artery and nerve
Dorsal branch of ulnar nerve
Flexor digitorum profundus muscle and tendons
Antebrachial fascia
Ulna
Extensor carpi ulnaris tendon
Pronator quadratus muscle and interosseous membrane
Extensor indicis muscle and tendon
Extensor digiti minimi tendon
Extensor digitorum tendons (common tendon to digits 4 and 5 at this level)

PLATE 432

UPPER LIMB

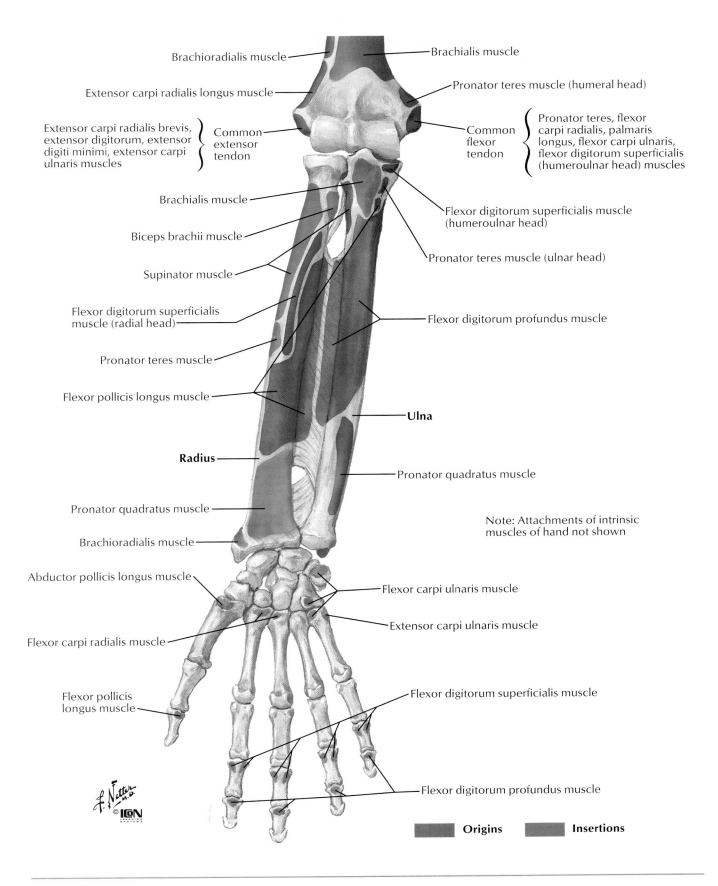

Brachioradialis muscle

Extensor carpi radialis longus muscle

Extensor carpi radialis brevis, extensor digitorum, extensor digiti minimi, extensor carpi ulnaris muscles

Common extensor tendon

Brachialis muscle

Biceps brachii muscle

Supinator muscle

Flexor digitorum superficialis muscle (radial head)

Pronator teres muscle

Flexor pollicis longus muscle

Radius

Pronator quadratus muscle

Brachioradialis muscle

Abductor pollicis longus muscle

Flexor carpi radialis muscle

Flexor pollicis longus muscle

Brachialis muscle

Pronator teres muscle (humeral head)

Common flexor tendon

Pronator teres, flexor carpi radialis, palmaris longus, flexor carpi ulnaris, flexor digitorum superficialis (humeroulnar head) muscles

Flexor digitorum superficialis muscle (humeroulnar head)

Pronator teres muscle (ulnar head)

Flexor digitorum profundus muscle

Ulna

Pronator quadratus muscle

Note: Attachments of intrinsic muscles of hand not shown

Flexor carpi ulnaris muscle

Extensor carpi ulnaris muscle

Flexor digitorum superficialis muscle

Flexor digitorum profundus muscle

Origins   **Insertions**

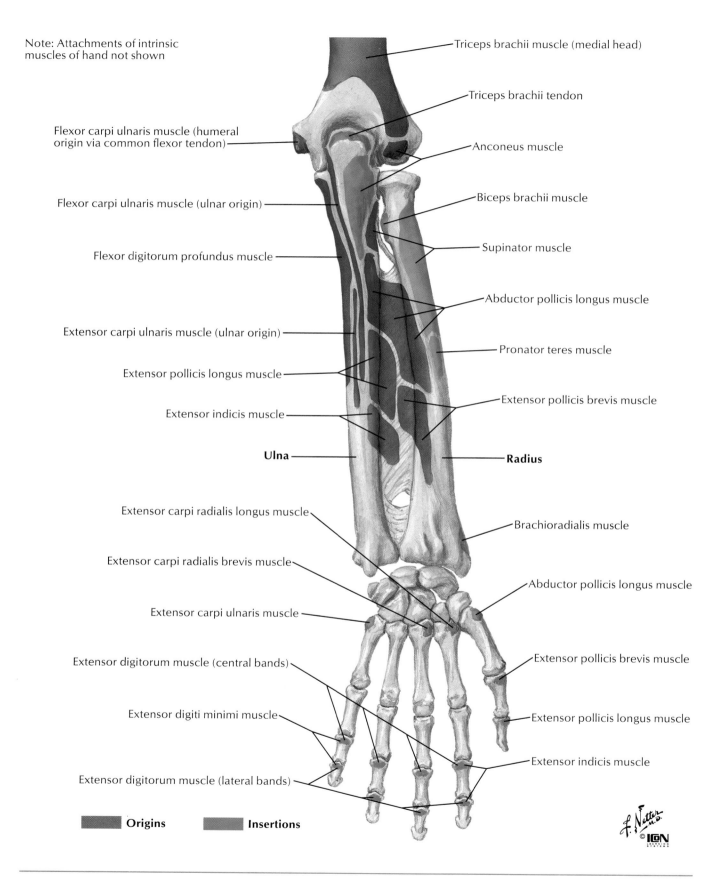

Note: Attachments of intrinsic muscles of hand not shown

Triceps brachii muscle (medial head)

Triceps brachii tendon

Flexor carpi ulnaris muscle (humeral origin via common flexor tendon)

Anconeus muscle

Flexor carpi ulnaris muscle (ulnar origin)

Biceps brachii muscle

Flexor digitorum profundus muscle

Supinator muscle

Abductor pollicis longus muscle

Extensor carpi ulnaris muscle (ulnar origin)

Pronator teres muscle

Extensor pollicis longus muscle

Extensor pollicis brevis muscle

Extensor indicis muscle

Ulna

Radius

Extensor carpi radialis longus muscle

Brachioradialis muscle

Extensor carpi radialis brevis muscle

Abductor pollicis longus muscle

Extensor carpi ulnaris muscle

Extensor digitorum muscle (central bands)

Extensor pollicis brevis muscle

Extensor digiti minimi muscle

Extensor pollicis longus muscle

Extensor indicis muscle

Extensor digitorum muscle (lateral bands)

Origins　**Insertions**

PLATE 434　　　　　　　　　　　　　　　　　　　　　　　　**UPPER LIMB**

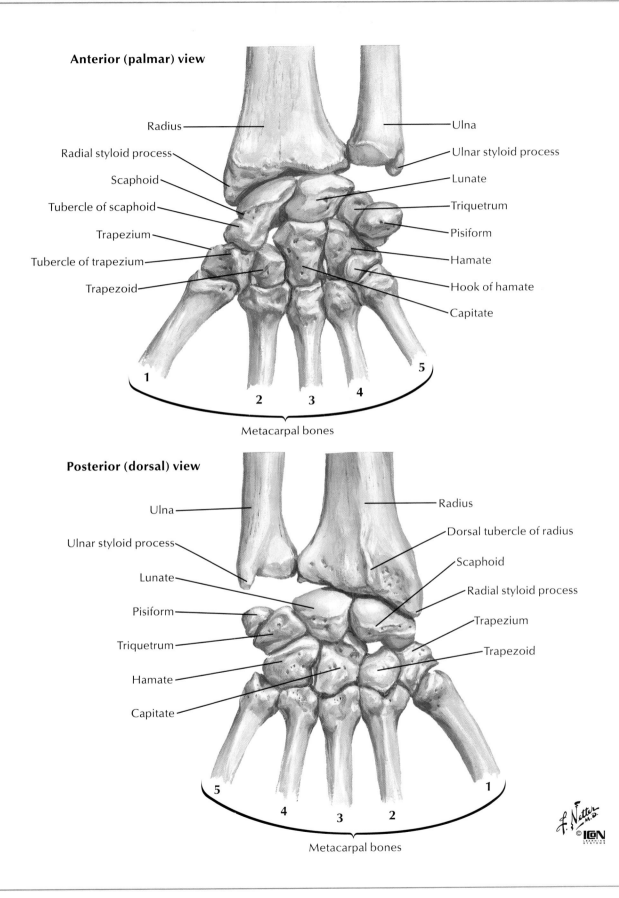

Anterior (palmar) view

Radius

Radial styloid process

Scaphoid

Tubercle of scaphoid

Trapezium

Tubercle of trapezium

Trapezoid

Ulna

Ulnar styloid process

Lunate

Triquetrum

Pisiform

Hamate

Hook of hamate

Capitate

1

2   3   4

5

Metacarpal bones

Posterior (dorsal) view

Ulna

Ulnar styloid process

Lunate

Pisiform

Triquetrum

Hamate

Capitate

Radius

Dorsal tubercle of radius

Scaphoid

Radial styloid process

Trapezium

Trapezoid

5

4   3   2

1

Metacarpal bones

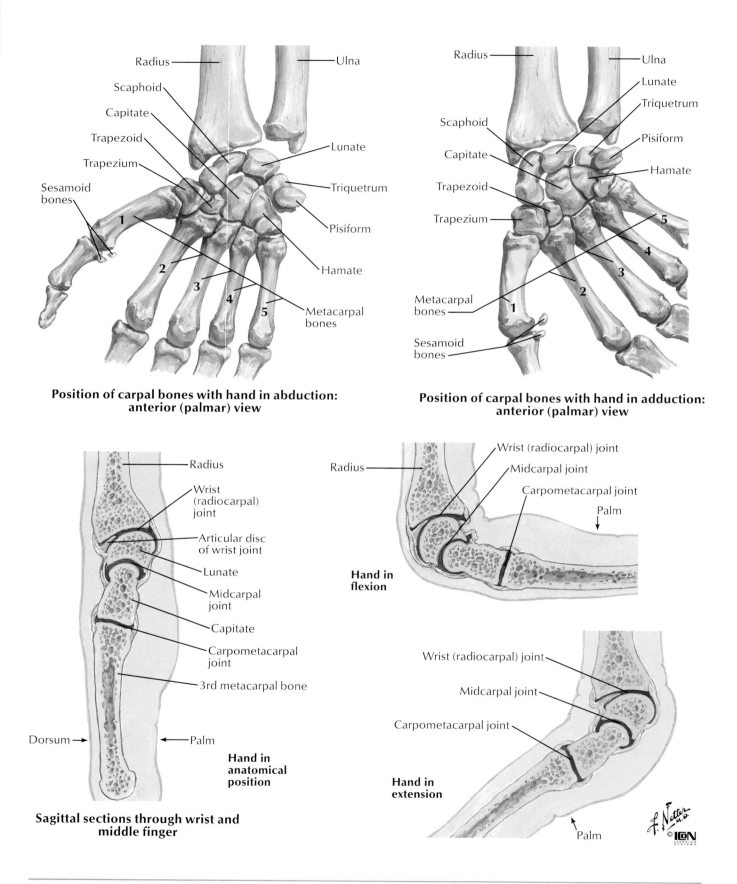

**Position of carpal bones with hand in abduction:
anterior (palmar) view**

**Position of carpal bones with hand in adduction:
anterior (palmar) view**

**Sagittal sections through wrist and
middle finger**

Hand in
flexion

Hand in
anatomical
position

Hand in
extension

PLATE 436   **UPPER LIMB**

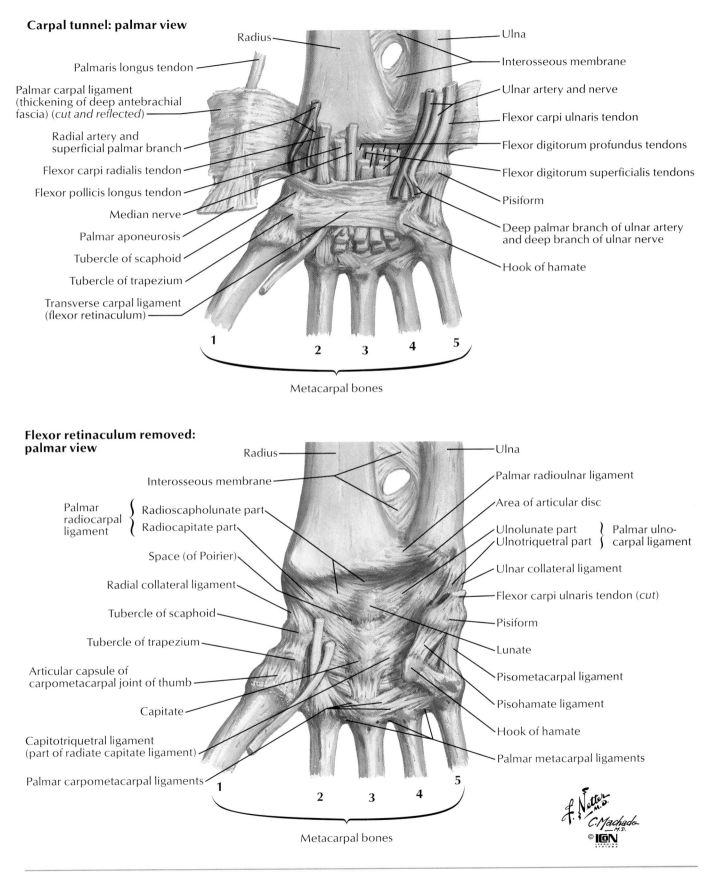

Carpal tunnel: palmar view

Radius

Palmaris longus tendon

Palmar carpal ligament (thickening of deep antebrachial fascia) (*cut and reflected*)

Radial artery and superficial palmar branch

Flexor carpi radialis tendon

Flexor pollicis longus tendon

Median nerve

Palmar aponeurosis

Tubercle of scaphoid

Tubercle of trapezium

Transverse carpal ligament (flexor retinaculum)

Ulna

Interosseous membrane

Ulnar artery and nerve

Flexor carpi ulnaris tendon

Flexor digitorum profundus tendons

Flexor digitorum superficialis tendons

Pisiform

Deep palmar branch of ulnar artery and deep branch of ulnar nerve

Hook of hamate

1   2   3   4   5

Metacarpal bones

Flexor retinaculum removed: palmar view

Radius

Interosseous membrane

Palmar radiocarpal ligament
{ Radioscapholunate part
  Radiocapitate part

Space (of Poirier)

Radial collateral ligament

Tubercle of scaphoid

Tubercle of trapezium

Articular capsule of carpometacarpal joint of thumb

Capitate

Capitotriquetral ligament (part of radiate capitate ligament)

Palmar carpometacarpal ligaments

Ulna

Palmar radioulnar ligament

Area of articular disc

Ulnolunate part
Ulnotriquetral part } Palmar ulno-carpal ligament

Ulnar collateral ligament

Flexor carpi ulnaris tendon (*cut*)

Pisiform

Lunate

Pisometacarpal ligament

Pisohamate ligament

Hook of hamate

Palmar metacarpal ligaments

1   2   3   4   5

Metacarpal bones

Ligaments of Wrist (continued)

Posterior (dorsal) view

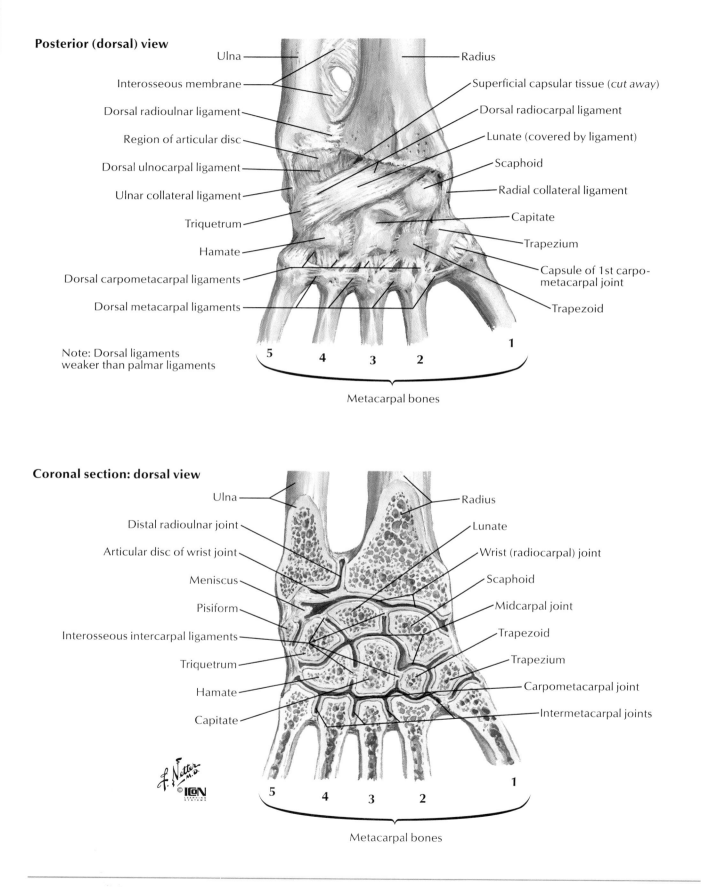

Ulna

Interosseous membrane

Dorsal radioulnar ligament

Region of articular disc

Dorsal ulnocarpal ligament

Ulnar collateral ligament

Triquetrum

Hamate

Dorsal carpometacarpal ligaments

Dorsal metacarpal ligaments

Radius

Superficial capsular tissue (*cut away*)

Dorsal radiocarpal ligament

Lunate (covered by ligament)

Scaphoid

Radial collateral ligament

Capitate

Trapezium

Capsule of 1st carpo-metacarpal joint

Trapezoid

Note: Dorsal ligaments weaker than palmar ligaments

5   4   3   2   1

Metacarpal bones

Coronal section: dorsal view

Ulna

Distal radioulnar joint

Articular disc of wrist joint

Meniscus

Pisiform

Interosseous intercarpal ligaments

Triquetrum

Hamate

Capitate

Radius

Lunate

Wrist (radiocarpal) joint

Scaphoid

Midcarpal joint

Trapezoid

Trapezium

Carpometacarpal joint

Intermetacarpal joints

5   4   3   2   1

Metacarpal bones

PLATE 438

UPPER LIMB

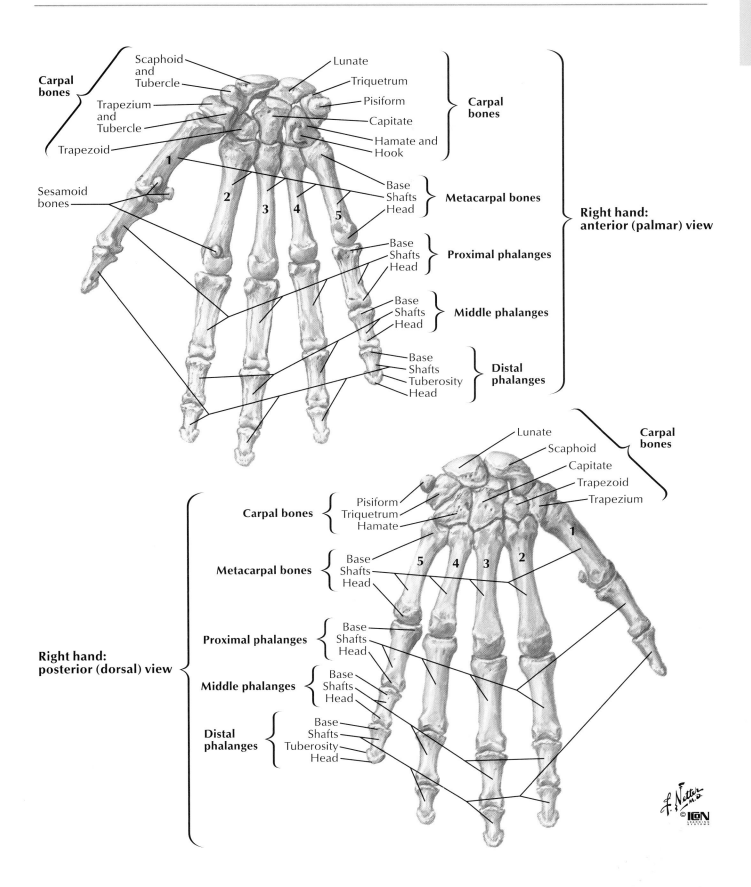

Carpal bones
Scaphoid and Tubercle
Trapezium and Tubercle
Trapezoid

Lunate
Triquetrum
Pisiform
Capitate
Hamate and Hook
Carpal bones

Sesamoid bones

1
2
3
4
5

Base
Shafts
Head
Metacarpal bones

Base
Shafts
Head
Proximal phalanges

Base
Shafts
Head
Middle phalanges

Base
Shafts
Tuberosity
Head
Distal phalanges

Right hand: anterior (palmar) view

Lunate
Scaphoid
Capitate
Trapezoid
Trapezium
Carpal bones

Carpal bones
Pisiform
Triquetrum
Hamate

Metacarpal bones
Base
Shafts
Head

5
4
3
2
1

Proximal phalanges
Base
Shafts
Head

Middle phalanges
Base
Shafts
Head

Distal phalanges
Base
Shafts
Tuberosity
Head

Right hand: posterior (dorsal) view

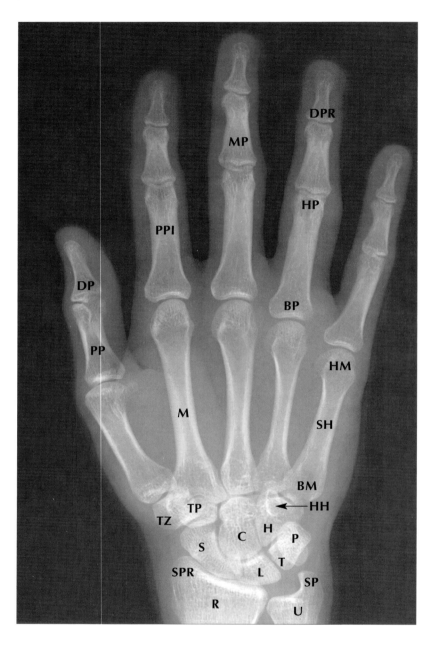

BM	Base of 5th metacarpal	**P**	Pisiform
BP	Base of 4th proximal phalanx	**PP**	Proximal phalanx of thumb
C	Capitate	**PPI**	Proximal phalanx of index finger
DP	Distal phalanx of thumb	**R**	Radius
DPR	Distal phalanx of ring finger	**S**	Scaphoid
H	Hamate	**SH**	Shaft of 5th metacarpal
HH	Hook of hamate	**SP**	Styloid process of ulna
HM	Head of 5th metacarpal	**SPR**	Styloid process of radius
HP	Head of proximal phalanx	**T**	Triquetrum
L	Lunate	**TP**	Trapezoid
M	Metacarpal of index finger	**TZ**	Trapezium
MP	Middle phalanx of middle finger	**U**	Ulna

PLATE 440

UPPER LIMB

Metacarpophalangeal and Interphalangeal Ligaments

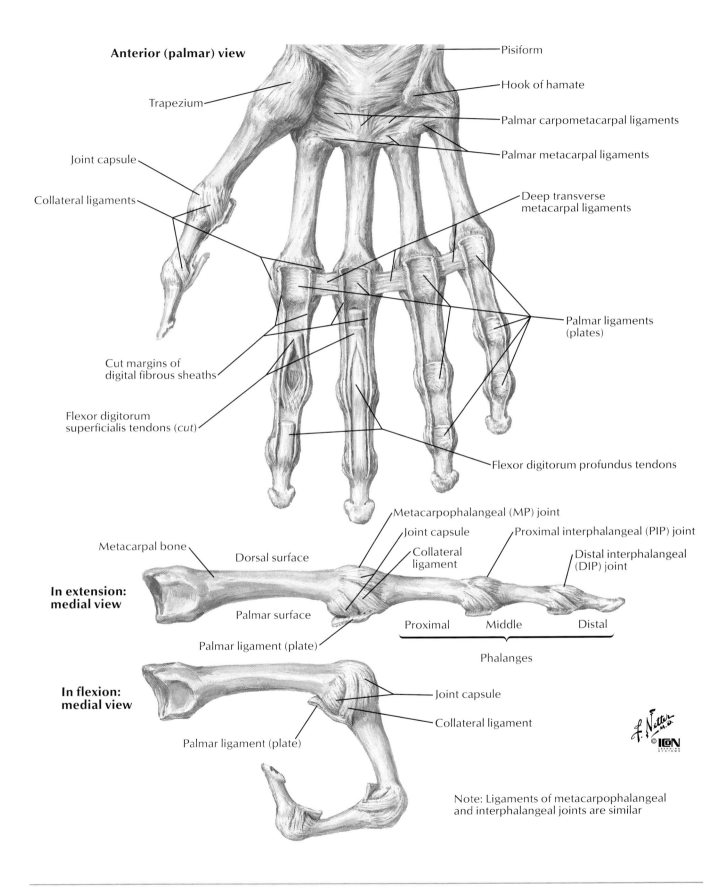

Anterior (palmar) view

Trapezium

Joint capsule

Collateral ligaments

Pisiform

Hook of hamate

Palmar carpometacarpal ligaments

Palmar metacarpal ligaments

Deep transverse metacarpal ligaments

Palmar ligaments (plates)

Cut margins of digital fibrous sheaths

Flexor digitorum superficialis tendons (*cut*)

Flexor digitorum profundus tendons

Metacarpophalangeal (MP) joint

Joint capsule

Collateral ligament

Proximal interphalangeal (PIP) joint

Distal interphalangeal (DIP) joint

Metacarpal bone

Dorsal surface

In extension: medial view

Palmar surface

Palmar ligament (plate)

Proximal   Middle   Distal

Phalanges

In flexion: medial view

Joint capsule

Collateral ligament

Palmar ligament (plate)

Note: Ligaments of metacarpophalangeal and interphalangeal joints are similar

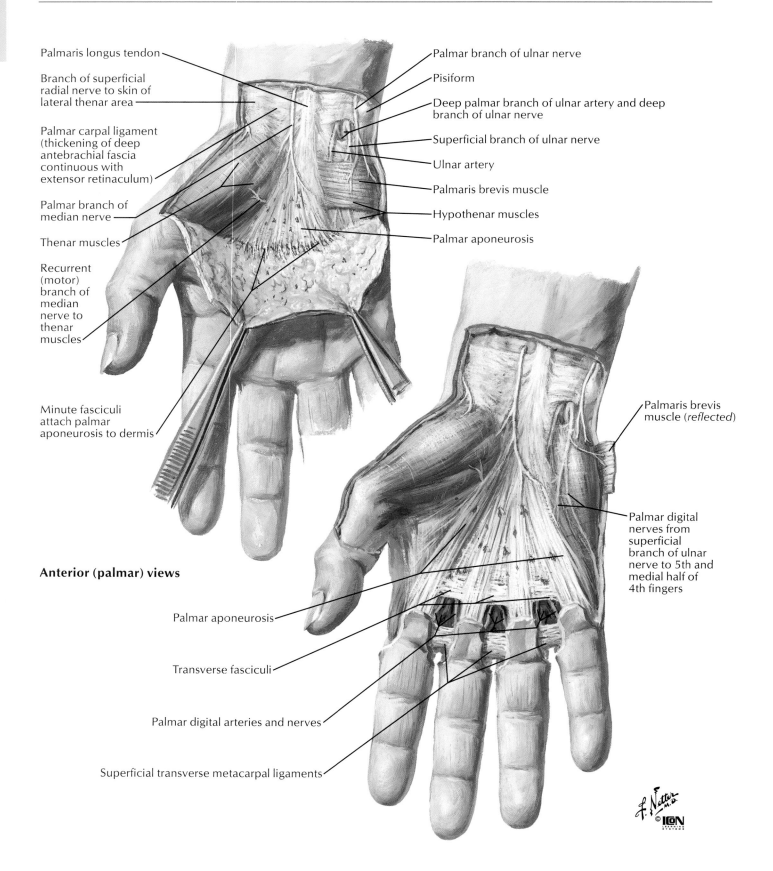

Palmaris longus tendon

Branch of superficial radial nerve to skin of lateral thenar area

Palmar carpal ligament (thickening of deep antebrachial fascia continuous with extensor retinaculum)

Palmar branch of median nerve

Thenar muscles

Recurrent (motor) branch of median nerve to thenar muscles

Minute fasciculi attach palmar aponeurosis to dermis

Palmar branch of ulnar nerve

Pisiform

Deep palmar branch of ulnar artery and deep branch of ulnar nerve

Superficial branch of ulnar nerve

Ulnar artery

Palmaris brevis muscle

Hypothenar muscles

Palmar aponeurosis

Anterior (palmar) views

Palmaris brevis muscle (*reflected*)

Palmar digital nerves from superficial branch of ulnar nerve to 5th and medial half of 4th fingers

Palmar aponeurosis

Transverse fasciculi

Palmar digital arteries and nerves

Superficial transverse metacarpal ligaments

PLATE 442

UPPER LIMB

Radial artery and venae comitantes

Flexor carpi radialis tendon

Tendinous sheath of flexor pollicis longus (radial bursa)

Median nerve

Palmaris longus tendon and palmar carpal ligament

Transverse carpal ligament (flexor retinaculum)

Thenar muscles

Proper palmar digital nerves of thumb

(Synovial) tendinous sheath of flexor pollicis longus (radial bursa)

Probe in 1st lumbrical fascial sheath

Common palmar digital artery

Proper palmar digital arteries

Septa from palmar aponeurosis forming canals

Palmar aponeurosis (*reflected*)

Anterior (palmar) views

Ulnar artery with venae comitantes and ulnar nerve

Flexor carpi ulnaris tendon

Common flexor sheath (ulnar bursa) containing superficialis and profundus flexor tendons

Pisiform

Deep palmar branch of ulnar artery and deep branch of ulnar nerve

Superficial branch of ulnar nerve

Palmar digital nerves to 5th finger and medial half of 4th finger

Median nerve

Common flexor sheath (ulnar bursa)

Superficial palmar arterial and venous arches

2nd, 3rd and 4th lumbrical muscles (in fascial sheaths)

(Synovial) flexor tendon sheaths of fingers

Superficial palmar branch of radial artery and recurrent branch of median nerve to thenar muscles

Ulnar artery and nerve

Common palmar digital branches of median nerve

Hypothenar muscles

Common flexor sheath (ulnar bursa)

5th finger (synovial) tendinous sheath

Probe in midpalmar space

Midpalmar space (deep to flexor tendons and lumbrical muscles)

Insertion of flexor digitorum superficialis tendon

Insertion of flexor digitorum profundus tendon

Proper palmar digital nerves of thumb

Fascia over adductor pollicis muscle

1st dorsal interosseous muscle

Probe in dorsal extension of thenar space deep to adductor pollicis muscle

Thenar space (deep to flexor tendons and 1st lumbrical muscle)

Septum separating thenar from midpalmar space

Common palmar digital artery

Proper palmar digital arteries and nerves

Anular and cruciform parts of fibrous sheath over (synovial) flexor tendon sheaths

Palmar view

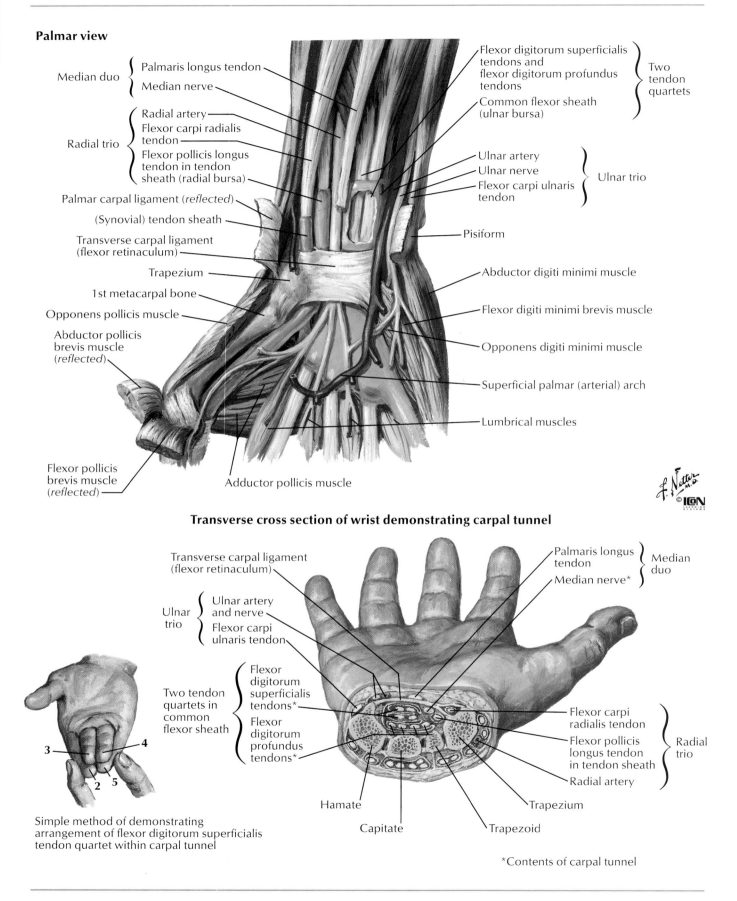

Median duo
- Palmaris longus tendon
- Median nerve

Radial trio
- Radial artery
- Flexor carpi radialis tendon
- Flexor pollicis longus tendon in tendon sheath (radial bursa)

Palmar carpal ligament (*reflected*)

(Synovial) tendon sheath

Transverse carpal ligament (flexor retinaculum)

Trapezium

1st metacarpal bone

Opponens pollicis muscle

Abductor pollicis brevis muscle (*reflected*)

Flexor pollicis brevis muscle (*reflected*)

Adductor pollicis muscle

Flexor digitorum superficialis tendons and flexor digitorum profundus tendons

Common flexor sheath (ulnar bursa)

Two tendon quartets

Ulnar artery
Ulnar nerve
Flexor carpi ulnaris tendon

Ulnar trio

Pisiform

Abductor digiti minimi muscle

Flexor digiti minimi brevis muscle

Opponens digiti minimi muscle

Superficial palmar (arterial) arch

Lumbrical muscles

Transverse cross section of wrist demonstrating carpal tunnel

Transverse carpal ligament (flexor retinaculum)

Ulnar trio
- Ulnar artery and nerve
- Flexor carpi ulnaris tendon

Two tendon quartets in common flexor sheath
- Flexor digitorum superficialis tendons*
- Flexor digitorum profundus tendons*

Palmaris longus tendon
Median nerve*

Median duo

Flexor carpi radialis tendon

Flexor pollicis longus tendon in tendon sheath

Radial artery

Radial trio

Hamate

Capitate

Trapezoid

Trapezium

3 4
2 5

Simple method of demonstrating arrangement of flexor digitorum superficialis tendon quartet within carpal tunnel

*Contents of carpal tunnel

PLATE 444   **UPPER LIMB**

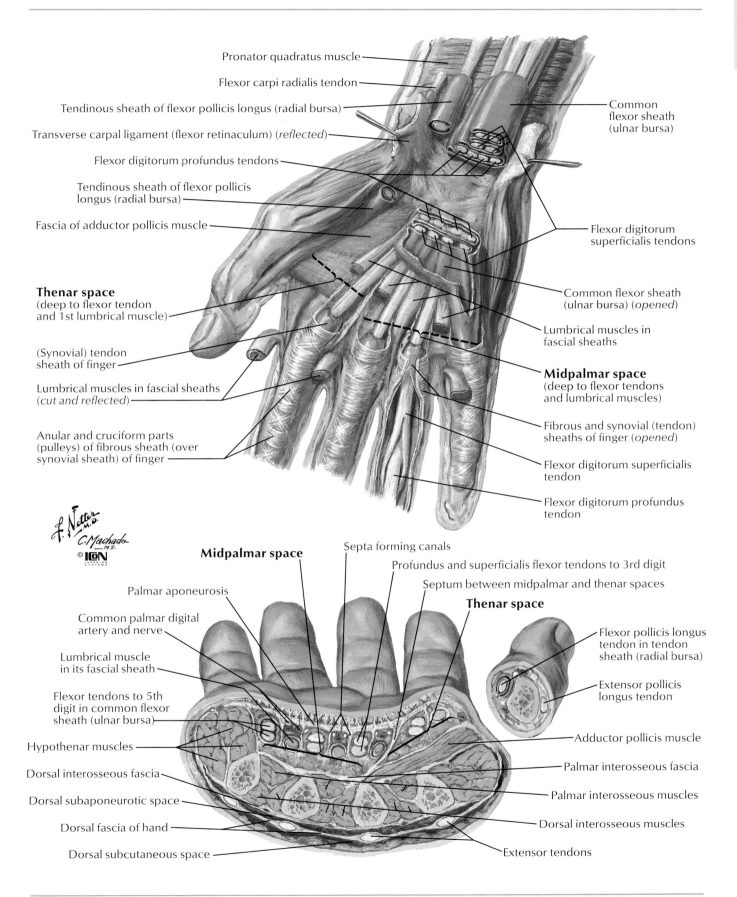

Pronator quadratus muscle

Flexor carpi radialis tendon

Tendinous sheath of flexor pollicis longus (radial bursa)

Transverse carpal ligament (flexor retinaculum) (*reflected*)

Flexor digitorum profundus tendons

Tendinous sheath of flexor pollicis longus (radial bursa)

Fascia of adductor pollicis muscle

Thenar space
(deep to flexor tendon
and 1st lumbrical muscle)

(Synovial) tendon
sheath of finger

Lumbrical muscles in fascial sheaths
(*cut and reflected*)

Anular and cruciform parts
(pulleys) of fibrous sheath (over
synovial sheath) of finger

Common
flexor sheath
(ulnar bursa)

Flexor digitorum
superficialis tendons

Common flexor sheath
(ulnar bursa) (*opened*)

Lumbrical muscles in
fascial sheaths

Midpalmar space
(deep to flexor tendons
and lumbrical muscles)

Fibrous and synovial (tendon)
sheaths of finger (*opened*)

Flexor digitorum superficialis
tendon

Flexor digitorum profundus
tendon

Midpalmar space

Septa forming canals

Profundus and superficialis flexor tendons to 3rd digit

Septum between midpalmar and thenar spaces

Thenar space

Palmar aponeurosis

Common palmar digital
artery and nerve

Lumbrical muscle
in its fascial sheath

Flexor tendons to 5th
digit in common flexor
sheath (ulnar bursa)

Hypothenar muscles

Dorsal interosseous fascia

Dorsal subaponeurotic space

Dorsal fascia of hand

Dorsal subcutaneous space

Flexor pollicis longus
tendon in tendon
sheath (radial bursa)

Extensor pollicis
longus tendon

Adductor pollicis muscle

Palmar interosseous fascia

Palmar interosseous muscles

Dorsal interosseous muscles

Extensor tendons

Lumbrical Muscles and Bursae, Spaces and Sheaths: Schema

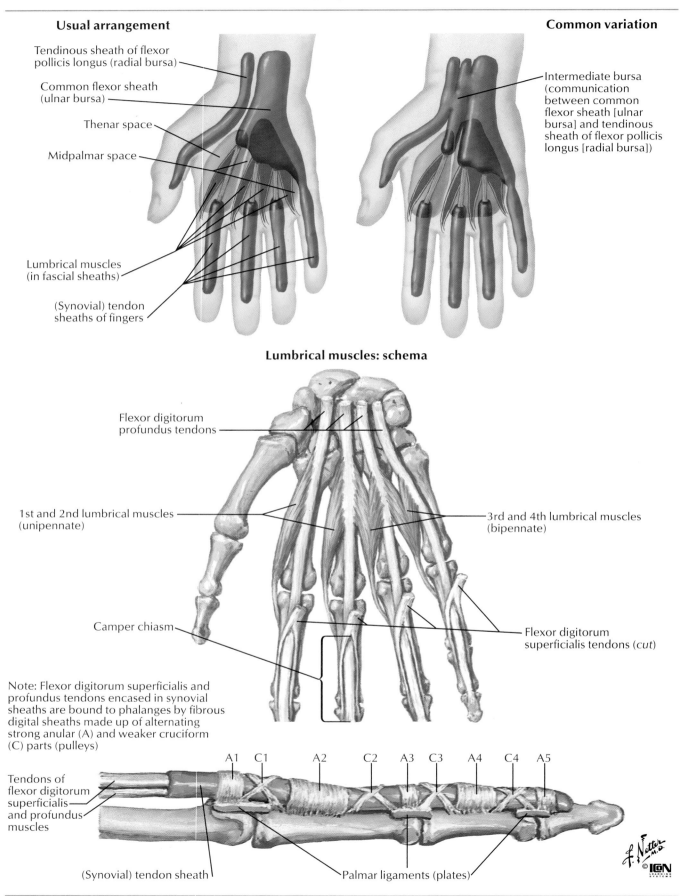

Usual arrangement

Tendinous sheath of flexor pollicis longus (radial bursa)

Common flexor sheath (ulnar bursa)

Thenar space

Midpalmar space

Lumbrical muscles (in fascial sheaths)

(Synovial) tendon sheaths of fingers

Common variation

Intermediate bursa (communication between common flexor sheath [ulnar bursa] and tendinous sheath of flexor pollicis longus [radial bursa])

Lumbrical muscles: schema

Flexor digitorum profundus tendons

1st and 2nd lumbrical muscles (unipennate)

3rd and 4th lumbrical muscles (bipennate)

Camper chiasm

Flexor digitorum superficialis tendons (*cut*)

Note: Flexor digitorum superficialis and profundus tendons encased in synovial sheaths are bound to phalanges by fibrous digital sheaths made up of alternating strong anular (A) and weaker cruciform (C) parts (pulleys)

A1 C1 A2 C2 A3 C3 A4 C4 A5

Tendons of flexor digitorum superficialis and profundus muscles

(Synovial) tendon sheath

Palmar ligaments (plates)

PLATE 446

UPPER LIMB

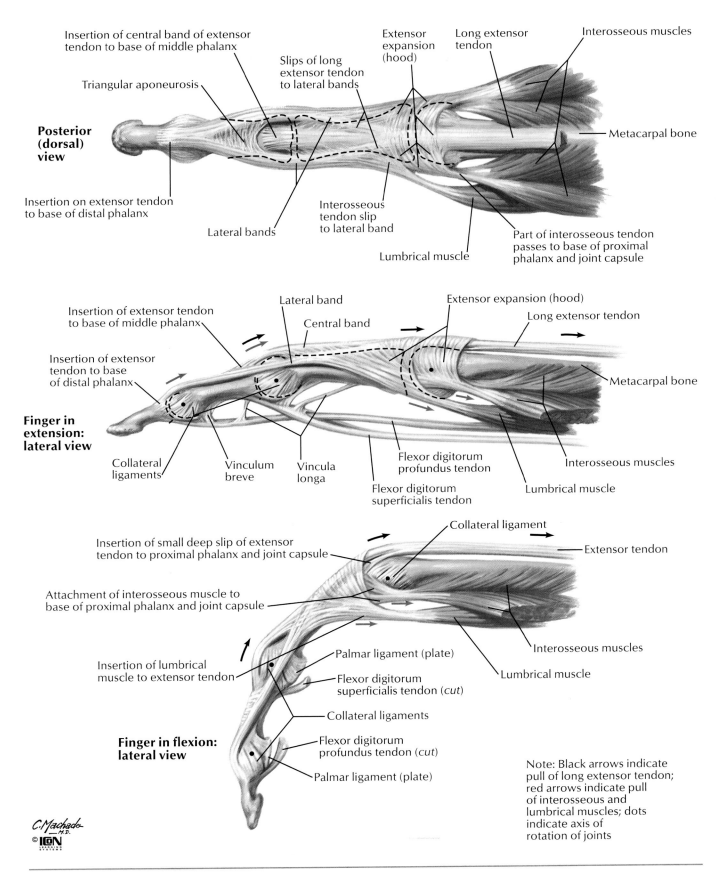

Posterior (dorsal) view

Insertion of central band of extensor tendon to base of middle phalanx

Slips of long extensor tendon to lateral bands

Extensor expansion (hood)

Long extensor tendon

Interosseous muscles

Triangular aponeurosis

Insertion on extensor tendon to base of distal phalanx

Metacarpal bone

Lateral bands

Interosseous tendon slip to lateral band

Lumbrical muscle

Part of interosseous tendon passes to base of proximal phalanx and joint capsule

Finger in extension: lateral view

Insertion of extensor tendon to base of middle phalanx

Lateral band

Central band

Extensor expansion (hood)

Long extensor tendon

Insertion of extensor tendon to base of distal phalanx

Metacarpal bone

Collateral ligaments

Vinculum breve

Vincula longa

Flexor digitorum profundus tendon

Flexor digitorum superficialis tendon

Interosseous muscles

Lumbrical muscle

Finger in flexion: lateral view

Insertion of small deep slip of extensor tendon to proximal phalanx and joint capsule

Collateral ligament

Extensor tendon

Attachment of interosseous muscle to base of proximal phalanx and joint capsule

Interosseous muscles

Lumbrical muscle

Insertion of lumbrical muscle to extensor tendon

Palmar ligament (plate)

Flexor digitorum superficialis tendon (cut)

Collateral ligaments

Flexor digitorum profundus tendon (cut)

Palmar ligament (plate)

Note: Black arrows indicate pull of long extensor tendon; red arrows indicate pull of interosseous and lumbrical muscles; dots indicate axis of rotation of joints

C. Machado M.D.

©ICN LEARNING SYSTEMS

Intrinsic Muscles of Hand

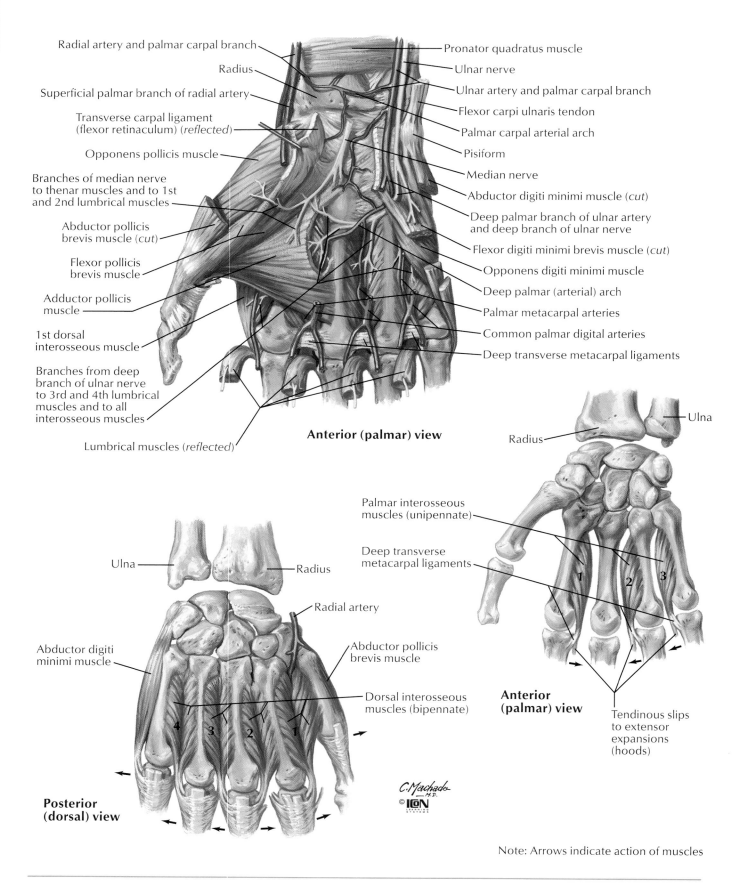

Radial artery and palmar carpal branch

Radius

Superficial palmar branch of radial artery

Transverse carpal ligament
(flexor retinaculum) (*reflected*)

Opponens pollicis muscle

Branches of median nerve
to thenar muscles and to 1st
and 2nd lumbrical muscles

Abductor pollicis
brevis muscle (*cut*)

Flexor pollicis
brevis muscle

Adductor pollicis
muscle

1st dorsal
interosseous muscle

Branches from deep
branch of ulnar nerve
to 3rd and 4th lumbrical
muscles and to all
interosseous muscles

Lumbrical muscles (*reflected*)

Pronator quadratus muscle

Ulnar nerve

Ulnar artery and palmar carpal branch

Flexor carpi ulnaris tendon

Palmar carpal arterial arch

Pisiform

Median nerve

Abductor digiti minimi muscle (*cut*)

Deep palmar branch of ulnar artery
and deep branch of ulnar nerve

Flexor digiti minimi brevis muscle (*cut*)

Opponens digiti minimi muscle

Deep palmar (arterial) arch

Palmar metacarpal arteries

Common palmar digital arteries

Deep transverse metacarpal ligaments

Anterior (palmar) view

Ulna

Radius

Palmar interosseous
muscles (unipennate)

Deep transverse
metacarpal ligaments

1   2   3

**Anterior
(palmar) view**

Tendinous slips
to extensor
expansions
(hoods)

Ulna

Radius

Abductor digiti
minimi muscle

Radial artery

Abductor pollicis
brevis muscle

Dorsal interosseous
muscles (bipennate)

4   3   2   1

**Posterior
(dorsal) view**

C. Machado
—M.D.

Note: Arrows indicate action of muscles

PLATE 448

UPPER LIMB

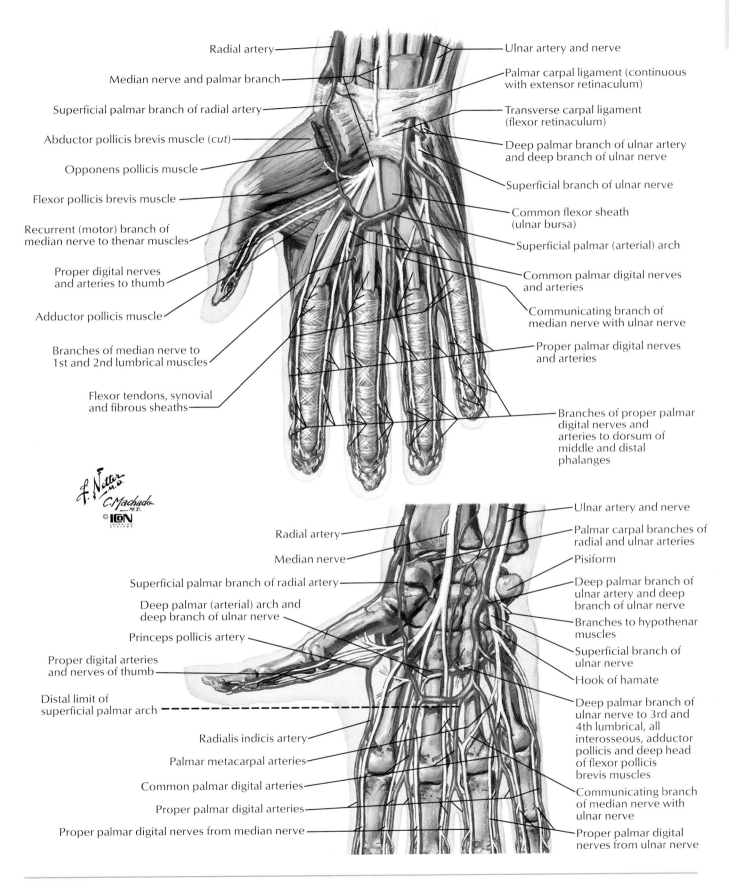

Radial artery

Median nerve and palmar branch

Superficial palmar branch of radial artery

Abductor pollicis brevis muscle (*cut*)

Opponens pollicis muscle

Flexor pollicis brevis muscle

Recurrent (motor) branch of median nerve to thenar muscles

Proper digital nerves and arteries to thumb

Adductor pollicis muscle

Branches of median nerve to 1st and 2nd lumbrical muscles

Flexor tendons, synovial and fibrous sheaths

Ulnar artery and nerve

Palmar carpal ligament (continuous with extensor retinaculum)

Transverse carpal ligament (flexor retinaculum)

Deep palmar branch of ulnar artery and deep branch of ulnar nerve

Superficial branch of ulnar nerve

Common flexor sheath (ulnar bursa)

Superficial palmar (arterial) arch

Common palmar digital nerves and arteries

Communicating branch of median nerve with ulnar nerve

Proper palmar digital nerves and arteries

Branches of proper palmar digital nerves and arteries to dorsum of middle and distal phalanges

Radial artery

Median nerve

Superficial palmar branch of radial artery

Deep palmar (arterial) arch and deep branch of ulnar nerve

Princeps pollicis artery

Proper digital arteries and nerves of thumb

Distal limit of superficial palmar arch

Radialis indicis artery

Palmar metacarpal arteries

Common palmar digital arteries

Proper palmar digital arteries

Proper palmar digital nerves from median nerve

Ulnar artery and nerve

Palmar carpal branches of radial and ulnar arteries

Pisiform

Deep palmar branch of ulnar artery and deep branch of ulnar nerve

Branches to hypothenar muscles

Superficial branch of ulnar nerve

Hook of hamate

Deep palmar branch of ulnar nerve to 3rd and 4th lumbrical, all interosseous, adductor pollicis and deep head of flexor pollicis brevis muscles

Communicating branch of median nerve with ulnar nerve

Proper palmar digital nerves from ulnar nerve

WRIST AND HAND

PLATE 449

Wrist and Hand: Superficial Radial Dissection

Lateral (radial) view

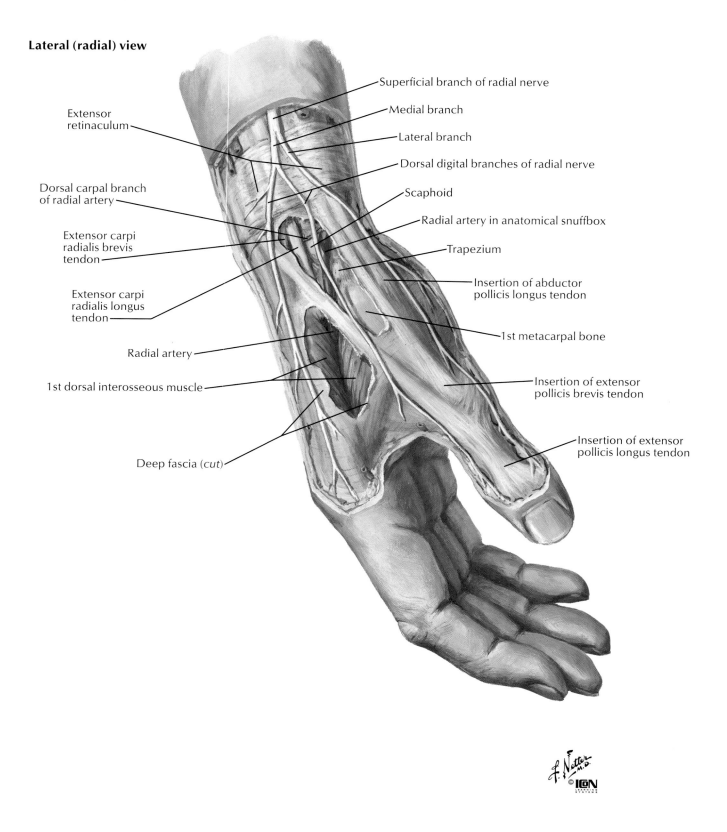

Extensor retinaculum

Dorsal carpal branch of radial artery

Extensor carpi radialis brevis tendon

Extensor carpi radialis longus tendon

Radial artery

1st dorsal interosseous muscle

Deep fascia (*cut*)

Superficial branch of radial nerve

Medial branch

Lateral branch

Dorsal digital branches of radial nerve

Scaphoid

Radial artery in anatomical snuffbox

Trapezium

Insertion of abductor pollicis longus tendon

1st metacarpal bone

Insertion of extensor pollicis brevis tendon

Insertion of extensor pollicis longus tendon

PLATE 450

UPPER LIMB

Posterior (dorsal) view

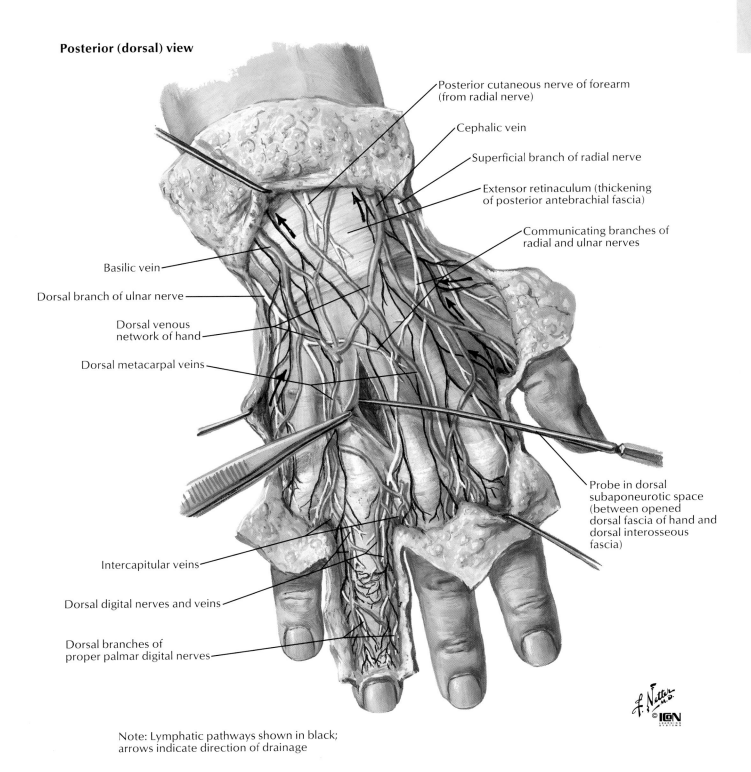

Posterior cutaneous nerve of forearm
(from radial nerve)

Cephalic vein

Superficial branch of radial nerve

Extensor retinaculum (thickening
of posterior antebrachial fascia)

Communicating branches of
radial and ulnar nerves

Basilic vein

Dorsal branch of ulnar nerve

Dorsal venous
network of hand

Dorsal metacarpal veins

Probe in dorsal
subaponeurotic space
(between opened
dorsal fascia of hand and
dorsal interosseous
fascia)

Intercapitular veins

Dorsal digital nerves and veins

Dorsal branches of
proper palmar digital nerves

Note: Lymphatic pathways shown in black;
arrows indicate direction of drainage

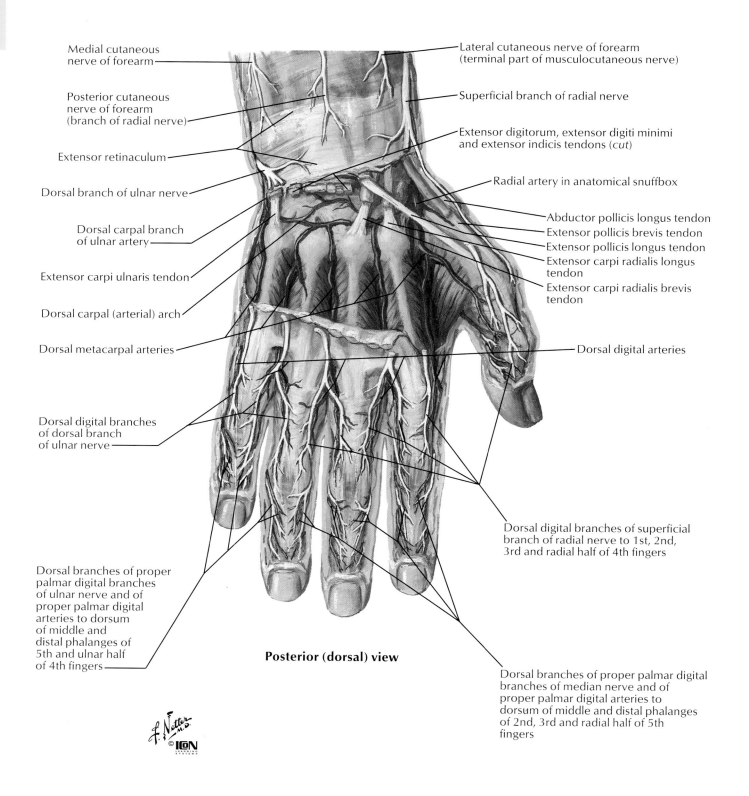

Medial cutaneous nerve of forearm

Posterior cutaneous nerve of forearm (branch of radial nerve)

Extensor retinaculum

Dorsal branch of ulnar nerve

Dorsal carpal branch of ulnar artery

Extensor carpi ulnaris tendon

Dorsal carpal (arterial) arch

Dorsal metacarpal arteries

Dorsal digital branches of dorsal branch of ulnar nerve

Dorsal branches of proper palmar digital branches of ulnar nerve and of proper palmar digital arteries to dorsum of middle and distal phalanges of 5th and ulnar half of 4th fingers

Lateral cutaneous nerve of forearm (terminal part of musculocutaneous nerve)

Superficial branch of radial nerve

Extensor digitorum, extensor digiti minimi and extensor indicis tendons (*cut*)

Radial artery in anatomical snuffbox

Abductor pollicis longus tendon
Extensor pollicis brevis tendon
Extensor pollicis longus tendon
Extensor carpi radialis longus tendon
Extensor carpi radialis brevis tendon

Dorsal digital arteries

Dorsal digital branches of superficial branch of radial nerve to 1st, 2nd, 3rd and radial half of 4th fingers

Dorsal branches of proper palmar digital branches of median nerve and of proper palmar digital arteries to dorsum of middle and distal phalanges of 2nd, 3rd and radial half of 5th fingers

Posterior (dorsal) view

PLATE 452

UPPER LIMB

Posterior (dorsal) view

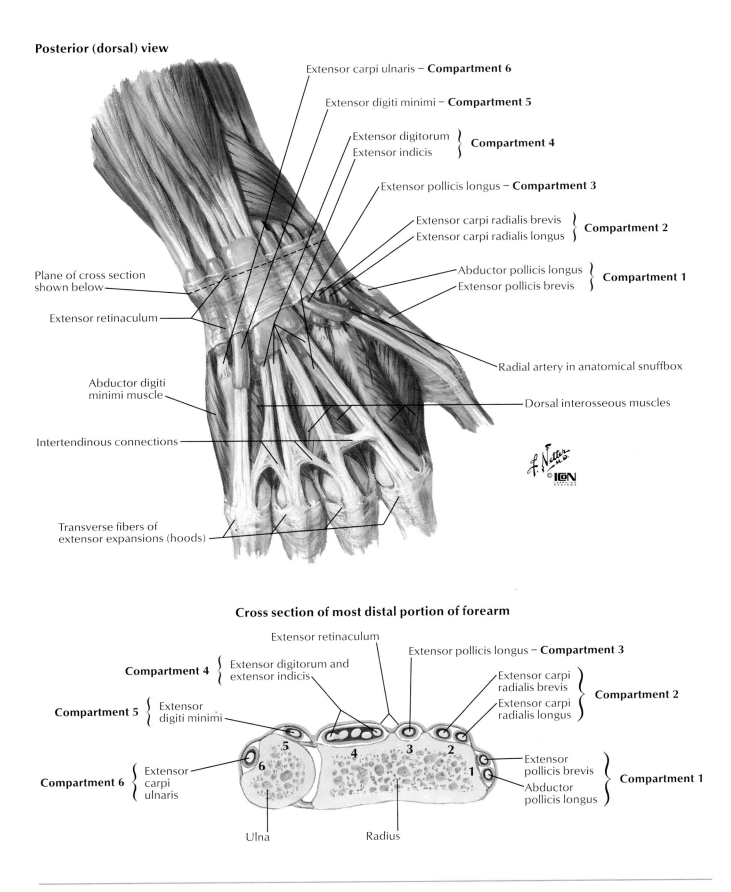

Extensor carpi ulnaris – **Compartment 6**

Extensor digiti minimi – **Compartment 5**

Extensor digitorum }
Extensor indicis } **Compartment 4**

Extensor pollicis longus – **Compartment 3**

Extensor carpi radialis brevis }
Extensor carpi radialis longus } **Compartment 2**

Abductor pollicis longus }
Extensor pollicis brevis } **Compartment 1**

Plane of cross section shown below

Extensor retinaculum

Radial artery in anatomical snuffbox

Abductor digiti minimi muscle

Dorsal interosseous muscles

Intertendinous connections

Transverse fibers of extensor expansions (hoods)

Cross section of most distal portion of forearm

Extensor retinaculum

Extensor pollicis longus – **Compartment 3**

Compartment 4 { Extensor digitorum and extensor indicis

Extensor carpi radialis brevis }
Extensor carpi radialis longus } **Compartment 2**

Compartment 5 { Extensor digiti minimi

Compartment 6 { Extensor carpi ulnaris

Extensor pollicis brevis }
Abductor pollicis longus } **Compartment 1**

5 6 4 3 2 1

Ulna

Radius

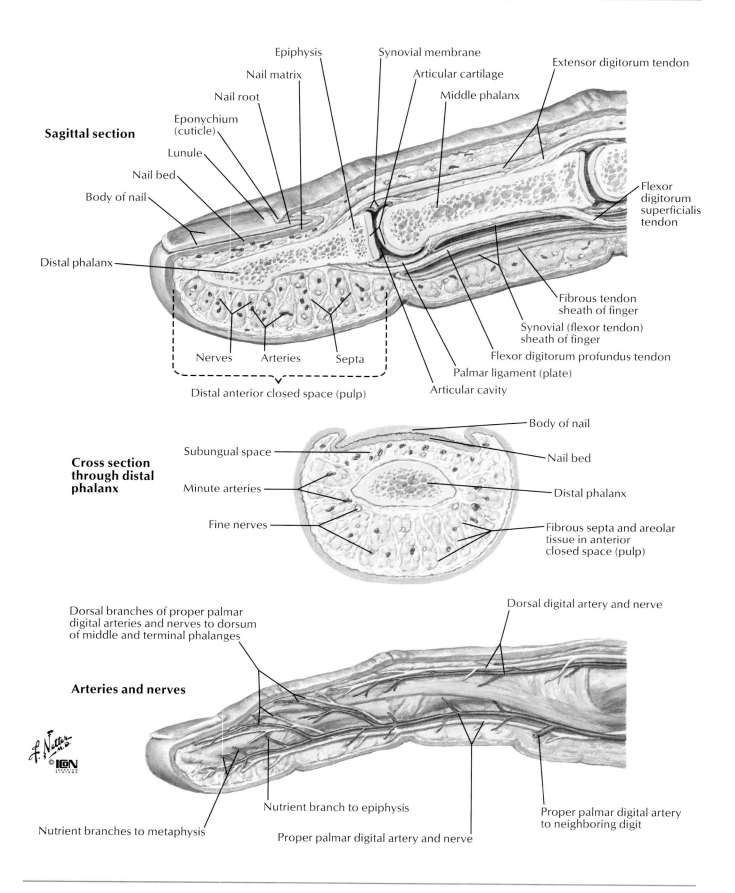

Sagittal section

Epiphysis

Synovial membrane

Nail matrix

Articular cartilage

Nail root

Middle phalanx

Eponychium (cuticle)

Extensor digitorum tendon

Lunule

Nail bed

Body of nail

Distal phalanx

Flexor digitorum superficialis tendon

Nerves

Arteries

Septa

Fibrous tendon sheath of finger

Synovial (flexor tendon) sheath of finger

Flexor digitorum profundus tendon

Palmar ligament (plate)

Articular cavity

Distal anterior closed space (pulp)

Cross section through distal phalanx

Subungual space

Body of nail

Nail bed

Minute arteries

Distal phalanx

Fine nerves

Fibrous septa and areolar tissue in anterior closed space (pulp)

Dorsal branches of proper palmar digital arteries and nerves to dorsum of middle and terminal phalanges

Dorsal digital artery and nerve

Arteries and nerves

Nutrient branches to metaphysis

Nutrient branch to epiphysis

Proper palmar digital artery and nerve

Proper palmar digital artery to neighboring digit

PLATE 454

UPPER LIMB

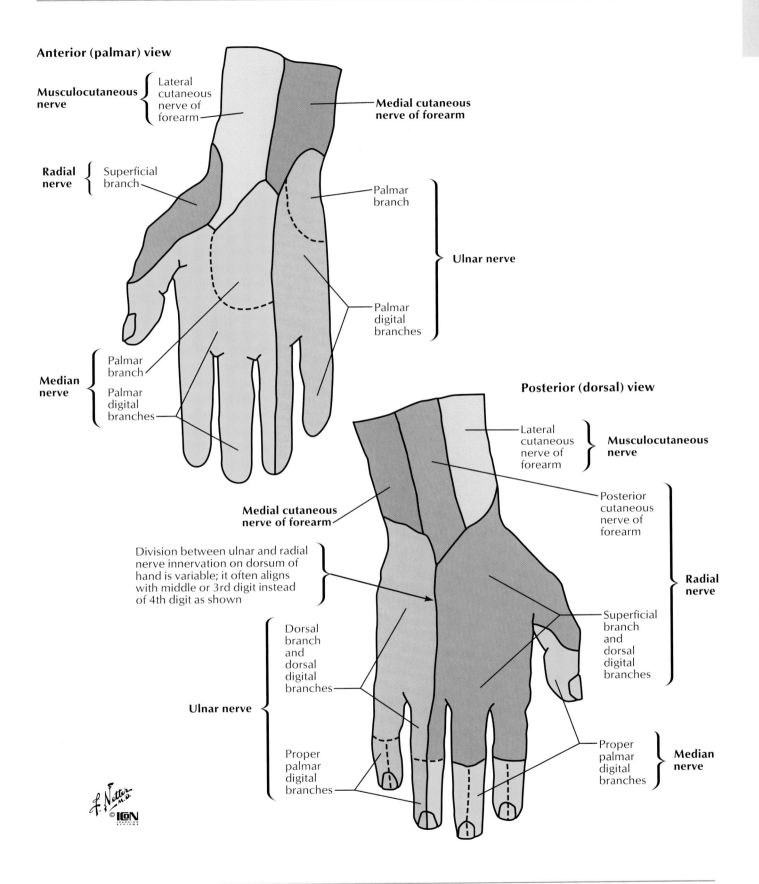

Anterior (palmar) view

Musculocutaneous nerve { Lateral cutaneous nerve of forearm

Medial cutaneous nerve of forearm

Radial nerve { Superficial branch

Palmar branch

Ulnar nerve

Palmar digital branches

Median nerve { Palmar branch

Palmar digital branches

Posterior (dorsal) view

Lateral cutaneous nerve of forearm — **Musculocutaneous nerve**

Medial cutaneous nerve of forearm

Posterior cutaneous nerve of forearm

Division between ulnar and radial nerve innervation on dorsum of hand is variable; it often aligns with middle or 3rd digit instead of 4th digit as shown

Radial nerve

Superficial branch and dorsal digital branches

Ulnar nerve { Dorsal branch and dorsal digital branches

Proper palmar digital branches

Proper palmar digital branches — **Median nerve**

Arteries and Nerves of Upper Limb

Anterior view

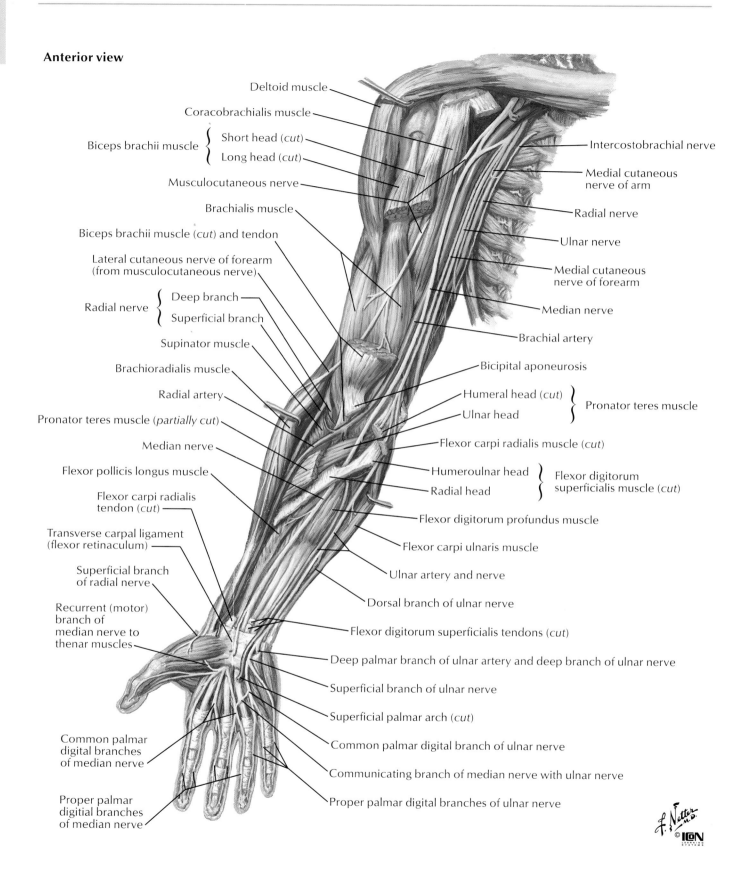

Deltoid muscle

Coracobrachialis muscle

Biceps brachii muscle { Short head (*cut*)
Long head (*cut*)

Musculocutaneous nerve

Brachialis muscle

Biceps brachii muscle (*cut*) and tendon

Lateral cutaneous nerve of forearm
(from musculocutaneous nerve)

Radial nerve { Deep branch
Superficial branch

Supinator muscle

Brachioradialis muscle

Radial artery

Pronator teres muscle (*partially cut*)

Median nerve

Flexor pollicis longus muscle

Flexor carpi radialis
tendon (*cut*)

Transverse carpal ligament
(flexor retinaculum)

Superficial branch
of radial nerve

Recurrent (motor)
branch of
median nerve to
thenar muscles

Common palmar
digital branches
of median nerve

Proper palmar
digitial branches
of median nerve

Intercostobrachial nerve

Medial cutaneous
nerve of arm

Radial nerve

Ulnar nerve

Medial cutaneous
nerve of forearm

Median nerve

Brachial artery

Bicipital aponeurosis

Humeral head (*cut*) } Pronator teres muscle
Ulnar head

Flexor carpi radialis muscle (*cut*)

Humeroulnar head } Flexor digitorum
superficialis muscle (*cut*)
Radial head

Flexor digitorum profundus muscle

Flexor carpi ulnaris muscle

Ulnar artery and nerve

Dorsal branch of ulnar nerve

Flexor digitorum superficialis tendons (*cut*)

Deep palmar branch of ulnar artery and deep branch of ulnar nerve

Superficial branch of ulnar nerve

Superficial palmar arch (*cut*)

Common palmar digital branch of ulnar nerve

Communicating branch of median nerve with ulnar nerve

Proper palmar digital branches of ulnar nerve

PLATE 456

UPPER LIMB

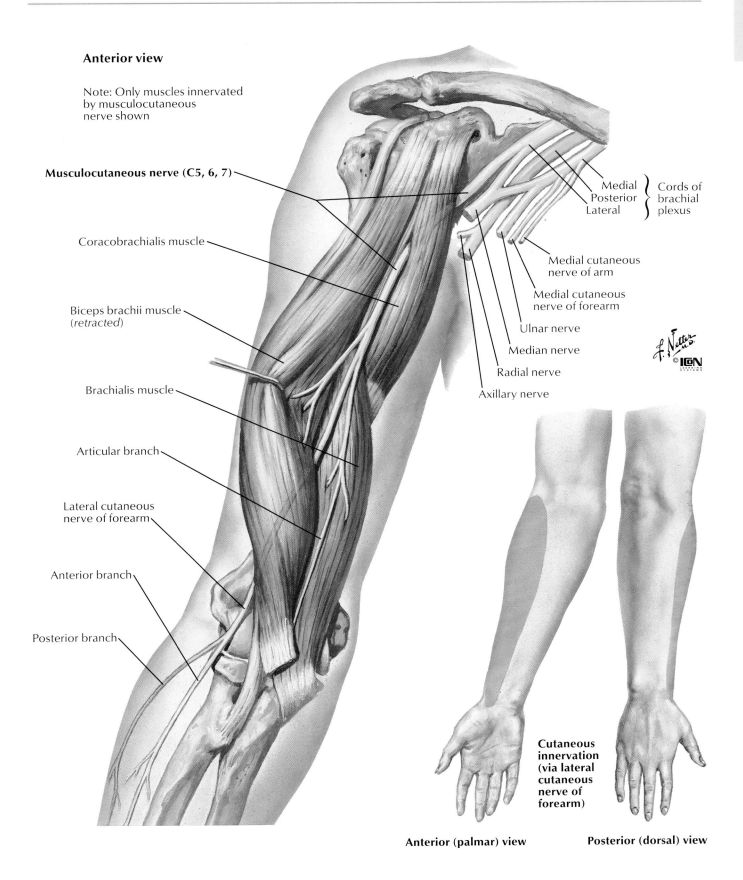

Anterior view

Note: Only muscles innervated by musculocutaneous nerve shown

Musculocutaneous nerve (C5, 6, 7)

Coracobrachialis muscle

Biceps brachii muscle (*retracted*)

Brachialis muscle

Articular branch

Lateral cutaneous nerve of forearm

Anterior branch

Posterior branch

Medial
Posterior } Cords of
Lateral } brachial plexus

Medial cutaneous nerve of arm

Medial cutaneous nerve of forearm

Ulnar nerve

Median nerve

Radial nerve

Axillary nerve

Cutaneous innervation (via lateral cutaneous nerve of forearm)

Anterior (palmar) view

Posterior (dorsal) view

Median Nerve

Note: Only muscles innervated by median nerve shown

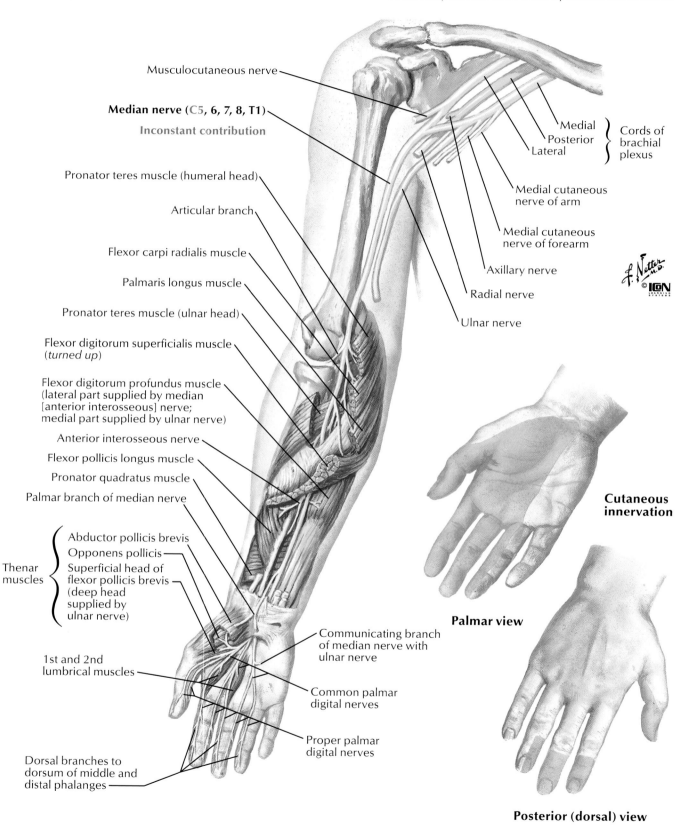

Musculocutaneous nerve

Median nerve (C5, 6, 7, 8, T1)
Inconstant contribution

Pronator teres muscle (humeral head)

Articular branch

Flexor carpi radialis muscle

Palmaris longus muscle

Pronator teres muscle (ulnar head)

Flexor digitorum superficialis muscle
(*turned up*)

Flexor digitorum profundus muscle
(lateral part supplied by median
[anterior interosseous] nerve;
medial part supplied by ulnar nerve)

Anterior interosseous nerve

Flexor pollicis longus muscle

Pronator quadratus muscle

Palmar branch of median nerve

Abductor pollicis brevis

Opponens pollicis

Thenar muscles

Superficial head of
flexor pollicis brevis
(deep head
supplied by
ulnar nerve)

1st and 2nd
lumbrical muscles

Dorsal branches to
dorsum of middle and
distal phalanges

Medial
Posterior
Lateral

Cords of
brachial
plexus

Medial cutaneous
nerve of arm

Medial cutaneous
nerve of forearm

Axillary nerve

Radial nerve

Ulnar nerve

**Cutaneous
innervation**

Palmar view

Communicating branch
of median nerve with
ulnar nerve

Common palmar
digital nerves

Proper palmar
digital nerves

Posterior (dorsal) view

PLATE 458

UPPER LIMB

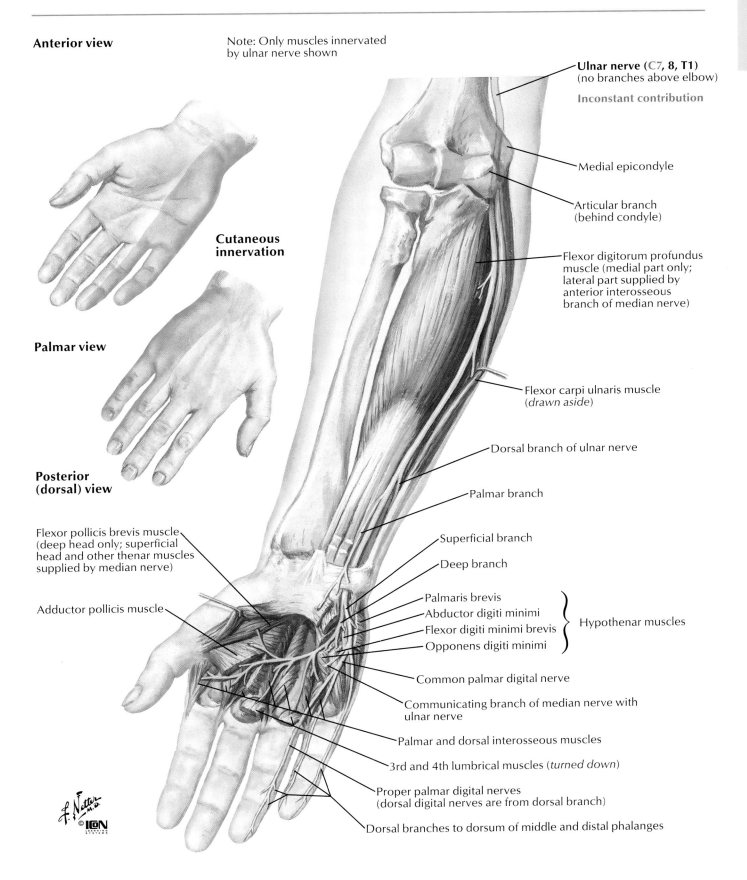

Anterior view

Note: Only muscles innervated by ulnar nerve shown

Ulnar nerve (C7, 8, T1)
(no branches above elbow)

Inconstant contribution

Medial epicondyle

Articular branch
(behind condyle)

Flexor digitorum profundus
muscle (medial part only;
lateral part supplied by
anterior interosseous
branch of median nerve)

Flexor carpi ulnaris muscle
(*drawn aside*)

Dorsal branch of ulnar nerve

Palmar branch

Superficial branch

Deep branch

Palmaris brevis
Abductor digiti minimi
Flexor digiti minimi brevis
Opponens digiti minimi
} Hypothenar muscles

Common palmar digital nerve

Communicating branch of median nerve with
ulnar nerve

Palmar and dorsal interosseous muscles

3rd and 4th lumbrical muscles (*turned down*)

Proper palmar digital nerves
(dorsal digital nerves are from dorsal branch)

Dorsal branches to dorsum of middle and distal phalanges

**Cutaneous
innervation**

Palmar view

**Posterior
(dorsal) view**

Flexor pollicis brevis muscle
(deep head only; superficial
head and other thenar muscles
supplied by median nerve)

Adductor pollicis muscle

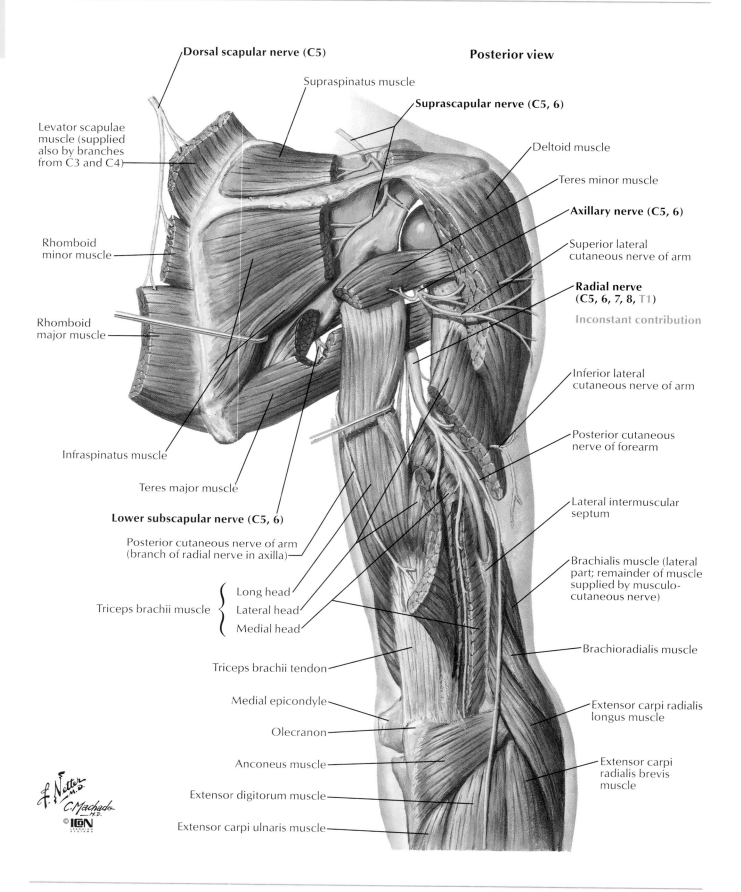

Dorsal scapular nerve (C5)

Posterior view

Supraspinatus muscle

Suprascapular nerve (C5, 6)

Levator scapulae muscle (supplied also by branches from C3 and C4)

Deltoid muscle

Teres minor muscle

Axillary nerve (C5, 6)

Superior lateral cutaneous nerve of arm

Rhomboid minor muscle

Radial nerve (C5, 6, 7, 8, T1)

Inconstant contribution

Rhomboid major muscle

Inferior lateral cutaneous nerve of arm

Posterior cutaneous nerve of forearm

Infraspinatus muscle

Teres major muscle

Lateral intermuscular septum

Lower subscapular nerve (C5, 6)

Posterior cutaneous nerve of arm (branch of radial nerve in axilla)

Brachialis muscle (lateral part; remainder of muscle supplied by musculo-cutaneous nerve)

Long head
Lateral head
Medial head

Triceps brachii muscle

Brachioradialis muscle

Triceps brachii tendon

Medial epicondyle

Extensor carpi radialis longus muscle

Olecranon

Anconeus muscle

Extensor carpi radialis brevis muscle

Extensor digitorum muscle

Extensor carpi ulnaris muscle

PLATE 460

UPPER LIMB

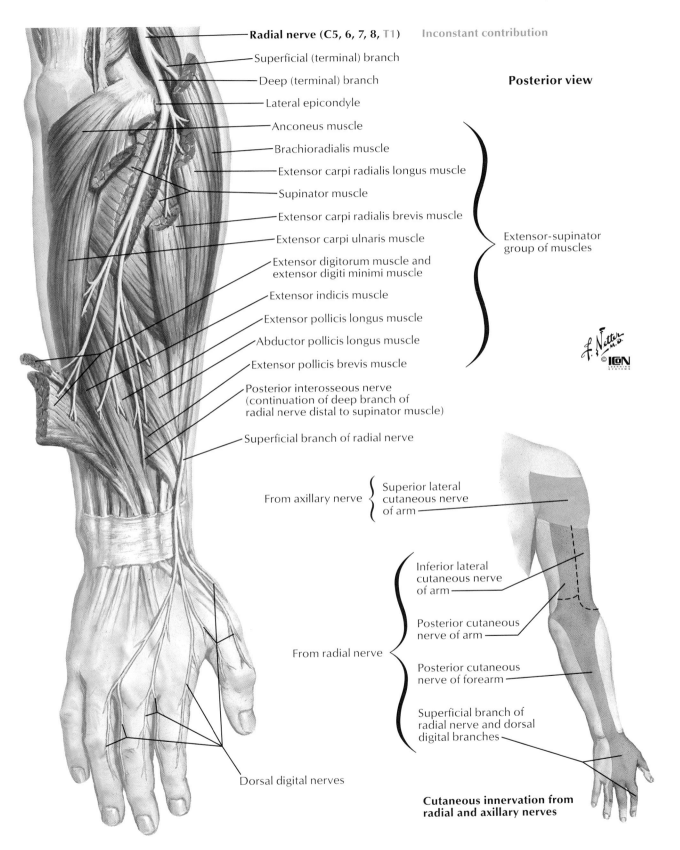

Radial nerve (C5, 6, 7, 8, T1)   Inconstant contribution

Superficial (terminal) branch

Deep (terminal) branch

Lateral epicondyle

Anconeus muscle

Brachioradialis muscle

Extensor carpi radialis longus muscle

Supinator muscle

Extensor carpi radialis brevis muscle

Extensor carpi ulnaris muscle

Extensor digitorum muscle and extensor digiti minimi muscle

Extensor indicis muscle

Extensor pollicis longus muscle

Abductor pollicis longus muscle

Extensor pollicis brevis muscle

Posterior interosseous nerve (continuation of deep branch of radial nerve distal to supinator muscle)

Superficial branch of radial nerve

Posterior view

Extensor-supinator group of muscles

Dorsal digital nerves

From axillary nerve

Superior lateral cutaneous nerve of arm

Inferior lateral cutaneous nerve of arm

From radial nerve

Posterior cutaneous nerve of arm

Posterior cutaneous nerve of forearm

Superficial branch of radial nerve and dorsal digital branches

Cutaneous innervation from radial and axillary nerves

Cutaneous Nerves and Superficial Veins of Shoulder and Arm

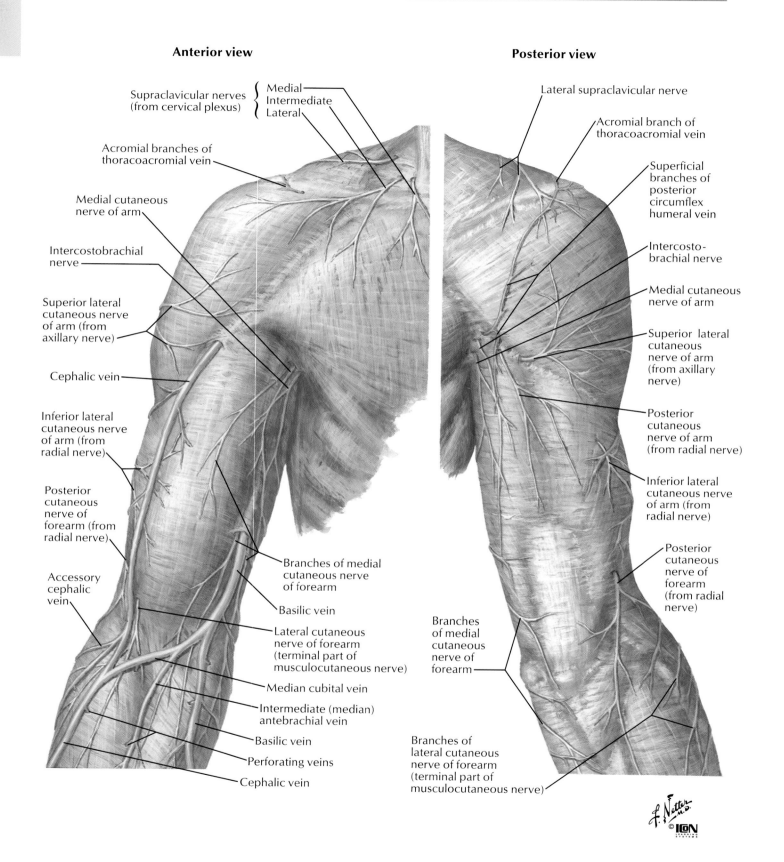

Anterior view

Supraclavicular nerves (from cervical plexus) { Medial — Intermediate — Lateral

Acromial branches of thoracoacromial vein

Medial cutaneous nerve of arm

Intercostobrachial nerve

Superior lateral cutaneous nerve of arm (from axillary nerve)

Cephalic vein

Inferior lateral cutaneous nerve of arm (from radial nerve)

Posterior cutaneous nerve of forearm (from radial nerve)

Accessory cephalic vein

Branches of medial cutaneous nerve of forearm

Basilic vein

Lateral cutaneous nerve of forearm (terminal part of musculocutaneous nerve)

Median cubital vein

Intermediate (median) antebrachial vein

Basilic vein

Perforating veins

Cephalic vein

Posterior view

Lateral supraclavicular nerve

Acromial branch of thoracoacromial vein

Superficial branches of posterior circumflex humeral vein

Intercosto-brachial nerve

Medial cutaneous nerve of arm

Superior lateral cutaneous nerve of arm (from axillary nerve)

Posterior cutaneous nerve of arm (from radial nerve)

Inferior lateral cutaneous nerve of arm (from radial nerve)

Posterior cutaneous nerve of forearm (from radial nerve)

Branches of medial cutaneous nerve of forearm

Branches of lateral cutaneous nerve of forearm (terminal part of musculocutaneous nerve)

f. Netter © ICON

PLATE 462

UPPER LIMB

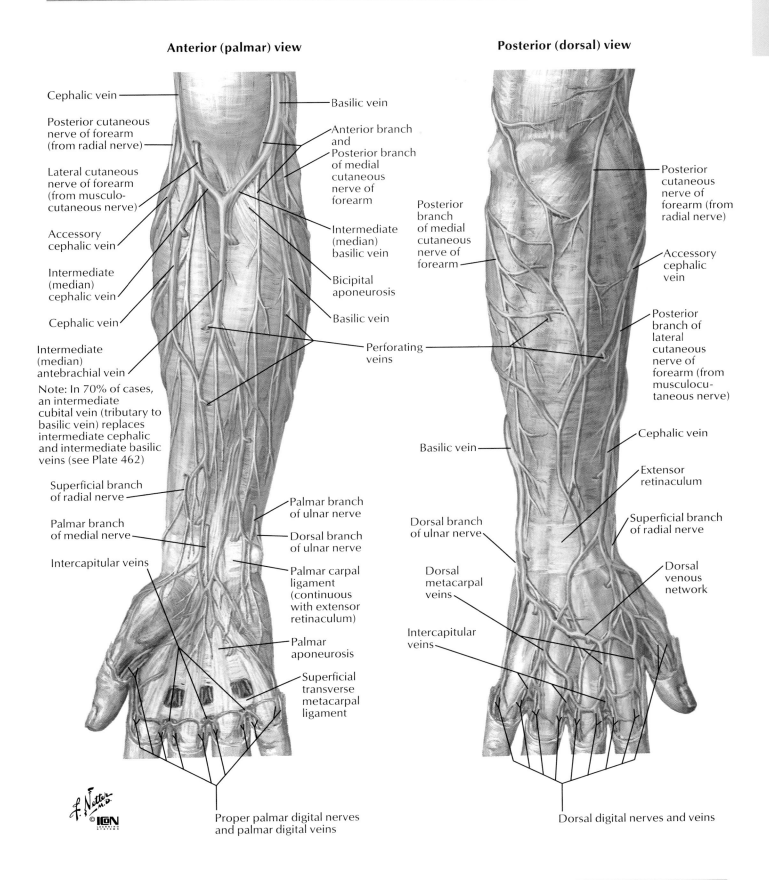

Anterior (palmar) view

Posterior (dorsal) view

Cephalic vein

Posterior cutaneous nerve of forearm (from radial nerve)

Lateral cutaneous nerve of forearm (from musculo-cutaneous nerve)

Accessory cephalic vein

Intermediate (median) cephalic vein

Cephalic vein

Intermediate (median) antebrachial vein

Note: In 70% of cases, an intermediate cubital vein (tributary to basilic vein) replaces intermediate cephalic and intermediate basilic veins (see Plate 462)

Superficial branch of radial nerve

Palmar branch of medial nerve

Intercapitular veins

Basilic vein

Anterior branch and Posterior branch of medial cutaneous nerve of forearm

Intermediate (median) basilic vein

Bicipital aponeurosis

Basilic vein

Perforating veins

Palmar branch of ulnar nerve

Dorsal branch of ulnar nerve

Palmar carpal ligament (continuous with extensor retinaculum)

Palmar aponeurosis

Superficial transverse metacarpal ligament

Proper palmar digital nerves and palmar digital veins

Posterior branch of medial cutaneous nerve of forearm

Posterior cutaneous nerve of forearm (from radial nerve)

Accessory cephalic vein

Posterior branch of lateral cutaneous nerve of forearm (from musculocutaneous nerve)

Cephalic vein

Extensor retinaculum

Superficial branch of radial nerve

Dorsal venous network

Basilic vein

Dorsal branch of ulnar nerve

Dorsal metacarpal veins

Intercapitular veins

Dorsal digital nerves and veins

Anterior (palmar) view

Posterior (dorsal) view

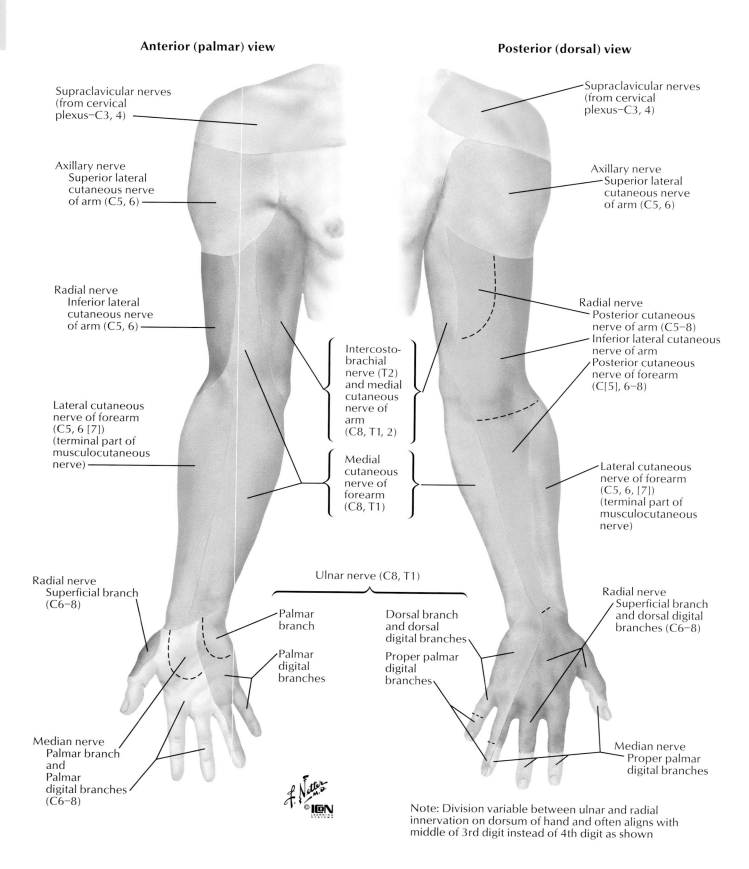

Supraclavicular nerves
(from cervical
plexus–C3, 4)

Axillary nerve
Superior lateral
cutaneous nerve
of arm (C5, 6)

Radial nerve
Inferior lateral cutaneous nerve
of arm (C5, 6)

Lateral cutaneous
nerve of forearm
(C5, 6 [7])
(terminal part of
musculocutaneous
nerve)

Radial nerve
Superficial branch
(C6–8)

Median nerve
Palmar branch
and
Palmar
digital branches
(C6–8)

Intercosto-
brachial
nerve (T2)
and medial
cutaneous
nerve of
arm
(C8, T1, 2)

Medial
cutaneous
nerve of
forearm
(C8, T1)

Ulnar nerve (C8, T1)

Palmar
branch

Palmar
digital
branches

Dorsal branch
and dorsal
digital branches

Proper palmar
digital
branches

Supraclavicular nerves
(from cervical
plexus–C3, 4)

Axillary nerve
Superior lateral
cutaneous nerve
of arm (C5, 6)

Radial nerve
Posterior cutaneous
nerve of arm (C5–8)
Inferior lateral cutaneous
nerve of arm
Posterior cutaneous
nerve of forearm
(C[5], 6–8)

Lateral cutaneous
nerve of forearm
(C5, 6, [7])
(terminal part of
musculocutaneous
nerve)

Radial nerve
Superficial branch
and dorsal digital
branches (C6–8)

Median nerve
Proper palmar
digital branches

Note: Division variable between ulnar and radial
innervation on dorsum of hand and often aligns with
middle of 3rd digit instead of 4th digit as shown

PLATE 464

UPPER LIMB

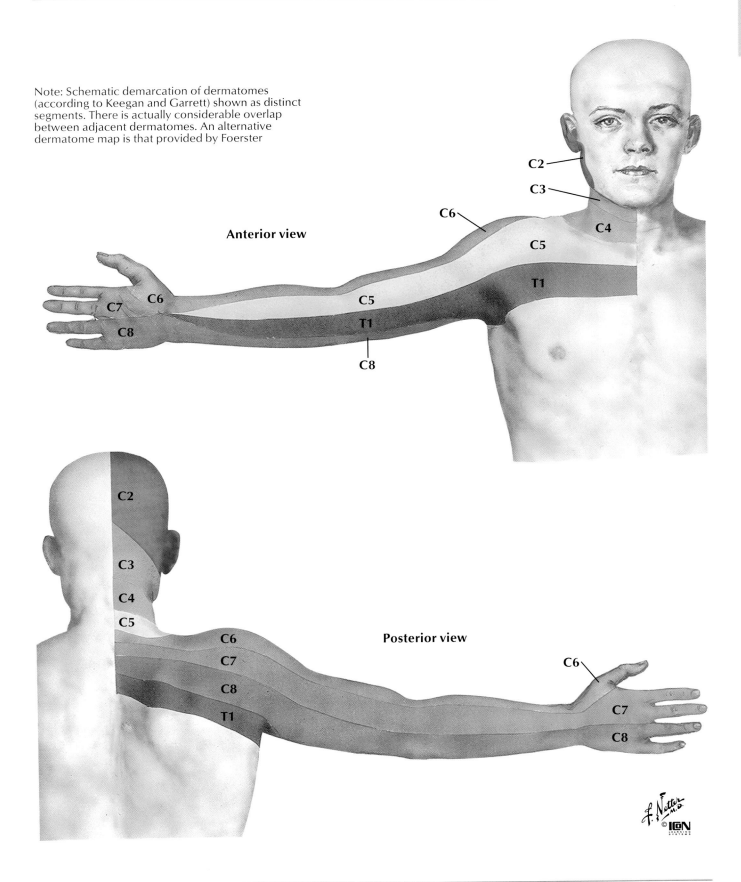

Note: Schematic demarcation of dermatomes (according to Keegan and Garrett) shown as distinct segments. There is actually considerable overlap between adjacent dermatomes. An alternative dermatome map is that provided by Foerster

Anterior view

C2
C3
C6
C4
C5
T1
C6
C5
C7
T1
C6
C8
C8
C8

C2
C3
C4
C5
C6
C7
C8
T1

Posterior view

C6
C7
C8

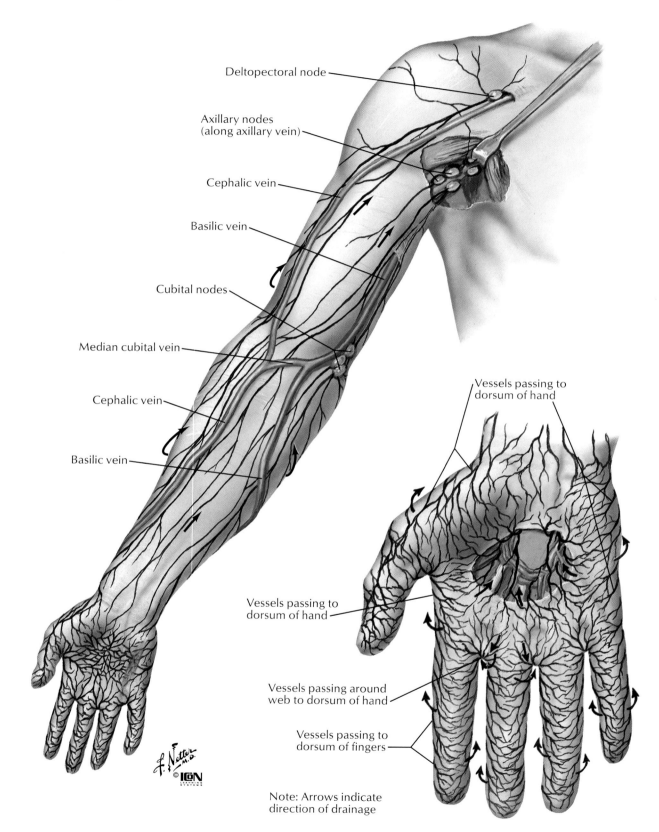

Deltopectoral node

Axillary nodes
(along axillary vein)

Cephalic vein

Basilic vein

Cubital nodes

Median cubital vein

Cephalic vein

Basilic vein

Vessels passing to
dorsum of hand

Vessels passing to
dorsum of hand

Vessels passing around
web to dorsum of hand

Vessels passing to
dorsum of fingers

Note: Arrows indicate
direction of drainage

PLATE 466

UPPER LIMB

Section VII
LOWER LIMB

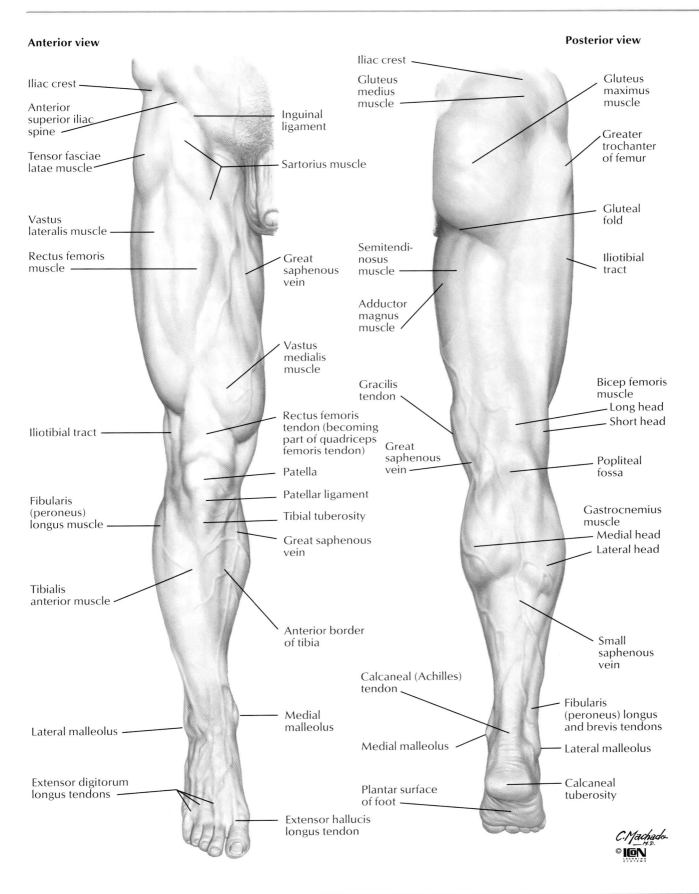

Anterior view

Iliac crest

Anterior superior iliac spine

Tensor fasciae latae muscle

Vastus lateralis muscle

Rectus femoris muscle

Iliotibial tract

Fibularis (peroneus) longus muscle

Tibialis anterior muscle

Lateral malleolus

Extensor digitorum longus tendons

Inguinal ligament

Sartorius muscle

Great saphenous vein

Vastus medialis muscle

Rectus femoris tendon (becoming part of quadriceps femoris tendon)

Patella

Patellar ligament

Tibial tuberosity

Great saphenous vein

Anterior border of tibia

Medial malleolus

Extensor hallucis longus tendon

Posterior view

Iliac crest

Gluteus medius muscle

Semitendinosus muscle

Adductor magnus muscle

Gracilis tendon

Great saphenous vein

Gluteus maximus muscle

Greater trochanter of femur

Gluteal fold

Iliotibial tract

Bicep femoris muscle
  Long head
  Short head

Popliteal fossa

Gastrocnemius muscle
  Medial head
  Lateral head

Small saphenous vein

Calcaneal (Achilles) tendon

Medial malleolus

Plantar surface of foot

Fibularis (peroneus) longus and brevis tendons

Lateral malleolus

Calcaneal tuberosity

C.Machado
—M.D.
© **ICON**
LEARNING SYSTEMS

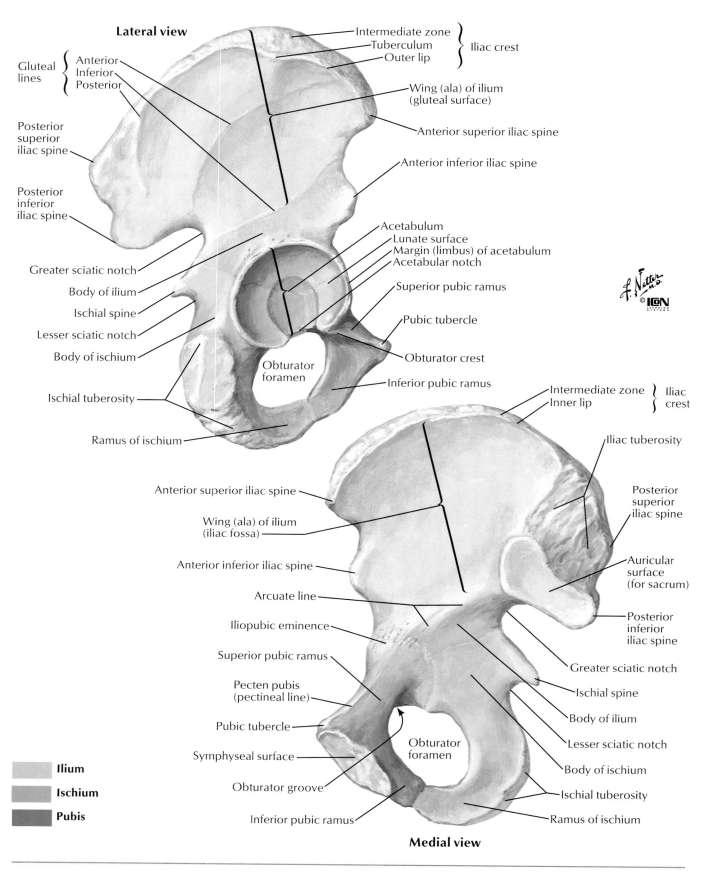

Lateral view

Iliac crest
- Intermediate zone
- Tuberculum
- Outer lip

Gluteal lines
- Anterior
- Inferior
- Posterior

Wing (ala) of ilium (gluteal surface)

Anterior superior iliac spine

Posterior superior iliac spine

Anterior inferior iliac spine

Posterior inferior iliac spine

Acetabulum
Lunate surface
Margin (limbus) of acetabulum
Acetabular notch

Greater sciatic notch

Body of ilium

Superior pubic ramus

Ischial spine

Pubic tubercle

Lesser sciatic notch

Body of ischium

Obturator crest

Ischial tuberosity

Obturator foramen

Inferior pubic ramus

Ramus of ischium

Iliac crest
- Intermediate zone
- Inner lip

Iliac tuberosity

Anterior superior iliac spine

Posterior superior iliac spine

Wing (ala) of ilium (iliac fossa)

Anterior inferior iliac spine

Auricular surface (for sacrum)

Arcuate line

Posterior inferior iliac spine

Iliopubic eminence

Greater sciatic notch

Superior pubic ramus

Ischial spine

Pecten pubis (pectineal line)

Body of ilium

Pubic tubercle

Lesser sciatic notch

Symphyseal surface

Body of ischium

Obturator foramen

Obturator groove

Ischial tuberosity

Inferior pubic ramus

Ramus of ischium

Medial view

- Ilium
- Ischium
- Pubis

PLATE 468

LOWER LIMB

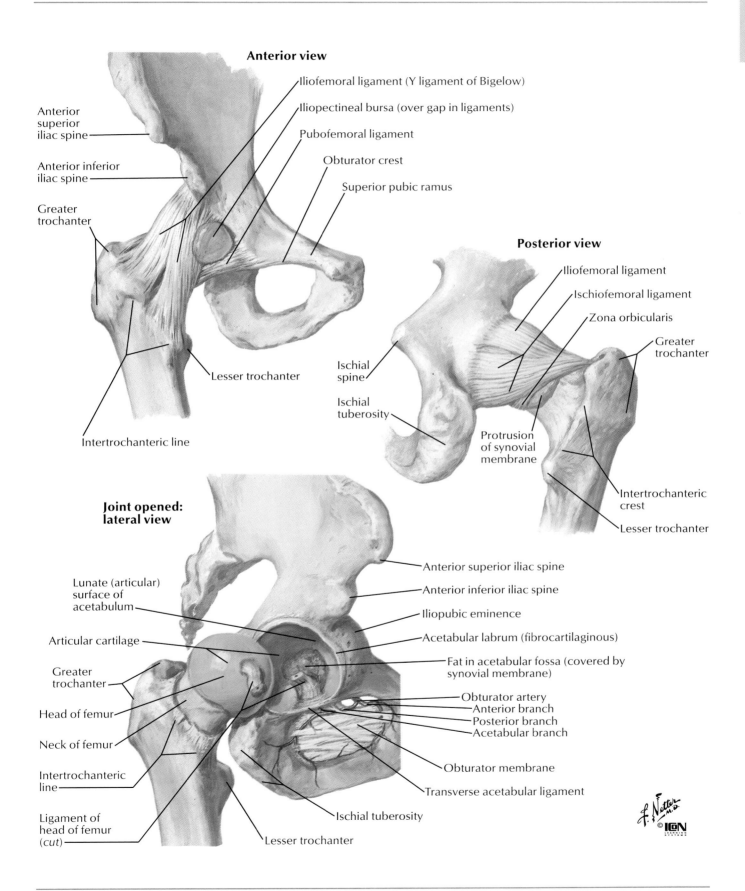

Anterior view

Iliofemoral ligament (Y ligament of Bigelow)

Iliopectineal bursa (over gap in ligaments)

Pubofemoral ligament

Obturator crest

Superior pubic ramus

Anterior superior iliac spine

Anterior inferior iliac spine

Greater trochanter

Lesser trochanter

Intertrochanteric line

Posterior view

Iliofemoral ligament

Ischiofemoral ligament

Zona orbicularis

Greater trochanter

Ischial spine

Ischial tuberosity

Protrusion of synovial membrane

Intertrochanteric crest

Lesser trochanter

Joint opened: lateral view

Lunate (articular) surface of acetabulum

Articular cartilage

Greater trochanter

Head of femur

Neck of femur

Intertrochanteric line

Ligament of head of femur (*cut*)

Anterior superior iliac spine

Anterior inferior iliac spine

Iliopubic eminence

Acetabular labrum (fibrocartilaginous)

Fat in acetabular fossa (covered by synovial membrane)

Obturator artery

Anterior branch

Posterior branch

Acetabular branch

Obturator membrane

Transverse acetabular ligament

Ischial tuberosity

Lesser trochanter

Hip Joint: Anteroposterior Radiograph

SEE ALSO PLATES 469, 471

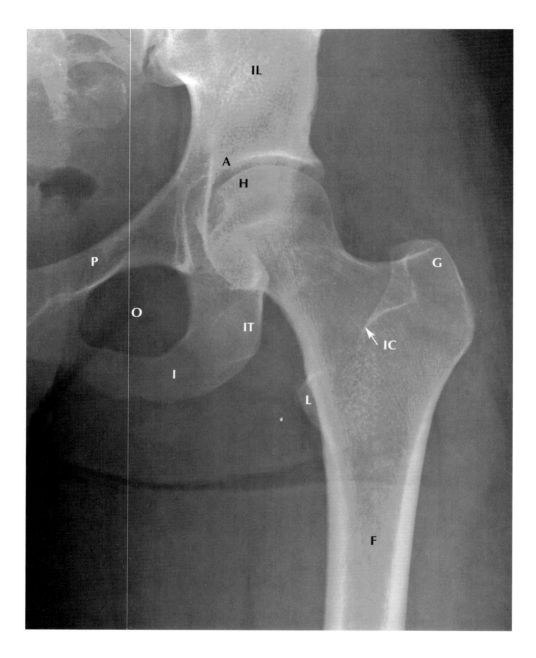

A	Acetabulum
F	Femur
G	Greater trochanter
H	Head of femur
I	Ischium
IC	Intertrochanteric crest
IL	Ileum
IT	Ischial tuberosity
L	Lesser trochanter
O	Obturator foramen
P	Pubis (superior ramus)

PLATE 470

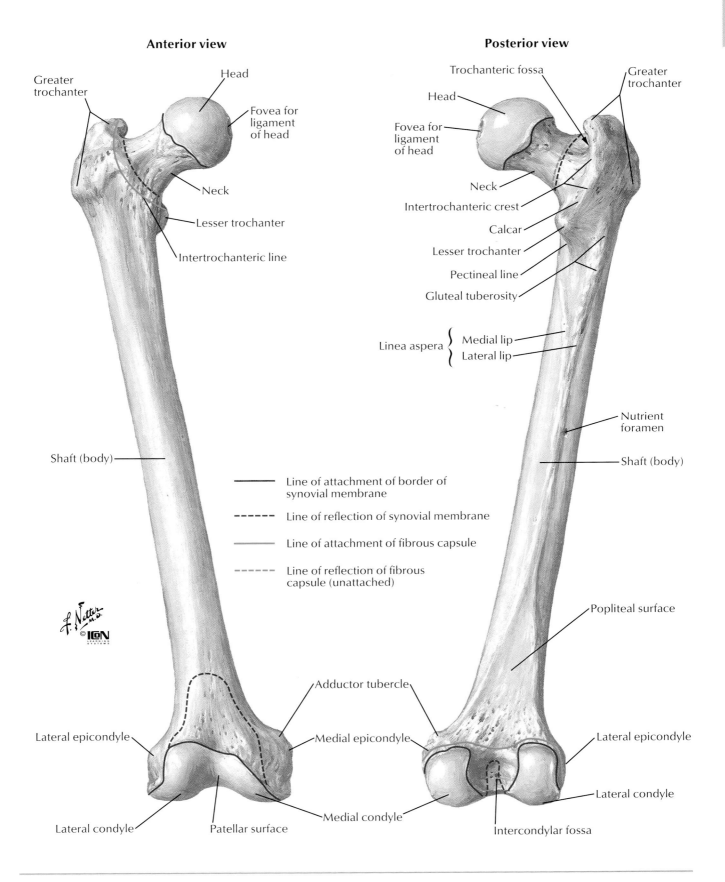

Anterior view

Greater trochanter

Head

Fovea for ligament of head

Neck

Lesser trochanter

Intertrochanteric line

Shaft (body)

Line of attachment of border of synovial membrane

Line of reflection of synovial membrane

Line of attachment of fibrous capsule

Line of reflection of fibrous capsule (unattached)

Lateral epicondyle

Adductor tubercle

Medial epicondyle

Lateral condyle

Patellar surface

Medial condyle

Posterior view

Trochanteric fossa

Greater trochanter

Head

Fovea for ligament of head

Neck

Intertrochanteric crest

Calcar

Lesser trochanter

Pectineal line

Gluteal tuberosity

Linea aspera { Medial lip
Lateral lip

Nutrient foramen

Shaft (body)

Popliteal surface

Lateral epicondyle

Lateral condyle

Intercondylar fossa

Bony Attachments of Muscles of Hip and Thigh: Anterior View

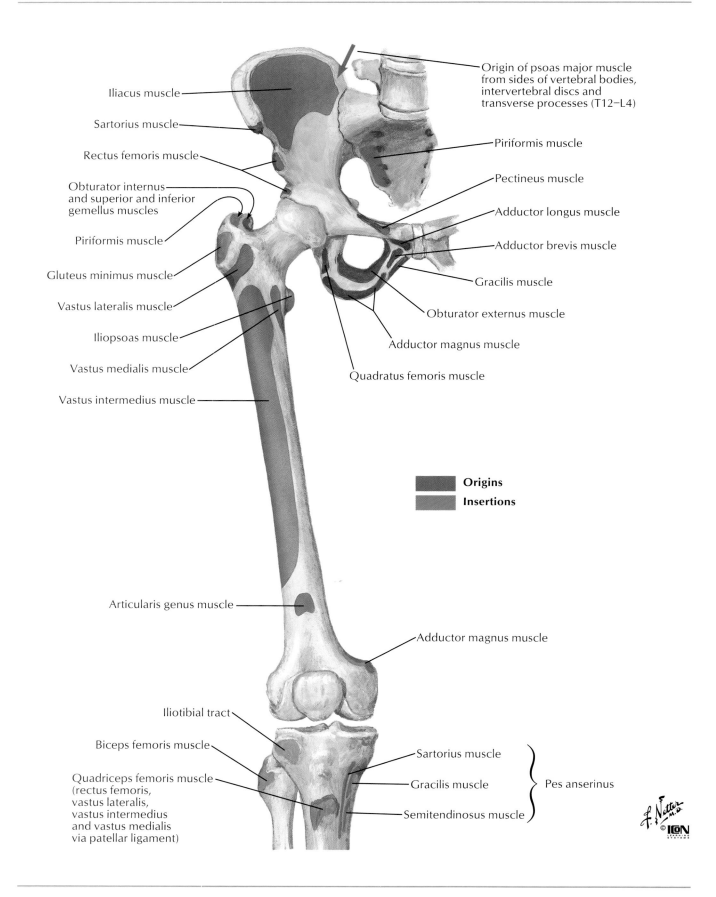

Iliacus muscle

Sartorius muscle

Rectus femoris muscle

Obturator internus and superior and inferior gemellus muscles

Piriformis muscle

Gluteus minimus muscle

Vastus lateralis muscle

Iliopsoas muscle

Vastus medialis muscle

Vastus intermedius muscle

Articularis genus muscle

Iliotibial tract

Biceps femoris muscle

Quadriceps femoris muscle (rectus femoris, vastus lateralis, vastus intermedius and vastus medialis via patellar ligament)

Origin of psoas major muscle from sides of vertebral bodies, intervertebral discs and transverse processes (T12–L4)

Piriformis muscle

Pectineus muscle

Adductor longus muscle

Adductor brevis muscle

Gracilis muscle

Obturator externus muscle

Adductor magnus muscle

Quadratus femoris muscle

Origins

Insertions

Adductor magnus muscle

Sartorius muscle

Gracilis muscle

Semitendinosus muscle

Pes anserinus

PLATE 472

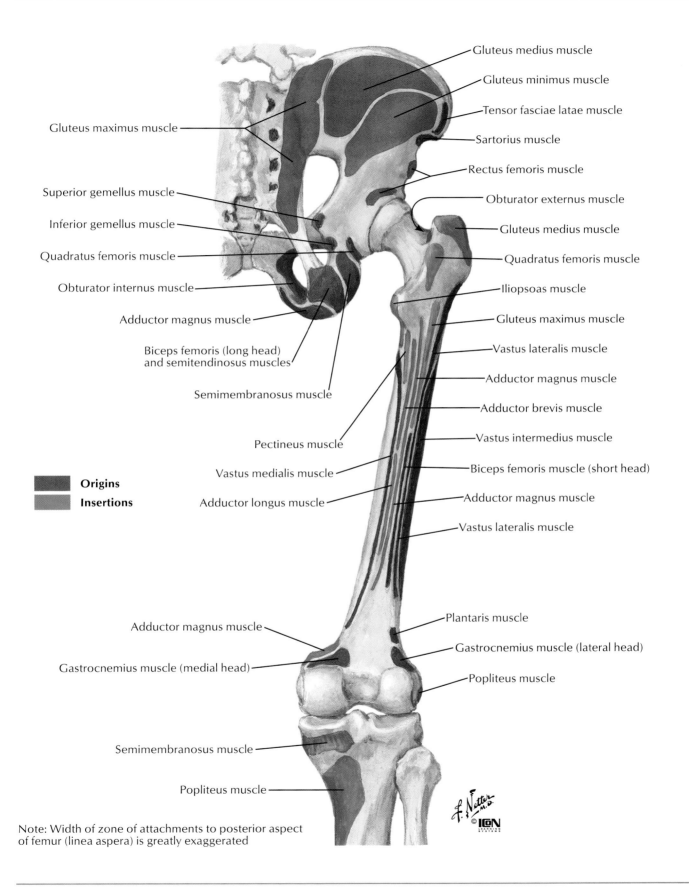

Gluteus medius muscle

Gluteus minimus muscle

Tensor fasciae latae muscle

Gluteus maximus muscle

Sartorius muscle

Rectus femoris muscle

Superior gemellus muscle

Obturator externus muscle

Inferior gemellus muscle

Gluteus medius muscle

Quadratus femoris muscle

Quadratus femoris muscle

Obturator internus muscle

Iliopsoas muscle

Gluteus maximus muscle

Adductor magnus muscle

Vastus lateralis muscle

Biceps femoris (long head)
and semitendinosus muscles

Adductor magnus muscle

Adductor brevis muscle

Semimembranosus muscle

Vastus intermedius muscle

Pectineus muscle

Biceps femoris muscle (short head)

Vastus medialis muscle

Adductor magnus muscle

Adductor longus muscle

Vastus lateralis muscle

Origins

Insertions

Adductor magnus muscle

Plantaris muscle

Gastrocnemius muscle (lateral head)

Gastrocnemius muscle (medial head)

Popliteus muscle

Semimembranosus muscle

Popliteus muscle

Note: Width of zone of attachments to posterior aspect
of femur (linea aspera) is greatly exaggerated

Muscles of Thigh: Anterior Views

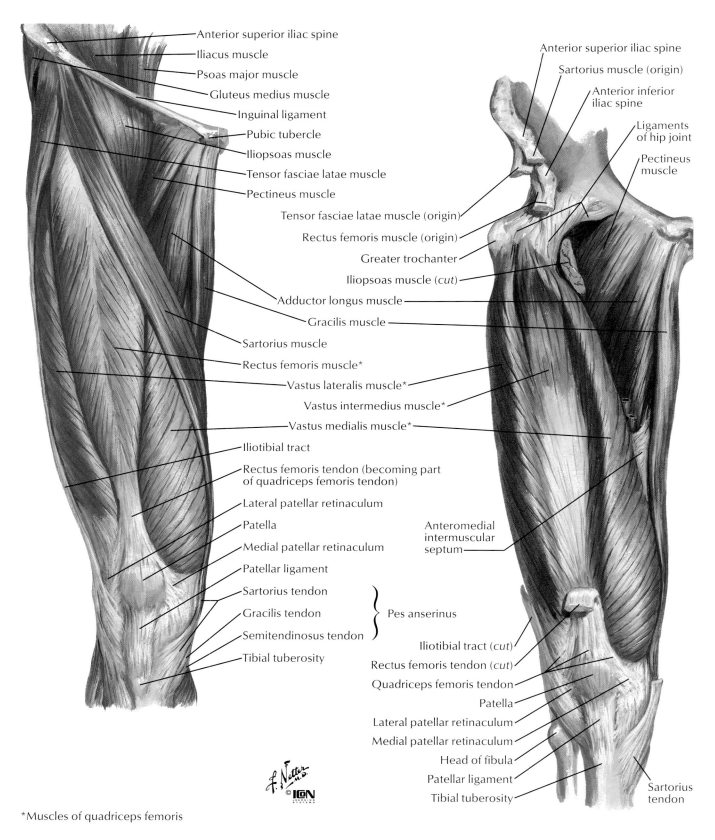

Anterior superior iliac spine

Iliacus muscle

Psoas major muscle

Gluteus medius muscle

Inguinal ligament

Pubic tubercle

Iliopsoas muscle

Tensor fasciae latae muscle

Pectineus muscle

Adductor longus muscle

Gracilis muscle

Sartorius muscle

Rectus femoris muscle*

Vastus lateralis muscle*

Vastus intermedius muscle*

Vastus medialis muscle*

Iliotibial tract

Rectus femoris tendon (becoming part of quadriceps femoris tendon)

Lateral patellar retinaculum

Patella

Medial patellar retinaculum

Patellar ligament

Sartorius tendon

Gracilis tendon

Semitendinosus tendon

Tibial tuberosity

} Pes anserinus

Anterior superior iliac spine

Sartorius muscle (origin)

Anterior inferior iliac spine

Ligaments of hip joint

Pectineus muscle

Tensor fasciae latae muscle (origin)

Rectus femoris muscle (origin)

Greater trochanter

Iliopsoas muscle (*cut*)

Anteromedial intermuscular septum

Iliotibial tract (*cut*)

Rectus femoris tendon (*cut*)

Quadriceps femoris tendon

Patella

Lateral patellar retinaculum

Medial patellar retinaculum

Head of fibula

Patellar ligament

Tibial tuberosity

Sartorius tendon

*Muscles of quadriceps femoris

PLATE 474

LOWER LIMB

Deep dissection

Anterior superior iliac spine

Anterior inferior iliac spine

Ligaments of hip joint

Greater trochanter of femur

Iliopsoas muscle (*cut*)

Pectineus muscle
(*cut and reflected*)

Adductor brevis muscle
(*cut and reflected*)

Vastus intermedius muscle

Adductor longus muscle
(*cut and reflected*)

Femoral artery and vein
passing through hiatus
of adductor magnus muscle

Vastus medialis muscle (*cut*)

Rectus femoris tendon (*cut as it
becomes part of quadriceps tendon*)

Vastus lateralis muscle (*cut*)

Lateral epicondyle of femur

Patella

Lateral patellar retinaculum

Fibular collateral ligament

Head of fibula

Patellar ligament

Tibial tuberosity

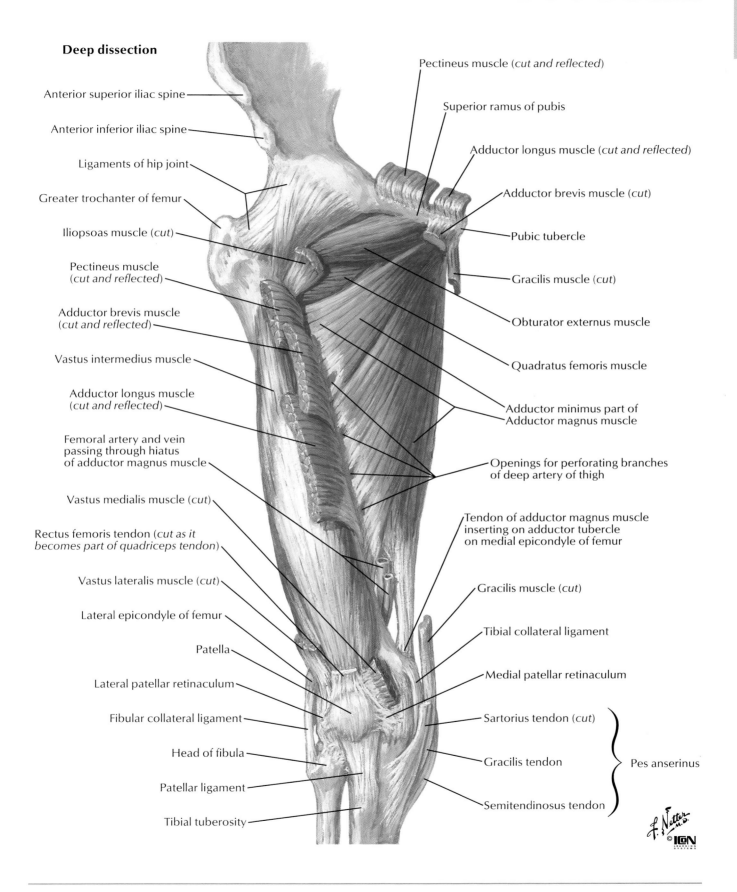

Pectineus muscle (*cut and reflected*)

Superior ramus of pubis

Adductor longus muscle (*cut and reflected*)

Adductor brevis muscle (*cut*)

Pubic tubercle

Gracilis muscle (*cut*)

Obturator externus muscle

Quadratus femoris muscle

Adductor minimus part of
Adductor magnus muscle

Openings for perforating branches
of deep artery of thigh

Tendon of adductor magnus muscle
inserting on adductor tubercle
on medial epicondyle of femur

Gracilis muscle (*cut*)

Tibial collateral ligament

Medial patellar retinaculum

Sartorius tendon (*cut*)

Gracilis tendon

Semitendinosus tendon

Pes anserinus

f. Netter
M.D.
©I⊂N
LEARNING
SYSTEMS

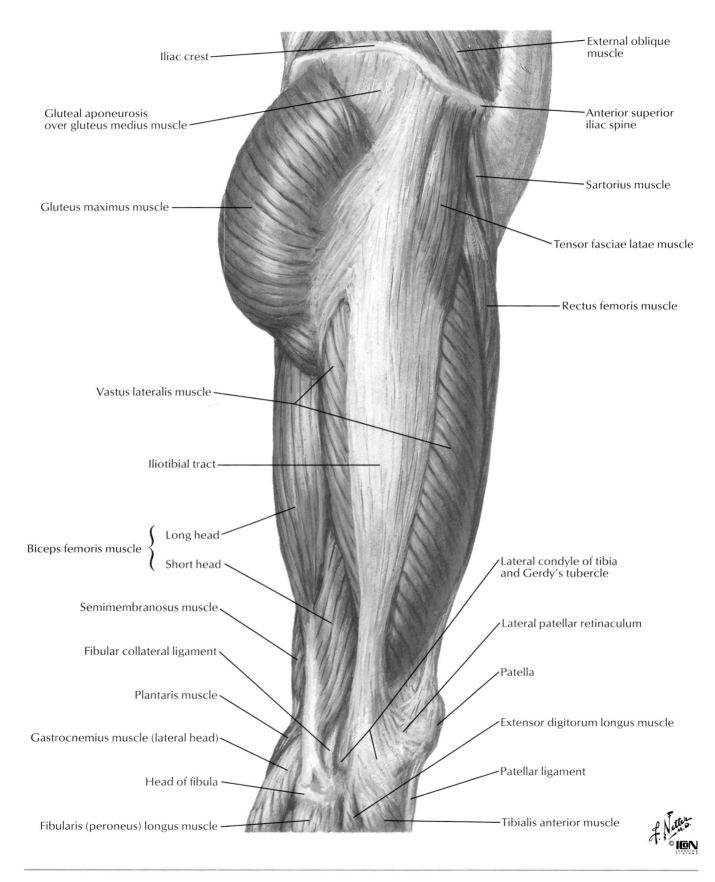

Iliac crest

External oblique muscle

Gluteal aponeurosis over gluteus medius muscle

Anterior superior iliac spine

Sartorius muscle

Gluteus maximus muscle

Tensor fasciae latae muscle

Rectus femoris muscle

Vastus lateralis muscle

Iliotibial tract

Biceps femoris muscle { Long head / Short head

Lateral condyle of tibia and Gerdy's tubercle

Lateral patellar retinaculum

Semimembranosus muscle

Fibular collateral ligament

Patella

Plantaris muscle

Extensor digitorum longus muscle

Gastrocnemius muscle (lateral head)

Patellar ligament

Head of fibula

Fibularis (peroneus) longus muscle

Tibialis anterior muscle

PLATE 476

LOWER LIMB

FOR PIRIFORMIS AND OBTURATOR INTERNUS SEE ALSO PLATES 343, 344; FOR OBTURATOR EXTERNUS SEE PLATE 483

Superficial dissection

Deeper dissection

Iliac crest

Gluteal aponeurosis over
Gluteus medius muscle

Gluteus minimus muscle

Gluteus maximus muscle

Piriformis muscle

Sciatic nerve

Sacrospinous ligament

Superior gemellus muscle

Obturator internus muscle

Inferior gemellus muscle

Sacrotuberous ligament

Quadratus femoris muscle

Ischial tuberosity

Semitendinosus muscle

Greater trochanter

Biceps femoris muscle (long head)

Adductor minimus part of
Adductor magnus muscle

Semimembranosus muscle

Iliotibial tract

Gracilis muscle

Biceps femoris muscle
Short head
Long head

Semimembranosus muscle

Semitendinosus muscle

Popliteal vessels and tibial nerve

Common fibular (peroneal) nerve

Plantaris muscle

Gastrocnemius muscle
Medial head
Lateral head

Sartorius muscle

Popliteus muscle

Tendinous arch of
Soleus muscle

Plantaris tendon (*cut*)

Psoas and Iliacus Muscles

SEE ALSO PLATE 255

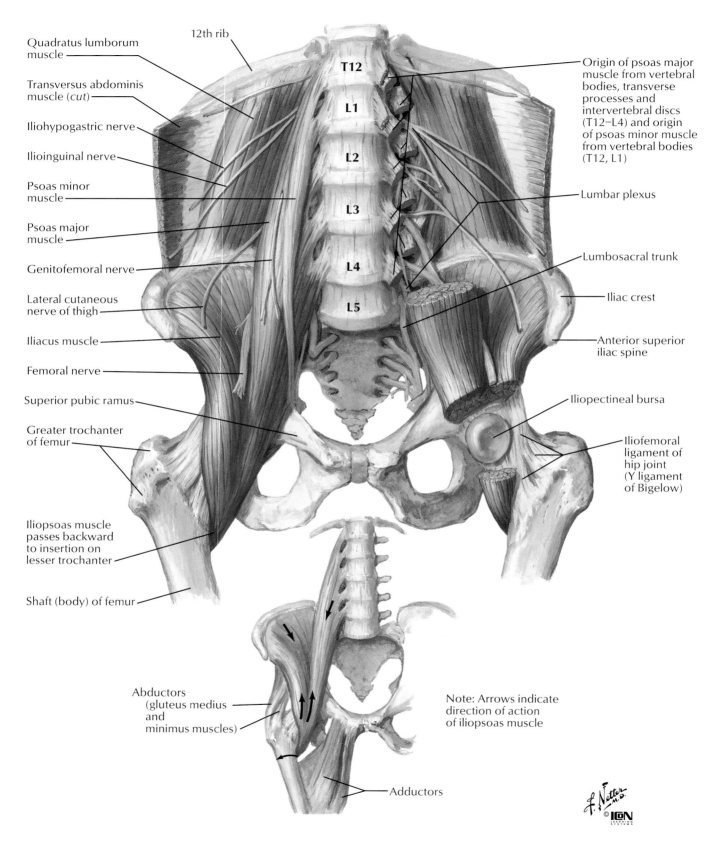

Quadratus lumborum muscle

12th rib

T12

Origin of psoas major muscle from vertebral bodies, transverse processes and intervertebral discs (T12–L4) and origin of psoas minor muscle from vertebral bodies (T12, L1)

Transversus abdominis muscle (*cut*)

L1

Iliohypogastric nerve

Ilioinguinal nerve

L2

Psoas minor muscle

Lumbar plexus

L3

Psoas major muscle

L4

Genitofemoral nerve

Lumbosacral trunk

L5

Lateral cutaneous nerve of thigh

Iliac crest

Iliacus muscle

Anterior superior iliac spine

Femoral nerve

Superior pubic ramus

Iliopectineal bursa

Greater trochanter of femur

Iliofemoral ligament of hip joint (Y ligament of Bigelow)

Iliopsoas muscle passes backward to insertion on lesser trochanter

Shaft (body) of femur

Abductors (gluteus medius and minimus muscles)

Note: Arrows indicate direction of action of iliopsoas muscle

Adductors

PLATE 478

LOWER LIMB

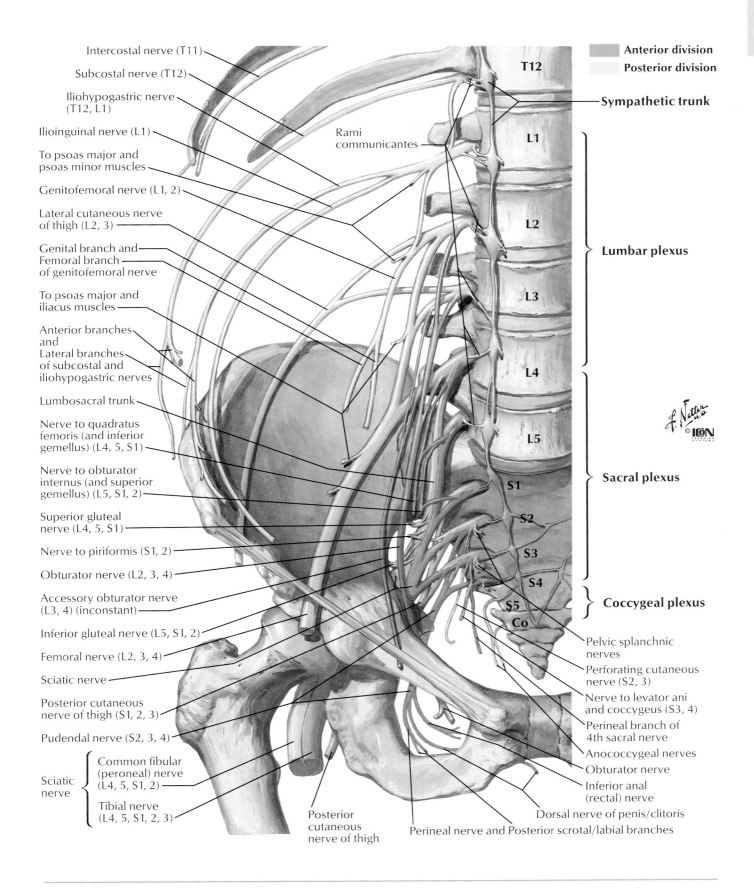

Intercostal nerve (T11)

Subcostal nerve (T12)

Iliohypogastric nerve
(T12, L1)

Ilioinguinal nerve (L1)

To psoas major and
psoas minor muscles

Genitofemoral nerve (L1, 2)

Lateral cutaneous nerve
of thigh (L2, 3)

Genital branch and
Femoral branch
of genitofemoral nerve

To psoas major and
iliacus muscles

Anterior branches
and
Lateral branches
of subcostal and
iliohypogastric nerves

Lumbosacral trunk

Nerve to quadratus
femoris (and inferior
gemellus) (L4, 5, S1)

Nerve to obturator
internus (and superior
gemellus) (L5, S1, 2)

Superior gluteal
nerve (L4, 5, S1)

Nerve to piriformis (S1, 2)

Obturator nerve (L2, 3, 4)

Accessory obturator nerve
(L3, 4) (inconstant)

Inferior gluteal nerve (L5, S1, 2)

Femoral nerve (L2, 3, 4)

Sciatic nerve

Posterior cutaneous
nerve of thigh (S1, 2, 3)

Pudendal nerve (S2, 3, 4)

Sciatic
nerve
{ Common fibular
(peroneal) nerve
(L4, 5, S1, 2)

Tibial nerve
(L4, 5, S1, 2, 3)

Rami
communicantes

Posterior
cutaneous
nerve of thigh

T12

L1

L2

L3

L4

L5

S1

S2

S3

S4

S5
Co

Anterior division
Posterior division

Sympathetic trunk

Lumbar plexus

Sacral plexus

Coccygeal plexus

Pelvic splanchnic
nerves

Perforating cutaneous
nerve (S2, 3)

Nerve to levator ani
and coccygeus (S3, 4)

Perineal branch of
4th sacral nerve

Anococcygeal nerves

Obturator nerve

Inferior anal
(rectal) nerve

Dorsal nerve of penis/clitoris

Perineal nerve and Posterior scrotal/labial branches

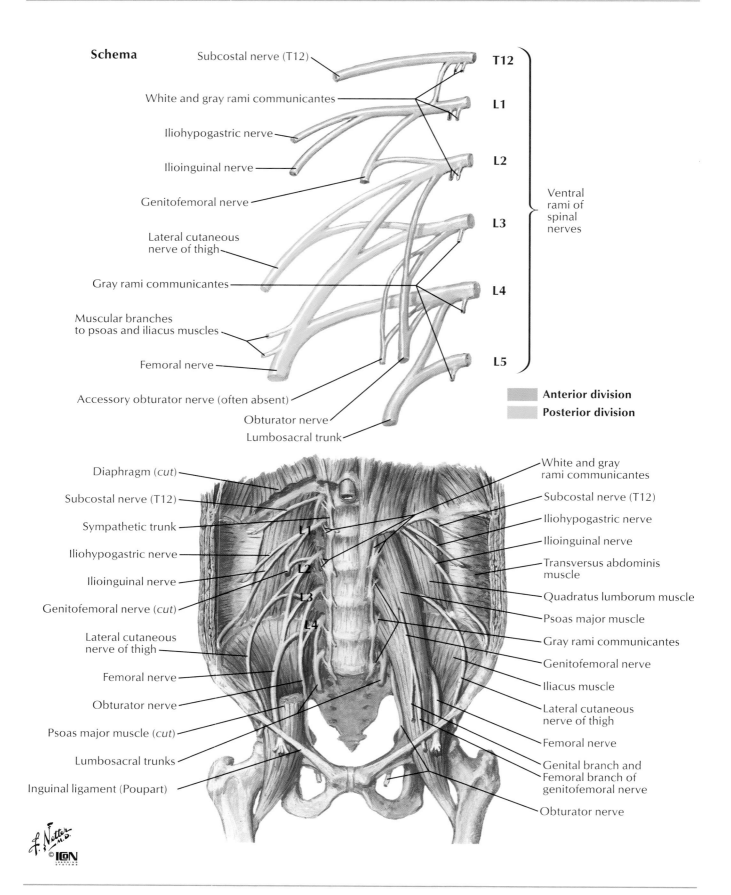

Schema

Subcostal nerve (T12)

White and gray rami communicantes

Iliohypogastric nerve

Ilioinguinal nerve

Genitofemoral nerve

Lateral cutaneous nerve of thigh

Gray rami communicantes

Muscular branches to psoas and iliacus muscles

Femoral nerve

Accessory obturator nerve (often absent)

Obturator nerve

Lumbosacral trunk

T12

L1

L2

L3

L4

L5

Ventral rami of spinal nerves

Anterior division
Posterior division

Diaphragm (cut)

Subcostal nerve (T12)

Sympathetic trunk

Iliohypogastric nerve

Ilioinguinal nerve

Genitofemoral nerve (cut)

Lateral cutaneous nerve of thigh

Femoral nerve

Obturator nerve

Psoas major muscle (cut)

Lumbosacral trunks

Inguinal ligament (Poupart)

White and gray rami communicantes

Subcostal nerve (T12)

Iliohypogastric nerve

Ilioinguinal nerve

Transversus abdominis muscle

Quadratus lumborum muscle

Psoas major muscle

Gray rami communicantes

Genitofemoral nerve

Iliacus muscle

Lateral cutaneous nerve of thigh

Femoral nerve

Genital branch and Femoral branch of genitofemoral nerve

Obturator nerve

PLATE 480

LOWER LIMB

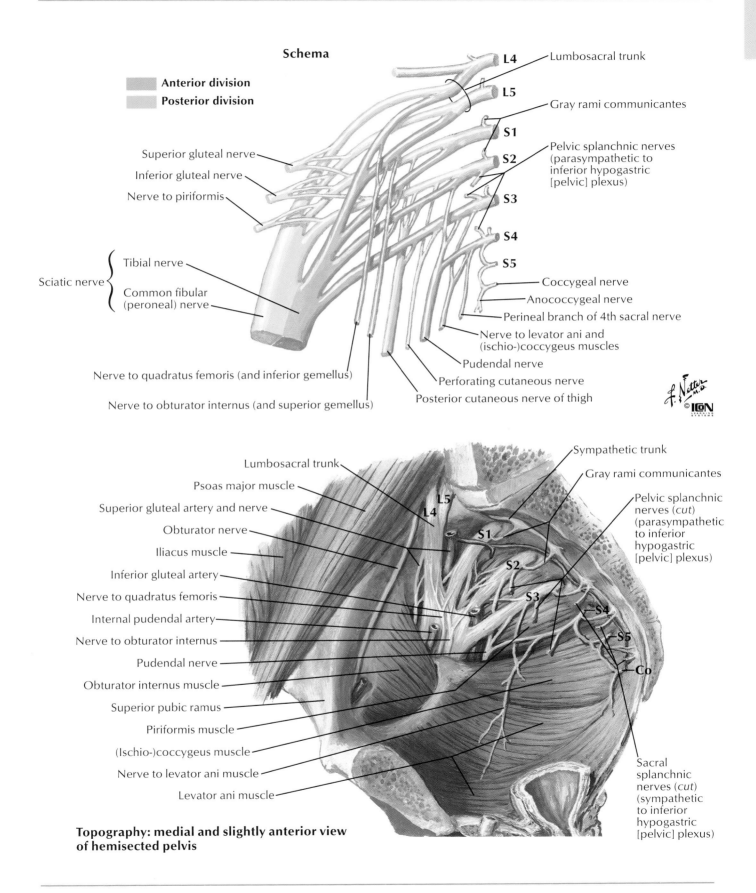

Schema

Anterior division
Posterior division

Superior gluteal nerve
Inferior gluteal nerve
Nerve to piriformis

L4 — Lumbosacral trunk
L5 — Gray rami communicantes
S1
S2 — Pelvic splanchnic nerves (parasympathetic to inferior hypogastric [pelvic] plexus)
S3
S4
S5
— Coccygeal nerve
— Anococcygeal nerve
— Perineal branch of 4th sacral nerve

Sciatic nerve {
Tibial nerve
Common fibular (peroneal) nerve
}

Nerve to levator ani and (ischio-)coccygeus muscles
Pudendal nerve
Perforating cutaneous nerve
Posterior cutaneous nerve of thigh

Nerve to quadratus femoris (and inferior gemellus)
Nerve to obturator internus (and superior gemellus)

Lumbosacral trunk
Psoas major muscle
Superior gluteal artery and nerve
Obturator nerve
Iliacus muscle
Inferior gluteal artery
Nerve to quadratus femoris
Internal pudendal artery
Nerve to obturator internus
Pudendal nerve
Obturator internus muscle
Superior pubic ramus
Piriformis muscle
(Ischio-)coccygeus muscle
Nerve to levator ani muscle
Levator ani muscle

Sympathetic trunk
Gray rami communicantes
Pelvic splanchnic nerves (*cut*) (parasympathetic to inferior hypogastric [pelvic] plexus)

L5
L4
S1
S2
S3
S4
S5
Co

Sacral splanchnic nerves (*cut*) (sympathetic to inferior hypogastric [pelvic] plexus)

Topography: medial and slightly anterior view of hemisected pelvis

Superficial dissections

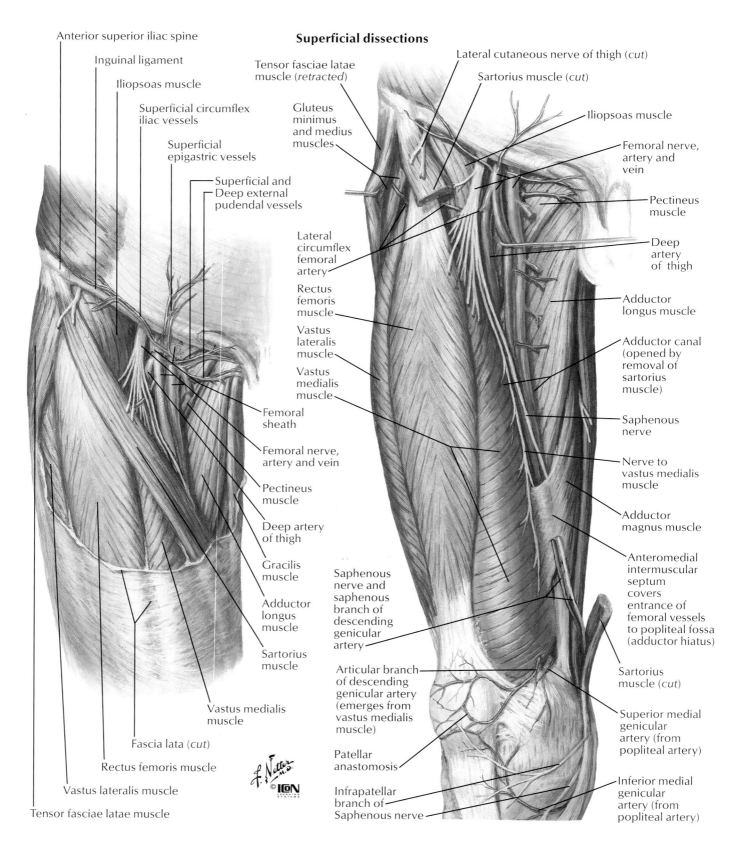

Anterior superior iliac spine

Inguinal ligament

Iliopsoas muscle

Superficial circumflex iliac vessels

Superficial epigastric vessels

Superficial and Deep external pudendal vessels

Tensor fasciae latae muscle (*retracted*)

Gluteus minimus and medius muscles

Lateral circumflex femoral artery

Rectus femoris muscle

Vastus lateralis muscle

Vastus medialis muscle

Lateral cutaneous nerve of thigh (*cut*)

Sartorius muscle (*cut*)

Iliopsoas muscle

Femoral nerve, artery and vein

Pectineus muscle

Deep artery of thigh

Adductor longus muscle

Adductor canal (opened by removal of sartorius muscle)

Saphenous nerve

Nerve to vastus medialis muscle

Adductor magnus muscle

Anteromedial intermuscular septum covers entrance of femoral vessels to popliteal fossa (adductor hiatus)

Sartorius muscle (*cut*)

Superior medial genicular artery (from popliteal artery)

Inferior medial genicular artery (from popliteal artery)

Femoral sheath

Femoral nerve, artery and vein

Pectineus muscle

Deep artery of thigh

Gracilis muscle

Adductor longus muscle

Sartorius muscle

Vastus medialis muscle

Fascia lata (*cut*)

Rectus femoris muscle

Vastus lateralis muscle

Tensor fasciae latae muscle

Saphenous nerve and saphenous branch of descending genicular artery

Articular branch of descending genicular artery (emerges from vastus medialis muscle)

Patellar anastomosis

Infrapatellar branch of Saphenous nerve

PLATE 482

LOWER LIMB

SEE ALSO PLATES 520, 521

Deep dissection

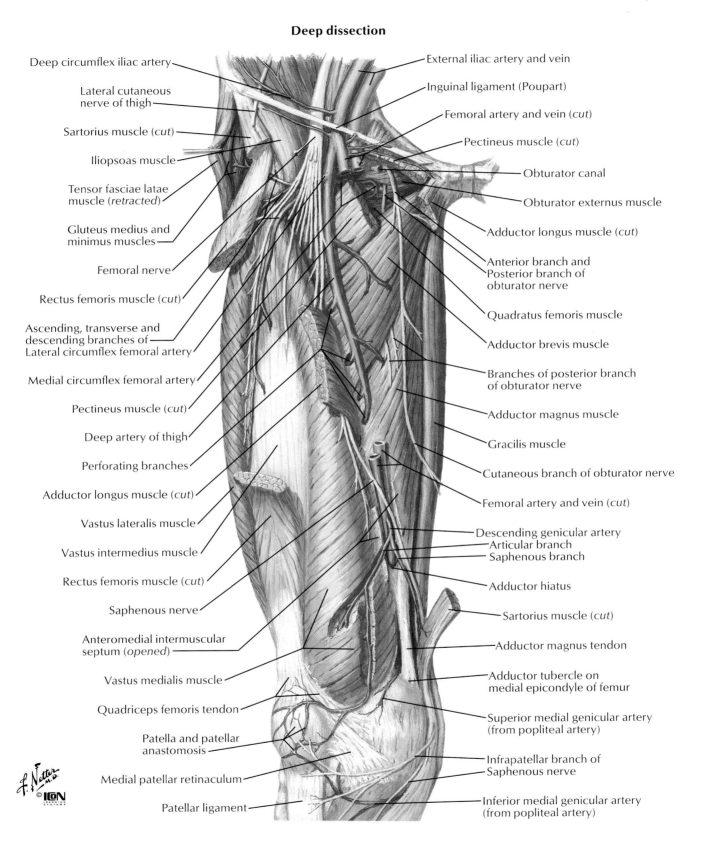

Deep circumflex iliac artery

Lateral cutaneous nerve of thigh

Sartorius muscle (*cut*)

Iliopsoas muscle

Tensor fasciae latae muscle (*retracted*)

Gluteus medius and minimus muscles

Femoral nerve

Rectus femoris muscle (*cut*)

Ascending, transverse and descending branches of Lateral circumflex femoral artery

Medial circumflex femoral artery

Pectineus muscle (*cut*)

Deep artery of thigh

Perforating branches

Adductor longus muscle (*cut*)

Vastus lateralis muscle

Vastus intermedius muscle

Rectus femoris muscle (*cut*)

Saphenous nerve

Anteromedial intermuscular septum (*opened*)

Vastus medialis muscle

Quadriceps femoris tendon

Patella and patellar anastomosis

Medial patellar retinaculum

Patellar ligament

External iliac artery and vein

Inguinal ligament (Poupart)

Femoral artery and vein (*cut*)

Pectineus muscle (*cut*)

Obturator canal

Obturator externus muscle

Adductor longus muscle (*cut*)

Anterior branch and Posterior branch of obturator nerve

Quadratus femoris muscle

Adductor brevis muscle

Branches of posterior branch of obturator nerve

Adductor magnus muscle

Gracilis muscle

Cutaneous branch of obturator nerve

Femoral artery and vein (*cut*)

Descending genicular artery
Articular branch
Saphenous branch

Adductor hiatus

Sartorius muscle (*cut*)

Adductor magnus tendon

Adductor tubercle on medial epicondyle of femur

Superior medial genicular artery (from popliteal artery)

Infrapatellar branch of Saphenous nerve

Inferior medial genicular artery (from popliteal artery)

Deep dissection

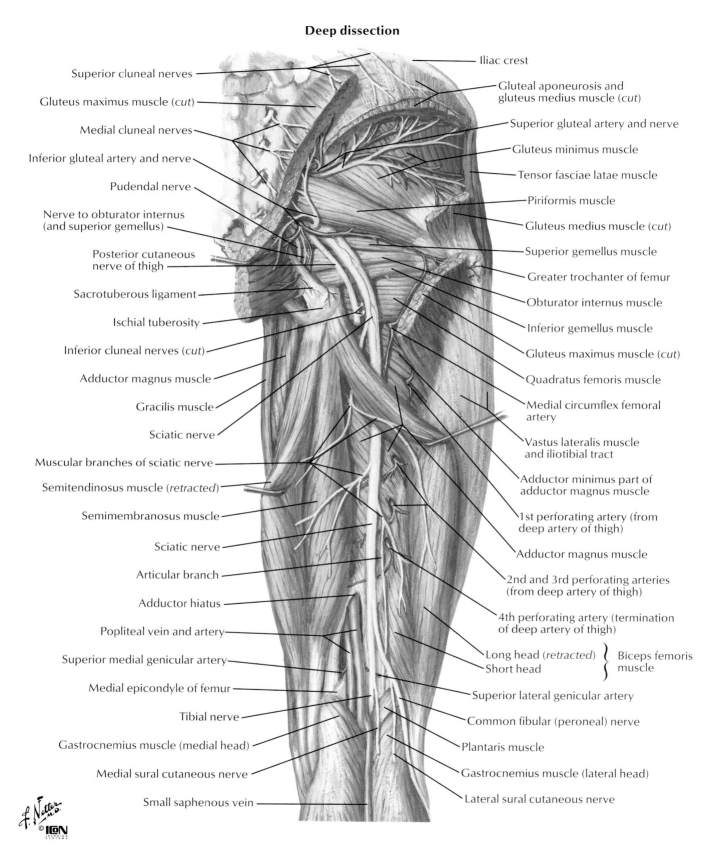

Superior cluneal nerves

Gluteus maximus muscle (*cut*)

Medial cluneal nerves

Inferior gluteal artery and nerve

Pudendal nerve

Nerve to obturator internus (and superior gemellus)

Posterior cutaneous nerve of thigh

Sacrotuberous ligament

Ischial tuberosity

Inferior cluneal nerves (*cut*)

Adductor magnus muscle

Gracilis muscle

Sciatic nerve

Muscular branches of sciatic nerve

Semitendinosus muscle (*retracted*)

Semimembranosus muscle

Sciatic nerve

Articular branch

Adductor hiatus

Popliteal vein and artery

Superior medial genicular artery

Medial epicondyle of femur

Tibial nerve

Gastrocnemius muscle (medial head)

Medial sural cutaneous nerve

Small saphenous vein

Iliac crest

Gluteal aponeurosis and gluteus medius muscle (*cut*)

Superior gluteal artery and nerve

Gluteus minimus muscle

Tensor fasciae latae muscle

Piriformis muscle

Gluteus medius muscle (*cut*)

Superior gemellus muscle

Greater trochanter of femur

Obturator internus muscle

Inferior gemellus muscle

Gluteus maximus muscle (*cut*)

Quadratus femoris muscle

Medial circumflex femoral artery

Vastus lateralis muscle and iliotibial tract

Adductor minimus part of adductor magnus muscle

1st perforating artery (from deep artery of thigh)

Adductor magnus muscle

2nd and 3rd perforating arteries (from deep artery of thigh)

4th perforating artery (termination of deep artery of thigh)

Long head (*retracted*) ⎫
Short head ⎬ Biceps femoris muscle

Superior lateral genicular artery

Common fibular (peroneal) nerve

Plantaris muscle

Gastrocnemius muscle (lateral head)

Lateral sural cutaneous nerve

PLATE 484

LOWER LIMB

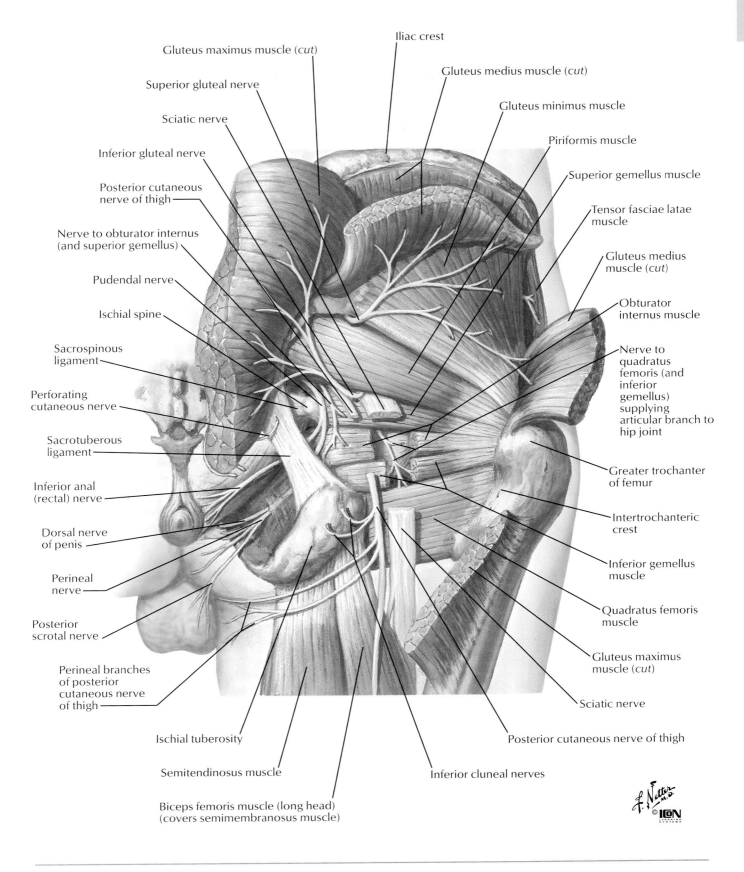

Gluteus maximus muscle (*cut*)

Iliac crest

Superior gluteal nerve

Gluteus medius muscle (*cut*)

Sciatic nerve

Gluteus minimus muscle

Inferior gluteal nerve

Piriformis muscle

Posterior cutaneous nerve of thigh

Superior gemellus muscle

Nerve to obturator internus (and superior gemellus)

Tensor fasciae latae muscle

Pudendal nerve

Gluteus medius muscle (*cut*)

Ischial spine

Obturator internus muscle

Sacrospinous ligament

Nerve to quadratus femoris (and inferior gemellus) supplying articular branch to hip joint

Perforating cutaneous nerve

Sacrotuberous ligament

Greater trochanter of femur

Inferior anal (rectal) nerve

Intertrochanteric crest

Dorsal nerve of penis

Inferior gemellus muscle

Perineal nerve

Quadratus femoris muscle

Posterior scrotal nerve

Gluteus maximus muscle (*cut*)

Perineal branches of posterior cutaneous nerve of thigh

Sciatic nerve

Ischial tuberosity

Posterior cutaneous nerve of thigh

Semitendinosus muscle

Inferior cluneal nerves

Biceps femoris muscle (long head) (covers semimembranosus muscle)

F. Netter M.D.

© ICON LEARNING SYSTEMS

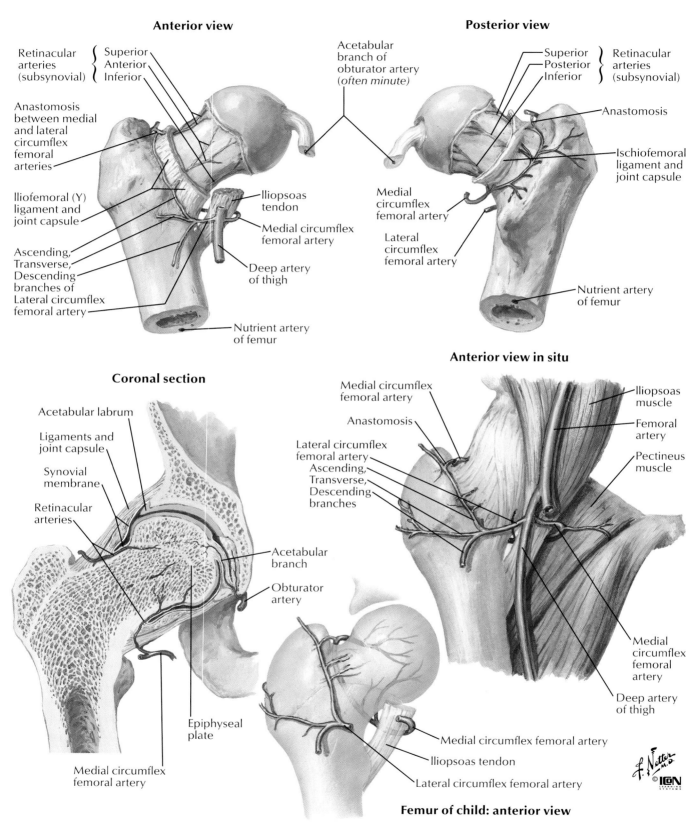

Anterior view

Retinacular arteries (subsynovial) { Superior / Anterior / Inferior

Anastomosis between medial and lateral circumflex femoral arteries

Iliofemoral (Y) ligament and joint capsule

Ascending, Transverse, Descending branches of Lateral circumflex femoral artery

Acetabular branch of obturator artery (often minute)

Iliopsoas tendon

Medial circumflex femoral artery

Deep artery of thigh

Nutrient artery of femur

Posterior view

Superior / Posterior / Inferior } Retinacular arteries (subsynovial)

Anastomosis

Ischiofemoral ligament and joint capsule

Medial circumflex femoral artery

Lateral circumflex femoral artery

Nutrient artery of femur

Coronal section

Acetabular labrum

Ligaments and joint capsule

Synovial membrane

Retinacular arteries

Acetabular branch

Obturator artery

Epiphyseal plate

Medial circumflex femoral artery

Anterior view in situ

Medial circumflex femoral artery

Anastomosis

Lateral circumflex femoral artery

Ascending, Transverse, Descending branches

Iliopsoas muscle

Femoral artery

Pectineus muscle

Medial circumflex femoral artery

Deep artery of thigh

Medial circumflex femoral artery

Iliopsoas tendon

Lateral circumflex femoral artery

Femur of child: anterior view

PLATE 486

LOWER LIMB

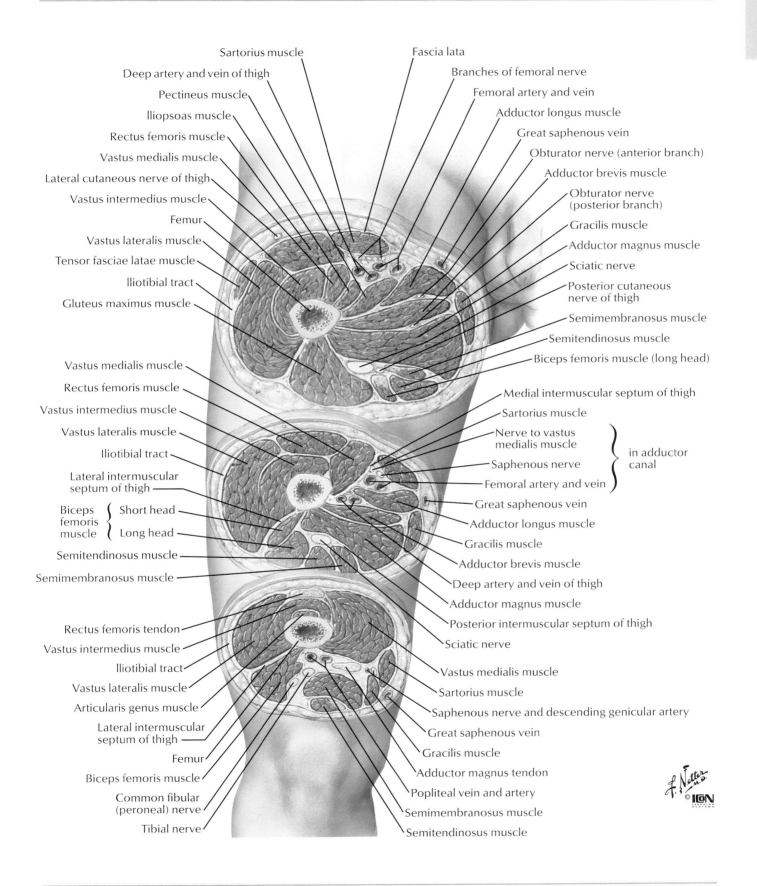

Sartorius muscle
Deep artery and vein of thigh
Pectineus muscle
Iliopsoas muscle
Rectus femoris muscle
Vastus medialis muscle
Lateral cutaneous nerve of thigh
Vastus intermedius muscle
Femur
Vastus lateralis muscle
Tensor fasciae latae muscle
Iliotibial tract
Gluteus maximus muscle

Fascia lata
Branches of femoral nerve
Femoral artery and vein
Adductor longus muscle
Great saphenous vein
Obturator nerve (anterior branch)
Adductor brevis muscle
Obturator nerve (posterior branch)
Gracilis muscle
Adductor magnus muscle
Sciatic nerve
Posterior cutaneous nerve of thigh
Semimembranosus muscle
Semitendinosus muscle
Biceps femoris muscle (long head)

Vastus medialis muscle
Rectus femoris muscle
Vastus intermedius muscle
Vastus lateralis muscle
Iliotibial tract
Lateral intermuscular septum of thigh
Biceps femoris muscle { Short head / Long head }
Semitendinosus muscle
Semimembranosus muscle

Medial intermuscular septum of thigh
Sartorius muscle
Nerve to vastus medialis muscle
Saphenous nerve
Femoral artery and vein
} in adductor canal
Great saphenous vein
Adductor longus muscle
Gracilis muscle
Adductor brevis muscle
Deep artery and vein of thigh
Adductor magnus muscle
Posterior intermuscular septum of thigh
Sciatic nerve

Rectus femoris tendon
Vastus intermedius muscle
Iliotibial tract
Vastus lateralis muscle
Articularis genus muscle
Lateral intermuscular septum of thigh
Femur
Biceps femoris muscle
Common fibular (peroneal) nerve
Tibial nerve

Vastus medialis muscle
Sartorius muscle
Saphenous nerve and descending genicular artery
Great saphenous vein
Gracilis muscle
Adductor magnus tendon
Popliteal vein and artery
Semimembranosus muscle
Semitendinosus muscle

Knee: Lateral and Medial Views

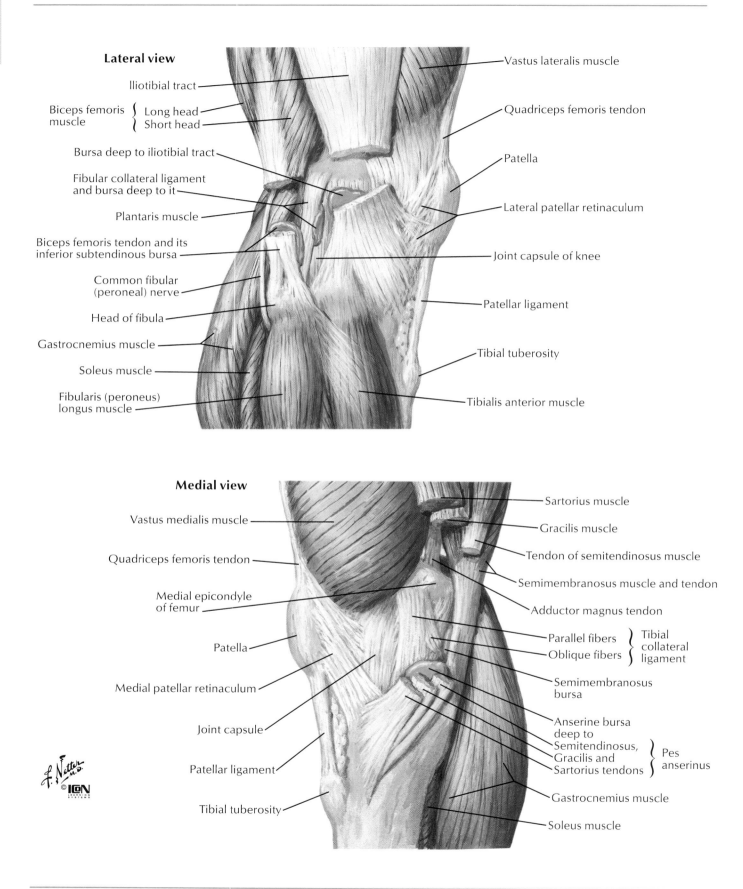

Lateral view

Iliotibial tract

Biceps femoris muscle { Long head / Short head

Bursa deep to iliotibial tract

Fibular collateral ligament and bursa deep to it

Plantaris muscle

Biceps femoris tendon and its inferior subtendinous bursa

Common fibular (peroneal) nerve

Head of fibula

Gastrocnemius muscle

Soleus muscle

Fibularis (peroneus) longus muscle

Vastus lateralis muscle

Quadriceps femoris tendon

Patella

Lateral patellar retinaculum

Joint capsule of knee

Patellar ligament

Tibial tuberosity

Tibialis anterior muscle

Medial view

Vastus medialis muscle

Quadriceps femoris tendon

Medial epicondyle of femur

Patella

Medial patellar retinaculum

Joint capsule

Patellar ligament

Tibial tuberosity

Sartorius muscle

Gracilis muscle

Tendon of semitendinosus muscle

Semimembranosus muscle and tendon

Adductor magnus tendon

Parallel fibers } Tibial collateral ligament
Oblique fibers }

Semimembranosus bursa

Anserine bursa deep to Semitendinosus, Gracilis and Sartorius tendons } Pes anserinus

Gastrocnemius muscle

Soleus muscle

PLATE 488

LOWER LIMB

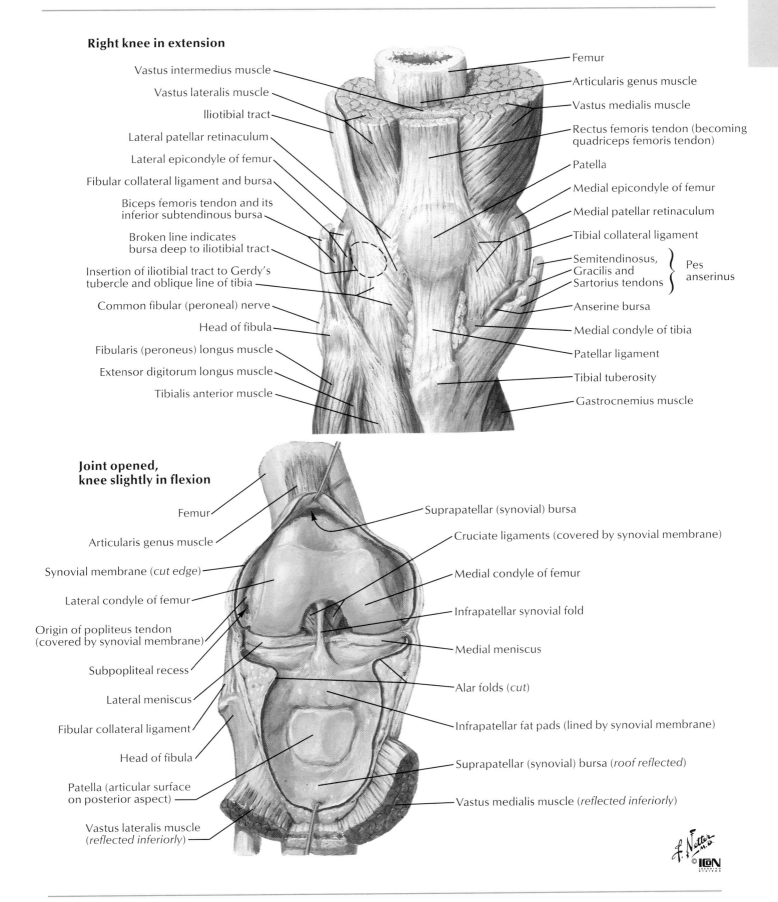

Right knee in extension

Vastus intermedius muscle

Vastus lateralis muscle

Iliotibial tract

Lateral patellar retinaculum

Lateral epicondyle of femur

Fibular collateral ligament and bursa

Biceps femoris tendon and its inferior subtendinous bursa

Broken line indicates bursa deep to iliotibial tract

Insertion of iliotibial tract to Gerdy's tubercle and oblique line of tibia

Common fibular (peroneal) nerve

Head of fibula

Fibularis (peroneus) longus muscle

Extensor digitorum longus muscle

Tibialis anterior muscle

Femur

Articularis genus muscle

Vastus medialis muscle

Rectus femoris tendon (becoming quadriceps femoris tendon)

Patella

Medial epicondyle of femur

Medial patellar retinaculum

Tibial collateral ligament

Semitendinosus, Gracilis and Sartorius tendons } Pes anserinus

Anserine bursa

Medial condyle of tibia

Patellar ligament

Tibial tuberosity

Gastrocnemius muscle

Joint opened, knee slightly in flexion

Femur

Articularis genus muscle

Synovial membrane (*cut edge*)

Lateral condyle of femur

Origin of popliteus tendon (covered by synovial membrane)

Subpopliteal recess

Lateral meniscus

Fibular collateral ligament

Head of fibula

Patella (articular surface on posterior aspect)

Vastus lateralis muscle (*reflected inferiorly*)

Suprapatellar (synovial) bursa

Cruciate ligaments (covered by synovial membrane)

Medial condyle of femur

Infrapatellar synovial fold

Medial meniscus

Alar folds (*cut*)

Infrapatellar fat pads (lined by synovial membrane)

Suprapatellar (synovial) bursa (*roof reflected*)

Vastus medialis muscle (*reflected inferiorly*)

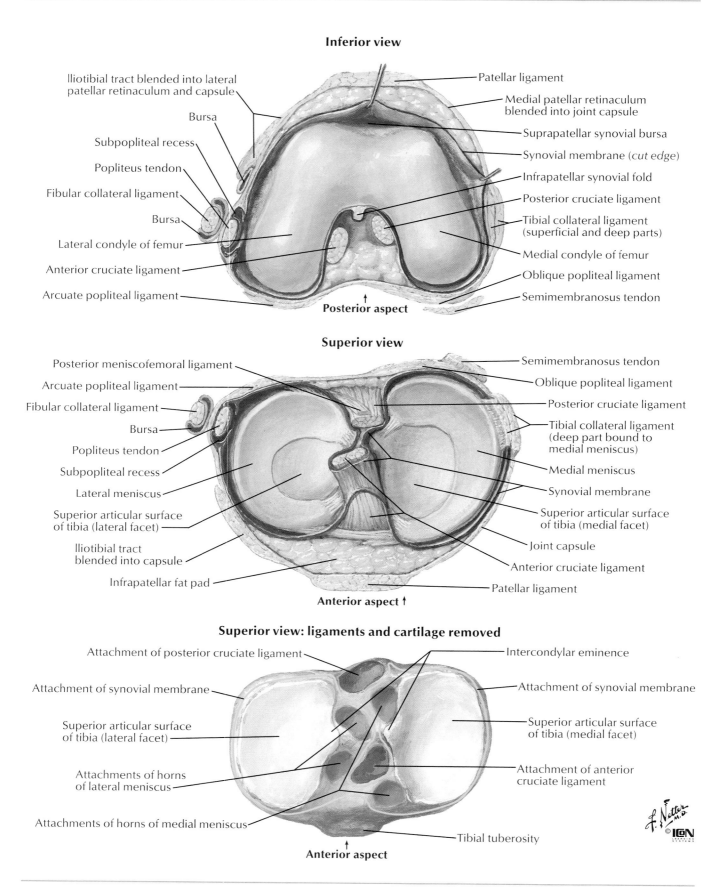

Inferior view

Iliotibial tract blended into lateral patellar retinaculum and capsule

Bursa

Subpopliteal recess

Popliteus tendon

Fibular collateral ligament

Bursa

Lateral condyle of femur

Anterior cruciate ligament

Arcuate popliteal ligament

Patellar ligament

Medial patellar retinaculum blended into joint capsule

Suprapatellar synovial bursa

Synovial membrane (*cut edge*)

Infrapatellar synovial fold

Posterior cruciate ligament

Tibial collateral ligament (superficial and deep parts)

Medial condyle of femur

Oblique popliteal ligament

Semimembranosus tendon

Posterior aspect ↑

Superior view

Posterior meniscofemoral ligament

Arcuate popliteal ligament

Fibular collateral ligament

Bursa

Popliteus tendon

Subpopliteal recess

Lateral meniscus

Superior articular surface of tibia (lateral facet)

Iliotibial tract blended into capsule

Infrapatellar fat pad

Semimembranosus tendon

Oblique popliteal ligament

Posterior cruciate ligament

Tibial collateral ligament (deep part bound to medial meniscus)

Medial meniscus

Synovial membrane

Superior articular surface of tibia (medial facet)

Joint capsule

Anterior cruciate ligament

Patellar ligament

Anterior aspect ↑

Superior view: ligaments and cartilage removed

Attachment of posterior cruciate ligament

Attachment of synovial membrane

Superior articular surface of tibia (lateral facet)

Attachments of horns of lateral meniscus

Attachments of horns of medial meniscus

Intercondylar eminence

Attachment of synovial membrane

Superior articular surface of tibia (medial facet)

Attachment of anterior cruciate ligament

Tibial tuberosity

Anterior aspect ↑

PLATE 490

LOWER LIMB

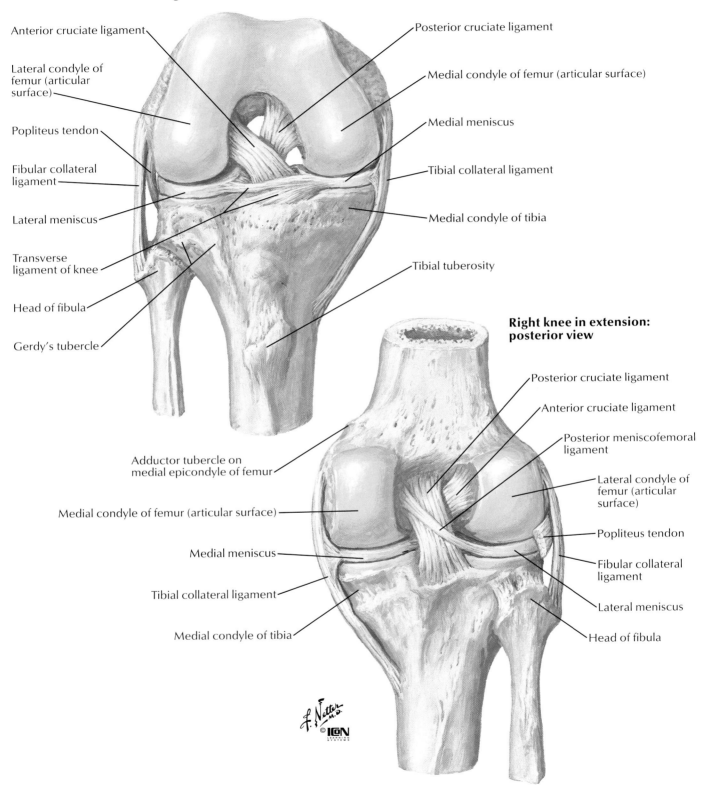

Right knee in flexion: anterior view

Anterior cruciate ligament

Lateral condyle of femur (articular surface)

Popliteus tendon

Fibular collateral ligament

Lateral meniscus

Transverse ligament of knee

Head of fibula

Gerdy's tubercle

Posterior cruciate ligament

Medial condyle of femur (articular surface)

Medial meniscus

Tibial collateral ligament

Medial condyle of tibia

Tibial tuberosity

Right knee in extension: posterior view

Adductor tubercle on medial epicondyle of femur

Medial condyle of femur (articular surface)

Medial meniscus

Tibial collateral ligament

Medial condyle of tibia

Posterior cruciate ligament

Anterior cruciate ligament

Posterior meniscofemoral ligament

Lateral condyle of femur (articular surface)

Popliteus tendon

Fibular collateral ligament

Lateral meniscus

Head of fibula

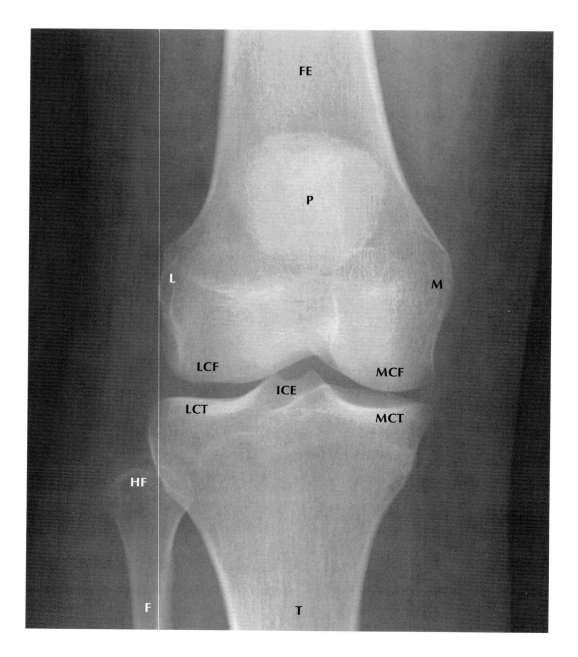

F	Fibula
FE	Femur
HF	Head of fibula
ICE	Intercondylar eminence
L	Lateral epicondyle
LCF	Lateral condyle of femur
LCT	Lateral condyle of tibia
M	Medial epicondyle
MCF	Medial condyle of femur
MCT	Medial condyle of tibia
P	Patella
T	Tibia

PLATE 492   **LOWER LIMB**

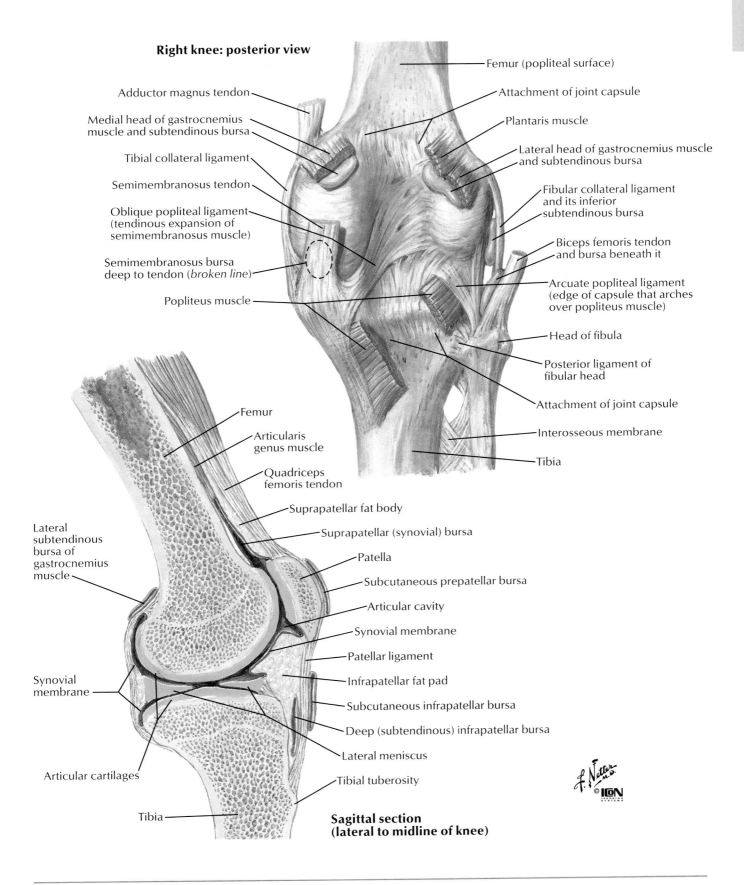

Right knee: posterior view

Adductor magnus tendon

Medial head of gastrocnemius muscle and subtendinous bursa

Tibial collateral ligament

Semimembranosus tendon

Oblique popliteal ligament (tendinous expansion of semimembranosus muscle)

Semimembranosus bursa deep to tendon (*broken line*)

Popliteus muscle

Femur (popliteal surface)

Attachment of joint capsule

Plantaris muscle

Lateral head of gastrocnemius muscle and subtendinous bursa

Fibular collateral ligament and its inferior subtendinous bursa

Biceps femoris tendon and bursa beneath it

Arcuate popliteal ligament (edge of capsule that arches over popliteus muscle)

Head of fibula

Posterior ligament of fibular head

Attachment of joint capsule

Interosseous membrane

Tibia

Femur

Articularis genus muscle

Quadriceps femoris tendon

Suprapatellar fat body

Suprapatellar (synovial) bursa

Patella

Subcutaneous prepatellar bursa

Articular cavity

Synovial membrane

Patellar ligament

Infrapatellar fat pad

Subcutaneous infrapatellar bursa

Deep (subtendinous) infrapatellar bursa

Lateral meniscus

Tibial tuberosity

Lateral subtendinous bursa of gastrocnemius muscle

Synovial membrane

Articular cartilages

Tibia

Sagittal section (lateral to midline of knee)

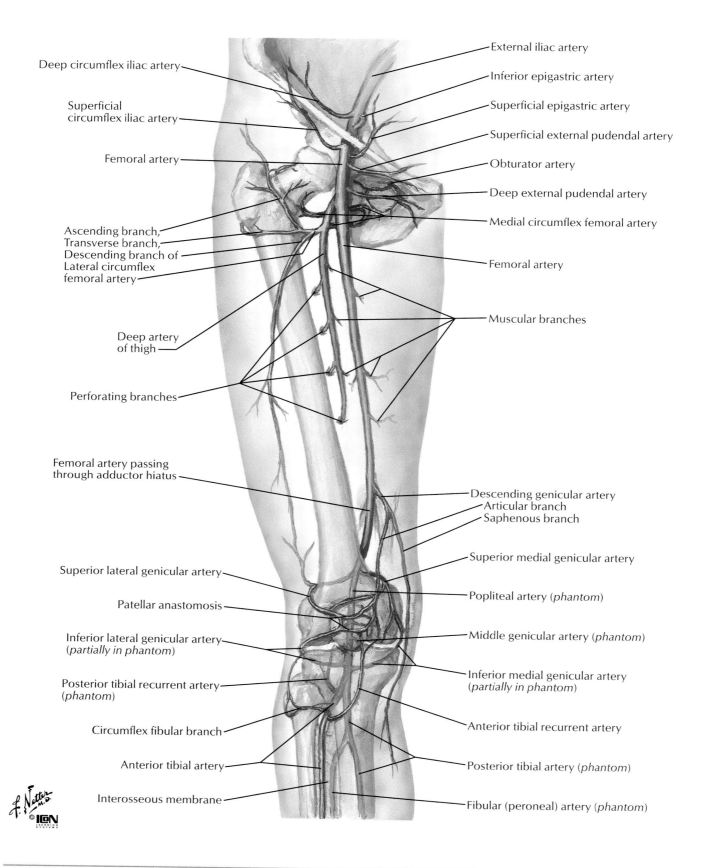

Deep circumflex iliac artery

Superficial circumflex iliac artery

Femoral artery

Ascending branch,
Transverse branch,
Descending branch of
Lateral circumflex
femoral artery

Deep artery of thigh

Perforating branches

Femoral artery passing through adductor hiatus

Superior lateral genicular artery

Patellar anastomosis

Inferior lateral genicular artery (partially in phantom)

Posterior tibial recurrent artery (phantom)

Circumflex fibular branch

Anterior tibial artery

Interosseous membrane

External iliac artery

Inferior epigastric artery

Superficial epigastric artery

Superficial external pudendal artery

Obturator artery

Deep external pudendal artery

Medial circumflex femoral artery

Femoral artery

Muscular branches

Descending genicular artery
Articular branch
Saphenous branch

Superior medial genicular artery

Popliteal artery (phantom)

Middle genicular artery (phantom)

Inferior medial genicular artery (partially in phantom)

Anterior tibial recurrent artery

Posterior tibial artery (phantom)

Fibular (peroneal) artery (phantom)

PLATE 494

LOWER LIMB

Bones of right leg

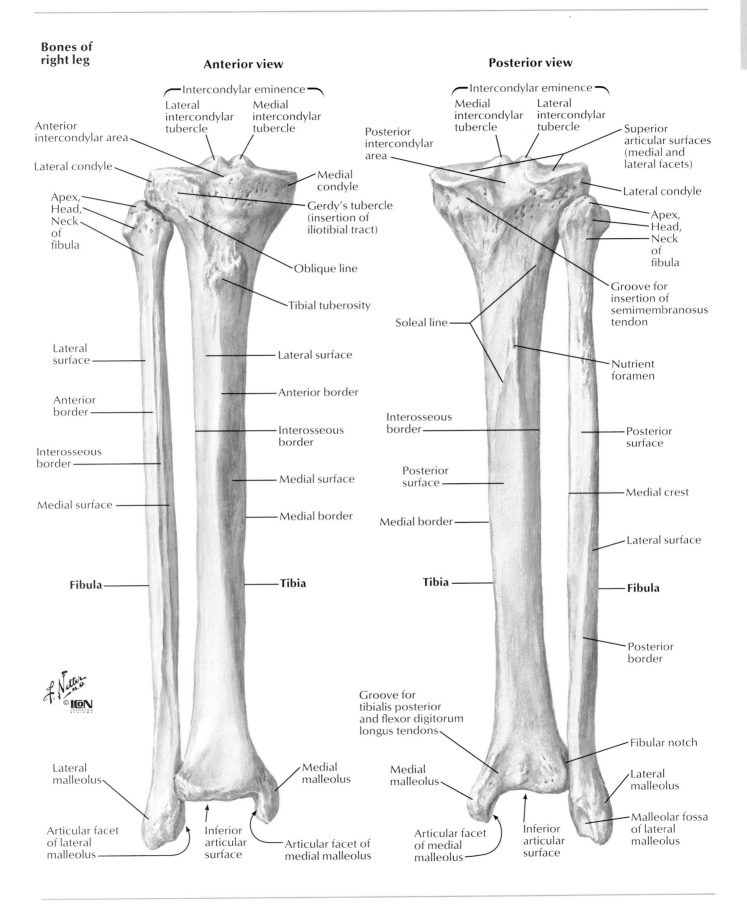

Anterior view

Intercondylar eminence

Lateral intercondylar tubercle

Medial intercondylar tubercle

Anterior intercondylar area

Lateral condyle

Medial condyle

Apex, Head, Neck of fibula

Gerdy's tubercle (insertion of iliotibial tract)

Oblique line

Tibial tuberosity

Lateral surface

Lateral surface

Anterior border

Anterior border

Interosseous border

Interosseous border

Medial surface

Medial surface

Medial border

Fibula

Tibia

Lateral malleolus

Medial malleolus

Articular facet of lateral malleolus

Inferior articular surface

Articular facet of medial malleolus

Posterior view

Intercondylar eminence

Medial intercondylar tubercle

Lateral intercondylar tubercle

Posterior intercondylar area

Superior articular surfaces (medial and lateral facets)

Lateral condyle

Apex, Head, Neck of fibula

Groove for insertion of semimembranosus tendon

Soleal line

Nutrient foramen

Interosseous border

Posterior surface

Posterior surface

Medial crest

Medial border

Lateral surface

Tibia

Fibula

Posterior border

Groove for tibialis posterior and flexor digitorum longus tendons

Fibular notch

Medial malleolus

Lateral malleolus

Malleolar fossa of lateral malleolus

Articular facet of medial malleolus

Inferior articular surface

Tibia and Fibula (continued)

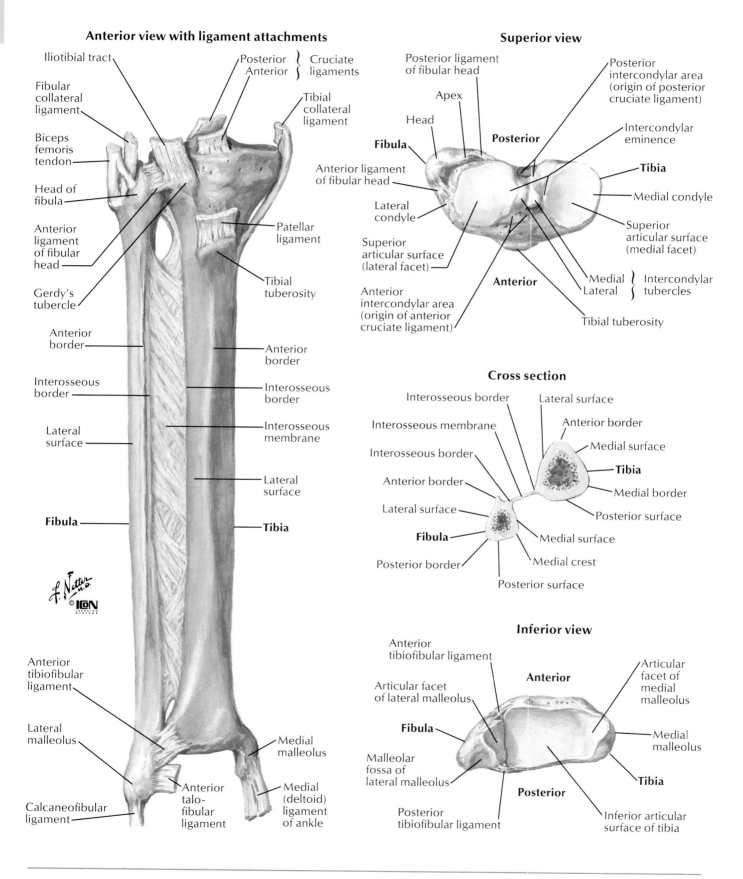

Anterior view with ligament attachments

Iliotibial tract

Fibular collateral ligament

Biceps femoris tendon

Head of fibula

Anterior ligament of fibular head

Gerdy's tubercle

Anterior border

Interosseous border

Lateral surface

Fibula

Posterior Anterior } Cruciate ligaments

Tibial collateral ligament

Patellar ligament

Tibial tuberosity

Anterior border

Interosseous border

Interosseous membrane

Lateral surface

Tibia

Anterior tibiofibular ligament

Lateral malleolus

Calcaneofibular ligament

Anterior talo-fibular ligament

Medial malleolus

Medial (deltoid) ligament of ankle

Superior view

Posterior ligament of fibular head

Apex

Head

Fibula

Anterior ligament of fibular head

Lateral condyle

Superior articular surface (lateral facet)

Anterior intercondylar area (origin of anterior cruciate ligament)

Posterior

Posterior intercondylar area (origin of posterior cruciate ligament)

Intercondylar eminence

Tibia

Medial condyle

Superior articular surface (medial facet)

Medial Lateral } Intercondylar tubercles

Tibial tuberosity

Anterior

Cross section

Interosseous border

Interosseous membrane

Interosseous border

Anterior border

Lateral surface

Fibula

Posterior border

Lateral surface

Anterior border

Medial surface

Tibia

Medial border

Posterior surface

Medial surface

Medial crest

Posterior surface

Inferior view

Anterior tibiofibular ligament

Articular facet of lateral malleolus

Fibula

Malleolar fossa of lateral malleolus

Posterior tibiofibular ligament

Anterior

Posterior

Articular facet of medial malleolus

Medial malleolus

Tibia

Inferior articular surface of tibia

PLATE 496

LOWER LIMB

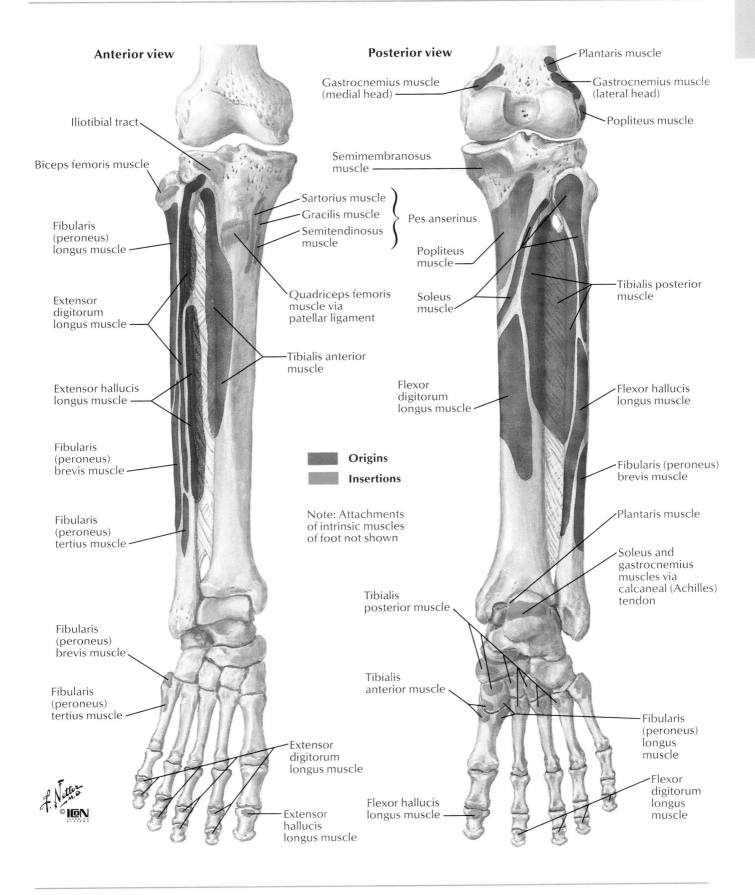

Anterior view

Iliotibial tract

Biceps femoris muscle

Fibularis (peroneus) longus muscle

Extensor digitorum longus muscle

Extensor hallucis longus muscle

Fibularis (peroneus) brevis muscle

Fibularis (peroneus) tertius muscle

Fibularis (peroneus) brevis muscle

Fibularis (peroneus) tertius muscle

Extensor digitorum longus muscle

Extensor hallucis longus muscle

Posterior view

Plantaris muscle

Gastrocnemius muscle (medial head)

Gastrocnemius muscle (lateral head)

Popliteus muscle

Semimembranosus muscle

Sartorius muscle
Gracilis muscle
Semitendinosus muscle
} Pes anserinus

Popliteus muscle

Quadriceps femoris muscle via patellar ligament

Soleus muscle

Tibialis posterior muscle

Tibialis anterior muscle

Flexor digitorum longus muscle

Flexor hallucis longus muscle

Fibularis (peroneus) brevis muscle

Plantaris muscle

Soleus and gastrocnemius muscles via calcaneal (Achilles) tendon

Tibialis posterior muscle

Tibialis anterior muscle

Fibularis (peroneus) longus muscle

Flexor hallucis longus muscle

Flexor digitorum longus muscle

Origins

Insertions

Note: Attachments of intrinsic muscles of foot not shown

Muscles of Leg (Superficial Dissection): Posterior View

SEE ALSO PLATE 522

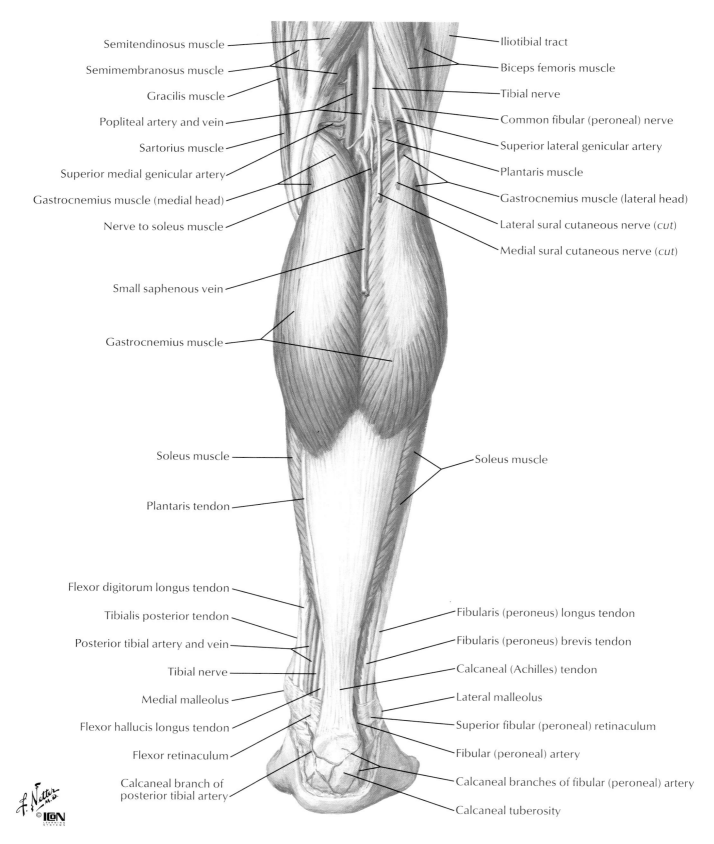

Semitendinosus muscle

Semimembranosus muscle

Gracilis muscle

Popliteal artery and vein

Sartorius muscle

Superior medial genicular artery

Gastrocnemius muscle (medial head)

Nerve to soleus muscle

Small saphenous vein

Gastrocnemius muscle

Soleus muscle

Plantaris tendon

Flexor digitorum longus tendon

Tibialis posterior tendon

Posterior tibial artery and vein

Tibial nerve

Medial malleolus

Flexor hallucis longus tendon

Flexor retinaculum

Calcaneal branch of
posterior tibial artery

Iliotibial tract

Biceps femoris muscle

Tibial nerve

Common fibular (peroneal) nerve

Superior lateral genicular artery

Plantaris muscle

Gastrocnemius muscle (lateral head)

Lateral sural cutaneous nerve (cut)

Medial sural cutaneous nerve (cut)

Soleus muscle

Fibularis (peroneus) longus tendon

Fibularis (peroneus) brevis tendon

Calcaneal (Achilles) tendon

Lateral malleolus

Superior fibular (peroneal) retinaculum

Fibular (peroneal) artery

Calcaneal branches of fibular (peroneal) artery

Calcaneal tuberosity

PLATE 498

LOWER LIMB

SEE ALSO PLATE 523

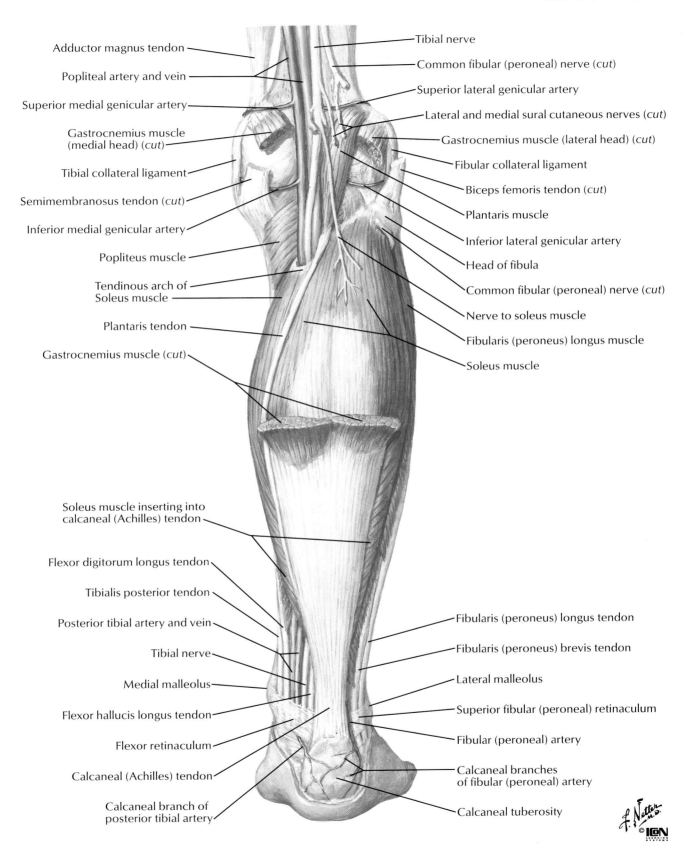

Adductor magnus tendon

Popliteal artery and vein

Superior medial genicular artery

Gastrocnemius muscle (medial head) (*cut*)

Tibial collateral ligament

Semimembranosus tendon (*cut*)

Inferior medial genicular artery

Popliteus muscle

Tendinous arch of Soleus muscle

Plantaris tendon

Gastrocnemius muscle (*cut*)

Soleus muscle inserting into calcaneal (Achilles) tendon

Flexor digitorum longus tendon

Tibialis posterior tendon

Posterior tibial artery and vein

Tibial nerve

Medial malleolus

Flexor hallucis longus tendon

Flexor retinaculum

Calcaneal (Achilles) tendon

Calcaneal branch of posterior tibial artery

Tibial nerve

Common fibular (peroneal) nerve (*cut*)

Superior lateral genicular artery

Lateral and medial sural cutaneous nerves (*cut*)

Gastrocnemius muscle (lateral head) (*cut*)

Fibular collateral ligament

Biceps femoris tendon (*cut*)

Plantaris muscle

Inferior lateral genicular artery

Head of fibula

Common fibular (peroneal) nerve (*cut*)

Nerve to soleus muscle

Fibularis (peroneus) longus muscle

Soleus muscle

Fibularis (peroneus) longus tendon

Fibularis (peroneus) brevis tendon

Lateral malleolus

Superior fibular (peroneal) retinaculum

Fibular (peroneal) artery

Calcaneal branches of fibular (peroneal) artery

Calcaneal tuberosity

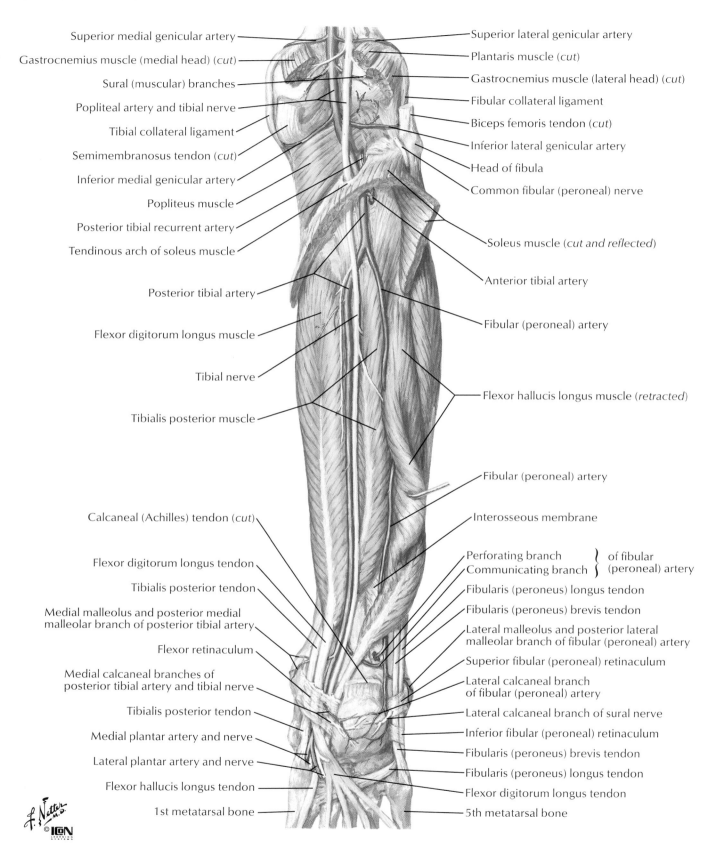

Superior medial genicular artery

Gastrocnemius muscle (medial head) (*cut*)

Sural (muscular) branches

Popliteal artery and tibial nerve

Tibial collateral ligament

Semimembranosus tendon (*cut*)

Inferior medial genicular artery

Popliteus muscle

Posterior tibial recurrent artery

Tendinous arch of soleus muscle

Posterior tibial artery

Flexor digitorum longus muscle

Tibial nerve

Tibialis posterior muscle

Calcaneal (Achilles) tendon (*cut*)

Flexor digitorum longus tendon

Tibialis posterior tendon

Medial malleolus and posterior medial malleolar branch of posterior tibial artery

Flexor retinaculum

Medial calcaneal branches of posterior tibial artery and tibial nerve

Tibialis posterior tendon

Medial plantar artery and nerve

Lateral plantar artery and nerve

Flexor hallucis longus tendon

1st metatarsal bone

Superior lateral genicular artery

Plantaris muscle (*cut*)

Gastrocnemius muscle (lateral head) (*cut*)

Fibular collateral ligament

Biceps femoris tendon (*cut*)

Inferior lateral genicular artery

Head of fibula

Common fibular (peroneal) nerve

Soleus muscle (*cut and reflected*)

Anterior tibial artery

Fibular (peroneal) artery

Flexor hallucis longus muscle (*retracted*)

Fibular (peroneal) artery

Interosseous membrane

Perforating branch } of fibular
Communicating branch } (peroneal) artery

Fibularis (peroneus) longus tendon

Fibularis (peroneus) brevis tendon

Lateral malleolus and posterior lateral malleolar branch of fibular (peroneal) artery

Superior fibular (peroneal) retinaculum

Lateral calcaneal branch of fibular (peroneal) artery

Lateral calcaneal branch of sural nerve

Inferior fibular (peroneal) retinaculum

Fibularis (peroneus) brevis tendon

Fibularis (peroneus) longus tendon

Flexor digitorum longus tendon

5th metatarsal bone

PLATE 500

LOWER LIMB

SEE ALSO PLATE 524

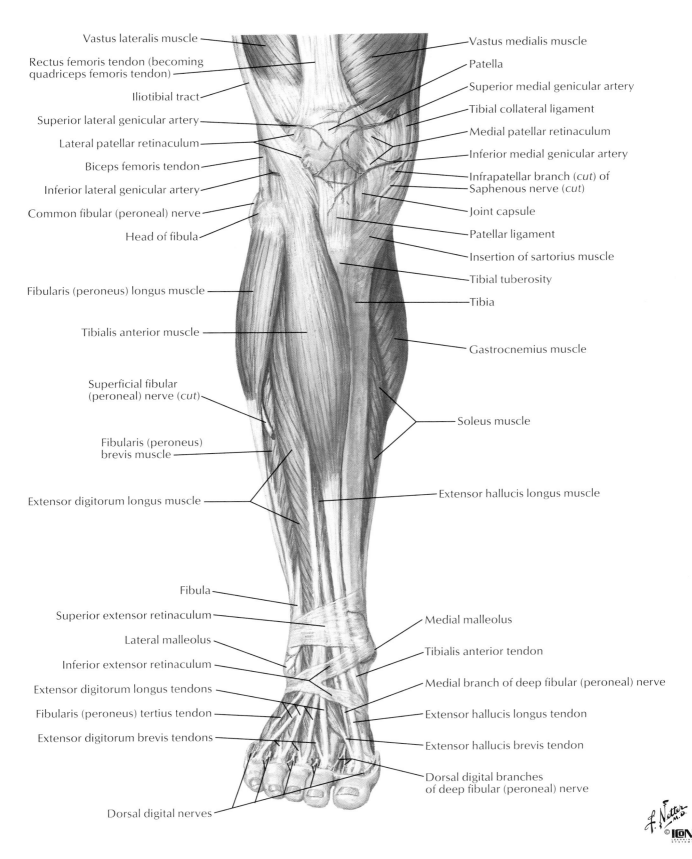

Vastus lateralis muscle

Rectus femoris tendon (becoming quadriceps femoris tendon)

Iliotibial tract

Superior lateral genicular artery

Lateral patellar retinaculum

Biceps femoris tendon

Inferior lateral genicular artery

Common fibular (peroneal) nerve

Head of fibula

Fibularis (peroneus) longus muscle

Tibialis anterior muscle

Superficial fibular (peroneal) nerve (*cut*)

Fibularis (peroneus) brevis muscle

Extensor digitorum longus muscle

Fibula

Superior extensor retinaculum

Lateral malleolus

Inferior extensor retinaculum

Extensor digitorum longus tendons

Fibularis (peroneus) tertius tendon

Extensor digitorum brevis tendons

Dorsal digital nerves

Vastus medialis muscle

Patella

Superior medial genicular artery

Tibial collateral ligament

Medial patellar retinaculum

Inferior medial genicular artery

Infrapatellar branch (*cut*) of Saphenous nerve (*cut*)

Joint capsule

Patellar ligament

Insertion of sartorius muscle

Tibial tuberosity

Tibia

Gastrocnemius muscle

Soleus muscle

Extensor hallucis longus muscle

Medial malleolus

Tibialis anterior tendon

Medial branch of deep fibular (peroneal) nerve

Extensor hallucis longus tendon

Extensor hallucis brevis tendon

Dorsal digital branches of deep fibular (peroneal) nerve

SEE ALSO PLATE 524

Superior lateral genicular artery

Fibular collateral ligament

Lateral patellar retinaculum

Iliotibial tract (cut)

Biceps femoris tendon (cut)

Inferior lateral genicular artery

Common fibular (peroneal) nerve

Head of fibula

Fibularis (peroneus) longus muscle (cut)

Anterior tibial artery

Extensor digitorum longus muscle (cut)

Superficial fibular (peroneal) nerve

Deep fibular (peroneal) nerve

Fibularis (peroneus) longus muscle

Extensor digitorum longus muscle

Fibularis (peroneus) brevis muscle and tendon

Fibularis (peroneus) longus tendon

Perforating branch of fibular (peroneal) artery

Anterior lateral malleolar artery

Lateral malleolus and arterial network

Lateral tarsal artery and lateral branch of deep fibular (peroneal) nerve

Extensor digitorum brevis and extensor hallucis brevis muscles (cut)

Fibularis (peroneus) brevis tendon

Posterior perforating branches from deep plantar arch

Extensor digitorum longus tendons (cut)

Extensor digitorum brevis tendons (cut)

Dorsal digital arteries

Branches of proper plantar digital arteries and nerves

Superior medial genicular artery

Quadriceps femoris tendon

Tibial collateral ligament

Medial patellar retinaculum

Infrapatellar branch of saphenous nerve (cut)

Inferior medial genicular artery

Saphenous nerve (cut)

Patellar ligament

Insertion of sartorius tendon

Anterior tibial recurrent artery and recurrent branch of deep peroneal nerve

Interosseous membrane

Tibialis anterior muscle (cut)

Gastrocnemius muscle

Soleus muscle

Tibia

Superficial fibular (peroneal) nerve (cut)

Extensor hallucis longus muscle and tendon (cut)

Interosseous membrane

Anterior medial malleolar artery

Medial malleolus and arterial network

Dorsalis pedis artery

Tibialis anterior tendon

Medial tarsal artery

Medial branch of deep fibular (peroneal) nerve

Arcuate artery

Deep plantar artery

Dorsal metatarsal arteries

Extensor hallucis longus tendon (cut)

Extensor hallucis brevis tendon (cut)

Dorsal digital branches of deep fibular (peroneal) nerve

PLATE 502

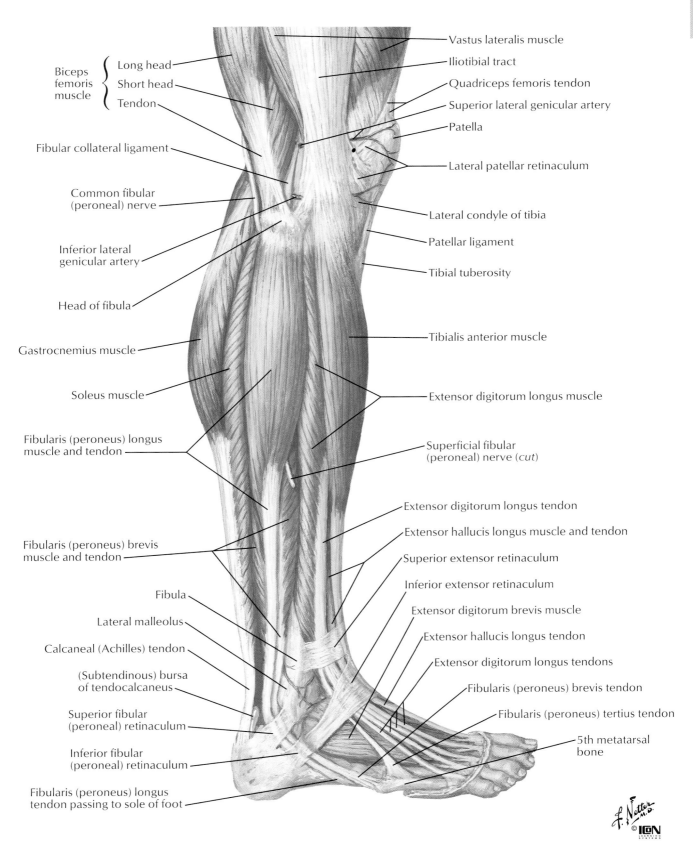

Biceps femoris muscle
- Long head
- Short head
- Tendon

Fibular collateral ligament

Common fibular (peroneal) nerve

Inferior lateral genicular artery

Head of fibula

Gastrocnemius muscle

Soleus muscle

Fibularis (peroneus) longus muscle and tendon

Fibularis (peroneus) brevis muscle and tendon

Fibula

Lateral malleolus

Calcaneal (Achilles) tendon

(Subtendinous) bursa of tendocalcaneus

Superior fibular (peroneal) retinaculum

Inferior fibular (peroneal) retinaculum

Fibularis (peroneus) longus tendon passing to sole of foot

Vastus lateralis muscle

Iliotibial tract

Quadriceps femoris tendon

Superior lateral genicular artery

Patella

Lateral patellar retinaculum

Lateral condyle of tibia

Patellar ligament

Tibial tuberosity

Tibialis anterior muscle

Extensor digitorum longus muscle

Superficial fibular (peroneal) nerve (*cut*)

Extensor digitorum longus tendon

Extensor hallucis longus muscle and tendon

Superior extensor retinaculum

Inferior extensor retinaculum

Extensor digitorum brevis muscle

Extensor hallucis longus tendon

Extensor digitorum longus tendons

Fibularis (peroneus) brevis tendon

Fibularis (peroneus) tertius tendon

5th metatarsal bone

Leg: Cross Sections and Fascial Compartments

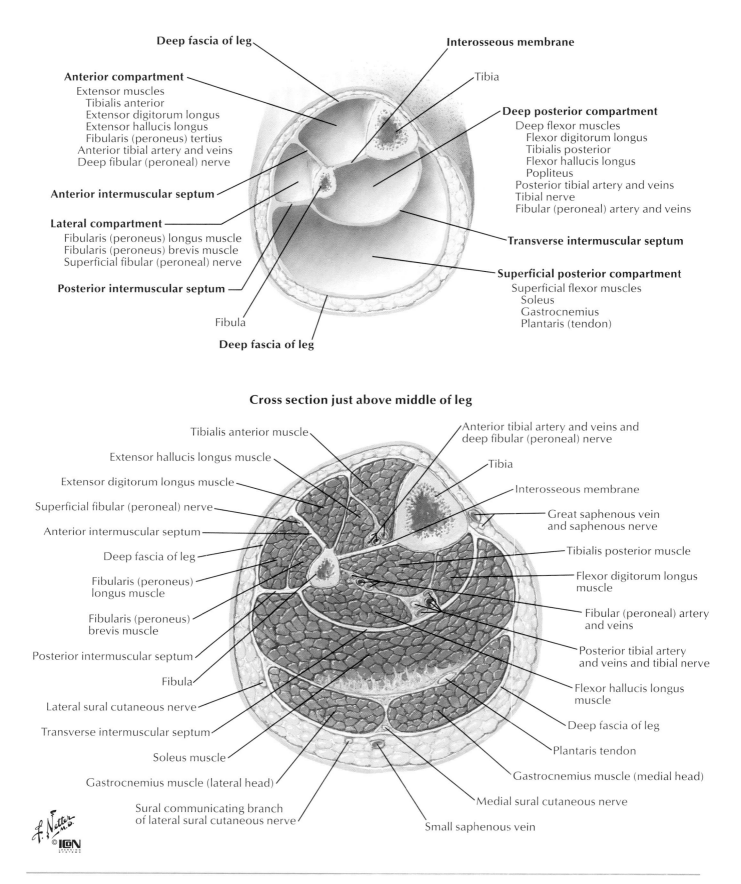

Deep fascia of leg

Anterior compartment
Extensor muscles
 Tibialis anterior
 Extensor digitorum longus
 Extensor hallucis longus
 Fibularis (peroneus) tertius
 Anterior tibial artery and veins
 Deep fibular (peroneal) nerve

Anterior intermuscular septum

Lateral compartment
Fibularis (peroneus) longus muscle
Fibularis (peroneus) brevis muscle
Superficial fibular (peroneal) nerve

Posterior intermuscular septum

Fibula

Deep fascia of leg

Interosseous membrane
Tibia

Deep posterior compartment
Deep flexor muscles
 Flexor digitorum longus
 Tibialis posterior
 Flexor hallucis longus
 Popliteus
Posterior tibial artery and veins
Tibial nerve
Fibular (peroneal) artery and veins

Transverse intermuscular septum

Superficial posterior compartment
Superficial flexor muscles
 Soleus
 Gastrocnemius
 Plantaris (tendon)

Cross section just above middle of leg

Tibialis anterior muscle
Extensor hallucis longus muscle
Extensor digitorum longus muscle
Superficial fibular (peroneal) nerve
Anterior intermuscular septum
Deep fascia of leg
Fibularis (peroneus) longus muscle
Fibularis (peroneus) brevis muscle
Posterior intermuscular septum
Fibula
Lateral sural cutaneous nerve
Transverse intermuscular septum
Soleus muscle
Gastrocnemius muscle (lateral head)
Sural communicating branch of lateral sural cutaneous nerve

Anterior tibial artery and veins and deep fibular (peroneal) nerve
Tibia
Interosseous membrane
Great saphenous vein and saphenous nerve
Tibialis posterior muscle
Flexor digitorum longus muscle
Fibular (peroneal) artery and veins
Posterior tibial artery and veins and tibial nerve
Flexor hallucis longus muscle
Deep fascia of leg
Plantaris tendon
Gastrocnemius muscle (medial head)
Medial sural cutaneous nerve
Small saphenous vein

PLATE 504

LOWER LIMB

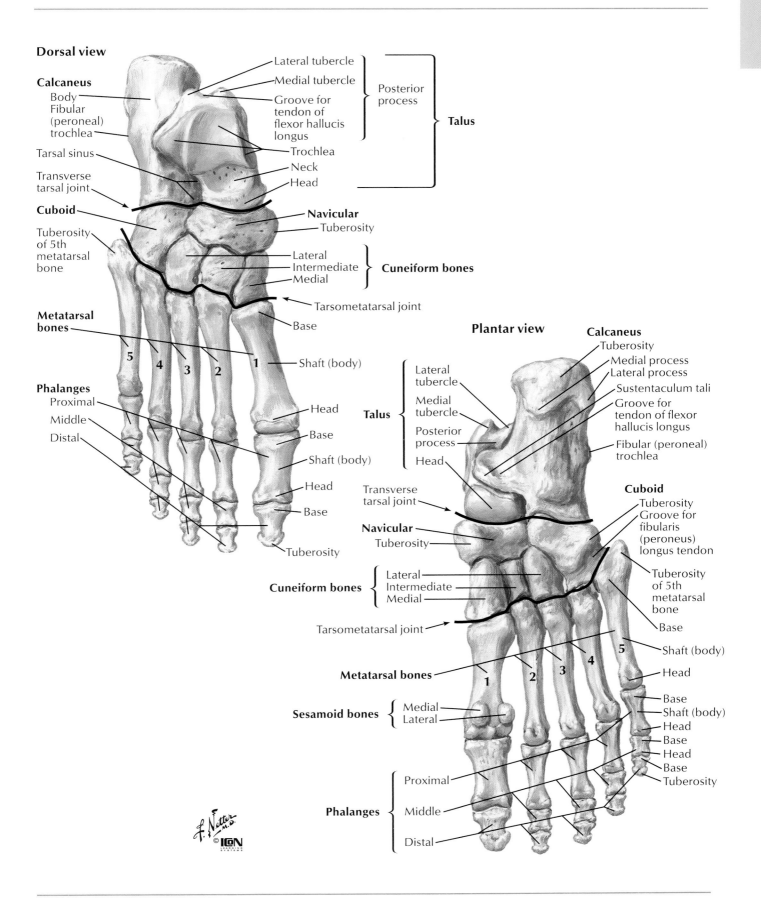

Dorsal view

Calcaneus
Body
Fibular (peroneal) trochlea
Tarsal sinus
Transverse tarsal joint
Cuboid
Tuberosity of 5th metatarsal bone

Lateral tubercle
Medial tubercle
Groove for tendon of flexor hallucis longus
Posterior process
Trochlea
Neck
Head
Talus

Navicular
Tuberosity

Lateral
Intermediate
Medial
Cuneiform bones

Tarsometatarsal joint
Base

Metatarsal bones

5 4 3 2 1

Shaft (body)

Phalanges
Proximal
Middle
Distal

Head
Base
Shaft (body)
Head
Base
Tuberosity

Plantar view

Calcaneus
Tuberosity
Medial process
Lateral process
Sustentaculum tali
Groove for tendon of flexor hallucis longus
Fibular (peroneal) trochlea

Lateral tubercle
Medial tubercle
Posterior process
Head
Talus

Transverse tarsal joint

Navicular
Tuberosity

Cuneiform bones
Lateral
Intermediate
Medial

Cuboid
Tuberosity
Groove for fibularis (peroneus) longus tendon
Tuberosity of 5th metatarsal bone
Base

Tarsometatarsal joint

Metatarsal bones

1 2 3 4 5

Shaft (body)
Head
Base
Shaft (body)
Head
Base
Head
Base
Tuberosity

Sesamoid bones
Medial
Lateral

Phalanges
Proximal
Middle
Distal

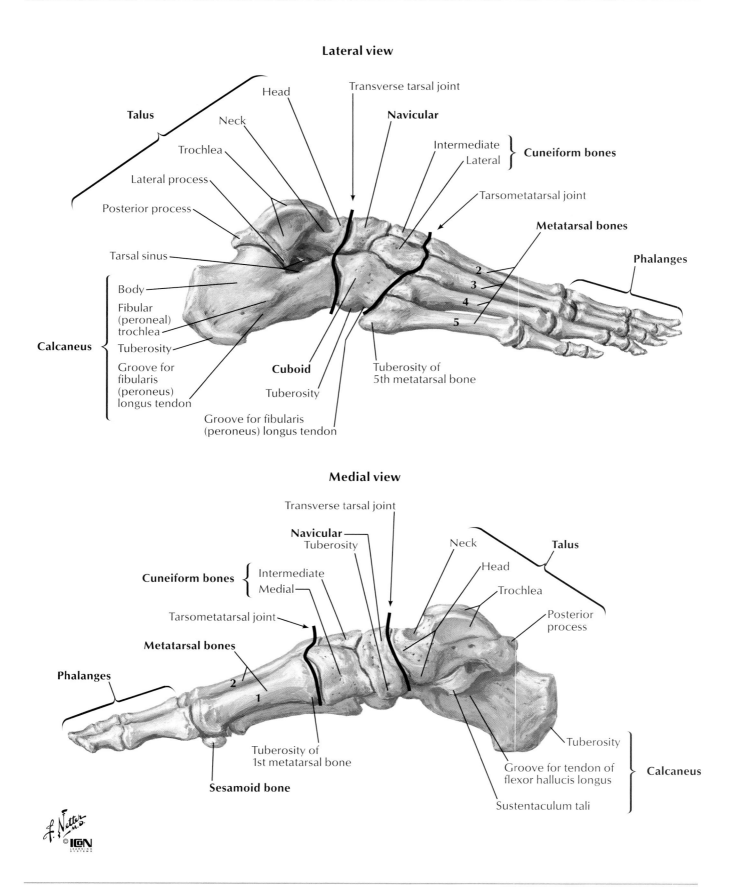

Lateral view

Transverse tarsal joint

Head

Talus

Neck

Navicular

Trochlea

Intermediate **Cuneiform bones**

Lateral process

Lateral

Posterior process

Tarsometatarsal joint

Tarsal sinus

Metatarsal bones

Body

Phalanges

2

Fibular
(peroneal)
trochlea

3

4

Calcaneus

Tuberosity

5

Groove for
fibularis
(peroneus)
longus tendon

Cuboid

Tuberosity of
5th metatarsal bone

Tuberosity

Groove for fibularis
(peroneus) longus tendon

Medial view

Transverse tarsal joint

Navicular

Tuberosity

Neck

Talus

Cuneiform bones

Intermediate

Head

Medial

Trochlea

Tarsometatarsal joint

Posterior
process

Metatarsal bones

Phalanges

2

1

Tuberosity

Tuberosity of
1st metatarsal bone

Groove for tendon of
flexor hallucis longus

Calcaneus

Sesamoid bone

Sustentaculum tali

PLATE 506

LOWER LIMB

Right foot

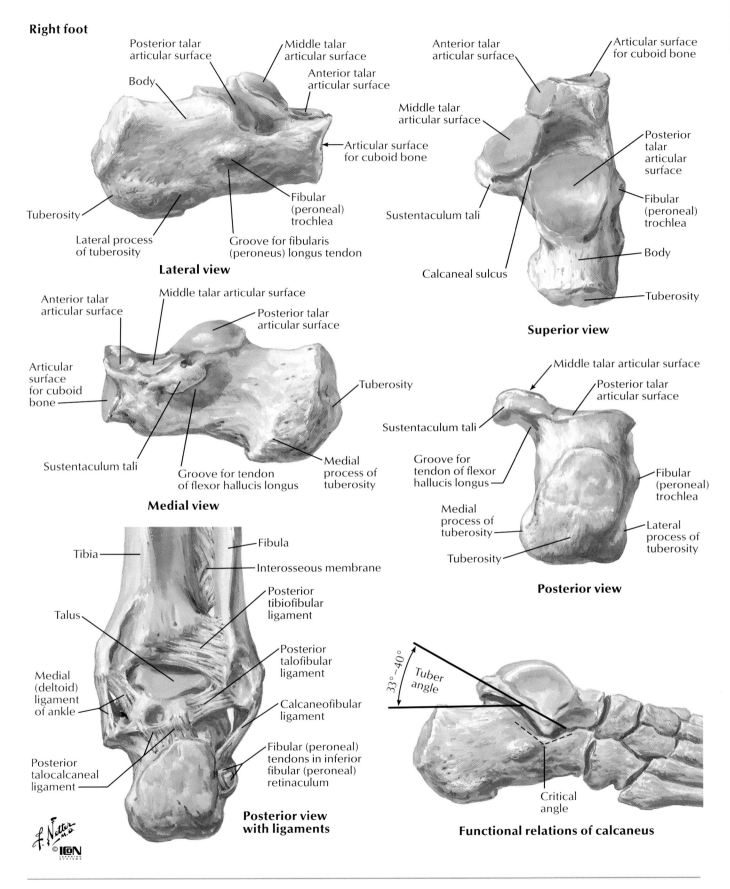

Posterior talar articular surface

Body

Posterior talar articular surface

Middle talar articular surface

Anterior talar articular surface

Articular surface for cuboid bone

Tuberosity

Lateral process of tuberosity

Fibular (peroneal) trochlea

Groove for fibularis (peroneus) longus tendon

Lateral view

Anterior talar articular surface

Middle talar articular surface

Posterior talar articular surface

Articular surface for cuboid bone

Tuberosity

Sustentaculum tali

Groove for tendon of flexor hallucis longus

Medial process of tuberosity

Medial view

Anterior talar articular surface

Articular surface for cuboid bone

Middle talar articular surface

Posterior talar articular surface

Sustentaculum tali

Fibular (peroneal) trochlea

Calcaneal sulcus

Body

Tuberosity

Superior view

Middle talar articular surface

Posterior talar articular surface

Sustentaculum tali

Groove for tendon of flexor hallucis longus

Medial process of tuberosity

Tuberosity

Fibular (peroneal) trochlea

Lateral process of tuberosity

Posterior view

Tibia

Talus

Medial (deltoid) ligament of ankle

Posterior talocalcaneal ligament

Fibula

Interosseous membrane

Posterior tibiofibular ligament

Posterior talofibular ligament

Calcaneofibular ligament

Fibular (peroneal) tendons in inferior fibular (peroneal) retinaculum

Posterior view with ligaments

33°–40°

Tuber angle

Critical angle

Functional relations of calcaneus

ANKLE AND FOOT

PLATE 507

Ankle: Radiographs

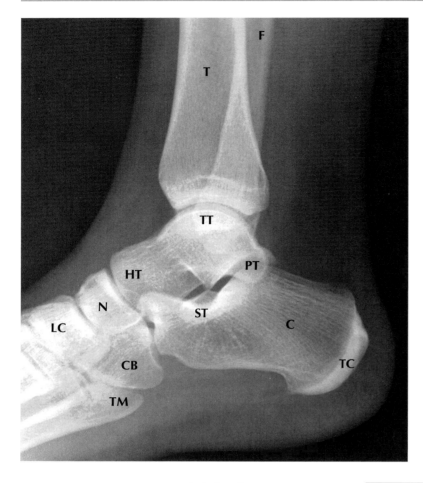

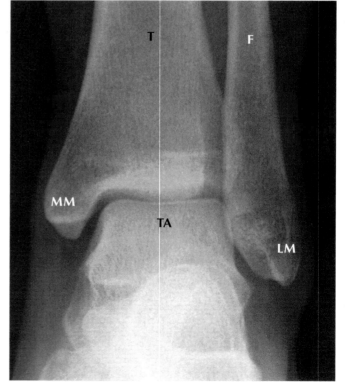

PLATE 508

LOWER LIMB

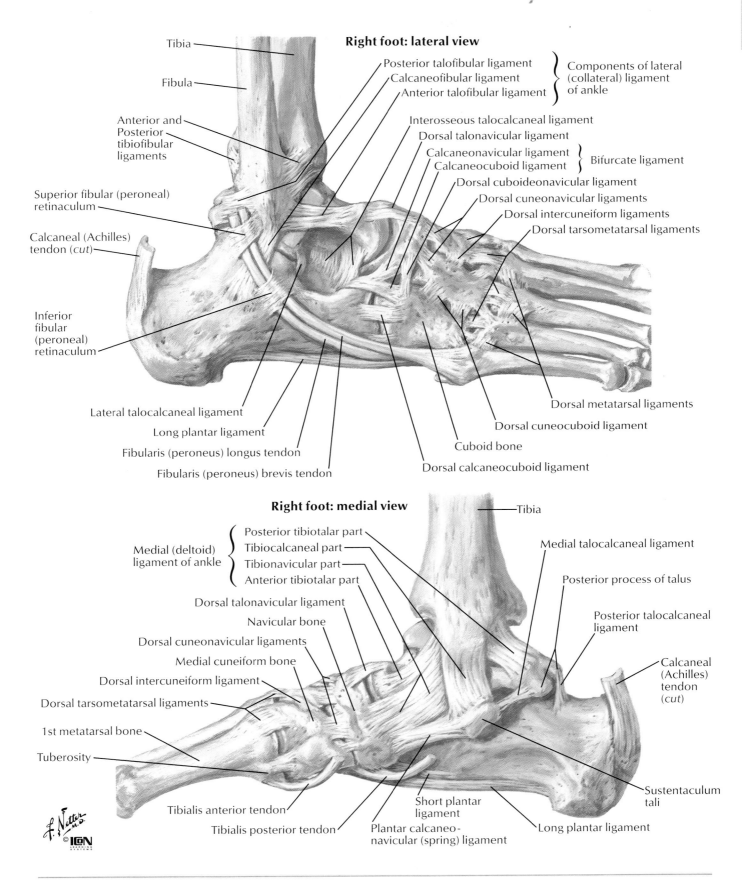

Right foot: lateral view

Tibia

Fibula

Anterior and Posterior tibiofibular ligaments

Superior fibular (peroneal) retinaculum

Calcaneal (Achilles) tendon (*cut*)

Inferior fibular (peroneal) retinaculum

Posterior talofibular ligament
Calcaneofibular ligament
Anterior talofibular ligament
} Components of lateral (collateral) ligament of ankle

Interosseous talocalcaneal ligament
Dorsal talonavicular ligament
Calcaneonavicular ligament
Calcaneocuboid ligament
} Bifurcate ligament
Dorsal cuboideonavicular ligament
Dorsal cuneonavicular ligaments
Dorsal intercuneiform ligaments
Dorsal tarsometatarsal ligaments

Lateral talocalcaneal ligament

Long plantar ligament

Fibularis (peroneus) longus tendon

Fibularis (peroneus) brevis tendon

Dorsal metatarsal ligaments

Dorsal cuneocuboid ligament

Cuboid bone

Dorsal calcaneocuboid ligament

Right foot: medial view

Medial (deltoid) ligament of ankle {
Posterior tibiotalar part
Tibiocalcaneal part
Tibionavicular part
Anterior tibiotalar part

Dorsal talonavicular ligament

Navicular bone

Dorsal cuneonavicular ligaments

Medial cuneiform bone

Dorsal intercuneiform ligament

Dorsal tarsometatarsal ligaments

1st metatarsal bone

Tuberosity

Tibia

Medial talocalcaneal ligament

Posterior process of talus

Posterior talocalcaneal ligament

Calcaneal (Achilles) tendon (*cut*)

Sustentaculum tali

Tibialis anterior tendon

Tibialis posterior tendon

Short plantar ligament

Plantar calcaneonavicular (spring) ligament

Long plantar ligament

f. Netter M.D.

© ICON

Ligaments and Tendons of Foot: Plantar View

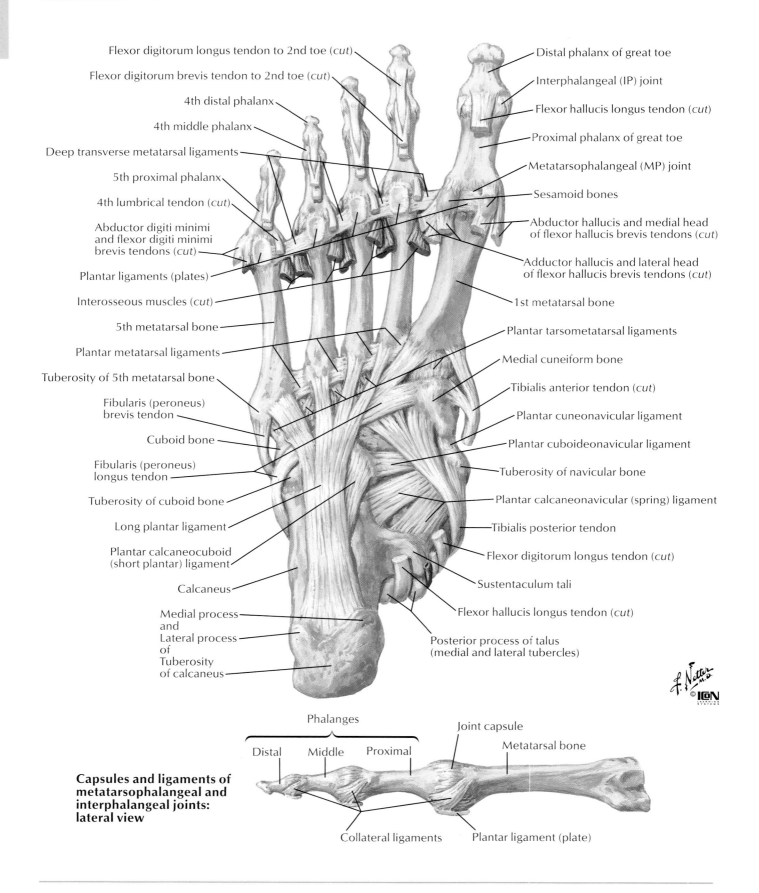

Flexor digitorum longus tendon to 2nd toe (*cut*)

Flexor digitorum brevis tendon to 2nd toe (*cut*)

4th distal phalanx

4th middle phalanx

Deep transverse metatarsal ligaments

5th proximal phalanx

4th lumbrical tendon (*cut*)

Abductor digiti minimi and flexor digiti minimi brevis tendons (*cut*)

Plantar ligaments (plates)

Interosseous muscles (*cut*)

5th metatarsal bone

Plantar metatarsal ligaments

Tuberosity of 5th metatarsal bone

Fibularis (peroneus) brevis tendon

Cuboid bone

Fibularis (peroneus) longus tendon

Tuberosity of cuboid bone

Long plantar ligament

Plantar calcaneocuboid (short plantar) ligament

Calcaneus

Medial process and Lateral process of Tuberosity of calcaneus

Distal phalanx of great toe

Interphalangeal (IP) joint

Flexor hallucis longus tendon (*cut*)

Proximal phalanx of great toe

Metatarsophalangeal (MP) joint

Sesamoid bones

Abductor hallucis and medial head of flexor hallucis brevis tendons (*cut*)

Adductor hallucis and lateral head of flexor hallucis brevis tendons (*cut*)

1st metatarsal bone

Plantar tarsometatarsal ligaments

Medial cuneiform bone

Tibialis anterior tendon (*cut*)

Plantar cuneonavicular ligament

Plantar cuboideonavicular ligament

Tuberosity of navicular bone

Plantar calcaneonavicular (spring) ligament

Tibialis posterior tendon

Flexor digitorum longus tendon (*cut*)

Sustentaculum tali

Flexor hallucis longus tendon (*cut*)

Posterior process of talus (medial and lateral tubercles)

Phalanges

Distal Middle Proximal

Joint capsule

Metatarsal bone

Capsules and ligaments of metatarsophalangeal and interphalangeal joints: lateral view

Collateral ligaments

Plantar ligament (plate)

PLATE 510

LOWER LIMB

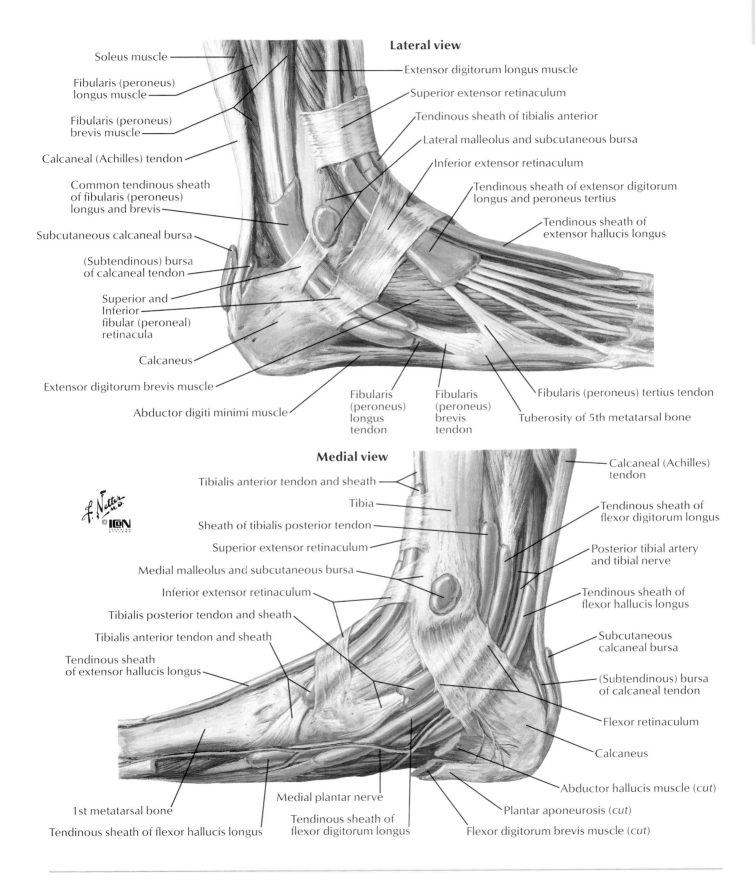

Lateral view

Soleus muscle

Fibularis (peroneus) longus muscle

Fibularis (peroneus) brevis muscle

Calcaneal (Achilles) tendon

Common tendinous sheath of fibularis (peroneus) longus and brevis

Subcutaneous calcaneal bursa

(Subtendinous) bursa of calcaneal tendon

Superior and Inferior fibular (peroneal) retinacula

Calcaneus

Extensor digitorum brevis muscle

Abductor digiti minimi muscle

Extensor digitorum longus muscle

Superior extensor retinaculum

Tendinous sheath of tibialis anterior

Lateral malleolus and subcutaneous bursa

Inferior extensor retinaculum

Tendinous sheath of extensor digitorum longus and peroneus tertius

Tendinous sheath of extensor hallucis longus

Fibularis (peroneus) longus tendon

Fibularis (peroneus) brevis tendon

Fibularis (peroneus) tertius tendon

Tuberosity of 5th metatarsal bone

Medial view

Tibialis anterior tendon and sheath

Tibia

Sheath of tibialis posterior tendon

Superior extensor retinaculum

Medial malleolus and subcutaneous bursa

Inferior extensor retinaculum

Tibialis posterior tendon and sheath

Tibialis anterior tendon and sheath

Tendinous sheath of extensor hallucis longus

1st metatarsal bone

Tendinous sheath of flexor hallucis longus

Medial plantar nerve

Tendinous sheath of flexor digitorum longus

Calcaneal (Achilles) tendon

Tendinous sheath of flexor digitorum longus

Posterior tibial artery and tibial nerve

Tendinous sheath of flexor hallucis longus

Subcutaneous calcaneal bursa

(Subtendinous) bursa of calcaneal tendon

Flexor retinaculum

Calcaneus

Abductor hallucis muscle (*cut*)

Plantar aponeurosis (*cut*)

Flexor digitorum brevis muscle (*cut*)

Muscles of Dorsum of Foot: Superficial Dissection

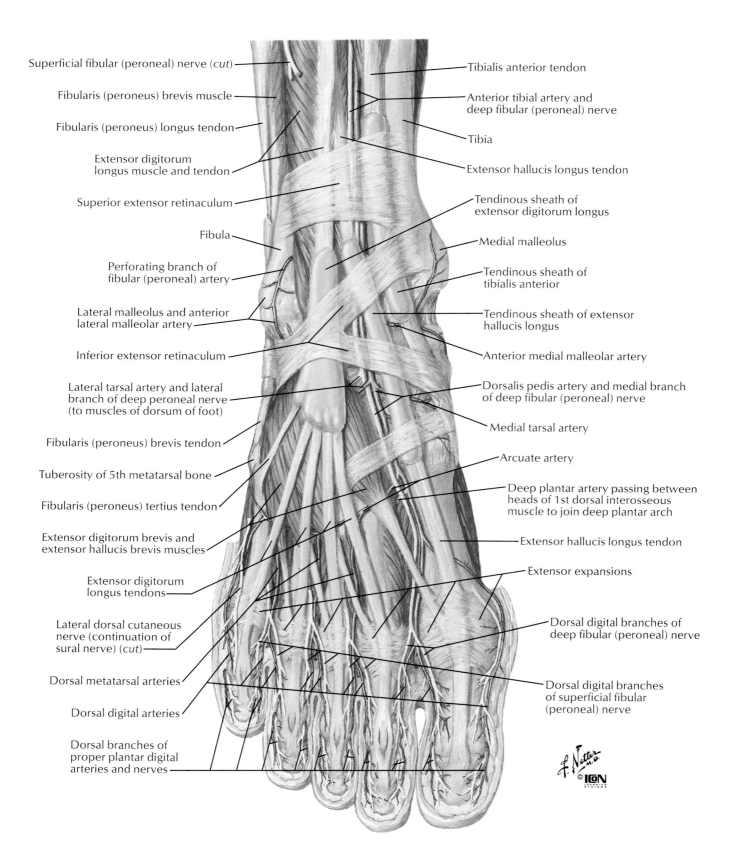

Superficial fibular (peroneal) nerve (*cut*)

Fibularis (peroneus) brevis muscle

Fibularis (peroneus) longus tendon

Extensor digitorum longus muscle and tendon

Superior extensor retinaculum

Fibula

Perforating branch of fibular (peroneal) artery

Lateral malleolus and anterior lateral malleolar artery

Inferior extensor retinaculum

Lateral tarsal artery and lateral branch of deep peroneal nerve (to muscles of dorsum of foot)

Fibularis (peroneus) brevis tendon

Tuberosity of 5th metatarsal bone

Fibularis (peroneus) tertius tendon

Extensor digitorum brevis and extensor hallucis brevis muscles

Extensor digitorum longus tendons

Lateral dorsal cutaneous nerve (continuation of sural nerve) (*cut*)

Dorsal metatarsal arteries

Dorsal digital arteries

Dorsal branches of proper plantar digital arteries and nerves

Tibialis anterior tendon

Anterior tibial artery and deep fibular (peroneal) nerve

Tibia

Extensor hallucis longus tendon

Tendinous sheath of extensor digitorum longus

Medial malleolus

Tendinous sheath of tibialis anterior

Tendinous sheath of extensor hallucis longus

Anterior medial malleolar artery

Dorsalis pedis artery and medial branch of deep fibular (peroneal) nerve

Medial tarsal artery

Arcuate artery

Deep plantar artery passing between heads of 1st dorsal interosseous muscle to join deep plantar arch

Extensor hallucis longus tendon

Extensor expansions

Dorsal digital branches of deep fibular (peroneal) nerve

Dorsal digital branches of superficial fibular (peroneal) nerve

PLATE 512

LOWER LIMB

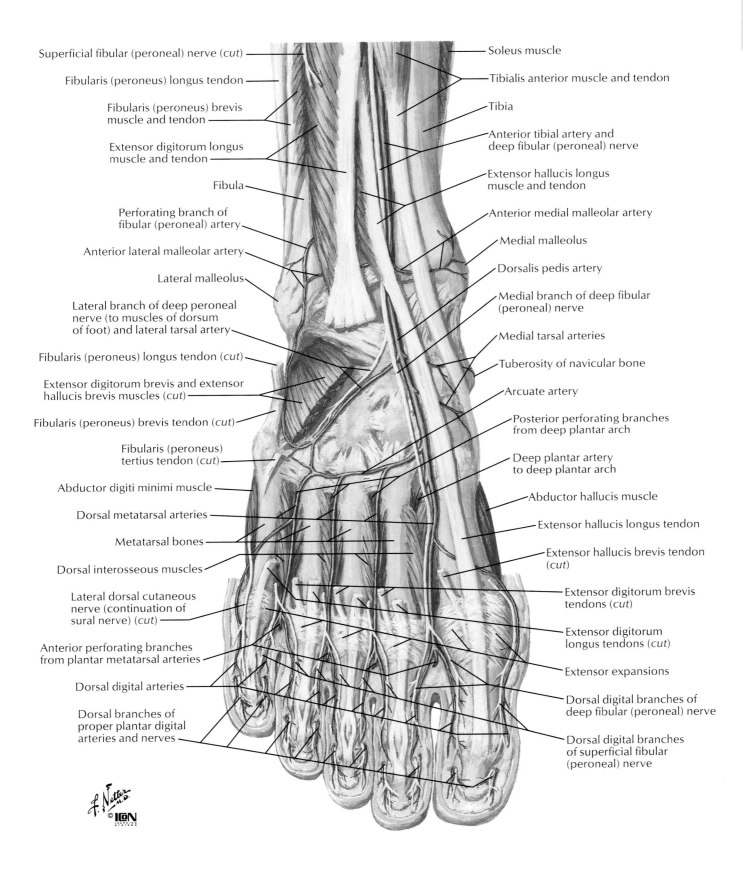

Superficial fibular (peroneal) nerve (*cut*)

Fibularis (peroneus) longus tendon

Fibularis (peroneus) brevis muscle and tendon

Extensor digitorum longus muscle and tendon

Fibula

Perforating branch of fibular (peroneal) artery

Anterior lateral malleolar artery

Lateral malleolus

Lateral branch of deep peroneal nerve (to muscles of dorsum of foot) and lateral tarsal artery

Fibularis (peroneus) longus tendon (*cut*)

Extensor digitorum brevis and extensor hallucis brevis muscles (*cut*)

Fibularis (peroneus) brevis tendon (*cut*)

Fibularis (peroneus) tertius tendon (*cut*)

Abductor digiti minimi muscle

Dorsal metatarsal arteries

Metatarsal bones

Dorsal interosseous muscles

Lateral dorsal cutaneous nerve (continuation of sural nerve) (*cut*)

Anterior perforating branches from plantar metatarsal arteries

Dorsal digital arteries

Dorsal branches of proper plantar digital arteries and nerves

Soleus muscle

Tibialis anterior muscle and tendon

Tibia

Anterior tibial artery and deep fibular (peroneal) nerve

Extensor hallucis longus muscle and tendon

Anterior medial malleolar artery

Medial malleolus

Dorsalis pedis artery

Medial branch of deep fibular (peroneal) nerve

Medial tarsal arteries

Tuberosity of navicular bone

Arcuate artery

Posterior perforating branches from deep plantar arch

Deep plantar artery to deep plantar arch

Abductor hallucis muscle

Extensor hallucis longus tendon

Extensor hallucis brevis tendon (*cut*)

Extensor digitorum brevis tendons (*cut*)

Extensor digitorum longus tendons (*cut*)

Extensor expansions

Dorsal digital branches of deep fibular (peroneal) nerve

Dorsal digital branches of superficial fibular (peroneal) nerve

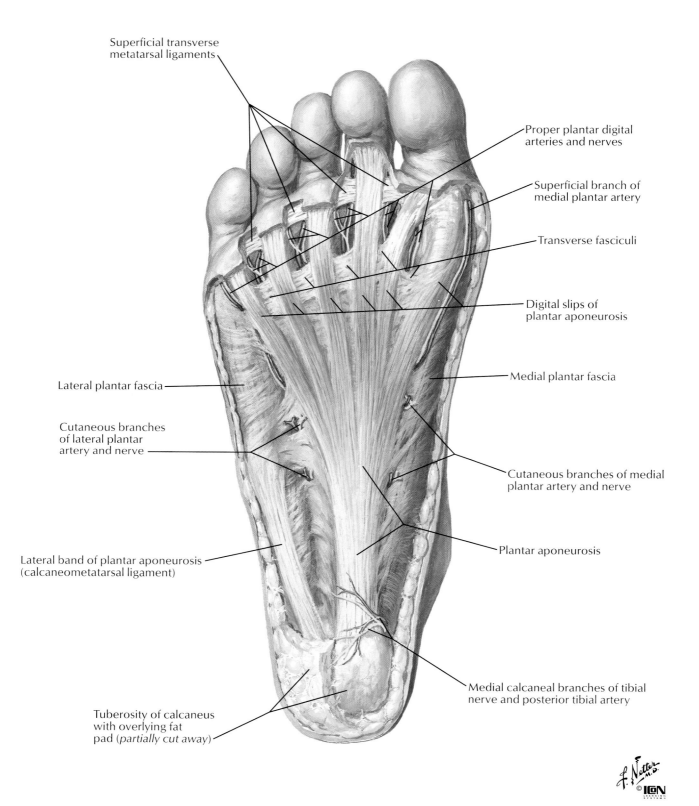

Superficial transverse
metatarsal ligaments

Proper plantar digital
arteries and nerves

Superficial branch of
medial plantar artery

Transverse fasciculi

Digital slips of
plantar aponeurosis

Medial plantar fascia

Lateral plantar fascia

Cutaneous branches
of lateral plantar
artery and nerve

Cutaneous branches of medial
plantar artery and nerve

Lateral band of plantar aponeurosis
(calcaneometatarsal ligament)

Plantar aponeurosis

Medial calcaneal branches of tibial
nerve and posterior tibial artery

Tuberosity of calcaneus
with overlying fat
pad (partially cut away)

PLATE 514

LOWER LIMB

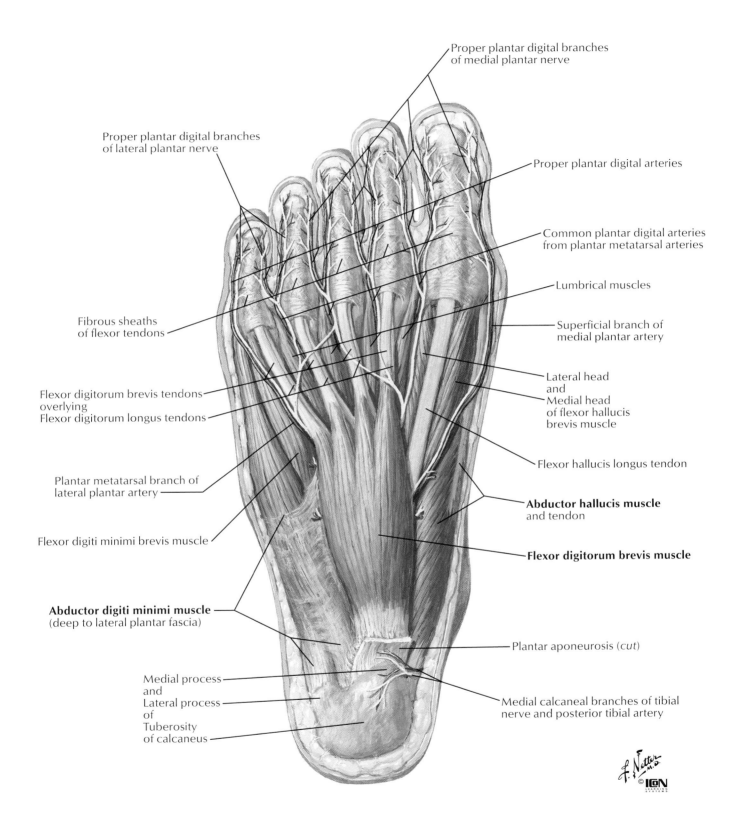

Proper plantar digital branches
of medial plantar nerve

Proper plantar digital branches
of lateral plantar nerve

Proper plantar digital arteries

Common plantar digital arteries
from plantar metatarsal arteries

Lumbrical muscles

Fibrous sheaths
of flexor tendons

Superficial branch of
medial plantar artery

Flexor digitorum brevis tendons
overlying
Flexor digitorum longus tendons

Lateral head
and
Medial head
of flexor hallucis
brevis muscle

Flexor hallucis longus tendon

Plantar metatarsal branch of
lateral plantar artery

Abductor hallucis muscle
and tendon

Flexor digiti minimi brevis muscle

Flexor digitorum brevis muscle

Abductor digiti minimi muscle
(deep to lateral plantar fascia)

Plantar aponeurosis (*cut*)

Medial process
and
Lateral process
of
Tuberosity
of calcaneus

Medial calcaneal branches of tibial
nerve and posterior tibial artery

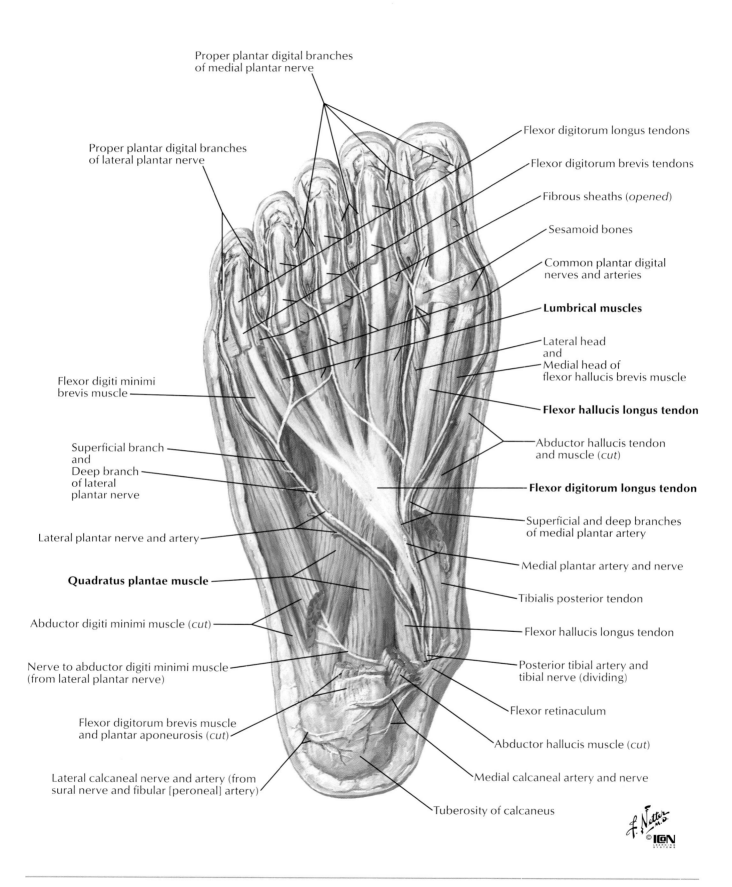

Proper plantar digital branches
of medial plantar nerve

Proper plantar digital branches
of lateral plantar nerve

Flexor digiti minimi
brevis muscle

Superficial branch
and
Deep branch
of lateral
plantar nerve

Lateral plantar nerve and artery

Quadratus plantae muscle

Abductor digiti minimi muscle (*cut*)

Nerve to abductor digiti minimi muscle
(from lateral plantar nerve)

Flexor digitorum brevis muscle
and plantar aponeurosis (*cut*)

Lateral calcaneal nerve and artery (from
sural nerve and fibular [peroneal] artery)

Flexor digitorum longus tendons

Flexor digitorum brevis tendons

Fibrous sheaths (*opened*)

Sesamoid bones

Common plantar digital
nerves and arteries

Lumbrical muscles

Lateral head
and
Medial head of
flexor hallucis brevis muscle

Flexor hallucis longus tendon

Abductor hallucis tendon
and muscle (*cut*)

Flexor digitorum longus tendon

Superficial and deep branches
of medial plantar artery

Medial plantar artery and nerve

Tibialis posterior tendon

Flexor hallucis longus tendon

Posterior tibial artery and
tibial nerve (dividing)

Flexor retinaculum

Abductor hallucis muscle (*cut*)

Medial calcaneal artery and nerve

Tuberosity of calcaneus

PLATE 516

LOWER LIMB

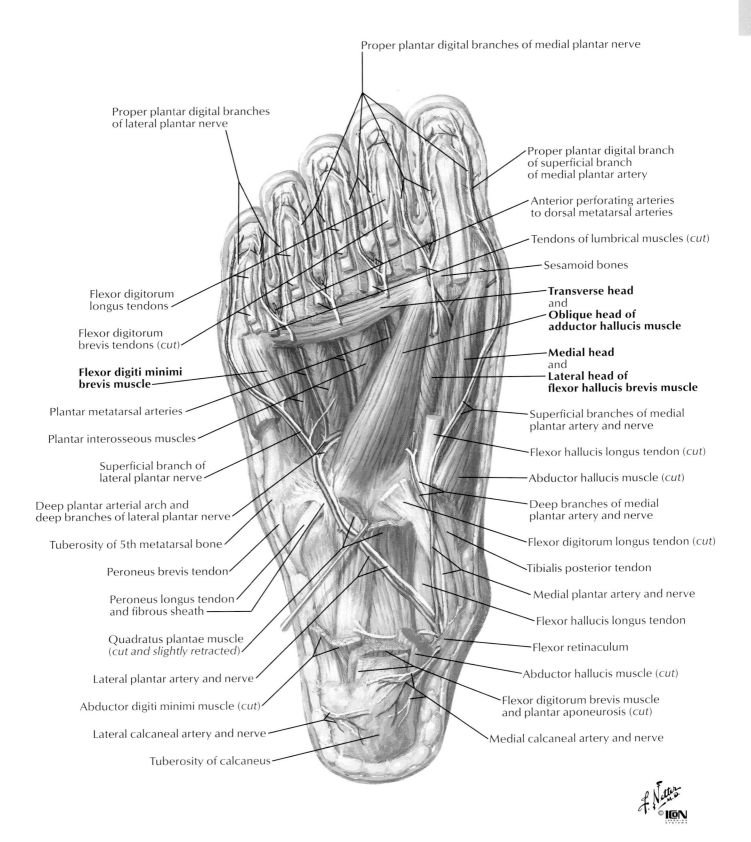

Proper plantar digital branches of medial plantar nerve

Proper plantar digital branches of lateral plantar nerve

Proper plantar digital branch of superficial branch of medial plantar artery

Anterior perforating arteries to dorsal metatarsal arteries

Tendons of lumbrical muscles (*cut*)

Sesamoid bones

Flexor digitorum longus tendons

Transverse head and **Oblique head of adductor hallucis muscle**

Flexor digitorum brevis tendons (*cut*)

Medial head and **Lateral head of flexor hallucis brevis muscle**

Flexor digiti minimi brevis muscle

Superficial branches of medial plantar artery and nerve

Plantar metatarsal arteries

Flexor hallucis longus tendon (*cut*)

Plantar interosseous muscles

Abductor hallucis muscle (*cut*)

Superficial branch of lateral plantar nerve

Deep branches of medial plantar artery and nerve

Deep plantar arterial arch and deep branches of lateral plantar nerve

Flexor digitorum longus tendon (*cut*)

Tuberosity of 5th metatarsal bone

Tibialis posterior tendon

Peroneus brevis tendon

Medial plantar artery and nerve

Peroneus longus tendon and fibrous sheath

Flexor hallucis longus tendon

Quadratus plantae muscle (*cut and slightly retracted*)

Flexor retinaculum

Lateral plantar artery and nerve

Abductor hallucis muscle (*cut*)

Abductor digiti minimi muscle (*cut*)

Flexor digitorum brevis muscle and plantar aponeurosis (*cut*)

Lateral calcaneal artery and nerve

Medial calcaneal artery and nerve

Tuberosity of calcaneus

Interosseous Muscles and Deep Arteries of Foot

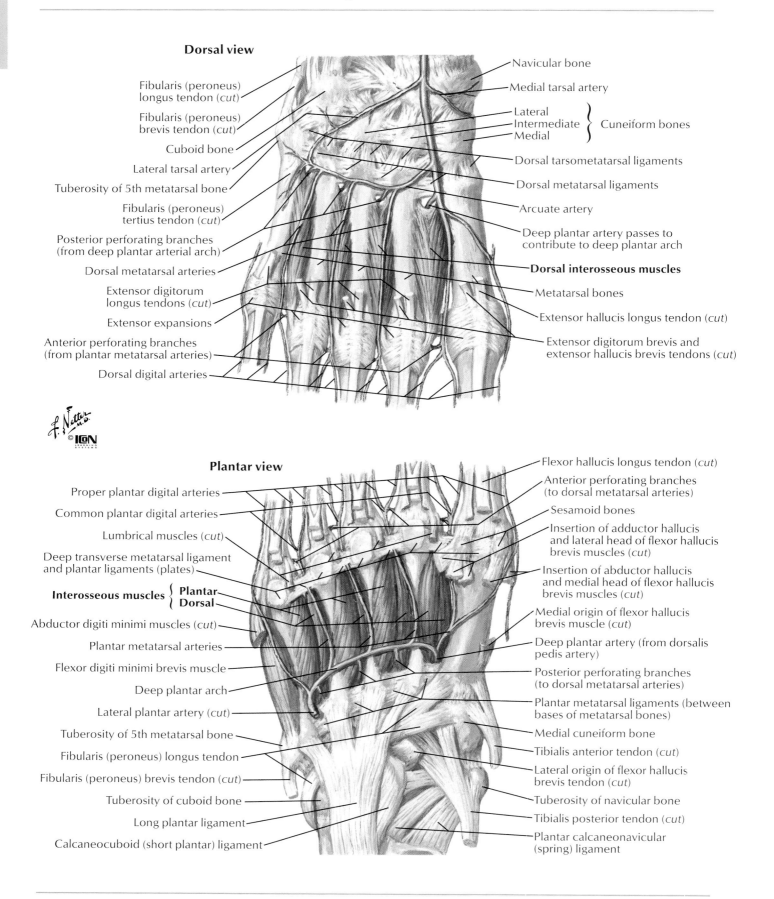

Dorsal view

Fibularis (peroneus) longus tendon (*cut*)

Fibularis (peroneus) brevis tendon (*cut*)

Cuboid bone

Lateral tarsal artery

Tuberosity of 5th metatarsal bone

Fibularis (peroneus) tertius tendon (*cut*)

Posterior perforating branches (from deep plantar arterial arch)

Dorsal metatarsal arteries

Extensor digitorum longus tendons (*cut*)

Extensor expansions

Anterior perforating branches (from plantar metatarsal arteries)

Dorsal digital arteries

Navicular bone

Medial tarsal artery

Lateral
Intermediate } Cuneiform bones
Medial

Dorsal tarsometatarsal ligaments

Dorsal metatarsal ligaments

Arcuate artery

Deep plantar artery passes to contribute to deep plantar arch

Dorsal interosseous muscles

Metatarsal bones

Extensor hallucis longus tendon (*cut*)

Extensor digitorum brevis and extensor hallucis brevis tendons (*cut*)

Plantar view

Proper plantar digital arteries

Common plantar digital arteries

Lumbrical muscles (*cut*)

Deep transverse metatarsal ligament and plantar ligaments (plates)

Interosseous muscles { **Plantar** **Dorsal**

Abductor digiti minimi muscles (*cut*)

Plantar metatarsal arteries

Flexor digiti minimi brevis muscle

Deep plantar arch

Lateral plantar artery (*cut*)

Tuberosity of 5th metatarsal bone

Fibularis (peroneus) longus tendon

Fibularis (peroneus) brevis tendon (*cut*)

Tuberosity of cuboid bone

Long plantar ligament

Calcaneocuboid (short plantar) ligament

Flexor hallucis longus tendon (*cut*)

Anterior perforating branches (to dorsal metatarsal arteries)

Sesamoid bones

Insertion of adductor hallucis and lateral head of flexor hallucis brevis muscles (*cut*)

Insertion of abductor hallucis and medial head of flexor hallucis brevis muscles (*cut*)

Medial origin of flexor hallucis brevis muscle (*cut*)

Deep plantar artery (from dorsalis pedis artery)

Posterior perforating branches (to dorsal metatarsal arteries)

Plantar metatarsal ligaments (between bases of metatarsal bones)

Medial cuneiform bone

Tibialis anterior tendon (*cut*)

Lateral origin of flexor hallucis brevis tendon (*cut*)

Tuberosity of navicular bone

Tibialis posterior tendon (*cut*)

Plantar calcaneonavicular (spring) ligament

PLATE 518

LOWER LIMB

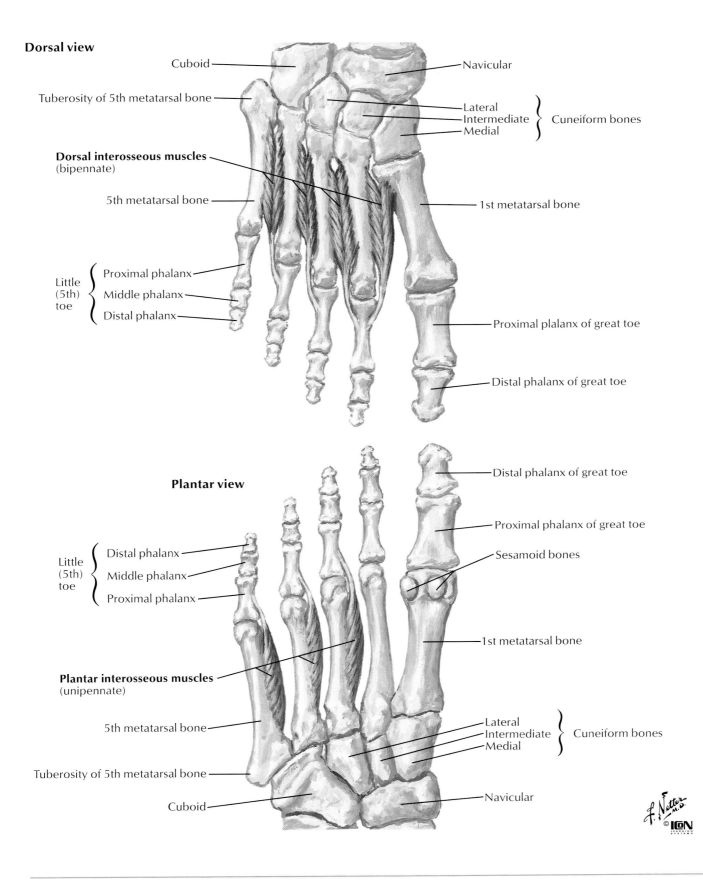

Dorsal view

Cuboid

Navicular

Tuberosity of 5th metatarsal bone

Lateral
Intermediate } Cuneiform bones
Medial

Dorsal interosseous muscles
(bipennate)

5th metatarsal bone

1st metatarsal bone

Little
(5th)
toe {
Proximal phalanx
Middle phalanx
Distal phalanx

Proximal plalanx of great toe

Distal phalanx of great toe

Plantar view

Distal phalanx of great toe

Proximal phalanx of great toe

Little
(5th)
toe {
Distal phalanx
Middle phalanx
Proximal phalanx

Sesamoid bones

1st metatarsal bone

Plantar interosseous muscles
(unipennate)

5th metatarsal bone

Lateral
Intermediate } Cuneiform bones
Medial

Tuberosity of 5th metatarsal bone

Navicular

Cuboid

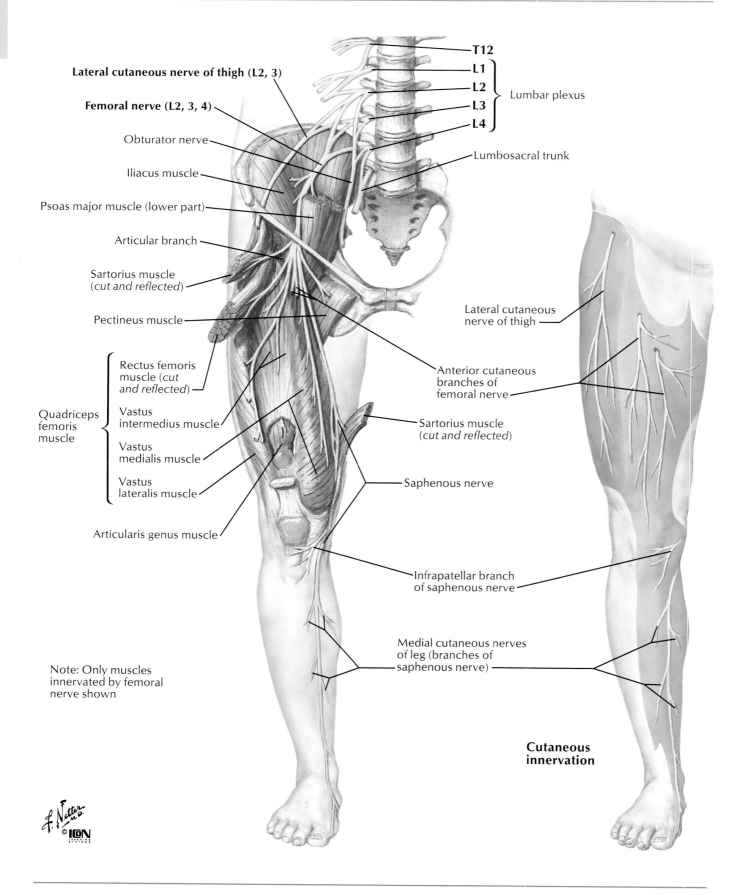

Lateral cutaneous nerve of thigh (L2, 3)

Femoral nerve (L2, 3, 4)

Obturator nerve

Iliacus muscle

Psoas major muscle (lower part)

Articular branch

Sartorius muscle
(*cut and reflected*)

Pectineus muscle

Rectus femoris
muscle (*cut
and reflected*)

Quadriceps
femoris
muscle

Vastus
intermedius muscle

Vastus
medialis muscle

Vastus
lateralis muscle

Articularis genus muscle

Note: Only muscles
innervated by femoral
nerve shown

T12
L1
L2
L3
L4

Lumbar plexus

Lumbosacral trunk

Lateral cutaneous
nerve of thigh

Anterior cutaneous
branches of
femoral nerve

Sartorius muscle
(*cut and reflected*)

Saphenous nerve

Infrapatellar branch
of saphenous nerve

Medial cutaneous nerves
of leg (branches of
saphenous nerve)

**Cutaneous
innervation**

PLATE 520

LOWER LIMB

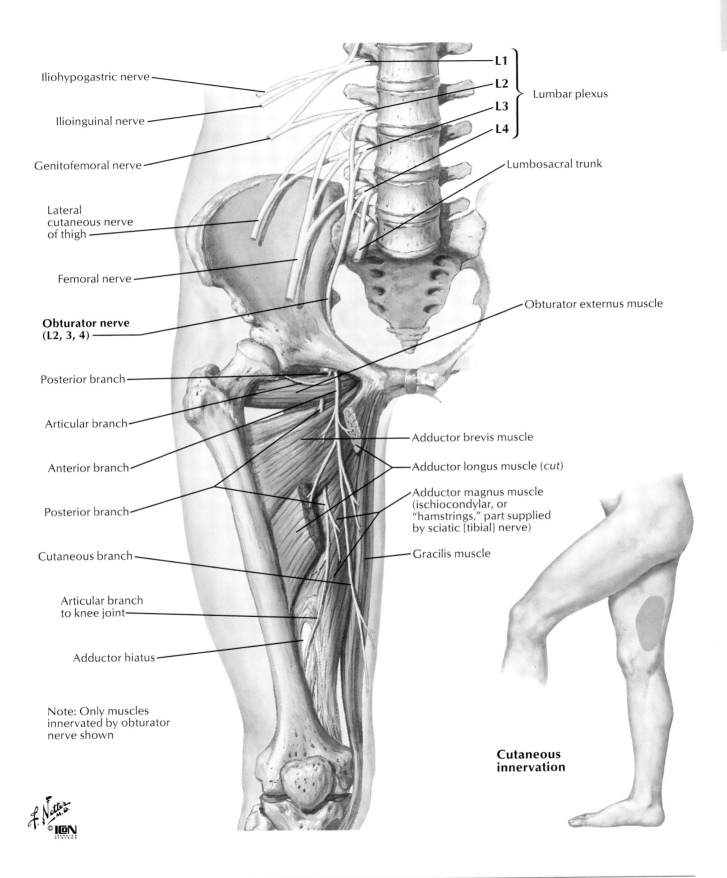

Iliohypogastric nerve

Ilioinguinal nerve

Genitofemoral nerve

Lateral cutaneous nerve of thigh

Femoral nerve

Obturator nerve (L2, 3, 4)

Posterior branch

Articular branch

Anterior branch

Posterior branch

Cutaneous branch

Articular branch to knee joint

Adductor hiatus

Note: Only muscles innervated by obturator nerve shown

L1
L2
L3
L4
} Lumbar plexus

Lumbosacral trunk

Obturator externus muscle

Adductor brevis muscle

Adductor longus muscle (*cut*)

Adductor magnus muscle (ischiocondylar, or "hamstrings," part supplied by sciatic [tibial] nerve)

Gracilis muscle

Cutaneous innervation

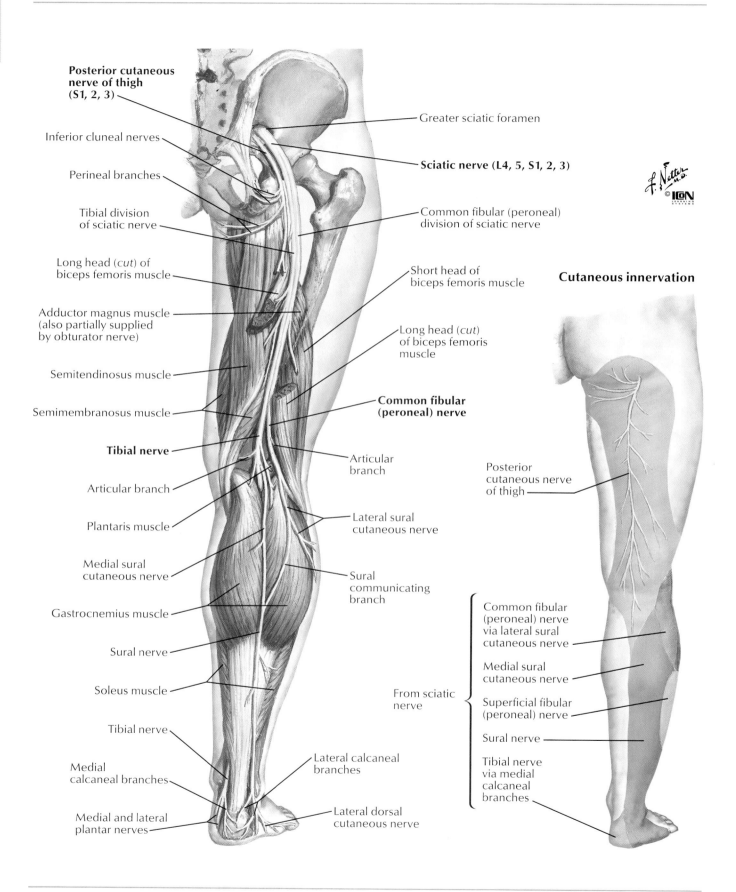

Posterior cutaneous nerve of thigh (S1, 2, 3)

Inferior cluneal nerves

Perineal branches

Tibial division of sciatic nerve

Long head (*cut*) of biceps femoris muscle

Adductor magnus muscle (also partially supplied by obturator nerve)

Semitendinosus muscle

Semimembranosus muscle

Tibial nerve

Articular branch

Plantaris muscle

Medial sural cutaneous nerve

Gastrocnemius muscle

Sural nerve

Soleus muscle

Tibial nerve

Medial calcaneal branches

Medial and lateral plantar nerves

Greater sciatic foramen

Sciatic nerve (L4, 5, S1, 2, 3)

Common fibular (peroneal) division of sciatic nerve

Short head of biceps femoris muscle

Long head (*cut*) of biceps femoris muscle

Common fibular (peroneal) nerve

Articular branch

Lateral sural cutaneous nerve

Sural communicating branch

Lateral calcaneal branches

Lateral dorsal cutaneous nerve

Cutaneous innervation

Posterior cutaneous nerve of thigh

From sciatic nerve

Common fibular (peroneal) nerve via lateral sural cutaneous nerve

Medial sural cutaneous nerve

Superficial fibular (peroneal) nerve

Sural nerve

Tibial nerve via medial calcaneal branches

PLATE 522

LOWER LIMB

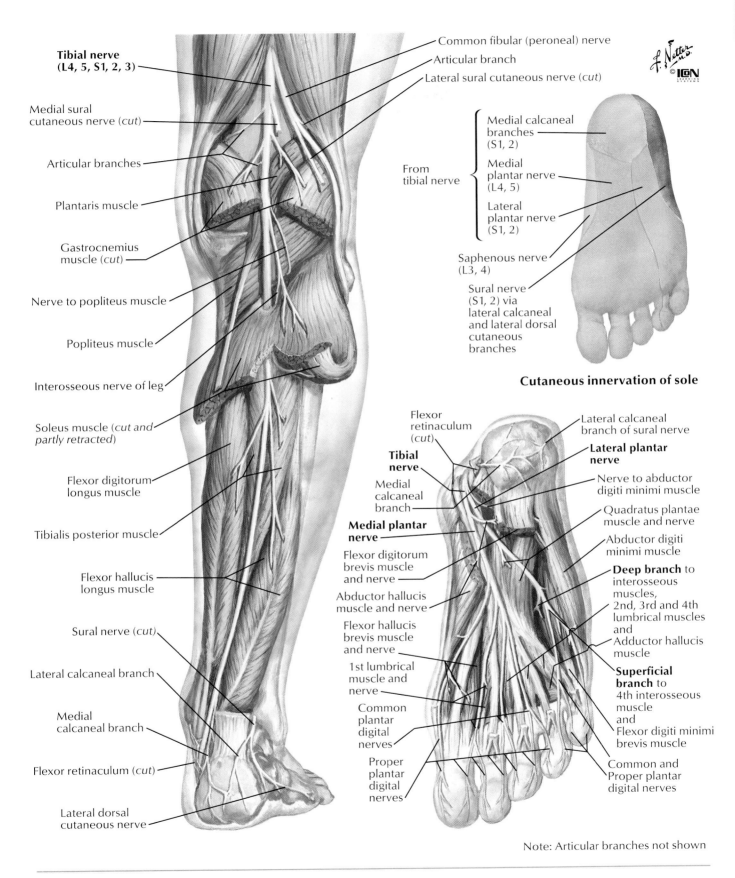

Tibial nerve (L4, 5, S1, 2, 3)

Medial sural cutaneous nerve (*cut*)

Articular branches

Plantaris muscle

Gastrocnemius muscle (*cut*)

Nerve to popliteus muscle

Popliteus muscle

Interosseous nerve of leg

Soleus muscle (*cut and partly retracted*)

Flexor digitorum longus muscle

Tibialis posterior muscle

Flexor hallucis longus muscle

Sural nerve (*cut*)

Lateral calcaneal branch

Medial calcaneal branch

Flexor retinaculum (*cut*)

Lateral dorsal cutaneous nerve

Common fibular (peroneal) nerve

Articular branch

Lateral sural cutaneous nerve (*cut*)

From tibial nerve:
- Medial calcaneal branches (S1, 2)
- Medial plantar nerve (L4, 5)
- Lateral plantar nerve (S1, 2)

Saphenous nerve (L3, 4)

Sural nerve (S1, 2) via lateral calcaneal and lateral dorsal cutaneous branches

Cutaneous innervation of sole

Flexor retinaculum (*cut*)

Tibial nerve

Medial calcaneal branch

Medial plantar nerve

Flexor digitorum brevis muscle and nerve

Abductor hallucis muscle and nerve

Flexor hallucis brevis muscle and nerve

1st lumbrical muscle and nerve

Common plantar digital nerves

Proper plantar digital nerves

Lateral calcaneal branch of sural nerve

Lateral plantar nerve

Nerve to abductor digiti minimi muscle

Quadratus plantae muscle and nerve

Abductor digiti minimi muscle

Deep branch to interosseous muscles, 2nd, 3rd and 4th lumbrical muscles and Adductor hallucis muscle

Superficial branch to 4th interosseous muscle and Flexor digiti minimi brevis muscle

Common and Proper plantar digital nerves

Note: Articular branches not shown

Common Fibular (Peroneal) Nerve

SEE ALSO PLATES 502, 503

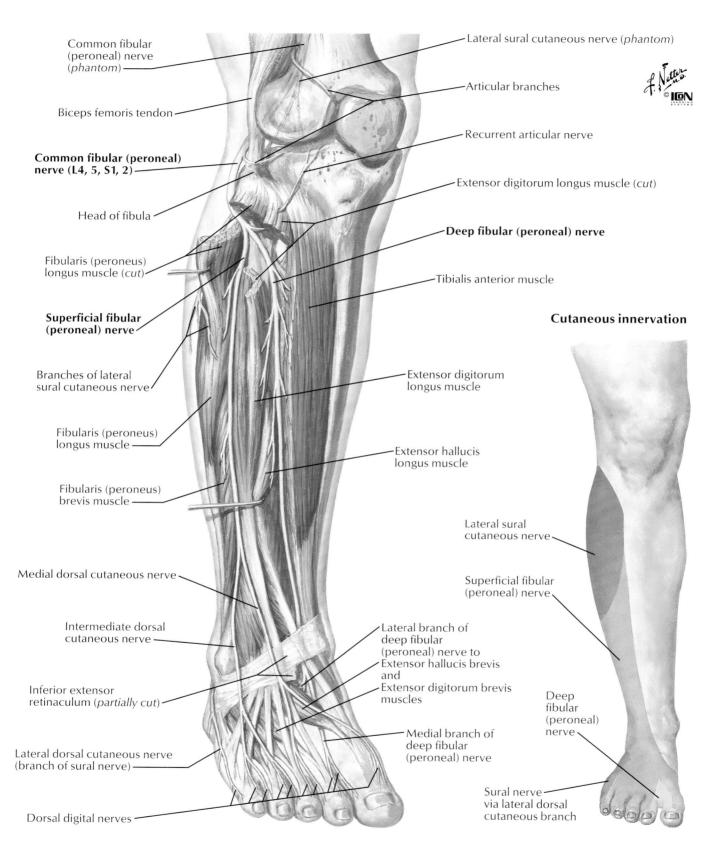

Common fibular (peroneal) nerve (*phantom*)

Biceps femoris tendon

Common fibular (peroneal) nerve (L4, 5, S1, 2)

Head of fibula

Fibularis (peroneus) longus muscle (*cut*)

Superficial fibular (peroneal) nerve

Branches of lateral sural cutaneous nerve

Fibularis (peroneus) longus muscle

Fibularis (peroneus) brevis muscle

Medial dorsal cutaneous nerve

Intermediate dorsal cutaneous nerve

Inferior extensor retinaculum (*partially cut*)

Lateral dorsal cutaneous nerve (branch of sural nerve)

Dorsal digital nerves

Lateral sural cutaneous nerve (*phantom*)

Articular branches

Recurrent articular nerve

Extensor digitorum longus muscle (*cut*)

Deep fibular (peroneal) nerve

Tibialis anterior muscle

Extensor digitorum longus muscle

Extensor hallucis longus muscle

Lateral branch of deep fibular (peroneal) nerve to Extensor hallucis brevis and Extensor digitorum brevis muscles

Medial branch of deep fibular (peroneal) nerve

Cutaneous innervation

Lateral sural cutaneous nerve

Superficial fibular (peroneal) nerve

Deep fibular (peroneal) nerve

Sural nerve via lateral dorsal cutaneous branch

PLATE 524

LOWER LIMB

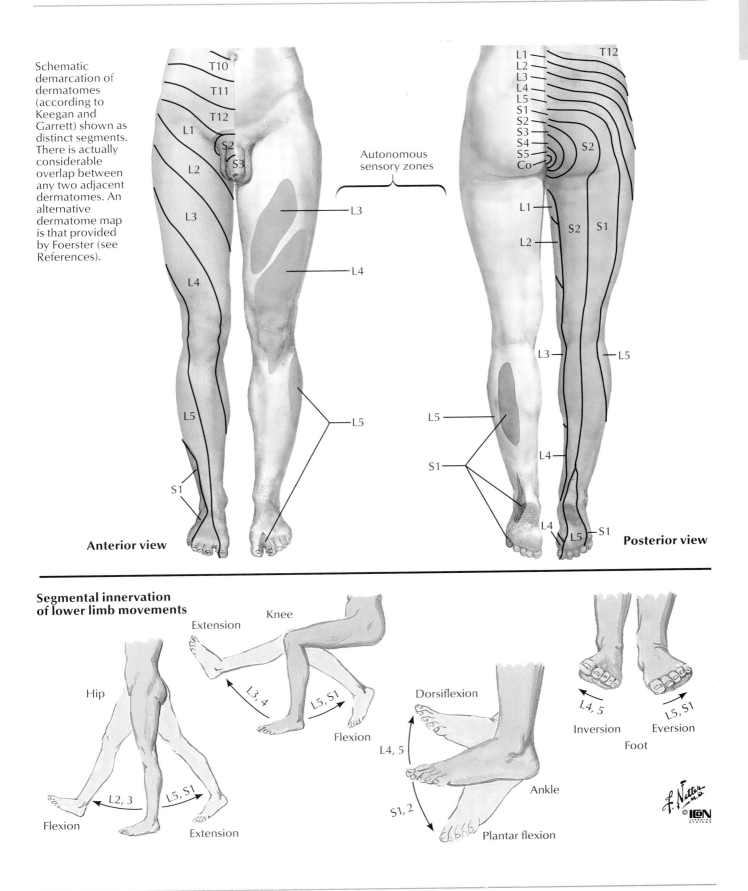

Schematic demarcation of dermatomes (according to Keegan and Garrett) shown as distinct segments. There is actually considerable overlap between any two adjacent dermatomes. An alternative dermatome map is that provided by Foerster (see References).

T10
T11
T12
L1
S2
S3
L2
L3
L4
L5
S1

Autonomous sensory zones

L3
L4
L5

Anterior view

L1
L2
L3
L4
L5
S1
S2
S3
S4
S5
Co
T12
S2
L1
S2
S1
L2
L3
L5
L5
S1
L4
L4
L5
S1

Posterior view

Segmental innervation of lower limb movements

Hip

Knee
Extension
L3, 4
L5, S1
Flexion

Dorsiflexion
L4, 5
S1, 2
Plantar flexion
Ankle

Flexion
L2, 3
L5, S1
Extension

L4, 5
Inversion
L5, S1
Eversion
Foot

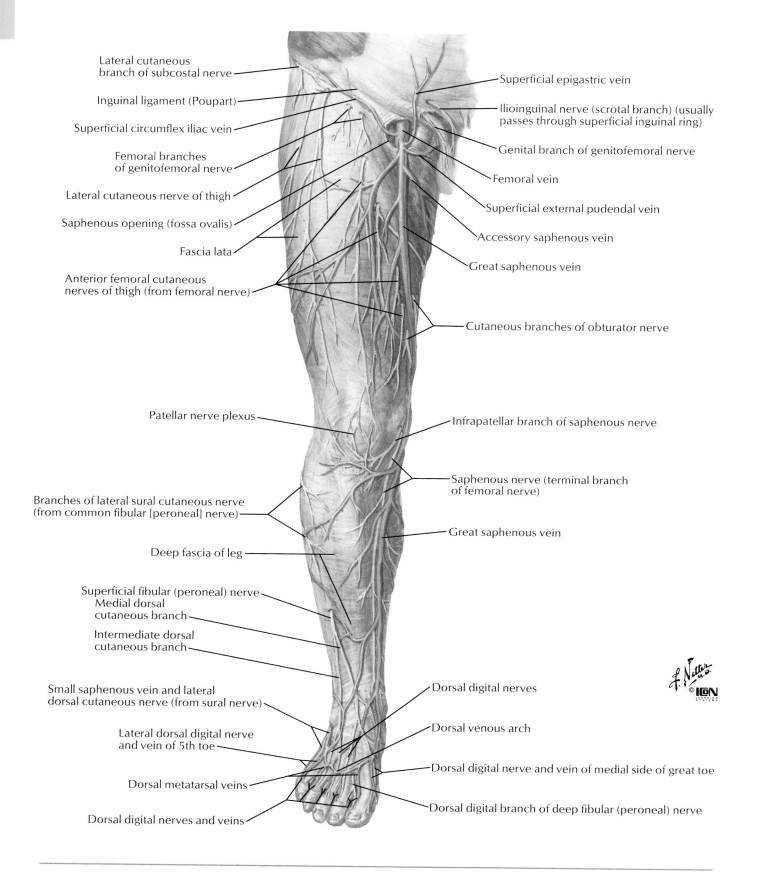

Lateral cutaneous branch of subcostal nerve

Inguinal ligament (Poupart)

Superficial circumflex iliac vein

Femoral branches of genitofemoral nerve

Lateral cutaneous nerve of thigh

Saphenous opening (fossa ovalis)

Fascia lata

Anterior femoral cutaneous nerves of thigh (from femoral nerve)

Patellar nerve plexus

Branches of lateral sural cutaneous nerve (from common fibular [peroneal] nerve)

Deep fascia of leg

Superficial fibular (peroneal) nerve
Medial dorsal cutaneous branch

Intermediate dorsal cutaneous branch

Small saphenous vein and lateral dorsal cutaneous nerve (from sural nerve)

Lateral dorsal digital nerve and vein of 5th toe

Dorsal metatarsal veins

Dorsal digital nerves and veins

Superficial epigastric vein

Ilioinguinal nerve (scrotal branch) (usually passes through superficial inguinal ring)

Genital branch of genitofemoral nerve

Femoral vein

Superficial external pudendal vein

Accessory saphenous vein

Great saphenous vein

Cutaneous branches of obturator nerve

Infrapatellar branch of saphenous nerve

Saphenous nerve (terminal branch of femoral nerve)

Great saphenous vein

Dorsal digital nerves

Dorsal venous arch

Dorsal digital nerve and vein of medial side of great toe

Dorsal digital branch of deep fibular (peroneal) nerve

PLATE 526

LOWER LIMB

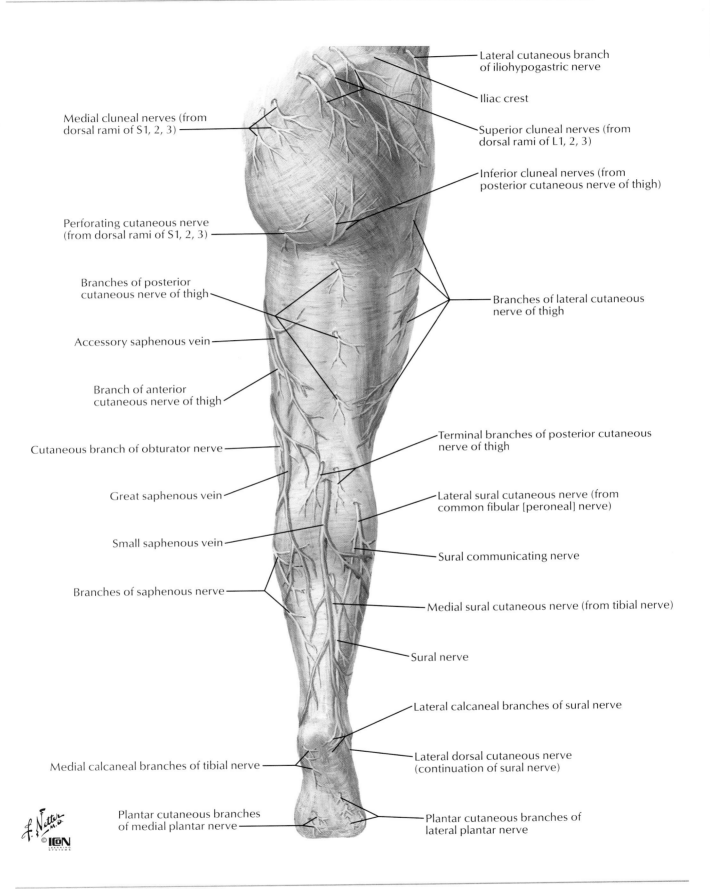

Lateral cutaneous branch of iliohypogastric nerve

Iliac crest

Medial cluneal nerves (from dorsal rami of S1, 2, 3)

Superior cluneal nerves (from dorsal rami of L1, 2, 3)

Inferior cluneal nerves (from posterior cutaneous nerve of thigh)

Perforating cutaneous nerve (from dorsal rami of S1, 2, 3)

Branches of posterior cutaneous nerve of thigh

Branches of lateral cutaneous nerve of thigh

Accessory saphenous vein

Branch of anterior cutaneous nerve of thigh

Cutaneous branch of obturator nerve

Terminal branches of posterior cutaneous nerve of thigh

Great saphenous vein

Lateral sural cutaneous nerve (from common fibular [peroneal] nerve)

Small saphenous vein

Sural communicating nerve

Branches of saphenous nerve

Medial sural cutaneous nerve (from tibial nerve)

Sural nerve

Lateral calcaneal branches of sural nerve

Medial calcaneal branches of tibial nerve

Lateral dorsal cutaneous nerve (continuation of sural nerve)

Plantar cutaneous branches of medial plantar nerve

Plantar cutaneous branches of lateral plantar nerve

SEE ALSO PLATES 387, 388

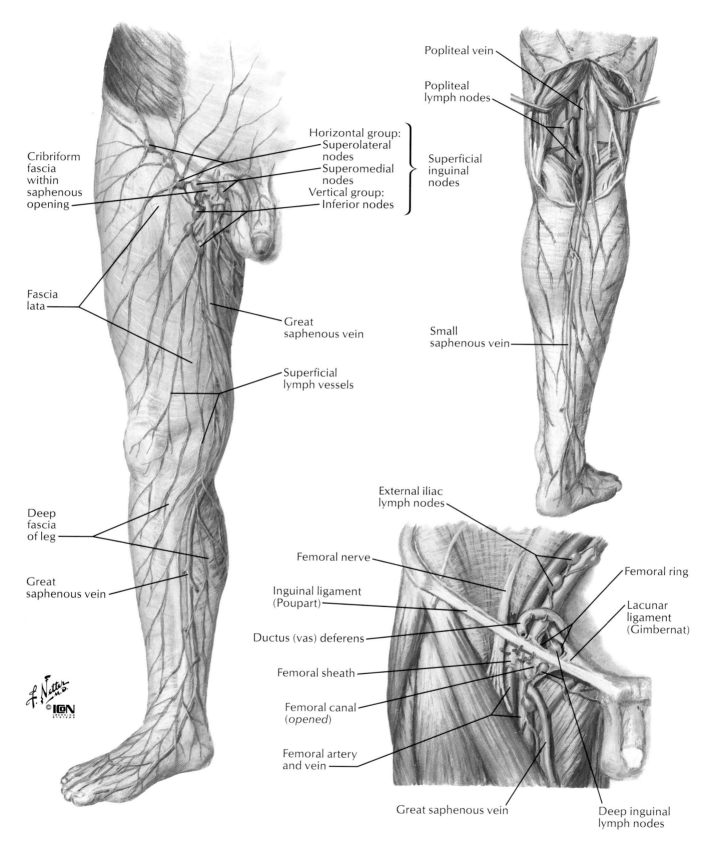

Cribriform fascia within saphenous opening

Horizontal group:
Superolateral nodes
Superomedial nodes
Vertical group:
Inferior nodes

Superficial inguinal nodes

Fascia lata

Great saphenous vein

Superficial lymph vessels

Deep fascia of leg

Great saphenous vein

Popliteal vein

Popliteal lymph nodes

Superficial inguinal nodes

Small saphenous vein

External iliac lymph nodes

Femoral nerve

Inguinal ligament (Poupart)

Ductus (vas) deferens

Femoral sheath

Femoral canal (*opened*)

Femoral artery and vein

Great saphenous vein

Femoral ring

Lacunar ligament (Gimbernat)

Deep inguinal lymph nodes

PLATE 528

LOWER LIMB

Section VIII
CROSS-SECTIONAL ANATOMY

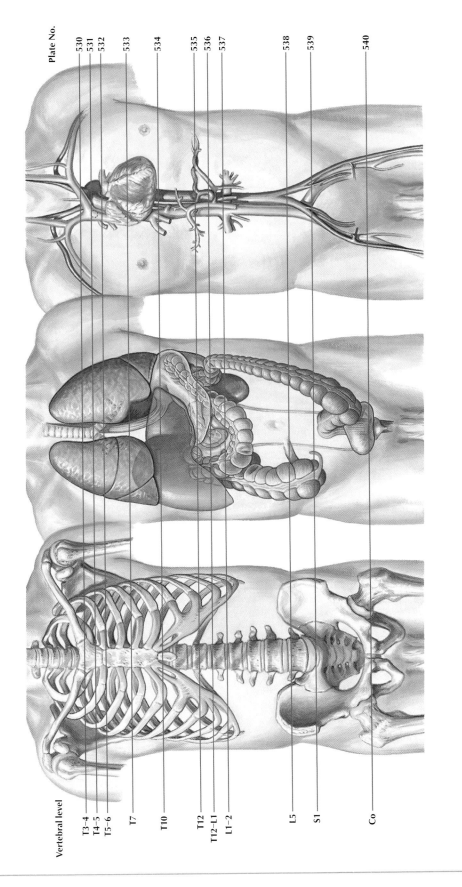

Plate No.

530
531
532

533

534

535
536
537

538

539

540

Vertebral level

T3–4
T4–5
T5–6

T7

T10

T12
T12–L1
L1–2

L5

S1

Co

Transverse Section: Upper Level of T4, Sternoclavicular Joint

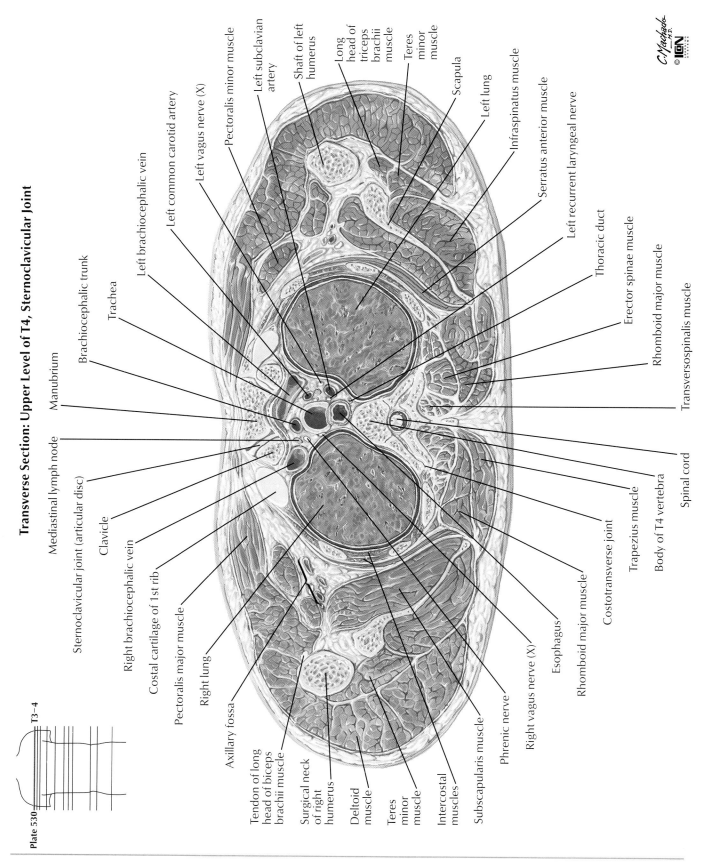

Pectoralis minor muscle

Left subclavian artery

Shaft of left humerus

Long head of triceps brachii muscle

Teres minor muscle

Scapula

Left lung

Infraspinatus muscle

Serratus anterior muscle

Left recurrent laryngeal nerve

Thoracic duct

Erector spinae muscle

Rhomboid major muscle

Transversospinalis muscle

Left vagus nerve (X)

Left common carotid artery

Left brachiocephalic vein

Brachiocephalic trunk

Trachea

Manubrium

Mediastinal lymph node

Sternoclavicular joint (articular disc)

Clavicle

Right brachiocephalic vein

Costal cartilage of 1st rib

Pectoralis major muscle

Right lung

Axillary fossa

Tendon of long head of biceps brachii muscle

Surgical neck of right humerus

Deltoid muscle

Teres minor muscle

Intercostal muscles

Subscapularis muscle

Phrenic nerve

Right vagus nerve (X)

Esophagus

Rhomboid major muscle

Costotransverse joint

Trapezius muscle

Body of T4 vertebra

Spinal cord

Plate 530

T3–4

PLATE 530

CROSS-SECTIONAL ANATOMY

Transverse Section: T4–5 Intervertebral Disc, Manubrium

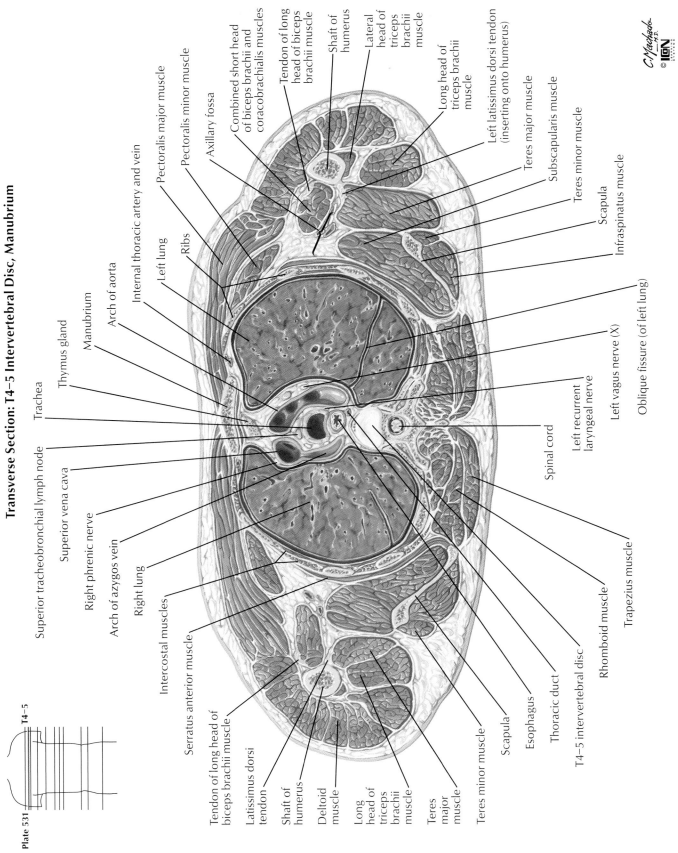

Pectoralis major muscle

Pectoralis minor muscle

Axillary fossa

Combined short head of biceps brachii and coracobrachialis muscles

Tendon of long head of biceps brachii muscle

Shaft of humerus

Lateral head of triceps brachii muscle

Long head of triceps brachii muscle

Left latissimus dorsi tendon (inserting onto humerus)

Teres major muscle

Subscapularis muscle

Teres minor muscle

Scapula

Infraspinatus muscle

Internal thoracic artery and vein

Left lung

Ribs

Arch of aorta

Manubrium

Thymus gland

Trachea

Superior tracheobronchial lymph node

Superior vena cava

Right phrenic nerve

Arch of azygos vein

Right lung

Intercostal muscles

Serratus anterior muscle

Tendon of long head of biceps brachii muscle

Latissimus dorsi tendon

Shaft of humerus

Deltoid muscle

Long head of triceps brachii muscle

Teres major muscle

Teres minor muscle

Scapula

Esophagus

Thoracic duct

T4–5 intervertebral disc

Rhomboid muscle

Trapezius muscle

Spinal cord

Left recurrent laryngeal nerve

Left vagus nerve (X)

Oblique fissure (of left lung)

C. Machado M.D.

© ICN

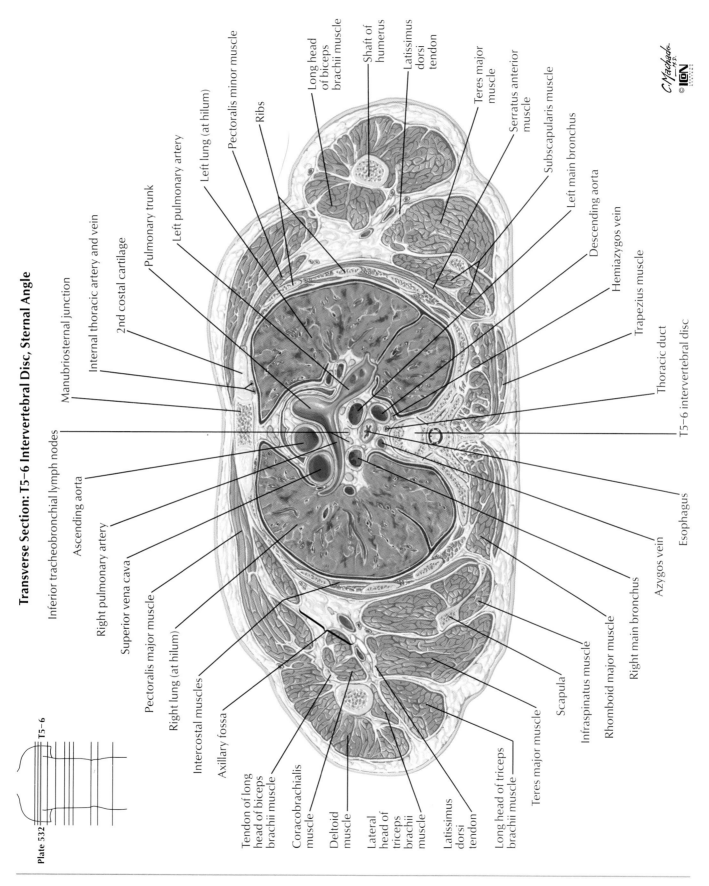

Transverse Section: T5–6 Intervertebral Disc, Sternal Angle

Inferior tracheobronchial lymph nodes

Manubriosternal junction

Internal thoracic artery and vein

2nd costal cartilage

Pulmonary trunk

Left lung (at hilum)

Left pulmonary artery

Pectoralis minor muscle

Ribs

Long head of biceps brachii muscle

Shaft of humerus

Latissimus dorsi tendon

Teres major muscle

Serratus anterior muscle

Subscapularis muscle

Left main bronchus

Descending aorta

Hemiazygos vein

Trapezius muscle

Thoracic duct

T5–6 intervertebral disc

Esophagus

Azygos vein

Right main bronchus

Rhomboid major muscle

Infraspinatus muscle

Scapula

Teres major muscle

Long head of triceps brachii muscle

Latissimus dorsi tendon

Lateral head of triceps brachii muscle

Deltoid muscle

Coracobrachialis muscle

Tendon of long head of biceps brachii muscle

Axillary fossa

Intercostal muscles

Right lung (at hilum)

Pectoralis major muscle

Superior vena cava

Right pulmonary artery

Ascending aorta

T5–6

Plate 532

PLATE 532

Transverse Section: Level of T7, 3rd Interchondral Space

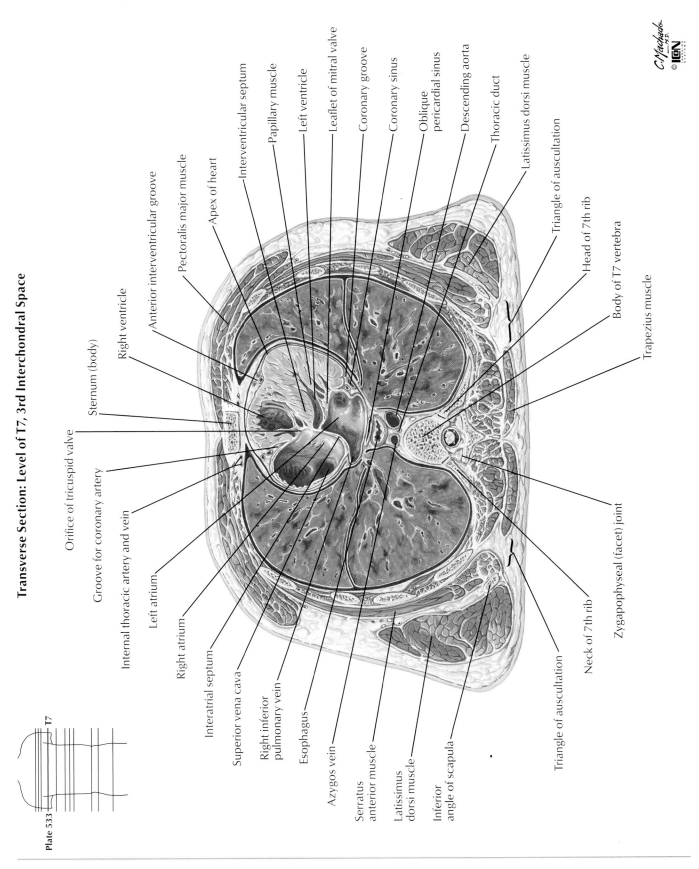

Orifice of tricuspid valve

Groove for coronary artery

Sternum (body)

Right ventricle

Anterior interventricular groove

Pectoralis major muscle

Apex of heart

Interventricular septum

Papillary muscle

Left ventricle

Leaflet of mitral valve

Coronary groove

Coronary sinus

Oblique pericardial sinus

Descending aorta

Thoracic duct

Latissimus dorsi muscle

Triangle of auscultation

Head of 7th rib

Body of T7 vertebra

Trapezius muscle

Internal thoracic artery and vein

Left atrium

Right atrium

Interatrial septum

Superior vena cava

Right inferior pulmonary vein

Esophagus

Azygos vein

Serratus anterior muscle

Latissimus dorsi muscle

Inferior angle of scapula

Triangle of auscultation

Neck of 7th rib

Zygapophyseal (facet) joint

T7

Plate 533

THORAX

PLATE 533

Transverse Section: Level of T10, Esophagogastric Junction

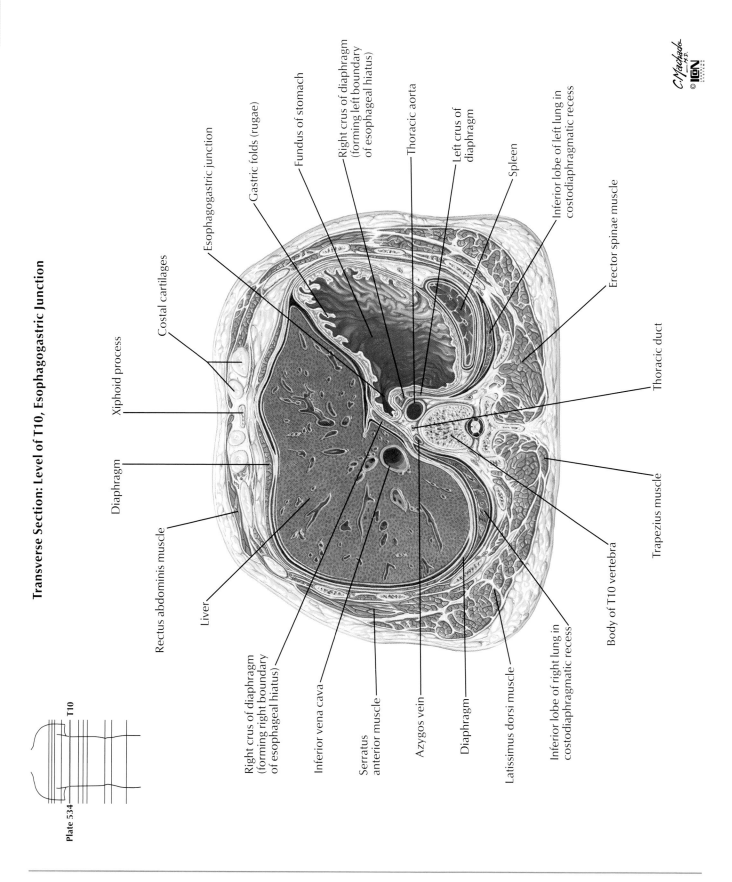

Plate 534

PLATE 534

CROSS-SECTIONAL ANATOMY

Transverse Section: Level of T12, Inferior to Xiphoid

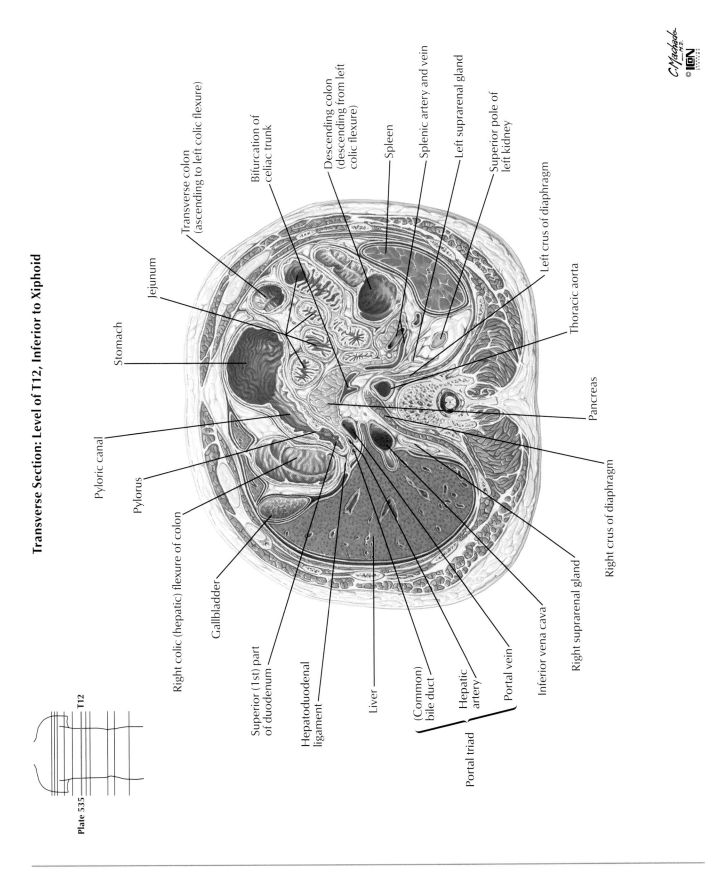

Transverse colon
(ascending to left colic flexure)

Bifurcation of
celiac trunk

Descending colon
(descending from left
colic flexure)

Spleen

Splenic artery and vein

Left suprarenal gland

Superior pole of
left kidney

Left crus of diaphragm

Thoracic aorta

Jejunum

Stomach

Pancreas

Pyloric canal

Pylorus

Right colic (hepatic) flexure of colon

Gallbladder

Superior (1st) part
of duodenum

Hepatoduodenal
ligament

Liver

(Common)
bile duct

Hepatic
artery

Portal vein

Portal triad

Inferior vena cava

Right suprarenal gland

Right crus of diaphragm

Plate 535

T12

Transverse Section: Level of T12–L1 Intervertebral Disc

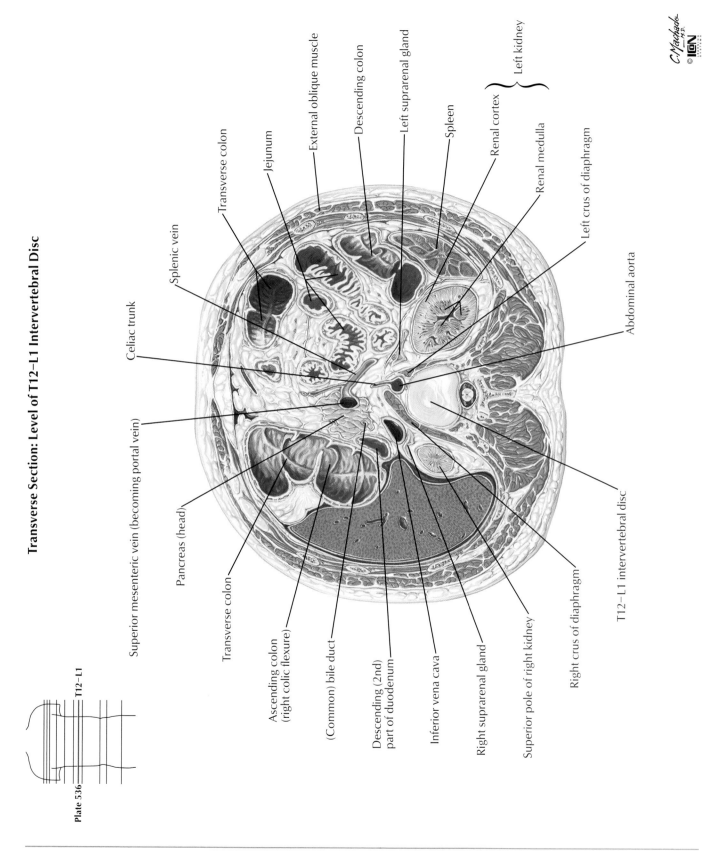

External oblique muscle

Descending colon

Left suprarenal gland

Spleen

Left kidney

Renal cortex

Renal medulla

Left crus of diaphragm

Jejunum

Transverse colon

Splenic vein

Celiac trunk

Abdominal aorta

Superior mesenteric vein (becoming portal vein)

Pancreas (head)

Transverse colon

Ascending colon (right colic flexure)

(Common) bile duct

Descending (2nd) part of duodenum

Inferior vena cava

Right suprarenal gland

Superior pole of right kidney

Right crus of diaphragm

T12–L1 intervertebral disc

T12–L1

Plate 536

PLATE 536

CROSS-SECTIONAL ANATOMY

Transverse Section: Level of L1–2 Intervertebral Disc

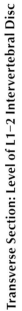

Plate 537

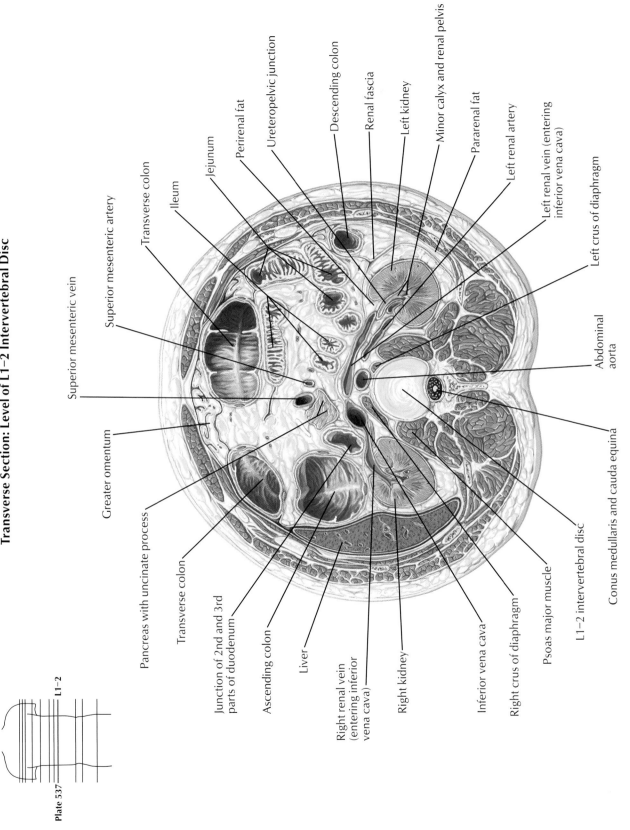

Superior mesenteric artery

Superior mesenteric vein

Transverse colon

Ileum

Jejunum

Perirenal fat

Ureteropelvic junction

Descending colon

Renal fascia

Left kidney

Minor calyx and renal pelvis

Pararenal fat

Left renal artery

Left renal vein (entering inferior vena cava)

Left crus of diaphragm

Abdominal aorta

Greater omentum

Pancreas with uncinate process

Transverse colon

Junction of 2nd and 3rd parts of duodenum

Ascending colon

Liver

Right renal vein (entering inferior vena cava)

Right kidney

Inferior vena cava

Right crus of diaphragm

Psoas major muscle

L1–2 intervertebral disc

Conus medullaris and cauda equina

Transverse Section: Level of L5, Near Transtubercular Plane

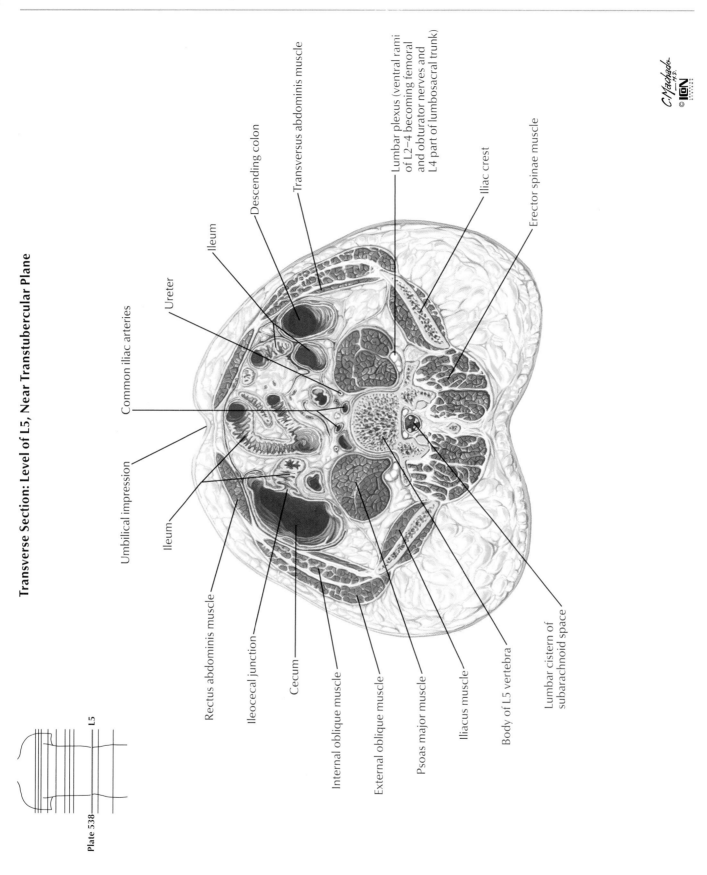

Descending colon

Transversus abdominis muscle

Lumbar plexus (ventral rami of L2–4 becoming femoral and obturator nerves and L4 part of lumbosacral trunk)

Iliac crest

Erector spinae muscle

Ileum

Ureter

Common iliac arteries

Umbilical impression

Ileum

Rectus abdominis muscle

Ileocecal junction

Cecum

Internal oblique muscle

External oblique muscle

Psoas major muscle

Iliacus muscle

Body of L5 vertebra

Lumbar cistern of subarachnoid space

L5

Plate 538

PLATE 538

CROSS-SECTIONAL ANATOMY

Transverse Section: Level of S1, Anterior Superior Iliac Spines

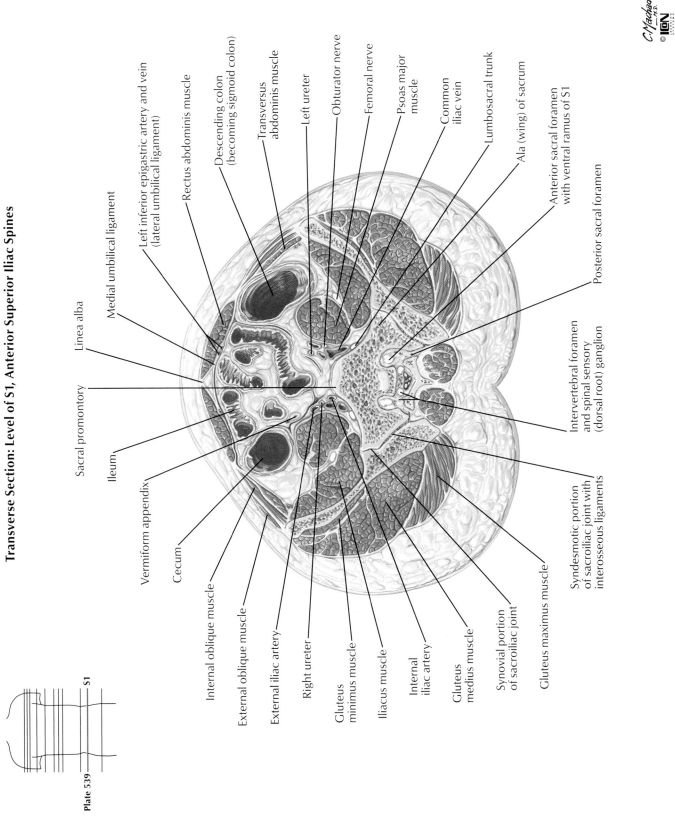

Left inferior epigastric artery and vein (lateral umbilical ligament)

Rectus abdominis muscle

Descending colon (becoming sigmoid colon)

Transversus abdominis muscle

Left ureter

Obturator nerve

Femoral nerve

Psoas major muscle

Common iliac vein

Lumbosacral trunk

Ala (wing) of sacrum

Anterior sacral foramen with ventral ramus of S1

Posterior sacral foramen

Medial umbilical ligament

Linea alba

Sacral promontory

Ileum

Vermiform appendix

Cecum

Internal oblique muscle

External oblique muscle

External iliac artery

Right ureter

Gluteus minimus muscle

Iliacus muscle

Internal iliac artery

Gluteus medius muscle

Synovial portion of sacroiliac joint

Gluteus maximus muscle

Syndesmotic portion of sacroiliac joint with interosseous ligaments

Intervertebral foramen and spinal sensory (dorsal root) ganglion

S1

Plate 539

Transverse Section: Pubic Crest, Femoral Heads, Coccyx

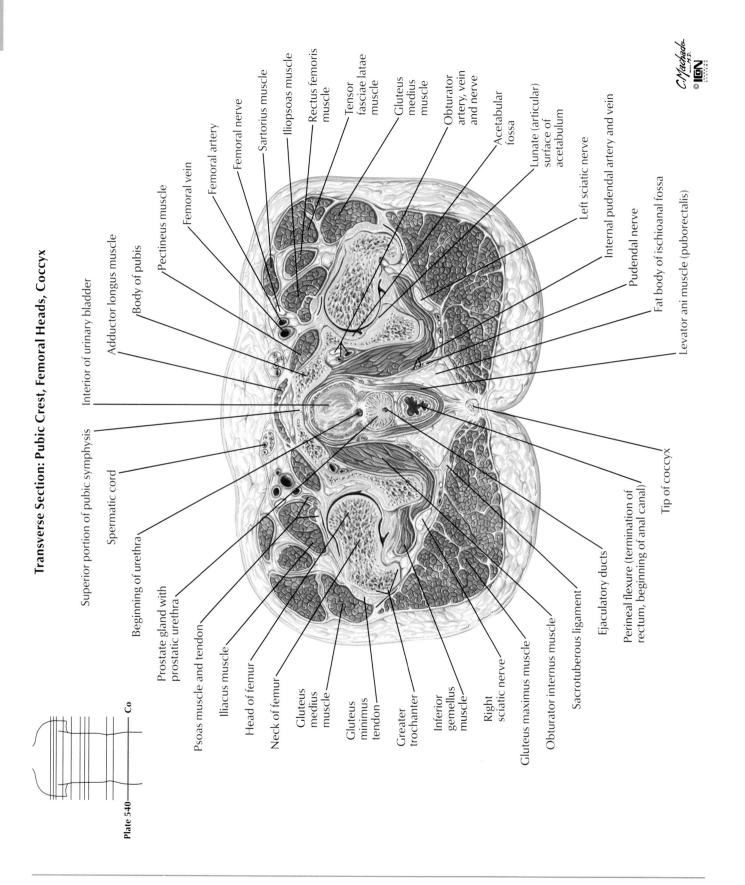

Femoral nerve

Sartorius muscle

Iliopsoas muscle

Rectus femoris muscle

Tensor fasciae latae muscle

Gluteus medius muscle

Obturator artery, vein and nerve

Acetabular fossa

Lunate (articular) surface of acetabulum

Left sciatic nerve

Internal pudendal artery and vein

Pudendal nerve

Fat body of ischioanal fossa

Levator ani muscle (puborectalis)

Femoral vein

Femoral artery

Pectineus muscle

Body of pubis

Adductor longus muscle

Interior of urinary bladder

Superior portion of pubic symphysis

Spermatic cord

Beginning of urethra

Prostate gland with prostatic urethra

Psoas muscle and tendon

Iliacus muscle

Head of femur

Neck of femur

Gluteus medius muscle

Gluteus minimus tendon

Greater trochanter

Inferior gemellus muscle

Right sciatic nerve

Gluteus maximus muscle

Obturator internus muscle

Sacrotuberous ligament

Ejaculatory ducts

Perineal flexure (termination of rectum, beginning of anal canal)

Tip of coccyx

Co

Plate 540

PLATE 540

CROSS-SECTIONAL ANATOMY

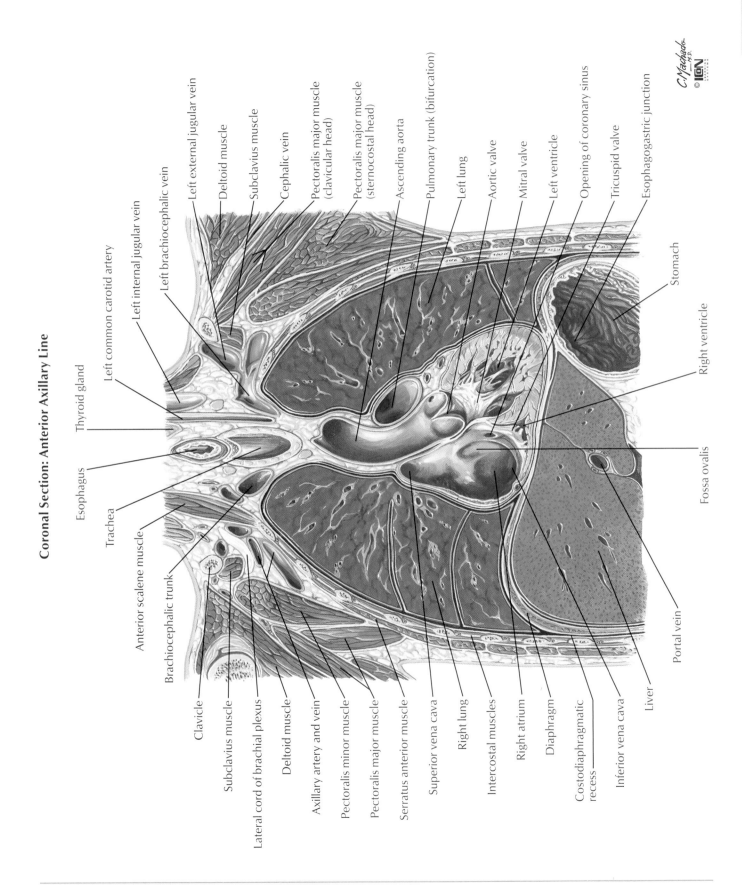

Coronal Section: Anterior Axillary Line

Left external jugular vein

Deltoid muscle

Subclavius muscle

Cephalic vein

Pectoralis major muscle (clavicular head)

Pectoralis major muscle (sternocostal head)

Ascending aorta

Pulmonary trunk (bifurcation)

Left lung

Aortic valve

Mitral valve

Left ventricle

Opening of coronary sinus

Tricuspid valve

Esophagogastric junction

Left brachiocephalic vein

Left internal jugular vein

Left common carotid artery

Thyroid gland

Esophagus

Trachea

Anterior scalene muscle

Brachiocephalic trunk

Stomach

Right ventricle

Fossa ovalis

Portal vein

Liver

Inferior vena cava

Costodiaphragmatic recess

Diaphragm

Right atrium

Intercostal muscles

Right lung

Superior vena cava

Serratus anterior muscle

Pectoralis major muscle

Pectoralis minor muscle

Axillary artery and vein

Deltoid muscle

Lateral cord of brachial plexus

Subclavius muscle

Clavicle

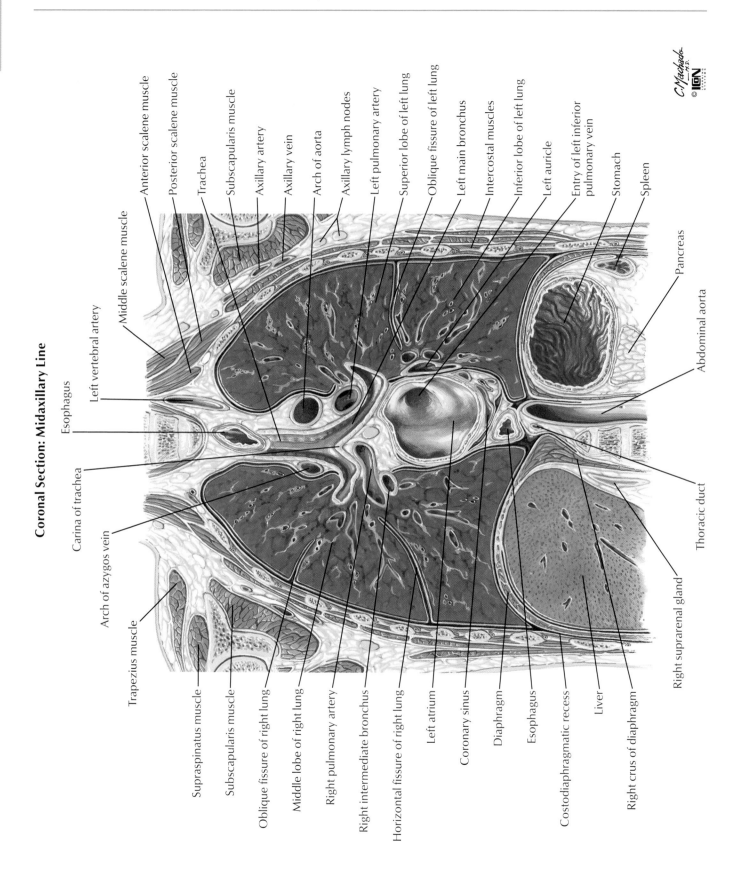

Coronal Section: Midaxillary Line

Anterior scalene muscle

Posterior scalene muscle

Trachea

Subscapularis muscle

Axillary artery

Axillary vein

Arch of aorta

Axillary lymph nodes

Left pulmonary artery

Superior lobe of left lung

Oblique fissure of left lung

Left main bronchus

Intercostal muscles

Inferior lobe of left lung

Left auricle

Entry of left inferior pulmonary vein

Stomach

Spleen

Middle scalene muscle

Left vertebral artery

Esophagus

Carina of trachea

Arch of azygos vein

Trapezius muscle

Pancreas

Abdominal aorta

Thoracic duct

Right suprarenal gland

Supraspinatus muscle

Subscapularis muscle

Oblique fissure of right lung

Middle lobe of right lung

Right pulmonary artery

Right intermediate bronchus

Horizontal fissure of right lung

Left atrium

Coronary sinus

Diaphragm

Esophagus

Costodiaphragmatic recess

Liver

Right crus of diaphragm

PLATE 542

CROSS-SECTIONAL ANATOMY

Frank H. Netter, M.D.

Frank H. Netter was born in 1906 in New York City. He studied art at the Art Student's League and the National Academy of Design before entering medical school at New York University, where he received his M.D. degree in 1931. During his student years, Dr. Netter's notebook sketches attracted the attention of the medical faculty and other physicians, allowing him to augment his income by illustrating articles and textbooks. He continued illustrating as a sideline after establishing a surgical practice in 1933, but he ultimately opted to give up his practice in favor of a full-time commitment to art. After service in the United States Army during World War II, Dr. Netter began his long collaboration with the CIBA Pharmaceutical Company (now Novartis Pharmaceuticals). This 45-year partnership resulted in the production of the extraordinary collection of medical art so familiar to physicians and other medical professionals worldwide.

Icon Learning Systems acquired the Netter Collection in July 2000 and continues to update Dr. Netter's original paintings and to add newly commissioned paintings by artists trained in the style of Dr. Netter.

Dr. Netter's works are among the finest examples of the use of illustration in the teaching of medical concepts. The 13-book Netter Collection of Medical Illustrations, which includes the greater part of the more than 20,000 paintings created by Dr. Netter, became and remains one of the most famous medical works ever published. The Netter Atlas of Human Anatomy, first published in 1989, presents the anatomical paintings from the Netter Collection. Now translated into 11 languages, it is the anatomy atlas of choice among medical and health professions students the world over.

The Netter illustrations are appreciated not only for their aesthetic qualities, but more importantly, for their intellectual content. As Dr. Netter wrote in 1949, ". . . clarification of a subject is the aim and goal of illustration. No matter how beautifully painted, how delicately and subtly rendered a subject may be, it is of little value as a medical illustration if it does not serve to make clear some medical point." Dr. Netter's planning, conception, point of view, and approach are what inform his paintings and what makes them so intellectually valuable.

Frank H. Netter, M.D., physician and artist, died in 1991.

REFERENCES

Plate 54

Braus H. Anatomie des Menschen. Berlin, Verlag von Julius Springer, 1924

Plate 85

Nishida S. The Structure of the Eye. New York, Elsevier North-Holland, 1982

Plates 110, 111, 121

Lachman N, Acland RD, Rosse C. Anatomical evidence for the absence of morphologically distinct cranial root of the accessory nerve in man. Clin Anat 2002;15:4

Plates 157, 465, 507, 525

Foerster O. The dermatomes in man. Brain 1933;56:1

Garrett FD. The segmental distribution of the cutaneous nerves in the limbs of man. Anat Rec 1948;102:409

Keegan JJ. J Neurosurg 1947;4:115

Plate 165

Turnbull IM. Blood supply of the spinal cord. In Vinken PJ, Bruyn GW (eds). Handbook of Clinical Neurology, XII. Amsterdam, North-Holland, 1972, pp 478-491

Plates 196, 197

Jackson CL, Huber JF. Correlated applied anatomy of the bronchial tree and lungs with a system of nomenclature. Dis Chest 1943;9:319

Plate 199

Ikeda S, Ono Y, Miyazawa S, et al. Flexible broncho-fiberscope. Otolaryngology (Tokyo) 1970;42:855

Plate 221

James TN. The internodal pathways of the human heart. Prog Cardiovas Dis 2001;43:495

Plates 245, 353, 355, 362, 366

Myers RP, King BF, Cahill DR. Deep perineal "space" as defined by magnetic resonance imaging. Presented at 14th Annual Scientific Session of the American Association of Clinical Anatomists, Honolulu, HI, 1997. (Abstract:Clin Anat 1998;11)

Plate 274

DiDio LJA. Anatomo-Fisiologia do Piloro ileo-ceco-colica no homen, Actas das Primeiras Jornadas Inter-universitarías Argentinas de Gastroenterologia, Rosario, 1954

———. Dados anatomicos sobre o "piloro" ileo-ceco-colico. (Com observacao direta in vivo de "papila" ileo-ceco-colica.) (English summary). Thesis, Fac Med, Univ de São Paulo, 1952

Plate 282

Healey JE Jr, Schroy. Anatomy of the biliary duct within the human liver; analysis of the prevailing pattern of branchings and the major variations of the biliary ducts. Arch Surg 1953;66:599

———, Sörensen. The intrahepatic distribution of the hepatic artery in man. J Int Coll Surg 1953;20:133

Plates 283, 284

Elias H. Liver morphology. Biol Rev 1955;30:263

———. Origin and early development of the liver in various vertebrates. Act Hepat 1955;3:1

———. Morphology of the liver. In "Liver Injury," Trans 11th Conference. New York, Macy Foundation, 1953

———. A re-examination of the structure of the mammalian liver; the hepatic lobule and its relation to the vascular and biliary system. Am J Anat 1949;85:379

————. A re-examination of the structure of the mammalian liver; parenchymal architecture. Am J Anat 1949;84:311

Plates 297, 298

Michels NA. Blood Supply and Anatomy of the Upper Abdominal Organs, With a Descriptive Atlas. Philadelphia, JB Lippincott, 1955

Plate 316

Thomas MD. In The Ciba Collection of Medical Illustrations, Vol 3, Part II. Summit NJ, CIBA, p 78

Plates 335, 348, 367, 377, 394

Stormont TJ, Cahill DR, King BF, Myers RP. Fascias of the male external genitalia and perineum. Clin Anat 1994;7:115

Plates 343, 347, 352, 355, 360, 361

Oelrich TM. The striated urogenital sphincter muscle in the female. Anat Rec 1983;205:223

Plates 346, 348

Myers RP, Goellner JR, Cahill DR. Prostate shape, external striated urethral sphincter and radical prostatectomy: the apical dissection. J Urol 1987;138:543

Plates 346, 348, 366, 367

Oelrich TM. The urethral sphincter muscle in the male. Am J Anat 1980;158:229

Plate 383

Flocks RH, Kerr HD, Elkins HB, et al. Treatment of carcinoma of the prostate by interstitial radiation with radio-active gold (Au 198):A preliminary report. J Urol 1952;68(2):510

Plate 465

Keegan JJ, Garrett FD. The segmental distribution of the cutaneous nerves in the limbs of man. Anat Rec 1948;102:409

Plate 525

Keegan JJ. Neurological interpretation of dermatome hypalgesia with herniation of the lumbar intervertebral disc. J Bone Joint Surg 1944;26:238

Last RJ. Innervation of the limbs. J Bone Joint Surg 1949;31(B):452

INDEX

References are to plate numbers; numbers in bold refer to primary sources. In most cases, structures are listed under singular nouns.

A

Abdomen
  autonomic nerves and ganglia of, 308
  axial CT images of, 338
  bony framework of, 240
  cross sections of, 534–539
    at L3, 4, 337
    at T12, 336
  innervation of, 308–318
  left lower quadrant of, 260
  left upper quadrant of, 260
  regions and planes of, 260
  right lower quadrant of, 260
  right upper quadrant of, 260
  subcutaneous tissue of, 241
  surface anatomy of, 239
  viscera of, 261
    median (sagittal) section of, 335
Abdominal aortic plexus. *See* Intermesenteric plexus
Abdominal muscles, 191
  transversus, 350
    aponeurosis of, 244
Abdominal wall
  anterior, 256, 257
    arteries of, 247
    deep dissection of, 243
    intermediate dissection of, 242
    internal view of, 245
    nerves of, 249
    superficial dissection of, 241
    veins of, 248
  median (sagittal) section of, 335
  posterior
    arteries of, 256
    internal view of, 255
    lymph vessels and nodes of, 258
    nerves of, 259
    peritoneum of, 266
    veins of, 257
  posterolateral, 246
Abdominalis muscle, transversus, 349
Abdominis aponeurosis, transversus, 337
Abdominis muscle
  aponeurosis of, 247
  rectus, 174, 182, 183, 187, 191, 239, 242, 243, 244, 245, 247, 249, 250, 251, 253, 335, 336, 337, 339, 348, 349, 350, 351, 360
    axial CT images of, 338
    cross section of, 534, 538
    sagittal MR images of, 400
    sheath of, 183
  transversus, 183, 184, 189, 243, 244, 245, 247, 249, 250, 251, 253, 255, 259, 319, 336, 337, 478, 480
    aponeurosis of, 320

cross section of, 539
  tendon of origin of, 185, 246, 332, 337
Abducent nerve (VI), 10, 79, 80, 82, 98, 108, 111, 115
  distribution of, 112
  schema of, 115
Abducent nucleus, 110, 111, 115
Abductor digiti minimi muscle, 444, 448, 453, 459, 511, 513, 515, 516, 517, 518, 523
  nerve to, 516, 523
Abductor digiti minimi tendon, 510
Abductor hallucis muscle, 511, 513, 515, 516, 517, 523
  insertion of, 518
  tendon of, 515
Abductor hallucis nerve, 523
Abductor hallucis tendon, 516
Abductor muscles, of thigh, 478
Abductor pollicis brevis muscle, 444, 448, 449, 458
Abductor pollicis brevis tendon, 453
Abductor pollicis longus muscle, 424, 427, 428, 432, 433, 434, 461
  area for, 422
Abductor pollicis longus tendon, 427, 431, 432, 452, 453
  insertion of, 450
Accessory muscle bundle, 63
Accessory nerve (XI), 10, 28, 30, 43, 67, 98, 108, 110, 111, 123, 170, 185, 186
  cranial root of, 120, 121
  distribution of, 112
  schema of, 121
  spinal nucleus of, 110, 111
  spinal roots of, 10, 121
Accessory oculomotor nucleus, 110, 111, 115, 126
Acetabular fossa
  fat in, 469
  transverse section of, 540
Acetabular labrum, 340, 469, 486
Acetabular ligament, transverse, 340, 469
Acetabular notch, 340, 468
Acetabulum, 340, 468
  anteroposterior radiograph of, 470
  lunate surface of, 340, 468, 469
    transverse section of, 540
  margin of, 340, 341, 345, 468
Achilles tendon. *See* Calcaneal tendon
Acinus, 200
Acoustic meatus
  external, 4, 8, 12, 87, 91
    auricular branch of vagus nerve to, 20
    axial CT images of, 143
    cartilaginous and osseous, 88
    coronal oblique section of, 88
  internal, 10, 87, 117, 118
Acoustic opening, internal, 92
Acromial anastomosis, 410
Acromial angle, 403, 404
Acromial plexus, 410
Acromioclavicular joint, 406, 408

capsule of, 406
Acromioclavicular ligament, 406
Acromion, 23, 177, 182, 186, 401, 403, 404, 406, 407, 408, 409, 410, 414, 415
  anteroposterior radiograph of, 405
Adamkiewicz, artery of, 164
Adductor brevis muscle, 475, 483, 487
  attachments of, 472, 473
  innervation of, 521
Adductor canal, 482, 487
Adductor hallucis muscle
  deep tibial nerve branch to, 523
  insertion of, 518
  oblique head of, 517
  transverse head of, 517
Adductor hiatus, 484, 521
  femoral artery passing through, 494
Adductor longus muscle, 474, 475, 482, 483, 487
  attachments of, 472, 473
  innervation of, 521
  transverse section of, 540
Adductor magnus muscle, 467, 482, 483, 484, 487
  adductor minimus part of, 475, 477, 484
  attachments of, 472, 473
  hiatus of, 475
  innervation of, 521, 522
  tendon of, 475
Adductor magnus tendon, 483, 488, 493, 499
Adductor muscles, thigh, 478
Adductor pollicis muscle, 445, 448, 449, 459
  fascia of, 443, 445
Adenohypophysis, 133, 140, 141
  cleft of, 140
Adnexa, 356
Adrenergic synapses, 161
Afferent fibers, olfactory bulb, 113
Afferent nerves
  of mouth and pharynx, 58
  from nose and sinuses, 206
Agger nasi, 33
Aglomerular arteriole, 326
Air cells, mastoid, 5, 43
Airway reflexes, nerves initiating, 206
Ala, 8, 240
  lateral part of, 150
  wing of, 150
Alar fibrofatty tissue, 32
Alar fold, 489
Alar ligament, 18
Albini's nodules, 219
Alcock canal. *See* Pudendal canal
Alveolar artery
  anterior superior, 36
  inferior, 36, 49, 56, 66
    lingual branch of, 65
    mental branch of, 36, 65
    mylohyoid branch of, 14, 65
  middle superior, 36
  posterior superior, 36, 65
Alveolar duct, 200
  opening of, 200